Enhancing Cognitive Fitness in Adults

Paula E. Hartman-Stein · Asenath La Rue
Editors

Enhancing Cognitive Fitness in Adults

A Guide to the Use and Development of Community-Based Programs

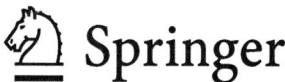

Editors
Paula E. Hartman-Stein, Ph.D.
Clinical Geropsychologist,
Center for Healthy Aging,
265 W. Main Street, Kent, 44240 Ohio
Adjunct Faculty, Department of Human
Development and Family Studies,
College of Education,
Health and Human Services,
Kent State University,
Kent, OH, USA
paula@centerforhealthyaging.com

Asenath La Rue, Ph.D.
Senior Research Scientist
Wisconsin Alzheimer's Institute
University of Wisconsin
Madison, WI, USA
larue@wisc.edu

ISBN 978-1-4419-0635-9 (Hardcover) e-ISBN 978-1-4419-0636-6
ISBN 978-1-4614-4767-2 (Softcover)
DOI 10.1007/978-1-4419-0636-6
Springer New York Dordrecht Heidelberg London

Library of Congress Control Number: 2011932488

© Springer Science+Business Media, LLC 2011
All rights reserved. This work may not be translated or copied in whole or in part without the written permission of the publisher (Springer Science+Business Media, LLC, 233 Spring Street, New York, NY 10013, USA), except for brief excerpts in connection with reviews or scholarly analysis. Use in connection with any form of information storage and retrieval, electronic adaptation, computer software, or by similar or dissimilar methodology now known or hereafter developed is forbidden.
The use in this publication of trade names, trademarks, service marks, and similar terms, even if they are not identified as such, is not to be taken as an expression of opinion as to whether or not they are subject to proprietary rights.
While the advice and information in this book are believed to be true and accurate at the date of going to press, neither the authors nor the editors nor the publisher can accept any legal responsibility for any errors or omissions that may be made. The publisher makes no warranty, express or implied, with respect to the material contained herein.

Printed on acid-free paper

Springer is part of Springer Science+Business Media (www.springer.com)

To Paula Hartman-Stein's mother, Pauline, and Asenath La Rue's father, Dale, who both experienced cognitive impairment in late life and who inspired their daughters to create novel yet practical ways of improving the quality of life of individuals who live with similar conditions.

Paula E. Hartman-Stein
Asenath La Rue

Foreword

To one degree or another we all face changes in our cognitive and emotional capacities as we age. As human beings and as professionals, we have a responsibility for thinking deeply and acting honestly to assist those who seek out our care for these challenges. Certainly we bring the power of our expertise to the therapeutic relationship but also our deepest human compassion.

The first editor of this volume, Dr. Paula Hartman-Stein, has exemplified these capabilities for me in our personal and professional relationships. She and her coeditor, Dr. Asenath La Rue, have assembled a group of experts to publish a most timely volume. The world of cognitive aging is changing radically as the challenges to the dominant medical models of brain aging mount, and the need for more positive, community-based approaches is recognized ever so more clearly. This volume addresses this need well.

As a geriatric neurologist, psychologist, cognitive neuroscientist, and environmental ethicist, I tried to take a broad perspective on how individuals, communities, and society at large should address the problems and opportunities of adult development and cognitive aging. It is a time to expand our horizons and cure our addiction to biological and medical approaches. The very survival of our species depends on framing problems correctly, creating opportunities together, and developing new sources of hope that draw us into the future.

Paula asked me to address in this foreword, which I am honored to contribute, why pills are not the answer to brain health. We see the crumbling of the pharmaceutically driven process of defining memory loss and cognitive decline as medical problems to be fixed. Yes, doctors can assist in assessing people as to whether medical conditions are contributing to loss of intellect. But their control over the full range of aging challenges is an example of the overreach of medicalization of social ills. The term *Alzheimer's disease* provokes fear and a longing for simplistic solutions to what can no longer be viewed as a molecular problem waiting for its magic solution. Few honest people are willing to claim that Alzheimer's disease is a singular condition. The heterogeneity at genetic, pathological, and clinical levels has become ever more evident. Many now share the skepticism that Dr. Alois Alzheimer himself demonstrated about what he described as being a single separate disease. Moreover, the intimate links between the biology of aging processes themselves and so-called Alzheimerization of the brain are apparent. Changes in synapses and neurons occur with age. Plaques and tangles are no longer seen as the specific characteristic of the single disorder.

The medical establishment has pushed recently for expensive biologically-based diagnostic tests whose reliability and validity have not been established. The emphasis on developing biomarkers is a result of desperation to better characterize Alzheimer's disease in life and create the probably unrealistic hope of discovering specific subtypes of disease hidden among the enormous clinical heterogeneity. Ever more expansive labels of unclear utility outside a limited research framework are being applied to the continuum of aging so that now we not only have early and late forms of mild cognitive impairment but subjective cognitive impairment as well. These efforts have been linked to the promise that effective therapies, which will prevent, slow the progression of, or even cure Alzheimer's disease, are just around the corner. Yet unfortunately, the number of failed therapeutic trials continues to grow. This is not surprising if one sees AD as a much more complex process intimately related to aging. Prominent CEOs of drug companies, molecular biologists, and even pioneers such as Robert Butler came to recognize the overly simplistic nature of our considering Alzheimer's as a single process.

However, the domination of reductionistic molecular approaches to chronic disease persists, in particular with the notion that genes hold the answers to most, if not all, health problems. Scientific leadership at the highest levels is obsessed by genes as causes and potential targets for therapy while relatively ignoring environmental science, public health, and prevention efforts. This is most evident in the pharmaceutical industry. Some physicians have allowed the pharmaceutical industry to not only manipulate them to prescribe new and often more expensive and less safe drugs and to invent entirely new categories of drugs and diseases to promote a sense of progress which is increasingly being seen as an illusion.

In my opinion, the promotion of "anti-aging medicine" represents the most malignant form of quackery yet seen in the long history of the attempts of healers to take advantage of those they strive to serve. We are moving towards an integrative health approach but are not yet there as we do not understand adequately what binds the healing traditions together. In my opinion, we need to focus on a personalized health approach not based on genes but on narrative. Every healer needs to co-create a healing story with the person suffering and seeking assistance. Moreover, this narrative needs to include greater attention to the relationships between the person and his social community and natural environment. We need to work with nature in our communities to foster healthy aging in all of us. Perhaps we need modern day shamans attentive to the interrelationships among individual, family, community, and environmental health!

Drs. Hartman-Stein and La Rue offer us a feast of authors and ideas under the title *Enhancing Cognitive Fitness in Adults: A Guide to the Use and Development of Community-Based Programs*. They focus on improving thinking and emotional life rather than treating disease. The editors recognize that most of the strategies outlined in the book should be implemented in community-based settings. No longer will the hospital or the doctor's office necessarily be seen as the exclusive locus of health. Rather we must embed health throughout community organizations, including schools as I will return to at the end of my foreword.

The beginning part of the book focuses on research foundations. The book strives for a balanced approach to brain versus cognitive fitness. Merely promoting concepts such as neuroplasticity or neurogenesis is not a game changer. Brain scientists must be challenged to improve our cognitive functioning and well-being in safe ways and help to bridge scientific discoveries with practical, humanistic interventions.

Part I of the book points out that exercise and cognitive engagement deserve a prominent place on the list of activities to do to keep the brain healthy. The editors have added a chapter that includes information about the role of meditation in not only improving cognition but also increasing compassion in caregivers of frail older adults.

Increasingly, information technology will play a greater role than biotechnology in improving our cognitive functioning. However, we must go beyond computer games to fully embracing the power of social networks and multimedia. It is not so important that we develop artificial intelligence in computers, but rather we should focus on how computers and other digital devices can help humans think and remember better as friendly aids to our cognition.

The second part of the book introduces us to some of the most successful community-based programs in the country. Multifaceted programs will likely be the most successful as they embrace the diversity of learning styles. My own particular interest is an intergenerational learning that fosters the greatest opportunities for co-creation of narratives that promote long-term thinking and valuing in human beings. Whether it be reading or writing poetry or prose, the power of story is gaining appropriate increased attention as a vehicle for promoting healthy individuals and communities. The role of competitive intellectual programs such as Odyssey of the Mind and an old fashioned spelling bee is also highlighted in this part of the volume. The final chapter in the second part focuses on nutrition, increasingly recognized as an important element of general and brain health.

Part III pays attention to creative artistic programming such as acting, creative dance, music composition done in groups, and viewing museum art work in small groups—all designed to enhance cognition in frail adults but perhaps more importantly, to enhance life's quality for the individuals and those who care for them, both paid caregivers and family.

Part IV of the book concentrates on wellness interventions for adults with cognitive impairment including biofeedback strategies for "brain brightening." My own attitude is that we should develop wellness approaches for learners of all ages that respect developmentally appropriate differences. In older adults these differences can be associated with loss of memory and ability to multitask. But just as with adults whose cognitive functioning is healthy, we need to look for opportunities for positive growth in those with dementia. This section of the book features community-based programs that strive to accomplish just that.

Positive psychology and positive aging have appeared on the scene as a counterbalance to the often negative language of clinical psychology and gerontology.

Yet a true wisdom of aging represents the need to balance the negative and positive aspects of aging. In fact, recognition of the limits of our individual human abilities as well as our life span is perhaps, etc. one of the sources for the kind of integrative knowledge that wisdom represents. We should not view wisdom as a rare occurrence in human society but rather see that each one of us has a little bit of wisdom that can be enhanced by working collectively with others.

The final chapters refer to two programs that focus on intergenerational learning. Danny George describes "The Intergenerational School" started by my wife Cathy and me ten years ago. This public charter school celebrates lifelong, experiential learning in-service of community. Its signature intergenerational reading, mentoring, computer, and gardening programs allow human beings of all ages to learn together. The school is nationally and internationally recognized as an innovative and effective model for educating children. Most of our children come from challenged urban areas and many are living with incomes below the poverty level." Yet, we have demonstrated, as Danny George describes, that such an environment can be life enhancing for elders with memory problems as well. The school is building on its decade-long commitment to environmental sustainability. If our societies are to survive the threats of global climate change, we need to develop more effective learning communities that can help us behave responsibly in the present to attempt to reverse the effect of destructive behaviors in the past.

Ultimately individuals need to ask what is their purpose in life, and what do they wish their legacy to be. As we age and become the elders, the baby boomers will need to find opportunities to remain cognitively fit and socially engaged. What better place to enhance one's own cognitive fitness than in a community serving the future by educating children? There is no greater purpose than the work shared in this book to enhance our cognitive fitness and our overall sense of well-being within sustainable communities.

Peter Whitehouse, M.D., Ph.D.

Preface

Older people across the world are embarking on an experiment in nature, adopting many different approaches to cognitive well-being, committing to physical exercise to benefit their brains as well as their hearts, changing their diets, managing stress more effectively, signing up for lifelong learning programs, participating in the arts, engaging in friendly academic competitions, and volunteering to advance causes beyond themselves, with the belief that these actions can improve their cognitive course. Research to guide choices about which activities may have the greatest benefit for late life cognitive function lags behind this popular movement, but as shown in the opening chapters, the scientific literature on what works, and what does not, is growing and can be spurred on in positive ways by the motivation to "be all you can be" in later life. This book brings together the exciting research underway on cognitive wellness interventions with the diverse and creative community-based programs being offered to stimulate cognition and well-being for older adults.

Another motivation fuels interest in cognitive wellness – the hope of avoiding Alzheimer's disease (AD) or other dementias. Researchers now recognize that the pathological substrates of AD develop across decades, and most view the clinical expression of this disease as a product of complex interactions of genetic, environmental, and lifestyle factors. As we have worked on this book, we recognize all too well that investigation to unravel the complex causes and clinical triggers for AD and other dementias is just beginning. Even at this early stage, however, animal research indicates that physical exercise can facilitate neurogenesis, synaptogenesis, and other aspects of brain structure and function important for learning and memory. Clinical trials of exercise interventions with humans show encouraging results for sustaining cognitive skills. Cognitive training interventions, some large-scale and well-controlled, are also showing positive outcomes, with training-related benefits lasting for months or even years in some cases. Epidemiological evidence continues to show that mentally active lifestyles are associated with slower rates of cognitive decline and later onset of dementia.

Concepts such as brain reserve and cognitive reserve are helping to provide a conceptual framework for why older persons are often able to sustain a high level of cognitive function despite having neuropathology of AD or other dementia. The general idea behind both of these concepts is that insults to the brain due to aging, strokes, or a host of other factors can be tolerated better by individuals with greater initial levels of critical brain resources (i.e., brain reserve) or more efficient or flexible cognitive coping mechanisms (i.e., cognitive reserve). We do not know yet whether lifestyle factors such as a sustained commitment to exercise or to cognitively stimulating activities in later life add to brain or cognitive reserve, but the possibility that they may is intriguing. Scaffolding theory and brain plasticity models provide an additional way of thinking about the characteristic cognitive changes of aging and about methods for supporting cognition.

Clinicians and program directors who work with older adults face practical and ethical challenges in deciding how best to help their clients sustain and maximize their cognitive skills. Both of us have worked in clinical settings and encountered older clients and their family members who looked to us for more than an accurate diagnosis followed by the message, "See your doctor for follow up for medication and come back for another evaluation in a year from now."

It is our hope that this book can inform clinical choices by demonstrating the breadth and scope of some of the cognitive support interventions that are available now, while at the same time recognizing that more work is needed to establish the efficacy of cognitive wellness interventions.

Part I covers research foundations for cognitive wellness interventions. Part II provides a rich sampling of the programs being offered to bolster emotional resilience and support cognitive function in normal aging older adults such as memory training courses taught by peers, to intergenerational and lifelong learning programs, friendly academic competitions, oral life review and creative writing, or nutritional and exercise recommendations. Part III describes programs for both frail and healthy older adults that promote immersion in the arts for cognitive fitness via acting courses for theatre and film, dance and movement, music composition, and exploring visual arts. Part IV provides examples of behavioral interventions tailored to older persons with cognitive impairment, and Part V shows how older adults' volunteering can benefit all concerned.

Work on this book has been important to us, too, on personal levels because of struggles with dementia in our families. Paula's mother, Pauline, suffered from probable mixed dementia that became apparent while she was in her late 70s. She lived at home with her husband, passing away in 2006 from a massive stroke at age 83. Paula remembers when she first recognized signs of possible early dementia in her mother. At that time the medical community placed a great deal of hope that individuals with mild cognitive impairment and early dementia would benefit from a cholinesterase inhibitor. After reviewing the available studies at the time, Paula agreed with the treatment plan recommended by her mother's primary care physician. But rather than stabilize her functioning, it appeared the medication contributed to a loss of her mother's vitality. Pauline experienced bradycardia (low heart rate), syncope, and multiple falls that led to frequent hospitalizations; symptoms later reported in population-based studies as potentially adverse side effects of cholinesterase inhibitors (Gill et al., 2009; Hernandez, Farwell, Cantor, & Lawler, 2009).

When Pauline was in her mid to late 70s, she was a witty, lively, very physically active woman, but her last few years were characterized by hours lying on the couch each day. Paula and her father were not as concerned about Pauline's memory loss as they were her inability to remain energetic enough to do simple household tasks, attend adult day care, or take walks. Understanding firsthand the helplessness felt by family caregivers in similar situations, Paula has developed interventions for her clients including meditation programs, memory enhancement and creative writing classes, spelling clubs, and other educational programs in the community. From the mid 1990s until her passing in 2006, Paula's major professor, Dr. Jeanette Reuter, stressed that she should not give up on her frail older adult clientele but strive to offer them opportunities for social and cognitive engagement.

Asenath's father, Dale, lived for many years with Lewy body dementia. In contrast to Paula's mother, Dale seemed to benefit from treatment from a cholinesterase inhibitor for at least a short time. More important over the long haul was the fact that he was able to "age in place," surrounded by a community of people familiar to him and his way of life, cared for by people whose dedication and compassion were appreciated by all of his family. Would he have benefited from more active engagement programs? There is no way to know. But having options for being involved and needed, to the extent of one's wishes and capacities, is what we wish for our loved ones and ourselves.

Finally, we realize that the topic of cognitive fitness for dementia prevention or amelioration of symptoms is fraught with controversy. The truth is that both pharmacological interventions to improve memory and cognition as well as cognitive training programs get modest effects at best. The "traditional" approaches of trying to recover function through drugs or training do not offer as much promise for living well with memory changes or dementia as do approaches that address quality of life. It is our sincere hope that this book will give attention to cognitive wellness support for older adults throughout the life course and inspire the creation of additional programs that provide social connections and pursuits that serve to keep older individuals positive and engaged during late life.

We want to acknowledge our many diverse contributors who were willing to provide their knowledge and expertise in this volume. Each chapter was written by highly skilled scientists, clinicians, artists, and educators. We thank them for their excellent work in synthesizing the literature as well as generating additional suggestions for future research, practice, and educational models.

We wish to heartily thank Janice Stern, Senior Editor, Health and Behavior, at Springer for her persistent belief that this volume would become a reality. Janice remained positive and cheerful, providing practical recommendations and generating positive energy throughout the project. Our thanks also goes to her assistant, Kathryn Hiler, for her detailed work to get to the finished product. We want to recognize the efforts of Jeanette Biermann, who served as a valuable research assistant and gave editorial support throughout the development of the book. We extend our thanks to Carolyn Smith, administrative assistant at the Center for Healthy Aging, who provided clerical support and worked long hours at the end of the process. Finally, thanks to Jim Bradshaw, an experienced correspondent for *The National Psychologist*, who was willing to give editorial assistance.

On a personal note, Paula wants to express her deep appreciation to her husband, Rob Stein, who encouraged her to undertake the project and who patiently supported her throughout its completion in countless ways. Paula also thanks her son, Eric Stein, who gave helpful words of support and encouragement during his mother's time and devotion towards completing the book.

Asenath would like to thank her husband, Art Montana, for support during writing and editing, and her colleagues at the Wisconsin Alzheimer's Institute for their encouragement of her interest in interventions of all types to support cognition in aging and dementia.

Kent, OH	Paula E. Hartman-Stein, Ph.D.
Madison, WI	Asenath La Rue, Ph.D.

References

Gill, S. S., Anderson, G. M., Fischer, H. D., et al. (2009). Syncope and its consequences in patients with dementia receiving cholinesterase inhibitors: A population-based cohort study. *Archives of Internal Medicine, 69,* 867–873.

Hernandez, R. K., Farwell, W., Cantor, M. D., & Lawler, E. V. (2009). Cholinesterase inhibitors and incidence of bradycardia in patients with dementia in the Veterans Affairs New England Healthcare System. *Journal of the American Geriatrics Society, 57,* 1997–2003.

Contents

Foreword vii

Preface xi

Contributors xix

Part I Research Foundations for Cognitive Wellness Interventions

1 **Memory Enhancement Strategies:
   What Works Best for Obtaining Memory Goals?** 3
   John Dunlosky, Heather Bailey, and Christopher Hertzog

2 **Mental and Physical Exercise as a Means
   to Reverse Cognitive Aging and Enhance Well-Being** 25
   Walter R. Boot and Daniel P. Blakely

3 **Consumer-Based Brain Fitness Programs** 45
   Elizabeth M. Zelinski, Sarah E. Dalton, and Glenn E. Smith

4 **Synapse: A Clinical Trial Examining the Impact
   of Actively Engaging the Aging Mind** 67
   Jennifer Lodi-Smith and Denise C. Park

5 **Meditation, Mindfulness, Cognition, and Emotion:
   Implications for Community-Based Older Adult Programs** 85
   Alfred W. Kaszniak

Part II Community-Based Programs to Enhance and Sustain Healthy Aging

6 **Keys to a Sharp Mind: Providing Choice and Quality Programming in a Retirement Community** 107
Jeanette S. Biermann and Paula E. Hartman-Stein

7 **Osher Lifelong Learning Institute at the University of Montana: A Model of Successful University and Community Partnerships** 125
Sharon Alexander, Cynthia Aten, Dannette Fadness, and Kali Lightfoot

8 **Closing the Generation Gap: Using Discussion Groups to Benefit Older Adults and College Students** 137
Kelly E. Cichy and Gregory C. Smith

9 **A Practical Guide to Senior Odyssey** 155
Elizabeth A.L. Stine-Morrow and Jeanine M. Parisi

10 **Spelling Clubs and Competitions for Older Adults: Language Boosting Within a Social Context** 169
Paula E. Hartman-Stein and Mary DeForest

11 **Oral Life Review in Older Adults: Principles for the Social Service Professional** 183
Thomas M. Meuser

12 **Creative Writing Groups: A Promising Avenue for Enhancing Working Memory and Emotional Well-Being** 199
Paula E. Hartman-Stein

13 **Peer-Led Memory Training Programs to Support Brain Fitness** 213
Linda M. Ercoli, Paul A. Cernin, and Gary W. Small

14 **Cognitive Wellness for Diverse Populations** 231
Stephanie R. Johnson

15 **The Role of Physical Activity in Cognitive Fitness: A General Guide for Community Programs** 239
Edward S. Potkanowicz

16 **Nutrition and Nutritional Supplements to Promote Brain Health** 249
Abhilash K. Desai, Joy Rush, Lakshmi Naveen, and Papan Thaipisuttikul

Contents

Part III Enhancing Cognition Through the Arts

17 Enhancing Healthy Cognitive Aging Through Theater Arts............ 273
Tony Noice and Helga Noice

18 Coming Alive: Kairos Dance Theatre's Dancing Heart™
– Vital Elders Moving in Community 285
Maria DuBois Genné and Cristopher Anderson

19 Art, Museums, and Culture 301
Sean Caulfield

20 The Songwriting Works™ Model: Enhancing Brain Health
and Fitness Through Collaborative Musical Composition
and Performance 325
Judith-Kate Friedman

**Part IV Cognitive Wellness Interventions for Adults
with Memory Impairment**

21 Supporting Cognition and Well-Being in Older Adults
with Mild Cognitive Impairment: A Pilot Intervention 361
Asenath La Rue

22 Early Memory Loss Clubs: A Novel Approach
for Stimulating and Sustaining Cognitive Function 381
Thomas Fritsch, Kathleen A. Smyth, Maggie S. Wallendal,
Kristin Einberger, and David S. Geldmacher

23 Implementing the "I'm Still Here"™ Approach:
Montessori-Based Methods for Engaging Persons
with Dementia 401
Cameron J. Camp, John Zeisel, and Vincent Antenucci

24 Kirtan Kriya Meditation: A Promising Technique
for Enhancing Cognition in Memory-Impaired Older Adults........... 419
Dharma Singh Khalsa and Andrew Newberg

25 Brain Brightening: Neurotherapy for Enhancing Cognition
in the Elderly 433
James Lawrence Thomas

**Part V Gaining Through Giving Back:
Programs with a Positive Societal Impact**

26 Neurons in Neighborhoods: How Purposeful Participation
in a Community-based Intergenerational Program Enhanced
Quality of Life for Persons Living with Dementia 447
Daniel R. George

27 **Experience Corps®: A Civic Engagement-Based
   Public Health Intervention in the Public Schools** 469
   George W. Rebok, Michelle C. Carlson, Jeremy S. Barron,
   Kevin D. Frick, Sylvia McGill, Jeanine M. Parisi,
   Teresa Seeman, Erwin J. Tan, Elizabeth K. Tanner,
   Paul R. Willging, and Linda P. Fried

Index 489

Contributors

Sharon Alexander, Ed.D. Osher Lifelong Learning Institute, University of Montana, Missoula, MT, USA

Cristopher Anderson Kairos Dance Theatre, Minneapolis, MN, USA

Cynthia Aten, M.D. Osher Lifelong Learning Institute, University of Montana, Missoula, MT, USA

Vincent Antenucci, M.A. Hearthstone Alzheimer Care, Woburn, MA, USA

Heather Bailey, Ph.D. Washington University, St. Louis, MO, USA

Jeremy S. Barron, M.D. School of Medicine, The Johns Hopkins University, Baltimore, MD, USA

Jeanette S. Biermann, Ph.D. Center for Healthy Aging, Kent, OH, USA; Counseling Psychology, University of Akron, Akron, OH, USA

Daniel P. Blakely, B.A. Department of Psychology, Florida State University, Tallahassee, FL, USA

Walter R. Boot, Ph.D. Department of Psychology, Florida State University, Tallahassee, FL, USA

Cameron J. Camp, Ph.D. Director of Research, Linda-&-Cameron, Inc., Solon, OH, USA

Michelle C. Carlson, Ph.D. Bloomberg School of Public Health, The Johns Hopkins University, Baltimore, MD, USA

Sean Caulfield ARTZ: Artists for Alzheimer's®, Hearthstone Alzheimer's Foundation, Woburn, MA, USA

Paul A. Cernin, Ph.D. University of California, Los Angeles, CA, USA

Kelly E. Cichy, Ph.D. Department of Human Development and Family Studies, College of Education, Health, and Human Services, Kent State University, Kent, OH, USA

Sarah E. Dalton Davis School of Gerontology, University of Southern California, Los Angeles, CA, USA

Mary DeForest Department of Modern Languages, University of Colorado at Denver, Denver, CO, USA

Abhilash K. Desai, M.D. Medical Director, Geriatric Psychiatry Director, Memory Clinic, Sheppard Pratt Health Systems, Associate Professor, Department of Neurology and Psychiatry, Division of Geriatric Psychiatry, Saint Louis University School of Medicine, Baltimore, MD, USA

John Dunlosky, Ph.D. Department of Psychology, Kent State University, Kent, OH, USA

Kristin Einberger Brain Boosters, Kristin Einberger Consulting, 11 Black Duck Court, Amerian Canyon, CA, USA

Linda M. Ercoli, Ph.D. University of California, Los Angeles, CA, USA

Dannette Fadness, M.S. University of Montana, Missoula, MT, USA

Kevin D. Frick, Ph.D. Bloomberg School of Public Health, The Johns Hopkins University, Baltimore, MD, USA

Linda P. Fried, M.D., M.P.H. Mailman School of Public Health, Columbia University, New York, NY, USA

Judith-Kate Friedman Songwriting Works™ Educational Foundation, Port Townsend, WA, USA

Thomas Fritsch, Ph.D. Parkinson Research Institute, Aurora Sinai Medical Center, Milwaukee, WI, USA;
University of Wisconsin-Milwaukee, Helen Bader School of Social Welfare, Milwaukee, WI, USA;
Department of Neurology, Case Western Reserve School of Medicine, Cleveland, OH, USA

David S. Geldmacher, M.D. Department of Neurology, Birmingham, AL, USA

Maria DuBois Genné, M.S.Ed. Kairos Dance Theatre, Minneapolis, MN, USA

Daniel R. George, Ph.D., M.Sc. Department of Humanities, College of Medicine Penn State Milton S. Hershey Medical Center, Hershey, PA, USA

Paula E. Hartman-Stein, Ph.D. Clinical Geropsychologist, Center for Healthy Aging, Kent, 44240 Ohio; Adjunct Faculty, Department of Human Development and Family Studies, College of Education, Health and Human Services, Kent State University, Kent, OH, USA

Christopher Hertzog, Ph.D. Georgia Institute of Technology, Atlanta, GA, USA

Contributors

Stephanie R. Johnson, Ph.D. Howard University School of Medicine, Washington, DC, USA

Alfred W. Kaszniak, Ph.D. Department of Psychology, University of Arizona, Tucson, AZ, USA

Dharma Singh Khalsa, M.D. Alzheimer's Research and Prevention Foundation, Tucson, AZ, USA

Asenath La Rue, Ph.D. Wisconsin Alzheimer's Institute, University of Wisconsin, Madison, WI, USA

Kali Lightfoot, M.S. National Resource Center, Osher Lifelong Learning Institutes, University of Southern Maine, Portland, ME, USA

Jennifer Lodi-Smith, Ph.D. Canisius College, Department of Psychology, Buffalo, NY, USA

Sylvia McGill, M.A. Greater Homewood Community Corporation, Baltimore, MD, USA

Thomas M. Meuser, Ph.D. Gerontology Graduate Program, University of Missouri – St. Louis, MO, USA

Lakshmi Naveen, M.D. Saint Louis University, St. Louis, MO, USA

Andrew Newberg, M.D. Myrna Brind Center of Integrative Medicine, Thomas Jefferson University and Hospital, Philadelphia, PA, USA

Helga Noice, Ph.D. Department of Psychology, Elmhurst College, Elmhurst, IL, USA

Tony Noice, Ph.D. Department of Theatre, Elmhurst College, Elmhurst, IL, USA

Jeanine M. Parisi, Ph.D. Bloomberg School of Public Health, The Johns Hopkins University, Baltimore, MD, USA

Denise C. Park, Ph.D. Center for Vital Longevity, University of Texas, Dallas, TX, USA

Edward S. Potkanowicz, Ph.D., ACSMHFS Assistant Professor of Exercise Physiology, Department of Human Performance and Sport Sciences, Ohio Northern University, Ada, OH, USA

George W. Rebok, Ph.D. Bloomberg School of Public Health, The Johns Hopkins University, Baltimore, MD, USA

Joy Rush, R.D. St. Louis University, St. Louis, MO, USA

Teresa Seeman, Ph.D. David Geffen School of Medicine, UCLA, Los Angeles, CA, USA

Gary W. Small, M.D. University of California, Los Angeles, CA, USA

Glenn E. Smith, Ph.D. Mayo College of Medicine, Rochester, MN, USA

Gregory C. Smith, Ph.D. Department of Human Development and Family Studies, College of Education, Health, and Human Services, Kent State University, Kent, OH, USA

Kathleen A. Smyth, Ph.D. Department of Epidemiology and Biostatistics, Case Western Reserve School of Medicine, Cleveland, OH, USA; Neurological Outcomes Center, University Hospitals Case Medical Center, Cleveland, OH, USA

Elizabeth A.L. Stine-Morrow, Ph.D. Psychology, and the Beckman Institute, University of Illinois at Urbana-Champaign, Champaign, IL, USA

Erwin J. Tan, M.D. School of Medicine, The Johns Hopkins University, Baltimore, MD, USA

Elizabeth K. Tanner, Ph.D., R.N. School of Nursing, The Johns Hopkins University, Baltimore, MD, USA

Papan Thaipisuttikul, M.D. Saint Louis University, St. Louis, MO, USA

James Lawrence Thomas, Ph.D. NYU Langone Medical Center, New York, NY, USA

Maggie S. Wallendal, M.S.W Parkinson Research Institute, Aurora Sinai Medical Center, Milwaukee, WI, USA; University of Wisconsin-Milwaukee, Helen Bader School of Social Welfare, Milwaukee, WI, USA

Peter J. Whitehouse, M.D., Ph.D. University Hospitals Case Medical Center, Neurological Institute Memory and Cognition Center, Beachwood, OH, USA

Paul R. Willging, Ph.D. Bloomberg School of Public Health, The Johns Hopkins University, Baltimore, MD, USA

Elizabeth M. Zelinski, Ph.D. Leonard Davis School of Gerontology, University of Southern California, Los Angeles, CA, USA

John Zeisel, Ph.D. Hearthstone Alzheimer Care, Woburn, MA, USA

Part I
Research Foundations for Cognitive Wellness Interventions

Chapter 1
Memory Enhancement Strategies: What Works Best for Obtaining Memory Goals?

John Dunlosky, Heather Bailey, and Christopher Hertzog

Abstract Adults of all ages experience difficulties remembering important information at times, and these difficulties occur more often as we grow older. Fortunately, a variety of easy-to-use strategies can be used to help people improve their learning and retention of a wide array of to-be-learned materials. In this chapter, we describe (a) many of these strategies, (b) why they work, and (c) how to apply basic principles of memory to adapt strategies to effectively learn and remember in novel contexts. Given that these strategies are often best suited for a single task or context, we also briefly discuss techniques that show promise for helping adults' memory (and cognition) function effectively across many contexts.

Almost everyone complains at times about forgetting an important name, idea, or event. For many younger adults, such failures may be frustrating but are often chalked up to a busy lifestyle or a forgetful personality. As we age, however, many people begin to blame aging itself for such forgetfulness. In the worst case, even healthy adults may become worried that they are showing the effects of getting older, and they may even fear that forgetting is an early sign of dementia. Even if such concerns are unfounded, it is true that as we grow older, learning and retrieving information typically become more challenging. Difficulties remembering needed information can be frustrating, because many contexts require that we learn, retain, and retrieve information to accomplish our goals. Some examples include remembering medical information or a new schedule for taking medications, learning names and procedures required to perform a new job or volunteer work, or even learning facts that are essential for enjoying a variety of past times – such as the names of birds for bird watching or the roster of the local franchise for spectator sports.

J. Dunlosky (✉)
Department of Psychology, Kent State University, Kent, OH 44242-0001, USA
e-mail: jdunlosk@kent.edu

Fortunately, numerous approaches are available to help improve people's memory and retention. Techniques to enhance learning and remembering have a range in their ease of use and overall efficacy. In this chapter, we highlight some strategies that are especially promising. To overview our chapter, we first consider some of the literature on how memory can be improved or trained. We pay special attention to the ultimate challenge of how skills or strategies that are trained can transfer to situations or contexts that differ from the training context. Although our chapter is written for a practitioner who may be seeking to improve his or her clients' memory, the strategies and ideas described herein can easily be adapted by anyone who is trying to overcome memory challenges.

Discovering the Magic Pill for Memory Rejuvenation

It would be great if just one thing were needed to ensure that people achieve their memory goals regardless of what memory obstacle they are trying to overcome. Are there any magic pills available to boost people's memory regardless of what they are trying to learn and remember? An older adult's wish list might include a painless dietary supplement, an easy-to-use memorization strategy that one simply had not heard about, or a lifestyle change that would restore memory function to what it was at age 20. Like Ponce de Leon's Fountain of Youth, the much-hoped for dietary supplement that restores memory has never been found. Although some dietary strategies for supporting cognitive health appear more promising than others (see Chap. 16), even the heralded ginkgo biloba (like other potentially memory enhancing supplements) has not fared well in controlled clinical trials (Einstein & McDaniel, 2004). There is at least some encouraging news, however, regarding cognitive and life-style interventions. Recent research involving recollection training and physical-fitness training has shown considerable promise for improving memory in old age. We briefly touch on this new wave of training research at the end of this chapter. Before doing so, we consider a critical issue in evaluating the effectiveness of an intervention: its breadth of transfer.

One critical aspect of this issue pertains specifically to the degree to which the benefits of a specific intervention – such as a cognitive mnemonic or a lifestyle change – will be broadly beneficial across a wide variety of tasks. In the context of intervention research, psychologists refer to the issue as involving the breadth of transfer of a trained skill to untrained contexts. For example, if one learns a specific memorization technique (often called a mnemonic), can this technique be effective for memorizing widely different kinds of information? Unfortunately, over 100 years of research have demonstrated that transfer is rather limited. Instead, people receive the greatest benefits of an intervention on only those tasks that the intervention was specifically devised to improve. In their chapters, Boot and Blakely (Chap. 2) as well as Zelinski and colleagues (Chap. 3) also address the transfer issue.

To get a sense of the transfer problem, consider the ambitious work by Ball et al. (2002), who had 2,832 older adults (65–94 years old) participate in a cognitive training program that included 4 groups. One group was a no-contact control group, and the other three groups had 10 training sessions that focused on one of three different kinds of cognition – either on memory, reasoning, or speed-of-processing. Adults in the memory-training group were taught to use a variety of mnemonic strategies (some of which we recommend below) for learning lists of words, such as organizing words into meaningful categories. Reasoning training involved learning strategies to identify patterns in stimuli that would support inductive reasoning (learning about the patterns inherent in information). Speed training involved practicing tasks that involved quickly identifying visual information. To evaluate whether the training worked, measures of the targeted cognitive abilities – memory, reasoning, and processing speed – were administered both before and after training. The training procedures boosted performance for the trained task. That is, adults trained to use memory strategies improved their performance on memory tasks, adults trained to solve abstract reasoning problems did better on similar reasoning problems, and adults trained to speed their visual processing showed improvements in these types of tasks as well. However, no evidence for transfer across types of cognition was found. Memory training did not improve reasoning or speed skills, reasoning training did not improve memory or speed skills, and speed training did not improve memory or reasoning skills. These findings are representative of a larger literature on training effects (e.g., Hertzog, Kramer, Wilson, & Lindenberger, 2009a; Lövdén, Bäckman, Lindenberger, Schaefer, & Schmiedek, 2010).

Even worse, numerous studies show that when older adults are trained to use a memory strategy for a specific kind of material (e.g., one is trained to organize words on a list to boost memory), this training does not transfer to other kinds of material (e.g., learning a list of paired associates). One difficulty in achieving transfer in such situations is that people may not realize that skills trained in one task can be adapted for use on other tasks.

In a recent study, Cavallini, Dunlosky, Bottiroli, Hertzog, and Vecchi (2010) trained older adults to use simple mnemonics (e.g., imagery, which is described in detail below); during training, the older adults practiced the mnemonics while learning paired associates and single words. When later asked to learn text materials, these older adults showed no improvement over their original baseline performance. By contrast, another group of older adults received the same mnemonic training, but they also were instructed how the mnemonics could be applied to other (nonpracticed) tasks. Although the application of the mnemonics to text learning was never mentioned, older adults in this transfer-instruction group did show significant increases in the learning of text materials after training. Even so, transfer was not found for all the uninstructed tasks. These results imply that individuals may not think carefully about how to perform in a task context, so that explicit instructions to do so may lead to a better use of available, appropriate strategies. Nevertheless, explicit instructions to consider these issues do not ensure widespread transfer.

One additional constraint is that many strategies devised to improve memory do not work well for all kinds of to-be-learned material. For instance, organizing a list of words into meaningful categories works well for remembering word lists, such as groceries to buy at a store, but would not be useful for learning the names of new acquaintances.

So, the bad news is that, even for cognitive interventions, no "magic pills" are available to boost people's learning and remembering across all possible tasks and situations (for a recent review reporting preliminary evidence that extensive training can produce transfer, see Zelinski, 2009). Instead, efforts must focus on building a larger repertoire of strategies and skills that can enhance memory and on training that will help an individual decide what strategy will help him or her most in a specific situation. In the next section, we describe some popular strategies that can be easily employed to improve learning and remembering specific tasks.

Approaches to Memory Improvement

Diagnosing the Problem

Given that a magic pill to boost learning across all tasks remains undiscovered, the desire to "improve one's memory" could be regarded as too general, and therefore somewhat misplaced. So, if an older adult is complaining about his or her memory and asks you, generically, "how can I improve it?" the implicit answer should be, "it depends!" In practice, first pose follow-up questions that define the client's perceived problem more narrowly. Exactly what are you trying to remember? In what contexts do you need to learn the information? Is there a time pressure to learn the information, or do you have plenty of time to study the target materials? What kinds of support will you have to help you when you remember – will there be cues in the environment to help you retrieve the sought after memories? Put differently, the best approach for providing practical advice about how to improve memory is a clinical model of differential diagnosis and treatment. Diagnose the problem and use this diagnosis to decide which memory-enhancement strategy will work best for the given context.

To strengthen this point, consider one of the most powerful strategies ever devised to improve memory. The *method of loci* involves teaching people to (a) visualize a series of familiar locations, (b) visualize an image representing each to-be-remembered item, and (c) mentally place each item into a corresponding location. A critical feature of this method is creating new associations between well-known locations and the set of to-be-remembered items. For instance, to memorize a grocery list, you could visualize specific rooms in your house and then place mental images of each grocery item into a room (for details, see Einstein & McDaniel, 2004). The method of loci can benefit adults of all ages because one knows where to begin item recall, knows how to monitor the accuracy of recall (one has forgotten an item when a room is empty), and knows when recall is completed. However, the success of the method of loci is typically constrained to concrete words (Baltes & Kliegl, 1992) and to serial learning paradigms (Herrmann, 1987). If someone is interested in improving memory for text materials or for the names of new acquaintances, then the method of loci will be less useful.

Thus, when clients are seeking to achieve a memory goal or want to improve their memory, a good way to begin is to figure out exactly what kinds of task need to be performed better, and then find (or develop) a strategy that will best match that task. In the remainder of this section, we discuss some general principles of memory that will help you understand why specific strategies tend to improve memory, so that you can choose (or develop) the best strategies for your clients' specific needs. We then use these principles to showcase some strategies and when they can be used to enhance performance.

Principles of Encoding and Retrieval

In general, our ability to retrieve previously studied information is related to (a) how well that information is organized in memory and (b) how well encoding strategies distinguish between the to-be-remembered information from other information in memory. In technical terms, *distinctive processing* involves processing differences among items in the context of some organizational framework (Hunt, 2003; see also, Hunt & McDaniel, 1993). The method of loci exemplifies the power of distinctive processing: the loci provide part of the organizational framework, and visualizing each item within a location provides cues that can be used at retrieval to distinguish the sought-after item from others stored in memory. So, imagine using this method to learn a list of groceries: You may take a mental walk to each location, and at the first one (the bedroom), you may remember that you visualized a green vegetable that looks like a forest. This distinguishing cue would lead you away from competitors (e.g., "cauliflower" or "carrots") and right toward "broccoli."

Besides distinctive processing, another principle is that memories will be easier to retrieve if the cues used to *study* the sought-after information are available at the time of retrieval. Again, part of the power of the method of loci can be attributed to the fact that the cues used at study (e.g., the locations) are subsequently available at retrieval (i.e., assuming one remembers the locations when they are needed – and that is why you should instruct clients to select highly familiar loci when using this method).

As we describe various mnemonics below, we discuss how each one draws on these principles in a manner that can enhance learning and retention. Before we get to these strategies, however, we want to stress what is perhaps the most essential principle of memory to remember: Memory is fallible regardless of what strategies are used, so when possible, make sure your clients don't rely on it – instead, encourage them to create an external reminder to get the job done.

Specific Strategies

External reminders. The following point cannot be stressed enough and deserves repeating: When any one really needs to remember something, they should not exclusively rely on memory but instead should support it through the use of an external aid. Fortunately, older adults do not appear to be averse to supporting their memory in this manner: They report using external memory aids more than do younger adults (Dixon & de Frias, 2007; Dixon, Hopp, Cohen, de Frias, & Bäckman, 2003), which is consistent with the argument that these aids can have a compensatory benefit.

External aids are most effective when they are used in a consistent manner. One cannot merely make a to-do list; one needs to check it at the appropriate time to support actually doing what is on the list. Thus, external aids work best if people develop the habit of using them effectively (Tobias, 2009). Consider the most obvious external aid: a written appointment schedule. If clients need to remember an appointment, train them both (a) to *write it down* in a schedule (on paper, a bulletin board, in an appointment book, or an electronic medium like a laptop computer, an intelligent cell phone, or another handheld device) and (b) to learn the habit of checking the schedule throughout the day. One effective technique is to get in the habit of reviewing tomorrow's schedule in the evening, before going to bed, and check it again in the morning before starting the day.

Routines, or habits of behaving, also can provide an important method for avoiding memory failures. People often complain about losing their car keys, and an easy way to lose them is to rely on remembering where they had been put every day. The same problem applies to parking a car in a large parking lot. In both cases, a routine can support memory. For keys, have your clients establish a "memory place" (e.g., a hook beside their door) and encourage them to consistently place their keys in that place when arriving home. For parking, instruct them to park their cars in the same general location in the parking lot every day, or mark down where they parked on a piece of paper put in a wallet or purse for this purpose. In these cases, however, if they failed to use the memory place and forget where something was put, one way to find it is to try to mentally recreate the initial episode. So, they might attempt to recall when they last saw their wallet (e.g., later last evening), and then attempt to recall what they were doing at the time (e.g., emptying their pockets as they watched television). Sometimes this method works (but not always) and its effectiveness has not been systematically investigated. Thus, encouraging your clients to get into the habit of using a memory place may provide better memory support.

A memory problem that we all struggle with is a failure to remember to do something in the future. Such prospective memory failures can be frustrating. For one embarrassing anecdote (feel free to share your own anecdote with your clients), the senior author of this paper was getting ready for a concert and thought to himself in the shower, "I can't forget to grab my ticket." After the hour drive to the venue (that involved going early to get the best seats), the junior author of the paper said, "Okay, take out your tickets for the Indigo Girls!" Needless to say, the drive back home for the ticket was not very pleasant. This problem is probably all too common: forgetting to take something when we leave home (e.g., umbrella, bills, books, mail, grocery lists, etc.), only later to realize one has forgotten to do so, usually when it is too late.

Fortunately, solving this problem is not difficult, as long as you can convince your clients to get into the habit of using the end of each evening to prepare for the next day. They should inspect their schedules for each activity that they need to accomplish the next day, and then they should place anything that needs to go with them in a place that cannot be missed. For the example above, the ticket could have been taped at eyelevel across the front door – no way to leave without it! One simple technique is to place a small table beside the door. Anything that needs to go the next day should be placed on the table, and just to make this fail safe, the table can even be nudged in front of the door. By getting in the habit of preparing each evening for the next day, this kind of forgetfulness can be easily mitigated (unless of course one regularly leaves the house from more than one door).

The best external reminders will not only ensure that you remember what you want, but they will also indicate that you actually remembered. Clients who take many pills and complain about forgetting them should immediately invest in any number of pill boxes available on the market, with the days of the week clearly displayed on each container. If they take the pills at night, then tell them to put the pill box on a pillow or in the bathroom sink; for those taken in the morning, then the pill box should be put beside a coffee pot or any object that is used every morning. Doing so will ensure that they remember to take them, and later in the day if they wonder whether they had, an empty container for that day will offer the best proof.

Sometimes we have numerous activities to attend to on a given day, and if these are not the ones we do often, some may be forgotten. To sidestep the anxiety of forgetting to do something important, older adults should be instructed to keep a calendar right beside the bed, and at night, to write down everything that needs to be accomplished the next day. If the calendar is checked in the morning (e.g., placing it in the bathroom sink will ensure that this check is remembered), they will be one step closer to a successful day.

If your clients can afford any of the new technologies that are hitting the market (e.g., iPhones with alarms, or e-calendars), then these can be used to help them sidestep prospective memory failures. The client (or their caregiver) can be easily trained to set up the device to remind them to do key activities each day. For instance, the iPhone alarm clock can be set to go off with different alarm sounds at various times of the day. Each different alarm can be matched with a different activity, and as important, the iPhone will even record a note that indicates the purpose of the alarm. Recently, Thöne-Otto and Walther (2009) discussed a variety of electronic memory aids that are clinically relevant, including advantages and disadvantages to each (for another critical review, see Kapur, Glisky, & Wilson, 2004). A common disadvantage – other than cost – is that adults who have cognitive impairments or difficulties with fine motor control may have problems programming some of the smaller devices; in this case, you (or a caregiver) will need to provide assistance.

Of course, occasionally we may need to remember something that we cannot write down – hilariously, we may record it on the iPhone, but merely forget to bring it with us when we leave the house. What to do? Well, if the activity is vital, then the best trick is to find a notepad to write the reminder on, and then put that in a place that cannot be missed. If that is not possible, they must rely on memory – and we offer many suggestions on how to improve it below. For prospective memory in particular, one strategy is to form an *implementation intention*. Although the term itself sounds foreboding, it merely means to think about doing what is intended at the right time, which can boost prospective memory performance.

To help one obtain a bird's-eye view on how all these external reminders can be combined, consider the following example: Remembering to take the laundry to the dry cleaners after work. In the evening, your clients should put the laundry in front of the door they use every morning. When they park at work, they should put a shirt on the steering wheel, which is a great external reminder for remembering the dry cleaners. If they need to keep the laundry in the trunk, only then should they turn to an implementation intention: Right before they leave the car to go to work, they should imagine themselves getting in the car after work and driving to the dry cleaners. This simple trick is not fail safe (relying on one's prospective memory rarely is), but some evidence suggests it does increase the chances of remembering (note, however, the technique is just now being widely investigated, and it may not work for adults of all ages, Schnitzspahn & Matthias, 2009).

In summary, the rule of thumb should be: If your clients can rely on an external reminder, then by all means have them do so. If they get into the habit of regularly using reminders and schedules, they may even gain the reputation of being a person who never forgets! However, if they must commit something to memory and cannot use an external reminder (or they just enjoy memorizing their grocery lists), one of the next strategies will likely help them increase the chances of remembering.

Method of loci. The *method of loci* involves teaching people to (a) visualize a series of familiar locations, (b) visualize an image representing each to-be-remembered item, and (c) mentally place each item into a corresponding location. A critical feature of this method is creating new associations between well-known locations and the set of to-be-remembered items. For instance, to memorize a grocery list, you could visualize specific rooms in your house and then place mental images of each grocery item into a room (for details, see Einstein & McDaniel, 2004). The method of loci can benefit adults of all ages because one knows where to begin item recall, knows how to monitor the accuracy of recall (one has forgotten an item when a room is empty), and knows when recall is completed. However, the success of the method of loci is typically constrained to concrete words (Baltes & Kliegl, 1992) and to serial learning paradigms (Herrmann, 1987). If someone is interested in improving memory for text materials or for the names of new acquaintances, then the method of loci will be less useful.

Explicit noticing and rehearsing. It is well known that remembering is, to a great degree, a byproduct of attending to information and processing its meaning. Often, we forget information because we do not attend to it in a meaningful way. Consider the example of forgetting where one's car is parked. This memory failure can occur because we are so absorbed in getting to where we are going and thinking about what we need to do, that we park the car without explicitly reflecting on where it is parked. Here again, writing down the location can be the best approach. But establishing the habit of explicitly encoding where the car is parked (e.g., Row 10, fifth car from the aisle) can also be effective. Moreover, it is often useful to pause before leaving the parking lot, stop and return one's gaze to the location of the parked car, noting its spatial location with reference to what one will encounter upon returning to the parking lot. In general, pausing one's routine to attend explicitly to important information lessens the chance that our tendency to behave on "auto-pilot" will prevent us from encoding the information distinctively.

Elaboration and imagery. Elaborative strategies involve using knowledge that people already have stored in memory to embellish (i.e., elaborate on) what they need to remember. When what needs to be remembered is largely arbitrary, elaboration is especially beneficial because it involves using what one already knows to make the arbitrary become meaningful. For instance, imagine a client – let's call her Betty – trying to remember a pin number for a new bank account (e.g., 3204). You should first help Betty find aspects of her life to elaborate on the number, so that it becomes meaningful to her. In this case, perhaps Betty has four children and the youngest is 32 years old, so she could use this mnemonic to help her remember: "my age (32) when I had my youngest son plus the number of my children (04)". Note how such embellishment makes the number meaningful in a manner that capitalizes on distinctive processing: the numbers are interrelated by the common theme of "information about my children," and using such self-relevant relational processing (or organization) is a powerful memory enhancer in its own right. As important, the power of relational processing is further enhanced by the use of item-specific processing. In this case, the two chunks of numbers (32 and 04) are given a specific meaning when they are processed as "my age when I had my youngest son" and "number of children." Thus, if Betty remembers her mnemonic (about children → age with youngest son and number of children), it would first allow her to reconstruct the general encoding context (it was about my children) and then would allow her to distinguish between the numbers she seeks vs. other numbers that may be relevant to her children (e.g., the age when she had her oldest daughter or son).[1] In this manner, the power of elaborative strategies often arises because they involve *distinctive* processing that entails identifying differences in the context of relational processes.

Many elaborative strategies exist, and we have already introduced one in detail – the method of loci, which has presumably been in use ever since Simonides (547-468 BCE) discovered its memory benefits about 2,500 years ago. The efficacy of this method partly relies on its use of imagery, or picturing to-be-remembered items interacting with the loci in the mind's eye. Similar to the elaborative strategy described above, interactive imagery that is personally meaningful also capitalizes on distinctive processing to enhance memory (Marschark, Richman, Yuille, & Hunt, 1987). To make this point concrete, consider another example. Let's say a client has been upset by repeated failures to remember the names of the various woodpeckers that feed in his backyard. For some reason, Tony cannot seem to remember which one is a Downy woodpecker. So, here is what he should do: Go to the picture of the bird, and identify an outstanding characteristic, such as the big red splotch on the back of its head.

---

[1] Admittedly, numbers are just difficult to remember and are best written down if possible. However, if you have some numbers that you need to memorize or if you are a number fanatic (e.g., you want to remember batting averages of your favorite players etc.), mnemonics have been developed specifically for learning numbers (e.g., Hill, Campbell, & Lindsay, 1997).

In this case, he might imagine the red splotch dripping *down* the woodpecker's back, so that each time Tony sees the red splotch he matches it with "down the back," which would then be linked to Downy. This visual image relates the to-be-remembered name (Downy) right to an obvious feature of the bird, and it helps to distinguish it from many other possible woodpeckers. When a Hairy woodpecker flies up to his window (who also dons the same red splotch), he will need to find other item-specific information to distinguish them. For instance, he could imagine a long ugly beak that is hairy to help him remember that the Hairy woodpecker tends to have a longer beak, whereas the Downy's beak is more petite and dainty.

The idea here is to use prominent features of information to associate, and then develop meaningful – and perhaps even exaggerated – images of those features interacting. By doing so, anyone can gain the power of both relational and item-specific processing, especially if their images are personally meaningful. In fact, imagery is just another form of elaboration, which can involve using any information – visual or verbal – to embellish what one is trying to remember. Just the added effort needed to elaborate on something is likely to boost learning, because it ensures attention is focused on what needs to be committed to memory (cf. Section on "Explicit Noticing and Rehearsing" above).

Structure analysis. When clients want to remember complex information (e.g., the gist of a news story or the pros and cons for a given health plan), they will likely need to use more than elaboration and imagery to obtain their learning goals. A well-written text may offer assistance, because texts that are well written often highlight the critical information using coherent sentence structures that make it easy to comprehend and remember (Britton & Gülgöz, 1991). Nevertheless, all writing is not made equal, so they may have their work cut out for them when they decide to commit a particular argument or story to memory.

To help out, Bonnie Meyer and her colleagues developed and tested a strategy that improves text memory and comprehension. A premise of their efforts is that we cannot remember everything from texts that we read – often, we do not even want to remember all of it anyway. Instead, the most critical information is by definition the most important to retain, and the *structure-strategy* intervention is meant to increase the chances that adults meet the goal of remembering the central information by training them to use signals in texts. While reading, these signals allow people to identify the writer's main goals and structure of the text, and the signals can later be used as a potent retrieval cue. For instance, a writer's main goal may be to discuss *causation* (e.g., what causes acid rain), which would be signaled by key words in the text (e.g., as a result, because, for the purpose of, etc.). Clients could be trained to identify the writer's goal by focusing on these signals, and when they surmise that the writer's goal is to discuss causation, they should then identify the causes and effects embedded in the text; for instance, acid rain (the effect: higher than normal levels of nitric and sulfuric acid in rain) has man-made causes (such as emissions from fossil fuel combustion) and natural causes (such as volcano and cow emissions). When later trying to remember details of the text, they would first identify the text structure (causal, about acid rain) and use that structure to help retrieve any causes and effects. In this case, an astute mnemonist may even use imagery to link acid rain, fuel combustion, and volcano emissions in an interactive visual image.

Another text structure involves comparisons, which are signaled with phrases such as "in contrast," "on the other hand," "whereas," "compared to," and so forth. When such signals are encountered, readers should identify the key issue(s) on which opposing views are being compared and then focus on identifying the differences and similarities of the views within the text. When later trying to recall the information, remembering that the text involved comparison will subsequently signal them to retrieve the issue(s) relevant to the comparison and then to attempt recalling the views on either side of the debate.

The structure-strategy intervention definitely improves people's retention of text materials, and it is likely to be effective for many reasons. Some reasons are that it encourages adults (a) to better attend to what the writer is discussing (because identifying text structures requires focused attention), (b) to organize the text material around one or more structures, and (c) to elaborate on the most pertinent information within that structure. Put differently, by using the structure-strategy intervention, your clients will be capitalizing on distinctive processing to retain and comprehend text materials. Meyer and her colleagues have identified six text structures, and each one is signaled by different text content, so relatively extensive training may be needed to master this strategy. For interested readers, Meyer, Young, and Bartlett (1989) provide detailed instructions on how clinicians and their clients can take advantage of this powerful strategy. Nevertheless, the larger point is that explicitly attending to the structure of ideas in the text and working with this structure to encode it (as opposed to merely reading the text in a more passive manner) can enhance memory for the important information in the text.

Self-testing. The mnemonics that we just discussed are limited in that they will not work for all tasks; the method of loci is great for memorizing lists but may be less useful for memorizing the details of a lengthy argument,[2] whereas structure analysis will not be useful for learning simple associations that are relevant to our day-to-day lives (e.g., remembering where you parked your car or even which evenings your favorite shows are airing). The next two devices that we discuss – self-testing and spaced practice – are more general in that they potentially could be adapted for use across many tasks.

Many people view testing as a way for teachers to evaluate how well their students have learned course content. Although tests do serve this purpose, the act of testing oneself can also have a potent influence on memory, particularly when one correctly recalls sought-after information from long-term memory (Roediger & Karpicke, 2006). Successfully retrieving information also increases the likelihood that this information can be retrieved at a later point in time. Although research has not fully unraveled why testing improves memory, one contributor is that recalling

---

[2] When books and paper were scarce (or just not available), orators would need to commit lengthy texts to memory, and adaptations of the method of loci were used to achieve phenomenal feats of remembering. No doubt, however, orators would use a variety of strategies to distinctively process stories to achieve their lofty goals (Yates, 1966). In our society, we no longer need to transfer the great works (or even lesser ones) by word of mouth, so if we really want to re-live a classic, one just needs to download it from Kindle or go to a local library for a copy.

sought-after information can boost the degree it is connected with other previously stored ideas in memory, and these ideas (or cues) can later be used to increase the likelihood of retrieval (Carpenter, 2009). The self-testing technique builds in part on this process. It involves waiting until sometime after study and trying to retrieve the sought-after information from memory. Afterward, feedback should be obtained by comparing what was retrieved to the correct answer, or if nothing was retrieved, the correct answer should be restudied.

Self-testing can boost memory via two routes. First, it can directly boost memory when the sought-out information is correctly retrieved, as just discussed. Second, self-testing can enhance memory by improving people's self-regulated learning. If people test themselves and cannot recall something now, the failed recall attempt will alert them to spend more time trying to learn the sought-after information. Not only could they spend more time restudying that information, but the failed recall attempt could also be a signal that they need to develop a different strategy to commit the information to memory. Sometimes one's original elaboration or strategy just does not work, and one of the best ways to find out is through self-testing (Bahrick & Hall, 2005).

We have been developing a training program aimed at getting older adults to use self-testing to regulate and improve their learning. Older adults in these programs learn about the benefits of self-testing and are also trained to (a) self-test after initial learning and (b) focus their relearning on information that they cannot currently retrieve. This regulation-training intervention has proved successful both when training occurred in the laboratory (Dunlosky, Kubat-Silman, & Hertzog, 2003) and when older adults trained themselves using a manual (Bailey, Dunlosky, & Hertzog, 2010). In fact, the impact of this self-testing intervention was relatively large when compared to a control group that did not receive self-testing instructions, and they were not appreciably different when older adults trained themselves at home than when they were trained in the laboratory.

Now let's consider how to adapt self-testing to a variety of tasks. Whenever clients meet someone new and care to remember his or her name, they should be trained to use the following strategy: Let's say that Robert introduces himself at a dinner party; immediately they should repeat his name, such as "Hello Robert – great to meet you." This immediate self-test will ensure that they actually attended to the name because if they did not attend and cannot immediately recall it, they are unlikely to remember the name later on. At least at this point, they can always chime in, "I'm sorry, I didn't quite hear what you said, it was…?" If they continue to talk with Robert, then self-tests could occur occasionally by trying to use "Robert" in conversation or by covertly recalling his name right before the conversation ends. If they can recall it then, their memory for the name will get a boost from the successful recall attempt. If they cannot recall it, they still have a chance to correct themselves by asking, "I'm sorry, it was great talking with you, but could you repeat your name again, my memory is a bit rusty."

Self-testing can play an even bigger role as we strive to meet our memory goals. Clients may be studying text materials for a state licensing exam; they may be getting ready to take a bird-watching vacation and want to have the likely candidates easily accessible from memory; or, as a burgeoning baseball fan, they may decide to memorize which teams belong to the leagues and various divisions. In each of these cases, they can use one of the strategies described above to initially study the to-be-remembered information. After finishing with study, they should then go back and test themselves by using the available cues to try to generate the correct answers. The cues they use should be as specific as possible. For instance, they should not simply say, what were the baseball teams? But rather, train them to create cues that map on to the specific information that they are trying to remember. For instance, they may start by learning the divisional structure of baseball and then ask themselves, "What are the teams of the American league, East division?" As we have already seen, organizing the information in a meaningful way (e.g., by league and division), by itself, can be an important part of effective learning.

To expand the illustration, the cues from the aforementioned examples could be the actual practice test questions for the licensing exam (e.g., a picture of each road hazard sign, while trying to retrieve what it signifies) or the pictures of birds (asking for each, what is its name). The critical feature here is not to view the cue and its answer (e.g., the picture of the bird and its name) while self-testing. To find out about what is learned and not yet learned, it is important to try to retrieve the information and use this act of remembering to decide how well the answer has been learned.

As mentioned previously, the very act of successful retrieval should help strengthen memory for that item. But as important, clients should be trained to use successful and unsuccessful retrievals to guide their further study efforts. Restudy should focus on what was not correctly recalled, and this process (study followed by self-testing) should be repeated until everything is correctly recalled at least once. At this point, they can be confident that their memory will be pretty good for what they are trying to remember, although memory will be even better if they continue to correctly recall the information more than once during a single study session (Pyc & Rawson, 2009). Of course, over time, everyone forgets some of what they had learned, so your clients should also allow for this possibility and not get discouraged by forgetting. To ensure very long-term retention of any material, they may even need to combine these elaborative strategies and self-testing with spaced retrieval practice. We consider this form of practice next, and then we discuss how it can be combined with other strategies to create enduring memories.

Spacing practice. Scheduling when and how often materials are studied can be just as important as which strategies are used to study them. A variety of schedules have been extensively investigated, but two are particularly popular. *Massed practice* involves studying a given to-be-remembered material until you are finished, without any intervening study of other materials. When studying Foreign-language vocabulary, one might repeat "chateau – castle" multiple times and then move onto the next item without ever returning to "chateau – castle." By contrast, *spaced practice* involves studying a given material, putting it down, and then coming back to it. For spaced practice, one might study "chateau – castle" for a brief period, study other vocabulary items, and then later go back to "chateau – castle." Research has repeatedly demonstrated the power of spaced practice: even when the amount of time studying is equivalent, subsequent memory performance is typically much higher after spaced than massed practice (for reviews and boundary conditions, see Cepeda, Pashler, Vul, Wixted, & Rohrer, 2006; Dempster, 1988; Donovan & Radosevich, 1999).

Spaced practice is not difficult to apply to many situations, especially with a little forethought. For example, when trying to remember someone's name, older adults should repeat it to themselves covertly as they are talking with the individual, but as important, those repetitions should be spaced, such as repeating the name after an occasional turn of the conversation. If a particular portion of a text is important to remember, then the best way to proceed is to begin by using the structure-strategy technique; afterward, the text should be put down and returned to later for a spaced booster, which involves attempting to recall the structure and the content (i.e., a self-testing attempt) and then rereading the text to make sure what was recalled matches the key points of the text. Such spaced self-testing (paired with restudy) can be easily adapted and highly effective for learning all kinds of material.

If used properly, spaced practice can lead to phenomenal levels of performance even after very long delays. To do so, however, one must have the time and be willing to space practice across multiple sessions that are separated by days and months. Harry Bahrick and his family (Bahrick, Bahrick, Bahrick, & Bahrick, 1993) demonstrated the power of spaced practice for retaining foreign-language vocabulary. Each Bahrick learned 300 vocabulary terms, but they studied only 50 words in any given session. During a session they repeatedly studied and tested themselves on each vocabulary item in a spaced fashion, until they correctly recalled each item one time. They then restudied each list, but at differing lags between practice sessions. For instance, for one deck of 50 words, practice occurred every 14 days for 12 more sessions; for another deck, practice occurred every 56 days for 12 more sessions. After the final practice session for each deck, a test occurred *5 years* later. Even after this long delay, they recalled 60% of the words when the spacing interval was 56 days and 35% when the interval was 14 days. The implication of this study is clear: If your clients want to retain important information over long periods of time, they should study that information until they initially can recall it, but then keep coming back to it from time to time, to make sure they still remember and to restudy what has been forgotten.

As impressive, spacing can actually improve concept learning and problem-solving. Concept learning involves understanding general concepts from experiencing specific examples, such as learning to identify the painting styles of painters (e.g., that a new painting is either by Monet, Renoir, or Pissarro) or learning to classify a new bird with respect to its family (e.g., that a new bird is a finch, a grosbeak, or a thrush). Intuitively, it seems that massing would be the best way to learn these and other concepts; that is, when learning birds, studying and comparing all the finches first, and then going to the grosbeaks second, and so on. By doing so, one might get a good sense of what it means to be "a finch" or "a grosbeak." On the contrary, recent research has shown that concept learning is actually better when practice is spaced (Kornell & Bjork 2008). In this case, one would study a finch, a grosbeak, a thrush, a vireo, a warbler, a thrasher, an oriole, and then begin again. Apparently, experiencing the contrast of how types of birds differ (a type of distinctiveness encoding) assists in classifying their similarity as well. By spacing (or interleaving) study of birds from the various families, it will be easier to identify the family to which a *novel* bird belongs (Wahlheim, Jacoby, & Dunlosky, in press).

Spacing also works for problem-solving. Rohrer and Taylor (2007) taught students to find the volume of four geometric solids (e.g., the volume of a wedge from a cylinder, a spheroid, a spherical cone, and a half cone). During practice, the students either solved each kind of problem en masse (e.g., practice finding the volume for the wedges, followed by practice finding the volume of spheroids) or other students practiced the problems in an interleaved and spaced fashion (e.g., practice with one wedge, then a spheroid). Performance during the *practice* session was better for the massed (89%) than for the spaced (63%) group, but a week after practice, performance on the final test was substantially better for spacers (63%) than for massers (20%)! So, when possible, your clients should space their practice because it can improve their memory for specific materials (e.g., for names, texts, medical information, etc.), their skill at learning new concepts (e.g., classifying paintings or birds), and even their skill to solve novel problems.

The power of combining strategies: Testing and spaced practice. Many of the strategies that we have described may work best when they are combined. In particular, two that seem to go hand-in-hand are testing and spaced practice. In fact, for testing to work well, it often should be delayed after initial study, so that the sought-after information is just not being regurgitated from short-term memory; thus, the testing strategy will often demand spaced practice. Nevertheless, questions do arise about (a) How much testing is necessary to achieve long-term retention, and (b) after a given self-testing attempt, when should the next test occur?

The best answers to these questions will likely be informed by what needs to be learned. The reason is that testing appears to benefit memory most when retrieval is successful. Of course, a failed retrieval attempt does provide valuable information about what has not been learned well enough. However, when the sought-after information is correctly retrieved, it can dramatically boost memory. Thus, for difficult-to-learn materials (e.g., arguments in texts), it may be best to start by trying to recall the argument soon after it is read, just to make sure that the critical arguments can be retrieved. If they can, then a good strategy is to wait longer (e.g., later that day or even the next day) to try to retrieve them again. For easier materials (e.g., Foreign-language vocabulary), most of them could probably be recalled after a short delay, so it is better to challenge memory by waiting until after a longer delay before the first self-test attempt (e.g., 30 min or an hour). The idea is to find a delay in which at least some of the material can be recalled. If nothing can be remembered, then the delay was too long. By contrast, if everything is recalled with ease, then either the test was too early or everything has been learned well enough to move on. Similarly, someone with memory problems (e.g., someone classified as having mild cognitive impairment) may need to begin with short delays between study and test (so that some information can be recalled), whereas a healthy older adult could potentially begin with longer delays.

You may be thinking to yourself, "Well, it could take quite a bit of effort to figure out the right testing schedule for each client who wants to remember different kinds of material." We agree, and no scientist today has a fail-safe prescription for how best to schedule practice to efficiently achieve the most durable learning. So, if clients want to master something important to them, then train them to use trial-and-error and to keep testing themselves (with restudy) at longer delays until they feel that they can fluently retrieve all that they need. One way to accomplish this feat is to create a schedule by using an external reminder (such as a reminder note in your appointment book or an alarm on an iPhone) to remember to keep self-testing until the important information is correctly and readily accessed across multiple test attempts.

This rationale also suggests that an expanding schedule of practice would often be most effective. For this schedule, the initial spacing of test (and restudy) trials is short; for instance, you may have clients study "chateau – castle" and then immediately ask, what does chateau mean? In this case, they are beginning with a test that is right after study, just to make sure that they attended to what they are studying. They should then wait for a longer interval (say enough time to study the rest of the vocabulary terms), self-test again, and then restudy any item they did not recall. The next interval should be even longer, and they should continue expanding the delays between each successive test-restudy trial.

This expanding practice schedule is more difficult to use than a fixed schedule of spaced practice in which the delays between each test-restudy trial are equal in length. Moreover, despite our arguments above, memory performance is not always better after an expanding than fixed schedule (for a recent demonstration involving older adults, see Balota, Duchek, Sergent-Marshall, & Roediger, 2006).

An expanding practice schedule may be ideal for some adults with cognitive impairments. For instance, Cameron Camp and his colleagues have been using a combination of testing (with feedback) and expanding practice to help individuals with dementia remember nurses' names and safe living habits (e.g., Camp & Stevens, 1990; Cherry, Simmons, & Camp, 1999; Brush & Camp, 1998). For these interventions, a trainer would assist the patient. The trainer may first present a picture of a nurse's face along with his name, and then immediately test the patient. If the patient cannot remember the name immediately after it was presented, then the face and name are presented again until they can recall it. Once the name is correctly recalled, then further testing occurs in which the trainer increases the length of the delays between subsequent tests in an expanding manner (e.g., 5 s delay, 10 s delay, 30 s and so forth). If a recall failure occurs at one interval (e.g., at a 30-s delay), then the name and face would be shown again, but the next delay would be the next shortest one (in this case, 10 s delay). If training occurs in an expanded manner during a session and is also repeated across sessions, even individuals with learning deficits can show long-term retention. For these special populations, the practitioner needs to take control away from the patient: the practitioner gives the tests, evaluates the patient's memory, and then makes a decision about when the next test (or restudy) trial should occur. By contrast, healthy older adults would likely be able to use these strategies – spaced retrieval and testing – on their own with relatively little practice (Bailey et al., 2010).

Adapting mnemonics to fit the task. Let's consider how the various strategies can be adapted to fit different task requirements. To illustrate, imagine that you are at the airport and parking in a lot relatively far away from the terminal; given that you travel often, you realize that sometimes you have a difficult time remembering where you parked for the current trip. Your Chevy is on the third floor of the west parking lot in space 12 of Row C. Unfortunately, you do not have a pencil or pen to write down your location, so what should you do? First, you could use imagery to imagine your car with a big C on the dashboard for "C" hevy and row C; this image will help you distinguish between your current row and other rows you have parked in during past trips. You still need to elaborate on third floor and space 12. Perhaps the date 3/12 (or 12/3) has personal meaning, and if it does, use that personal connection to elaborate on the numbers. Perhaps you decide that the space does not matter (you can just walk up the row when the time comes), so you only need to remember 3-West, Row C. For 3-West, you could use imagery by envisioning your car flying west over a field with a big number "3" sewn into it.

To ease your mind, you may decide to combine the imaginal strategy with testing at spaced intervals. You walk to the elevator, and right before getting in, you take a test: if you see a big C on your dash as you are flying west (perhaps the sun is going down) over a field with a "3" on it, then walk onto the elevator. However, if your retrieval attempt at the elevator fails and the image does not come to mind quickly, you have time to check the location again and try to come up with an alternative elaboration to help you remember. Thus, to remember where you parked, you first relied on imagery and then on spaced testing to enhance your memory. When you finally make it to check-in, test yourself again, and if you are on the ball, write down the location and put that external reminder in the same place that you *always* put your car keys when you travel. When you later search for the keys, you will find your note and a sure-fire way to make it back to where you parked. The major recommendation here is that whenever a client takes on a new learning task, you should help them develop the best combination of strategies to use. These should include organizing the to-be-remembered information and processing each piece of information in a manner that will distinguish it from other memories.

Our discussion of strategies above is not exhaustive. Instead we chose to highlight a few strategies that research has shown can improve older adults' memory across relatively common tasks. With a little creativity, these strategies can be adapted to fit any task to improve the likelihood that your clients will learn effectively and remember what they learned. If you are interested in exploring these and other strategies in more depth, we recommend reading Einstein and McDaniel's book, *Memory Fitness: A Guide for Successful Aging*, or the edited volume by Hill, Stigsdotter Neely, and Bäckman (2000), *Cognitive Rehabilitation in Old Age*.

Maybe Some Magic Exists After All

Although no mnemonic strategy will work for *all* learning contexts and tasks, we hope it is clear that many of the mnemonics discussed above can be adapted to fit several tasks. For instance, self-testing often can be used successfully for learning many kinds of material, and in many contexts, spacing practice will also be an option. Also, much of what we want to learn can benefit through the use of elaboration. Thus, even though there is no magic pill per se, many of these strategies will have relatively wide applicability. As important, despite the previous lack of evidence that a given intervention will produce *general* transfer, recent advances in intervention science have uncovered two strategies that show promise for relatively general transfer: training one's recollection and exercising. We briefly touch on each one, and for an extensive review of these (and a few other) new and promising strategies, see Hertzog et al. (2009a).

Training recollection. Some older adults (and even not-so old adults) have problems recollecting specific information, such as remembering whether one turned off the coffee pot or shut the garage door before leaving the house. By recollection, we mean having a vivid and specific memory about the relevant context. For example, when someone asks, "did I turn off the coffee pot," he or she may specifically remember "returning to the kitchen to put a glass in the dishwasher" and "turning the coffee pot off right afterward." Getting older reduces the likelihood of having strong recollective experiences, which could have some negative consequences. For instance, imagine a situation in which an older adult was taking two medications with similar names, such as Celebrex for arthritis pain and Celexa for depression. If she cannot recollect taking Celexa, but the name immediately sounds familiar because she already had taken Celebrex, she might accidentally skip a dose of the depression medication.

Recollection can be trained, in part by using the kinds of powerful methods for learning new information we described earlier in this chapter. For example, Jennings and Jacoby (2003) devised an intervention that enhances recollection and that also seems to transfer to different task contexts. They improved older adults' recollection by having them remember the source of information across increasingly long intervals. This procedure has a study phase and a test phase. In the study phase, people are given a list of words (e.g., house, book, dog…), and in the test phase, they are given studied words (e.g., book) as well as new words (e.g., tree). Critically, the new words are presented twice during the test phase (e.g., tree, iron, dog, bike, tree) after an increasing amount of intervening words, and the second presentation of new words likely elicits a feeling of familiarity. Thus, when people see a repeated new word, they must decide whether it is familiar because they had originally *studied* it or because they saw it recently during the test. That is, they must accurately decide which source (study or test) is responsible for their familiarity with a repeated item. If they respond correctly, the number of items between the first and second presentation of repeated words is increased (e.g., from 1 up to 28 intervening items). Following 7 h of training, older adults were able to remember information as well as young adults with up to 28 intervening items, and these improvements were maintained for up to 3 months. Most importantly, Jennings and Jacoby (2003) found transfer: Improvements after training were not limited to the task on which they were trained. They also improved on a wide variety of cognitive tasks, including those that measure working memory, long-term memory, sustained attention, and processing speed.

Beyond its benefits to recognition memory and many other cognitive processes, another advantage of recollection training is that it can be implemented outside of the laboratory. For instance, to-be-remembered information (e.g., words, names, and pictures) can be printed on note cards. Each card consists of the target information (e.g., a picture) on one side and a label (e.g., "studied" or "new") on the other side. Each "new" item would need to have two cards – one for each presentation. Presentation order during the test phase depends on the desired difficulty. In the beginning, only 1 or 2 cards should separate the first and second presentation of a new item. The number of intervening items should be increased if performance is accurate (e.g., 0 or 1 error). Although self-administered versions of recollection training need to be empirically evaluated, this training is promising because anyone can use it while learning material that matters to them.

Exercising for a fit mind and better memory. Another type of intervention that improves cognitive ability involves aerobic exercise (for a recent review, see Hertzog et al., 2009a). One study tracked older adults who completed either aerobic (i.e., walking) or anaerobic (stretching and toning) exercise (Kramer et al., 1999). After 6 months, the aerobic group was in better shape and demonstrated better performance on a variety of executive function measures as compared to the anaerobic group. Aerobic exercise also has been linked to better cognitive flexibility, long-term memory, and even lower levels of depression. Importantly, all of these cognitive benefits can be enjoyed after as little as 45 min of brisk walking 3 times per week (see Chaps. 2 and 15).

Although physical fitness is not a memory strategy, it seems to benefit memory. But more generally, it can be pursued easily by anyone who wants to improve his or her cognitive and physical well-being (Hertzog, Kramer, Wilson, & Lindenberger, 2009b). A fitness program does not have to be strenuous to provide benefit; a regular walking program that increases heart rate has been shown to have benefits for well-being, physical health, and cognition. Many health maintenance organizations offer programs with graded levels of demand to accommodate to the current capabilities of their members. A cautionary note is in order, however, because if older clients want to reap these benefits of aerobic exercise, they should definitely consult their physician before they begin, particularly if they currently have a sedentary lifestyle.

Final Comments

The strategies described above definitely can promote better memory. At times, they may take a lot of work to master and apply, and even when they are used properly, memory rarely will be perfect – especially if the strategies are used during only a single session of study. Our recommendation is that clients should be trained to use them. With a little creativity, the strategies can be combined and adapted to produce distinctive and relatively durable memories. However, remember that these strategies should be used only when clients absolutely need to remember something. The best way to remember something is not to rely solely on memory. So, an essential aspect of helping your clients meet their memory goals will involve training them to use external reminders and to adapt them to meet any new memory challenge.

Acknowledgments This research was supported by a grant from the National Institute on Aging, one of the National Institutes of Health (R37 AG13148).

References

Bahrick, H. P., Bahrick, L. E., Bahrick, A. S., & Bahrick, P. E. (1993). Maintenance of foreign language vocabulary and the spacing effect. *Psychological Science, 4*, 316–321.

Bahrick, H. P., & Hall, L. K. (2005). The importance of retrieval failures to long-term retention: A metacognitive explanation of the spacing effect. *Journal of Memory and Language, 52*, 566–577.

Bailey, H., Dunlosky, J., & Hertzog, C. (2010). Metacognitive training at home: Does it improve older adults' learning? *Gerontology., 56*, 414–20.

Ball, K., Berch, D. B., Helmers, K. F., Jobe, J. B., Leveck, M. D., Marsiske, M., et al. (2002). Effects of cognitive training interventions with older adults: A randomized controlled trial. *JAMA, 288*, 2271–2281.

Balota, D. A., Duchek, J. M., Sergent-Marshall, S. D., & Roediger, H. L. (2006). Does expanded retrieval produce benefits over equal-interval spacing? Explorations of spacing effects in healthy aging and early stage Alzheimer's disease. *Psychology and Aging, 21*, 19–31.

Baltes, P. B., & Kliegl, R. (1992). Further testing of limits of cognitive plasticity: Negative age differences in a mnemonic skill are robust. *Developmental Psychology, 28*, 121–125.

Britton, B. K., & Gülgöz, S. (1991). Using Kintsch's computational model to improve instructional text: Effects of repairing inference calls on recall and cognitive structures. *Journal of Educational Psychology, 83*, 329–345.

Brush, J. A., & Camp, C. J. (1998). Spaced retrieval during dysphagia therapy: A case study. *Clinical Gerontologist: The Journal of Aging and Mental Health, 19*, 96–99.

Camp, C. J., & Stevens, A. G. (1990). Spaced-retrieval: A memory intervention for dementia of the Alzheimer's type. *Clinical Gerontologist, 10*, 58–61.

Carpenter, S. K. (2009). Cue strength as a moderator of the testing effect: The benefits of elaborative retrieval. *Journal of Experimental Psychology: Learning, Memory, and Cognition, 35*, 1563–1569.

Cavallini, E., Dunlosky, J., Bottiroli, S., Hertzog, C., & Vecchi, T. (2010). Promoting transfer in memory training for older adults. *Aging Clinical and Experimental Research., 22*, 314–323.

Cepeda, N. J., Pashler, H., Vul, E., Wixted, J., & Rohrer, D. (2006). Distributed practice in verbal recall tasks: A review and quantitative synthesis. *Psychological Bulletin, 132*, 354–380.

Cherry, K. E., Simmons, S. S., & Camp, C. J. (1999). Spaced retrieval enhances memory in older adults with probable Alzheimer's disease. *Journal of Clinical Geropsychology, 5*, 159–175.

Dempster, F. N. (1988). The spacing effect: A case study in the failure to apply the results of psychological research. *American Psychologist, 43*, 627–634.

Dixon, R. A., & de Frias, C. M. (2007). Mild memory deficits differentially affect 6-year changes in compensatory strategy use. *Psychology & Aging, 3*, 632–638.

Dixon, R. A., Hopp, G. A., Cohen, A. L., De Frias, C. M., & Bäckman, L. (2003). *Journal of Clinical and Experimental Neuropsychology, 25*, 382–390.

Donovan, J. J., & Radosevich, D. J. (1999). A meta-analytic review of the distribution of practice effect: Now you see it, now you don't. *Journal of Applied Psychology, 84*, 795–805.

Dunlosky, J., Kubat-Silman, A. K., & Hertzog, C. (2003). Training monitoring skills improves older adults' self-paced associative learning. *Psychology and Aging, 18*, 340–345.

Einstein, G., & McDaniel, M. (2004). *Memory fitness: A guide for successful aging*. New Haven: Yale University Press.

Herrmann, D. J. (1987). Task appropriateness of mnemonic techniques. *Perceptual and Motor Skills, 64*, 171–178.

Hertzog, C., Kramer, A. F., Wilson, R. S., & Lindenberger, U. (2009a). Enrichment effects on adult cognitive development: Can the functional capacity of older adults be preserved and enhanced? *Psychological Science in the Public Interest, 9*, 1–65.

Hertzog, C., Kramer, A. F., Wilson, R. S., & Lindenberger, U. (2009b). Fit body, fit mind? Your workout makes you smarter. *Scientific American, 20*, 24–31.

Hill, R. D., Campbell, B. W., & Lindsay, S. (1997). The effectiveness of the number-consonant mnemonic for retention of numeric material in community-dwelling older adults. *Experimental Aging Research, 23*, 275–286.

Hill, R. D., Stigsdotter Neely, A., & Bäckman, L. (2000). *Cognitive Rehabilitation in Old Age*. New York: NY: Oxford University Press.

Hunt, R. R. (2003). Two contributions of distinctive processing to accurate memory. *Journal of Memory and Language, 48*, 811–825.

Hunt, R. R., & McDaniel, M. A. (1993). The enigma of organization and distinctiveness. *Journal of Memory and Language, 32*, 421–445.

Jennings, J. M., & Jacoby, L. L. (2003). Improving memory in older adults: Training recollection. *Neuropsychological Rehabilitation, 14*, 417–440.

Kapur, N., Glisky, E. L., & Wilson, B. A. (2004). Technological memory aids for people with memory deficits. *Nueropsychological Rehabilitation, 14*, 41–60.

Kornell, N., & Bjork, R. A. (2008). Learning concepts and categories: Is spacing the enemy of induction? *Psychological Science, 19*, 585–592.

Kramer, A. F., Hahn, S., Cohen, N., Banich, M., McAuley, E., Harrison, C., et al. (1999). Aging, fitness, and neurocognitive function. *Nature, 400*, 418–419.

Lövdén, M., Bäckman, L., Lindenberger, U., Schaefer, S., & Schmiedek, F. (2010). A theoretical framework for adult plasticity. *Psychological Bulletin, 136*, 659–676.

Marschark, M., Richman, C. L., Yuille, J. C., & Hunt, R. R. (1987). The role of imagery in memory: On shared and distinctive information. *Psychological Bulletin, 102*, 28–41.

Meyer, B. J. F., Young, C. J., & Bartlett, B. J. (1989). *Memory improved: Reading and memory enhancement across the life span through strategic text structure*. Hillsdale, NJ: Erlbaum.

Pyc, M., & Rawson, K. (2009). Testing the retrieval effort hypothesis: Does greater difficulty correctly recalling information lead to higher levels of memory? *Journal of Memory and Language, 60*, 437–447.

Roediger, H. L., & Karpicke, J. D. (2006). Test-enhanced learning: Taking memory tests improves long-term retention. *Psychological Science, 17*, 249–255.

Rohrer, D., & Taylor, K. (2007). The shuffling of mathematics problems improves learning. *Instructional Science, 35*, 481–498.

Schnitzspahn, K. M., & Matthia, K. (2009). Age effects in prospective memory performance within older adults: The paradoxical impact of implementation intentions. *European Jouranl of Ageing, 6*, 147–155.

Thöne-Otto, A. I., & Walther, K. (2009). Assessment and treatment of prospective memory disorders in clinical practice. In M. Kliegel, M. A. McDaniel, & G. Einstein (Eds.), *Prospective memory: Cognitive, neuroscience, developmental, and applied perspectives* (pp. 321–345). New York: Lawrence Erlbaum Associates.

Tobias, R. (2009). Changing behavior by memory aids: A social psychological model of prospective memory and habit development tested with dynamic field data. *Psychological Review, 116*, 408–438.

Wallheim, C., Jacoby, L. L., & Dunlosky, J. (in press) Spacing enhances the learning of natural concepts: *An investigation of mechanisms, metacognition, and aging*. Memory & Cognition.

Yates, F. A. (1966). *The art of memory*. Routledge and Kegan Paul: UK.

Zelinski, E. M. (2009). Far transfer in cognitive training of older adults. *Restorative Neurology and Neuroscience, 27*, 455–471.

Chapter 2
Mental and Physical Exercise as a Means to Reverse Cognitive Aging and Enhance Well-Being

Walter R. Boot and Daniel P. Blakely

Abstract This chapter examines the current data on cognitive interventions, as well as physical fitness interventions, as means of improving cognitive functioning, including a review of the most recent behavioral and brain data. We present evidence that cognitive interventions involving complex video game training are especially promising. Special attention is devoted to the discussion of transfer of training from these interventions to important real-world activities performed every day. Recommendations and future directions are discussed.

Introduction

Numerous studies over the years have detailed age-related changes in basic perceptual and cognitive abilities. These changes include declines in long and short-term memory, attentional control, dual-tasking and task-switching ability, processing speed, and reasoning ability (e.g., Park et al., 2002; Salthouse, 2004; Verhaeghen & Cerella, 2002). Declines occur, in part, as a result of normative age-related changes in brain structure and function (Dennis & Cabeza, 2008; Raz, 2000). Critically, these changes are associated with difficulties performing everyday activities important for functional independence (e.g., Royall, Palmer, Chiodo, & Polk, 2004). In other words, declines in cognition appear to be related to an individual's inability to perform the everyday tasks that allow for independent living without the need for assistance from others (e.g., driving, shopping, finance management, cooking, and housekeeping).

W.R. Boot (✉)
Department of Psychology, Florida State University, Tallahassee, FL, USA
e-mail: boot@psy.fsu.edu

The demonstrated relationship between cognitive abilities and functional independence strongly suggests that interventions capable of improving cognition have the potential to prolong functional independence and provide a better quality of life for seniors. Effective interventions may also provide peace of mind and improved well-being to older adults worried about failing abilities and loss of independence. In addition to benefits to the individual, interventions capable of boosting cognitive functioning have the potential to reduce the societal burden of caring for individuals when functional independence is lost. This may be an especially critical line of research as industrialized nations face dramatic population aging (an increased proportion of the population made up of older adults). It is estimated that by the middle of this century, the proportion of the population composed of individuals 60 years of age or older will more than double in these nations (Cohen, 2003; Lutz, Sanderson, & Scherbov, 2008). Effective methods to support cognition and preserve function may be able to substantially reduce the investment of resources required to confront this challenge, which some have referred to as the "silver tsunami."

New technology may be able to substitute for decreased perceptual and cognitive functioning, and technology designers are beginning to design technology products with age-related changes in mind (Charness & Boot, 2009). For example, cell phones are currently being marketed to older adults taking into account age-related ability changes in vision and hearing. While these approaches are promising and necessary, the current chapter focuses on another approach to assisting older adults in maintaining independence, well-being, and cognitive vitality: the potential of cognitive training and aerobic fitness interventions to ameliorate or reverse cognitive aging and preserve cognitive vitality.

We specifically address normative age-related changes and not cognitive decline associated with dementia, although this is an interesting and important line of research as well. We begin by reviewing evidence that demonstrates older adults can substantially improve their performance on cognitively demanding and challenging tasks with training and practice. We then discuss issues of transfer of skill from trained to untrained tasks; a critical issue to understand if our goal is to improve general cognitive abilities that might augment performance on a variety of important everyday tasks. We then critically review evidence for the ability of cognitive and physical fitness interventions to improve cognition, well-being, and ultimately functional independence. Special focus will be placed on emerging evidence that interventions involving complex video games might improve a number of cognitive abilities. Finally, we wrap up by summarizing not only what we know about the possibility of reversing cognitive aging but also gaps in our knowledge and potential future research directions.

Cognitive Training

Contrary to the often repeated adage that you can't teach an old dog new tricks, there is ample evidence that adult humans maintain a high degree of cognitive plasticity throughout their lifespan. A review of the literature indicates that performance measures on a number of challenging perceptual and cognitive tasks show extensive improvement with practice and training, both for younger and older adults. Although skill acquisition of older adults is slower compared to younger adults, the degree of benefit derived from training is often quite similar (Charness, 2006). For example, Bherer et al. (2005) trained participants (younger and older adults) to perform a difficult task requiring two concurrent discrimination judgments. Both age groups improved to a similar degree with practice, and both benefited to the same degree from individualized adaptive training. Older and younger adults also showed a similar degree of cognitive flexibility when properties of the task were changed. Similar training effects were obtained by Kramer, Larish, and Strayer (1995), who found that performance on a challenging monitoring and arithmetic dual-task substantially improved for both younger and older adults. Although space limitations prevent a detailed discussion, numerous other examples can be observed in the literature. With practice, skilled memory search becomes faster and more efficient for younger and older adults, although automaticity (fast, accurate, and effortless performance) takes longer for older adults to achieve (Hertzog, Cooper, & Fisk, 1996). Older adults and younger adults also benefit greatly in terms of memory training involving mnemonic techniques (Baltes & Kliegl, 1992). Even in an extremely difficult visual search task, older adults can improve as much or more than younger adults in terms of response speed and accuracy with practice, and demonstrate the same degree of transfer of skill to novel search targets (Becic, Boot, & Kramer, 2008; Neider, Boot, & Kramer, 2010). However, even after extensive practice absolute performance of older adults often does not match that of their younger counterparts, suggesting limits to what can be achieved through practice and training. Nonetheless, performance improvements of older adults are robust and impressive, and often match or exceed improvements observed in younger adults.

Overall, results suggest that large improvements on cognitively demanding tasks (at least on tasks that individuals received practice and training on) are possible for older adults. This is encouraging news in terms of designing training interventions that target specific tasks an older adult might be experiencing difficulty with. However, when it comes to improving perceptual and cognitive abilities on a more general level, there is reason to be skeptical that such improvements are possible. This is related to the often studied issue of transfer of acquired skill from trained tasks to untrained tasks.

Training and Transfer of Training

In recent years, numerous brain fitness software packages have been marketed to older adults that make implicit or explicit claims of being able to slow or reverse the cognitive aging process. Nintendo®'s Brain Age™ game is one particularly popular recent example; over 17 million copies of Brain Age™ have been sold worldwide as of 2009 (Nintendo, 2009). As part of the Brain Age™ game, players are assigned a "Brain Age" after a series of tests. A player's "Brain Age" decreases as performance on these tests improve. Brain fitness software packages marketed by companies such as Posit Science® and CogniFit® are also becoming increasingly popular, and many independent and assisted living facilities now provide their residents with access to computer-based cognitive training.

The assumption underlying each of these brain fitness games and software packages is that training benefits obtained on the specific tasks trained within the program will transfer to untrained tasks (specifically, tasks of significance such as driving, remembering important dates, maintaining concentration and preventing distraction in order to follow a conversation, etc.). In other words, the ultimate goal of these interventions is to impact performance of everyday tasks related to independent living and quality of life. However, there is a long history of examining training benefits and transfer of training benefits to untrained tasks in the field of cognitive psychology that gives reason to be critical of these claims. For example, early work by Edward Thorndike (1874-1949) found that training individuals (in this case, younger adults) to estimate the area of rectangles improved performance on that specific task, but did not improve estimates of the areas of other shapes, nor did it transfer to estimates of other dimensions such as weight (Thorndike & Woodworth, 1901a, 1901b). In other words, participants learned a very specific skill that did not generalize to other tasks similar to the task they were trained on. Thorndike also found that training participants to read passages of text and mark words containing a particular letter combination (e.g., words containing both an e and s) did not improve speed or accuracy of marking words containing other letters or marking misspelled words (Thorndike & Woodworth, 1901c). Finally, Thorndike examined the once popular notion that learning Latin would lead to a disciplined mind, thus having broad transfer to a number of different domains (Thorndike, 1923). However, no evidence of such a benefit was found. These early studies set the stage for future research suggesting that broad transfer is difficult to achieve and that there is a great deal of specificity in training and learning.

More recent work in a number of different domains supports the notion of limited transfer of training. Narrow transfer of skills such as problem-solving is a major issue with regard to education (e.g., Mayer, 1987). The ideal in education is to teach skills that are broadly useful, but this has proven to be a difficult task. Consistent with Thorndike's study of Latin training, learning computer programming does not appear to improve general problem-solving abilities (Pea & Kurland, 1984). Learning the solution to a problem does not guarantee that the same solution will be applied to solve similar problems in other contexts (Catrambone & Holyoak, 1989). Expertise in one domain does not necessarily transfer to other domains or tasks (e.g., Chase & Simon, 1973, Larkin, McDermott, Simon, & Simon, 1980). In general, although practice within a domain and on specific tasks can lead to substantially improved performance, this by no means guarantees better performance on other tasks, even tasks that may seem superficially similar to the learned tasks. As an example, take the case of master chess players. When asked to memorize the location of pieces on a chess board, chess masters can quickly and nearly perfectly replicate the presented pattern of pieces from memory as long as the chess pieces are arranged in such a way that they could have come from an actual game. However, if the presented chess boards show pieces arranged randomly, the performance of master chess players is sometimes indistinguishable from that of novice players (Chase & Simon, 1973).

Perceptual learning also appears to be particularly specific. Learning to discriminate vertical waveforms does not transfer to horizontal waveforms (Fiorentini & Berardi, 1980). Learning to discriminate motion in one pair of directions does not transfer to other directions (Ball & Sekuler, 1982). Training in a discrimination task may not fully transfer from one eye to another (Fahle, Edelman, & Poggio, 1995) and may not transfer from one retinal location to another within the same eye (Shiu & Pashler, 1992). These results suggest that even in fairly simple tasks broad transfer of training (transfer from one task to multiple other dissimilar tasks) is the exception rather than the rule. It is likely that difficulties in obtaining transfer of skills in more complex tasks may result both from the limited transfer of perceptual learning, as well as limited transfer of higher level cognitive skills such as problem-solving and reasoning (see Owen et al., 2010 for another interesting example of lack of transfer). These findings highlight the challenge of using computer-based training interventions to improve perceptual and cognitive abilities that can and will be transferred to everyday tasks critical for functional independence. However, many researchers have confronted this challenge, partly due to observational studies in humans and experimental studies in animals that have served as the basis for the *cognitive enrichment hypothesis*. These findings suggest that engagement in complex physical and cognitive activities can improve and maintain cognitive vitality.

The Cognitive Enrichment Hypothesis

A common finding is that individuals who maintain a higher degree of cognitive engagement throughout life and into old age fare better in terms of cognitive aging (e.g., Hultsch, Hertzog, Small, & Dixon, 1999; Schooler & Mulatu, 2001). It may not be possible to draw strong causal conclusions from these studies, but they are suggestive that a lifetime of mentally stimulating work and activities can function to preserve cognition. Furthermore, work with animals suggests that more complex living environments that include opportunities to exercise, socialize, and explore can improve memory and result in various positive changes to brain structure and function (van Praag, Kempermann, & Gage, 2000). Early attempts to improve cognitive abilities in older adult humans focused on improving specific abilities with targeted training interventions rather than trying to improve general abilities that might impact multiple tasks (Schaie & Willis, 1986; Willis & Nesselroade, 1990). However, nonexperimental human studies and experimental animal studies appear to suggest the possibility of improving function generally. Experimentally, researchers have tried to demonstrate the efficacy of various training programs to impact cognitive functioning to varying degrees of success. Next, we review evidence of the effectiveness of a number of cognitive training interventions, including a detailed discussion of the largest randomized trial to examine this issue.

The ACTIVE Trial

The Advanced Cognitive Training for Independent and Vital Elderly (ACTIVE) randomized trial represents, to date, one of the largest and most carefully conducted investigations into the effects of cognitive training on measures of basic cognitive abilities and everyday functioning (Ball et al., 2002). In total, over 2,800 participants were randomly assigned to complete one of three training interventions or were assigned to a control group that received no cognitive training. Training interventions were tested that had shown promise in smaller-scale studies. The *memory training group* received training that focused on teaching strategies to improve verbal memory. The *reasoning training group* practiced recognizing and utilizing patterns to solve problems. Finally, the *speed-of-processing training group* received training on a divided-attention visual search task. Outcome measures included tests of basic abilities as well as measures of everyday functioning, which were assessed at baseline, after 10 h of training, and multiple years afterward (with some participants receiving booster training). Everyday functioning outcome measures tested participants' ability to react to road signs, count change, and remember and interpret information on food labels and medication bottles, in addition to a number of other everyday activities requiring speed, memory, and reasoning ability.

For each training intervention, participants demonstrated impressive gains on the specific tasks on which they were trained, consistent with the existing literature on aging and cognitive plasticity. Encouragingly, training benefits were maintained for years afterward. However, little to no improvement in real-world outcome measures was observed, at least in the initial 2 years post-training. Transfer of training results were largely consistent with the extant literature on learning and training finding limited transfer of acquired skills to nontrained tasks. Although initial reports of the outcome of the ACTIVE trial were disappointing with respect to improving performance on everyday tasks, follow-up assessments of participants who received training were more encouraging. It may be important to consider that participants indicating signs of functional or cognitive decline were not admitted into the trial, and even the control group demonstrated little functional decline over the 2-year period initially reported. Thus lack of improvement could be attributable to ceiling effects.

The framework proposed by Hertzog, Kramer, Wilson, and Lindenberger (2009) posits that intervention effects may not be apparent immediately, but instead may postpone the age at which an individual crosses the threshold at which functional independence is lost. With respect to the ACTIVE trial, 5-year follow-up assessments indicated milder self-reported declines in ability to perform instrumental activities of daily living for the group receiving reasoning training (Willis et al., 2006). Participants in the speed-of-processing training group self-reported fewer health problems at 2 and 5-year follow-up assessments, as did participants in the memory and reasoning training groups after 5 years, although these effects were smaller in magnitude (Wolinsky, Unverzagt, Smith, Jones, Stoddard, et al., 2006; Wolinsky, Unverzagt, Smith, Jones, Wright, et al., 2006b). Furthermore, the speed-of-processing group was less likely to demonstrate clinically relevant increases in depressive symptoms 1 and 5 years post-training compared to the control group (Wolinsky, Mahncke, et al., 2009; Wolinsky, Weg, et al., 2009). Thus, the ACTIVE trial suggests that cognitive training of highly functional older adults may build reserve capacity which can function to ameliorate declines later in life, potentially postponing the loss of functional independence.

The IMPACT Trial

The IMPACT (Improvement in Memory with Plasticity-based Adaptive Cognitive Training) study provides evidence for more immediate gains as a result of cognitive training (Smith et al., 2009). The IMPACT study was a randomized, double-blind clinical trial in which older adults were assigned to either a cognitive training intervention or an "active control" group, in which participants watched educational DVDs. Compared to the control group, the cognitive intervention group engaged in tasks that focused on improving performance in auditory discrimination and memory tasks, based on the idea that age-related declines in cognition depend in part on the quality of the sensory information passed along to higher cognitive processes. Additional information about the IMPACT study intervention is provided in Chap. 3.

Differential improvement by the cognitive intervention group was observed on a number of neuropsychological tests of auditory memory and attention. Reliable differences were also observed in self-reported cognitive functioning, unlike the ACTIVE trial in which transfer of training effects were not observed until years after the conclusion of the intervention. The results of the IMPACT trial are encouraging in that the observed transfer was immediate. However, interpretation of the effectiveness of the intervention is somewhat limited. First, objective outcome measures assessing everyday abilities, functional status, and well-being were not included in the trial. Additionally, other cognitive abilities that experience large age-related declines (e.g., reasoning and executive control) were not measured, thus it is uncertain how broad transfer of training actually was. Finally, it is uncertain how long the achieved gains might last as no follow-up assessments were conducted.

Internet and Computer Use Interventions

Positive results of some forms of cognitive engagement do not necessarily bode well for all interventions promoting cognitive enrichment. A notable instance of cognitive engagement intervention failing to provide observable benefits to cognition and well-being comes from an intervention examining the influence of computer and Internet use on cognitive aging. Slegers, Boxtel, & Jolles (2008, 2009) conducted a dual-purpose study to assess the effects of computer and Internet use on the subjective well-being and quality of life of older adults as well as its potential to decelerate, halt, or reverse cognitive decline. Past research in this area has found positive effects of such interventions on both psychosocial (e.g., McConatha,

McConatha, & Dermigny, 1994; McConatha, McConatha, Deaner, & Dermigny, 1995; Sherer, 1996) and cognitive measures (McConatha, McConatha, & Dermigny, 1994), but Slegers et al. argued that these studies lacked proper control, selected samples poorly, or utilized imprecise assessments. Their goal was to implement rigorous randomization and control that would lend their investigation a more methodologically sound approach than previous endeavors in this area.

Two-hundred and forty older adults ranging in age from 64 to 75 participated. For those in the intervention, Internet-capable computers were installed in their homes for 1 year. The remaining participants comprised three different control groups in order to eliminate confounding effects that might be attributable to the initial training program and participants' willingness to use computers. Quality of life and cognitive ability measurements were administered at the beginning of the experiment and again at 4 and 12 months.

In order to assess the effects of computer and Internet use on the well-being and quality of life of older adults, Slegers et al. used measures of subjective physical well-being, subjective activity, social network and perceived loneliness, psychological functioning, mood, neuroticism and extraversion, activity level, satisfaction with life, activities of daily living, and perceived autonomy. These measures were chosen in accordance with Felce and Perry's (1995) theory of the five dimensions of well-being fundamental for quality of life: physical, material, social, and emotional well-being as well as development and activity. After comparing differences in scores of the intervention group over time to those of the control groups, Slegers et al. were unable to find evidence to support the hypothesis that computer and Internet use improves older adults' well-being and quality of life.

Following Swaab's (1991) argument that neural use prolongs neural efficiency, Slegers et al. also hypothesized that habitual computer and Internet use might elicit this effect in older adults since it is an activity that often requires one to employ many different cognitive abilities in order to complete a complex task. The effect of their intervention on cognition was assessed through a battery of tasks that examined verbal memory, psychomotor speed, general cognitive speed, cognitive flexibility, and attention. A subjective measure of cognitive failure was also used. Unfortunately, similar to well-being measures, no meaningful improvement was observed as a function of the intervention.

While these results may initially seem damaging to the hypothesis that computer and Internet use may be beneficial for older adults, Slegers et al. grant that some aspects of this study may have led to the null findings. Like the ACTIVE trial, participants were all healthy, community-dwelling older adults who were largely independent and performed at the average of their cohort on many of the measures. Therefore, their results may not be representative of the possible effects computer and Internet use could have on those experiencing a more dramatic decline in cognition or well-being. Additionally, the measures of both dimensions in question were not necessarily exhaustive. The intervention may have had an impact on aspects of quality of life or cognitive ability that were not evaluated. With respect to subjective measures of well-being, the participants' self-assessments only represent their views at a particular moment, not necessarily their average view over time. Finally, it may be possible that 1 year of computer and Internet use may not be enough for these effects to be evident. Although Slegers and colleagues question the likelihood of effects to manifest themselves at longer intervention durations when they were not found after an entire year of use, they propose the intriguing question of whether a suitable preventive intervention of computer and Internet use would be beneficial to older adults at the point when they begin to experience age-related disabilities in both the psychosocial and cognitive domains.

Video Games as Cognitive Interventions

Despite cited evidence of limited transfer of training, intriguing new data suggest that training involving complex, commercially available video games may be an exception to this general rule. Cognitive aging interventions involving video game play may be a promising approach to enhance failing perceptual and cognitive abilities. As we will discuss later, such an approach, if effective, has a number of potential advantages over more traditional approaches.

Much attention has been devoted to improving functional field of view in older adults given that this measure appears to be related to driving safety (e.g., Ball et al., 1988; Ball & Owsley, 1991; Roenker et al., 2003). However, equivalent gains in useful field of view appear to be engendered by engagement in action video game play in young adults. Green and Bavelier (2003) found that habitual video game players demonstrated superior visual and attentional abilities compared to nonvideo game players, including a wider useful field of view. Furthermore, nonvideo game players demonstrated substantial gains in visual and attentional abilities after just 10 h of action video game play compared to a control group that played a nonaction game (Tetris, a game that has similar motor demands but substantially different visual and attentional demands). Subsequent studies have found that action video game play can improve both visual acuity and contrast sensitivity and that effects are long-lasting (Green, & Bavelier, 2007; Li, et al., 2009). Boot and colleagues (2008) demonstrated that compared to nongamers, habitual gamers have a greater memory capacity for objects and can manage multiple tasks more efficiently, suggesting game benefits may extend beyond the realm of vision and visual attention. Thus, interventions involving complex video game play appear to be a promising direction of investigation when it comes to slowing or reversing age-related declines in perceptual and cognitive abilities (Achtman, Green, & Bavelier, 2008; Green & Bavelier, 2008).

This hypothesis was initially tested using the relatively visually sparse and simple games of the 1980s and early 1990s (Dustman et al., 1992; Goldstein et al., 1997). In general, although older adults improved in response time tasks with training on these early video games, transfer of training was otherwise fairly limited and did not include improvements in measures of inhibition, reasoning, or planning. However, based on the results of Green and Bavelier using more complex, modern video games that include a much greater amount of complexity, Basak, Boot, Voss, and Kramer (2008) examined the idea that a short-term video game intervention might improve a variety of cognitive abilities in older adults.

Older adults were randomly assigned to a video game training condition or control condition in which they received no treatment, and perceptual and cognitive abilities were assessed before, during, and after training. Participants assigned to the video game condition were required to play a complex real-time strategy game called *Rise of Nations* for approximately 23 h over the course of 8 weeks. This game situates players on a large map along with one or more computer players. At first the player is in control of a primitive stone-age civilization. As resources are collected and allocated, and as new structures and towns are built, the civilization advances toward the modern age. The game is won when a player controls 70% of the map, when all other players are defeated through battle, or when one player builds all "Wonders of the World." This game was specifically chosen based on its demands on memory, reasoning, and executive control. *Rise of Nations* involves maintaining and switching between multiple goals (e.g., building new cities, fighting attacking armies, collecting and managing resources). It also involves planning and places a high demand on working memory (remembering where your own cities are on a large map, where enemy forces are located, etc.). Based on these demands, it was expected that executive control and memory would be improved.

Confirming this prediction, participants who played *Rise of Nations* differentially improved on measures of reasoning ability, task-switching, working memory, and spatial ability. Furthermore, larger gains were observed for participants who improved the most on the game. Note that compared to the ACTIVE trial, this transfer of training was immediate. However, important caveats are that transfer to everyday tasks was not assessed, and participants were not assessed again after the secession of training, so it is unclear how durable the cognitive gains were (although work with young adults finds lasting benefits; Li et al., 2009). Results are suggestive, though, that gaming interventions involving complex strategy games can improve performance on a number of different tasks.

The appeal of such interventions is obvious. Video games are specifically designed to be enjoyable and rewarding, and they are inherently motivating. Thus, adherence to a gaming intervention might exceed adherence to more traditional computer-based cognitive interventions. With advances in hand-held gaming technologies, video game interventions can be made to be highly portable and convenient (training can occur anywhere, on a bus or in a doctor's waiting room). However, the issue of transfer of training is still somewhat of a concern even in the case of video game training. To date, little convincing experimental data exists demonstrating the ability of video game play to improve performance on everyday tasks performed outside of the laboratory (although see Gopher, Weil, & Bareket, 1994 for a notable exception). Future research will be able to determine whether the exceptionally broad transfer of training engendered by video games extends to performance of everyday tasks.

Physical Fitness Training

We have thus far reviewed the evidence that cognitive training interventions can improve cognitive functioning in older adults. However, a growing body of evidence now suggests that *physical* exercise may be a particularly effective means of improving cognition and enhancing brain structure and function. For example, in adult animals (mostly mice and rats) research has found that a number of beneficial changes occur in the brain as a result of exercise. Specifically, aerobic exercise is associated with increased neuron survival, neurogenesis (growth of new neurons), angiogenesis (growth of new vasculature), higher concentrations of neuroprotective molecules, and changes in neurotransmitter systems (see Kramer, Erickson, and McAuley (2008) and Vaynman and Gomez-Pinilla (2006) for recent reviews). The results obtained by Nichol, Parachikova, and Cotman (2007) are particularly interesting. Nichol and colleagues examined the effects of exercise on cognitive functioning in a mouse model of Alzheimer's disease. A 3-week running intervention reversed cognitive declines in older animals already experiencing significant cognitive impairment. This finding implies that exercise interventions may serve not just as a preventive measure but also as a treatment for cognitive decline. The sum of the animal literature examining the relationship between brain, cognition, and exercise suggests that exercise interventions might serve to preserve cognitive functioning in humans if these changes also occur as a result of exercise in the adult human brain.

Aerobic exercise interventions with humans confirm the influence of physical fitness on cognition and brain structure and function. Kramer et al. (1999) examined the effect of fitness interventions on cognition in a sample of 124 sedentary older adults. Participants were randomly assigned to participate in either an aerobic exercise intervention or a stretching and toning intervention. For 6 months, participants engaged in the activity they were assigned 3 times a week, for approximately 1 h each session. Not surprisingly, aerobic fitness (as measured by VO_2 peak, an indicator of cardiorespiratory endurance) improved for the participants assigned to the aerobic exercise intervention. However, compared to the nonaerobic stretching and toning group, the aerobic exercise group also demonstrated improved performance on a number of cognitive tasks and tests measuring executive control, inhibition, and selective attention. These results are significant for a number of reasons. First, the amount and intensity of aerobic exercise (walking) needed to induce improved cognition were relatively modest. Second, the cognitive abilities that demonstrated improvement were those that decline most with age. A meta-analysis conduced by Colcombe and Kramer (2003) found both broad and specific effects of aerobic exercise on cognitive functioning. Eighteen intervention studies examining the effects of aerobic exercise on cognition published from 1966 to 2001 were included in this meta-analysis. Significant exercise effects were observed in tasks measuring processing speed (e.g., simple reaction time tasks), spatial ability (e.g., mental rotation), controlled processing (e.g., choice reaction time), and executive control (e.g., flanker task). Although exercise influences cognition broadly, the largest exercise effects were observed in tasks measuring executive control (planning, scheduling multiple tasks and responses, inhibition, etc.). Several moderating variables were found to be important as well. Interventions that combined aerobic training and strength training produced greater improvement compared to aerobic fitness training alone. Training session duration also mattered. Exercise sessions of less than 30 min had little effect on cognition.

Similar to effects observed in nonhuman animals, improved cognition may be a result of beneficial effects of exercise on brain structure and functioning. Colcombe et al. (2003) assessed cardiovascular fitness in a sample of 55 healthy older adults who were at least 55 years of age. Using anatomical MRI scans, Colcombe et al. observed previously observed age-related declines in gray and white matter density. However, cardiovascular fitness moderated declines such that age-related declines in gray and white matter density were reduced for individuals demonstrating higher aerobic fitness. Even stronger evidence that brain structure and function can be influenced by aerobic exercise comes from intervention studies. For example, a 6-month aerobic fitness intervention is capable of increasing gray and white matter density in older adults (Colcombe et al., 2006). A similar intervention can change brain function during an attentional control task such that older adults demonstrated a pattern of brain activation similar to younger adults (Colcombe et al., 2004). Thus, in terms of improving cognitive ability and brain structure and function, numerous animal studies, human cross-sectional, and human longitudinal studies implicate aerobic exercise as producing the largest, most reliable, and robust effects.

Future Directions and Recommendations

From the evidence reviewed here, it is clear that older adults, while vulnerable to cognitive decline, are capable of acquiring new skills and exhibiting a high degree of neural plasticity. However, the greatest concern encompassing these findings is how well training can successfully improve the performance of meaningful, everyday activities in order to provide perceivable benefits. In general, training involving simple, unimodal, process-specific tasks typically results in improved performance that does not generalize beyond the specific tasks trained. This is a major obstacle if our goal is to improve cognition generally. As an alternative to this view, the cognitive enrichment hypothesis proposes that exposure to complex, multimodal interventions involving physical and cognitive activities may be the key to combating age-related declines in perceptual and cognitive abilities and prolonging functional independence. Within this promising framework, a number of important questions still remain to be answered (see Table 2.1).

General vs. Targeted Training: Effectiveness and Training Efficiency

In addition to training effectiveness, we believe that training efficiency should receive greater attention. One potential measure of intervention success is the amount of benefit gained per unit of time invested. The advantage of general interventions designed with the purpose of encouraging broad transfer of training is that performance improvements on many different tasks can be engendered

Table 2.1 Unresolved issues and future directions

Issue	Question	Potential future direction
General vs. task specific training	Should training target specific tasks (e.g., driving) or try to improve cognition generally?	Identify performance improvements that would be most meaningful and compare benefits of each approach using the same measures
Comparative effectiveness	Which activities produce the largest benefit with the least investment of time, effort, and money?	Contrast interventions in terms of training time, compliance, financial cost, effect size, and breadth of transfer
Individualized training	Can we develop individualized, adaptive training methods that target specific needs?	Develop interventions that take into account baseline ability and adjust the nature of training activities based on the deficits of the individual
Combination interventions	Can maximum improvement be achieved through an intervention that combines aspects of multiple approaches?	Compare cognitive training programs (including video game training) that include aspects of physical exercise to physical or mental exercise alone

simultaneously. However, if the goal is to improve performance on one or a handful of specific everyday tasks, a critical question is this: how does a general, nontask-specific training approach compare to a targeted intervention offering training on specific everyday tasks, in terms of both effectiveness and efficiency? For example, one can ask how many hours of brain fitness software training are necessary to meaningfully improve older driver safety compared to the number of hours needed to improve driving performance to the same degree using a targeted intervention focused on driving skill. Such trade-offs need to be considered in evaluating the overall value of an intervention.

Comparative Effectiveness

Currently, older adults concerned about cognitive aging are confronted with a number of products on the market claiming to be able to slow the cognitive aging process (some of which require hundreds of dollars in software costs alone). Which products are worth the investment in terms of time and money and which are not? Moreover, how do these interventions compare to other forms of cognitive engagement that are less costly and may have other positive effects associated with them? One possibility is that alternate forms of cognitive engagement such as learning a new language, musical instrument, or hobby may produce similar benefits compared to brain fitness software packages. If this is the case, then older adults may have more enjoyable and readily available options to boost their brain power.

However, if contrary to the encouraging data presented here, commercially available brain fitness software packages and alternative activities of cognitive engagement fail to produce large effects on functional independence, one can argue that these alternative activities are still worthwhile in terms of personal enjoyment and gaining a potentially useful skill. Returning to the large body of evidence that aerobic exercise improves cognition, it is known that exercise has a number of noncognitive health benefits. It is possible that a free exercise intervention (walking) may be more effective than commercially available software packages in preserving cognitive vitality, in addition to improving overall physical health. Comparative effectiveness of different interventions with the purpose of improving cognition is thus an open and important question to consider.

Individualized Training

Related to the idea of training effectiveness and efficiency, it is clear that individuals differ in ability. Thus, a "one-size-fits-all" strategy to boosting perceptual and cognitive abilities of older adults may be ill-advised. Future intervention studies might examine the effect of adapting the intervention to the specific needs of the individual. Thus more time is devoted to training abilities that are deficient, and less time is devoted to training skills that are intact. With respect to video game training, although improvements appear to be broad, some games appear to improve certain abilities better than others (e.g., action games tend to improve visual abilities while strategy games improve higher-level cognitive functioning). In the future, it may be possible to "prescribe" video game interventions based on individual needs.

The Future of Video Game Interventions

Although video game interventions appear highly promising, there may still be a number of obstacles to overcome in order for these interventions to reach their fullest potential in addressing the problem of cognitive aging. These issues are discussed next.

Issues Regarding Aging and Gaming

Currently, it appears video game companies are marketing games to older adults based largely on older adults' fears of declining ability. Other than this, little effort is being made in designing the types of games that older adults may *enjoy* playing, and, according to Pearce (2008), older gamers are taking notice. This trend may not be wise given the growing numbers in this demographic. Pearce's study investigating the video game preferences of adults ranging from 40 to 65 years of age suggests that those verging on older adulthood prefer video games that are intellectually challenging and include role-playing, mystery, or adventure. The participants in this study largely preferred video game elements involving exploration, puzzle-solving, "questing," and socializing. Preference for combat and shooting games was more evenly split, while fighting, racing, and sports games were generally disliked. When considering possible intervention programs that utilize this medium, knowledge of the likes and dislikes of typical older adults in the realm of video games will be crucial in obtaining optimal motivation and compliance.

The Future of Combined Physical and Mental Exercise

There is ample evidence to suggest that exercise can improve various cognitive abilities in older adults, including executive control, inhibition, selective attention, processing speed, and spatial abilities. We have also discussed existing research indicating that gaming can improve attentional and spatial abilities, visual acuity, contrast sensitivity, working memory capacity, executive control, and reasoning. Could a combination of these two promising interventions maximally counteract the effects of cognitive decline in older adults? Arguably, the most contemporary and prevalent device that incorporates both of these activities is the Nintendo Wii™. This video game console utilizes motion sensing technology through an infrared sensor and accelerometers in the controllers, thereby allowing players to manipulate actions occurring on-screen. The system also offers an optional balance board accessory that detects the user's foot placement, shifts in weight distribution, and center of gravity, and it is often used in conjunction with exercise-oriented games.

The potential of this type of system to provide users with a combination of video game playing and exercise is readily apparent, but there is little to no research assessing its potential effects on cognitive abilities, especially in older adults. Therefore, this is an avenue of research that is ripe for exploration. In order to explore the potential of this and similar devices as possible intervention tools for confronting age-related cognitive decline, there are a number of factors that must be considered concerning the nature of the video games to be used. As mentioned previously, in order for an intervention to be maximally effective, the games will need to appeal to older adults. The exercise literature indicates that games will need to produce a level of activity deemed aerobic to impact cognition. So far, conclusions regarding the effectiveness of "exergames" in providing sufficient aerobic activity, at least in children and adolescents, are mixed (Graves et al., 2007; Lanningham-Foster et al., 2006; Maddison et al., 2007). Safety issues, such as preventing injury and falls, need to be addressed as well. Finally, although a game may produce aerobic activity, it may not have the visual and psychomotor complexity to engender broad transfer of training. Taking each of these points into consideration, the designer of an intervention using exergames faces the challenge of finding video games that are appealing to older adults, intellectually stimulating, and also involve action and elicit aerobic activity. Though this may be difficult, the outcome of such a study is theoretically promising.

Practical Recommendations

Physical exercise is worthwhile for its physical health benefits alone, but evidence reviewed demonstrates positive cognitive effects as well. However, physical activity is not solitary in providing such gains as researchers have shown that video game playing as well as other forms of cognitive engagement can lead to improvements in a number of cognitive skills. While brain-fitness software packages show promise as cognitive enhancement tools for older adults, there is work yet to be done in evaluating their effectiveness with respect to objective measures of everyday performance. Primarily, this class of intervention needs to demonstrate a robust ability to improve scores on measures of everyday functioning, particularly actual or simulated everyday tasks. After all, what is the true benefit of a cognitive intervention to the individual older adult if the only perceivable effects are improved scores on laboratory task? Given the current evidence, the best practical recommendations that can be made for confronting cognitive decline in older adults are as follows:

Physical Exercise. Demonstrated to promote brain structure and function

- Considerations:
  - Aerobic exercise produces maximum benefit
  - Even moderate levels of exercise are effective (walking 3 times a week for 40 min each time)
  - Initial physical fitness and health status must be considered before an exercise program is implemented

Cognitive Engagement. Promising data indicate potential cognitive benefits

- Considerations:
  - Complex, multimodel activities produce maximum benefit
  - Evidence suggests promise of complex video game training
  - Cognitive activity must be engaging enough to maintain interest and enhance compliance

In conclusion, the current state of the literature indicates steps that an individual can take to reduce the effects of cognitive aging (see Hertzog, Kramer, Wilson, and Lindenberger, 2009; Lustig, Shah, Seidler, & Reuter-Lorenz, 2009; Park & Reuter-Lorenz, 2009 for similar but slightly different conclusions based on the current state of the literature). Future research must elaborate on the nature, duration, and relative effectiveness and efficiency of different approaches.

References

Achtman, R. L., Green, C. S., & Bavelier, D. (2008). Video games as a tool to train visual skills. *Restorative Neurology and Neuroscience, 26*(4–5), 435–446.

Ball, K. K., Beard, B. L., Roenker, D. L., & Miller, R. L. (1988). Age and visual search: Expanding the useful field of view. *Journal of the Optical Society of America, A, Optics, Image & Science, 5*(12), 2210–~.

Ball, K., Berch, D. B., Helmers, K. F., Jobe, J. B., Leveck, M. D., Marsiske, M., et al. (2002). Effects of cognitive training interventions with older adults: A randomized controlled trial. *JAMA: Journal of the American Medical Association, 288*(18), 2271–2281.

Ball, K., & Owsley, C. (1991). Identifying correlates of accident involvement for the older driver. *Human Factors. Special Issue: Safety and Mobility of Elderly Drivers: Part I, 33*(5), 583–595.

Ball, K., & Sekuler, R. (1982). A specific and enduring improvement in visual motion discrimination. *Science, 218*, 697–698.

Baltes, P. B., & Kliegl, R. (1992). Further testing of limits of cognitive plasticity: Negative age differences in a mnemonic skill are robust. *Developmental Psychology, 28*(1), 121–125.

Basak, C., Boot, W. R., Voss, M. W., & Kramer, A. F. (2008). Can training in a real-time strategy video game attenuate cognitive decline in older adults? *Psychology and Aging, 23*(4), 765–777.

Becic, E., Boot, W. R., & Kramer, A. F. (2008). Training older adults to search more effectively: Scanning strategy and visual search in dynamic displays. *Psychology and Aging, 23*(2), 461–466.

Bherer, L., Kramer, A. F., Peterson, M. S., Colcombe, S., Erickson, K., & Becic, E. (2005). Training effects on dual-task performance: Are there age-related differences in plasticity of attentional control? *Psychology and Aging Special Issue: Emotion-Cognition Interactions and the Aging Mind, 20*(4), 695–709.

Boot, W. R., Kramer, A. F., Simons, D. J., Fabiani, M., & Gratton, G. (2008). The effects of video game playing on attention, memory, and executive control. *Acta Psychologica, 129*(3), 387–398.

Catrambone, R., & Holyoak, K. J. (1989). Overcoming contextual limitations on problem-solving transfer. *Journal of Experimental Psychology: Learning, Memory and Cognition, 15*, 1147–1156.

Charness, N. (2006). The influence of work and occupation on brain development. In P. B. Baltes, P. A. Reuter-Lorenz, & F. Rösler (Eds.), *Lifespan development and the brain: The perspective of biocultural co-constructivism* (pp. 306–325). New York: Cambridge University Press.

Charness, N., & Boot, W. R. (2009). Aging and information technology use: Potential and barriers. *Current Directions in Psychological Science, 18*(5), 253–258.

Chase, W. G., & Simon, H. A. (1973). Perception in chess. *Cognitive Psychology, 4*, 55–81.

Cohen, J. E. (2003). Human population: the next half century. *Science, 302*(5648), 1172–1175.

Colcombe, S. J., Erickson, K. I., Raz, N., Webb, A. G., Cohen, N. J., McAuley, E., et al. (2003). Aerobic fitness reduces brain tissue loss in aging humans. *Journal of Gerontology: Medical Sciences, 58*, 176–180.

Colcombe, S. J., Erickson, K. I., Scalf, P., Kim, J., Wadhwa, R., McAuley, E., et al. (2006). Aerobic exercise training increases brain volume in aging humans: Evidence from a randomized clinical trial. *Journal of Gerontology: Medical Sciences, 61B*, M1166–M1170.

Colcombe, S., & Kramer, A. F. (2003). Fitness effects on the cognitive function of older adults: A meta-analytic study. *Psychological Science, 14*, 125–130.

Colcombe, S. J., Kramer, A. F., Erickson, K. I., Scalf, P., McAuley, E., Cohen, N. J., et al. (2004). Cardiovascular fitness, cortical plasticity, and aging. *Proceedings of the National Academy of Sciences, USA, 101*, 3316–3321.

Dennis, N. A., & Cabeza, R. (2008). Neuroimaging of healthy cognitive aging. In F. I. M. Craik & T. A. Salthouse (Eds.), *The handbook of aging and cognition* (3rd ed., pp. 1–54). New York: Psychology Press.

Dustman, R. E., Emmerson, R. Y., Steinhaus, L. A., Shearer, D. E., & Dustman, T. J. (1992). The effects of videogame playing on neuropsychological performance of elderly individuals. *Journal of Gerontology, 47*, 168–171.

Fahle, M., Edelman, S., & Poggio, T. (1995). Fast perceptual learning in hyperacuity. *Vision Research, 35*, 3003–3013.

Felce, D., & Perry, J. (1995). Quality of life: Its definition and measurement. *Research in Developmental Disabilities, 16*, 51–74.

Fiorentini, A., & Berardi, N. (1980). Perceptual learning specific for orientation and spatial frequency. *Nature, 287*, 43–44.

Goldstein, J., Cajko, L., Oosterbroek, M., Michielsen, M., Van Houten, O., & Salvedera, F. (1997). Videogames and the elderly. *Social Behavior and Personality, 25*, 345–352.

Gopher, D., Weil, M., & Bareket, T. (1994). Transfer of skill from a computer game trainer to flight. *Human Factors, 36*(3), 387–405.

Graves, L., Stratton, G., Ridgers, N. D., & Cable, N. T. (2007). Comparison of energy expenditure in adolescents when playing new generation and sedentary computer games: Cross sectional study. *British Medical Journal, 335*, 1282–1284.

Green, C. S., & Bavelier, D. (2003). Action video game modifies visual selective attention. *Nature, 423*(6939), 534–537.

Green, C. S., & Bavelier, D. (2007). Action-video-game experience alters the spatial resolution of vision. *Psychological Science, 18*(1), 88–94.

Green, C. S., & Bavelier, D. (2008). Exercising your brain: A review of human brain plasticity and training-induced learning. *Psychology and Aging, 23*(4), 692–701.

Hertzog, C., Cooper, B. P., & Fisk, A. D. (1996). Aging and individual differences in the development of skilled memory search performance. *Psychology and Aging, 11*(3), 497–520.

Hertzog, C., Kramer, A. F., Wilson, R. S., & Lindenberger, U. (2009). Enrichment effects on adult cognitive development. *Psychological Science in the Public Interest, 9*, 1–65.

Hultsch, D. F., Hertzog, C., Small, B. J., & Dixon, R. A. (1999). Use it or lose it: Engaged lifestyle as a buffer of cognitive decline in aging? *Psychology and Aging, 14*(2), 245–263.

Kramer, A. F., Erickson, K. I., & McAuley, E. (2008). Effects of physical activity on cognition and brain. In D. T. Stuss, G. Winocur, & I. H. Robertson (Eds.), *Cognitive Neurorehabilitation: Evidence and Applications (2nd Edition)* (pp. 417–434). United Kingdom: Cambridge University Press.

Kramer, A. F., Hahn, S., Cohen, N. J., Banich, M. T., McAuley, E., Harrison, C. R., et al. (1999). Ageing, fitness and neurocognitive function. *Nature, 400*, 418–419.

Kramer, A. F., Larish, J. F., & Strayer, D. L. (1995). Training for attentional control in dual task settings: A comparison of young and old adults. *Journal of Experimental Psychology: Applied, 1*(1), 50–76.

Lanningham-Foster, L., Jensen, T. B., Foster, R. C., Redmond, A. B., Walker, B. A., Heinz, D., et al. (2006). Energy expenditure of sedentary screen time compared with active screen time for children. *Pediatrics, 118*, 1831–1835.

Larkin, J., McDermott, J., Simon, D. P., & Simon, H. A. (1980). Expert and novice performance in solving physics problems. *Science, 208*, 1335–1342.

Li, R., Polat, U., Makous, W., & Bavelier, D. (2009). Enhancing the contrast sensitivity function through action video game playing. *Nature Neuroscience, 12*, 549–551.

Lustig, C., Shah, P., Seidler, R., & Reuter-Lorenz, P. A. (2009). Aging, training, and the brain: a review and future directions. *Neuropsychological Review, 19*, 504–522.

Lutz, W., Sanderson, W., & Scherbov, S. (2008). The coming acceleration of global population ageing. *Nature, 451*, 716–719.

Maddison, R., Mhurchu, C. N., Jull, A., Jiang, Y., Prapavessis, H., & Rodgers, A. (2007). Energy expended playing video console games: An opportunity to increase children's physical activity? *Pediatric Exercise Science, 19*, 334–343.

Mayer, R. E. (1987). The elusive search for teachable aspects of problem solving. In J. A. Glover & R. R. Ronning (Eds.), *Historical Foundations of Educational Psychology* (pp. 327–347). New York: Plenum Press.

McConatha, J. T., McConatha, D., Deaner, S. L., & Dermigny, R. (1995). A computer-based intervention for the education and therapy of institutionalized older adults. *Educational Gerontology, 21*, 129–138.

McConatha, D., McConatha, J. T., & Dermigny, R. (1994). The use of computer services to enhance the quality of life for long term care residents. *The Gerontologist, 34*, 553–556.

Neider, M. B., Boot, W. R., & Kramer, A. F. (2010). Visual search for real world targets under conditions of high target–background similarity: Exploring training and transfer in younger and older adults. *Acta Psychologica, 134*(1), 29–39.

Nichol, K. E., Parachikova, A. I., & Cotman, C. W. (2007). Three weeks of running wheel exposure improves cognitive performance in the aged Tg2576 mouse. *Behavioural Brain Research, 184*, 124–132.

Nintendo (2009). Financial results briefing for fiscal year ended March 2009: Supplementary Information (PDF). Retrieved June 21, 2009, from http://www.nintendo.co.jp/ir/pdf/2009/090508e.pdf#page=6.

Owen, A. M., Hampshire, A., Grahn, J. A., Stenton, R., Dajani, S., Burns, A. S., et al. (2010). Putting brain training to the test. *Nature, 465*, 775–779.

Park, D. C., Lautenschlager, G., Hedden, T., Davidson, N. S., Smith, A. D., & Smith, P. K. (2002). Models of visuospatial and verbal memory across the adult life span. *Psychology and Aging, 17*(2), 299–320.

Park, D. C., & Reuter-Lorenz, P. A. (2009). The adaptive brain: Aging and Neurocognitive Scaffolding. *Annual Review of Psychology, 60*, 173–196.

Pea, R. D., & Kurland, D. M. (1984). On the cognitive effects of learning computer programming. *New Ideas in Psychology, 2*, 137–168.

Pearce, C. (2008). The truth about baby boomer gamers: A study of over-forty computer game players. *Games and Culture: A Journal of Interactive Media, 3*(2), 142–174.

Raz, N. (2000). Aging of the brain and its impact on cognitive performance: Integration of structural and functional findings. In F. I. M. Craik & T. A. Salthouse (Eds.), *The handbook of aging and cognition* (2nd ed., pp. 1–90). Mahwah, NJ: Lawrence Erlbaum Associates.

Roenker, D. L., Cissell, G. M., Ball, K. K., Wadley, V. G., & Edwards, J. D. (2003). Speed-of-processing and driving simulator training result in improved driving performance. *Human Factors, 45*(2), 218–233.

Royall, D. R., Palmer, R., Chiodo, L. K., & Polk, M. J. (2004). Declining executive control in normal aging predicts change in functional status: The freedom house study. *Journal of the American Geriatrics Society, 52*(3), 346–352.

Salthouse, T. A. (2004). What and when of cognitive aging. *Current Directions in Psychological Science, 13*(4), 140–144.

Schaie, K. W., & Willis, S. L. (1986). Can decline in adult intellectual functioning be reversed. *Developmental Psychology, 22*(2), 223–232.

Schooler, C., & Mulatu, M. S. (2001). The reciprocal effects of leisure time activities and intellectual functioning in older people: A longitudinal analysis. *Psychology and Aging, 16*(3), 466–482.

Sherer, M. (1996). The impact of using personal computers on the lives of nursing home residents. *Physical & Occupational Therapy in Geriatrics, 14*, 13–31.

Shiu, L. P., & Pashler, H. (1992). Improvement in line orientation discrimination is retinally local but dependent on cognitive set. *Perception and Psychophysics, 52*, 582–588.

Slegers, K., Van Boxtel, M. P. J., & Jolles, J. (2008). Effects of computer training and internet usage on the well-being and quality of life of older adults: A randomized, controlled study. *The Journals of Gerontology: Series B: Psychological Sciences and Social Sciences, 63B*(3), 176–184.

Slegers, K., Van Boxtel, M. P. J., & Jolles, J. (2009). Effects of computer training and internet usage on cognitive abilities of older adults: A randomized controlled study. *Aging, Clinical and Experimental Research, 21*(1), 43–54.

Smith, G. E., Housen, P., Yaffee, K., Ruff, R., Kennison, R. F., Mahncke, H. W., et al. (2009). A cognitive training program based on principles of brain plasticity: Results from the Improvement in Memory with Plasticity-based Adaptive Control Training (IMPACT) study. *Journal of the American Geriatrics Society., 57*, 594–603.

Swaab, D. F. (1991). Brain aging and Alzheimer's disease: 'wear and tear' versus 'use it or lose it'. *Neurobiology of Aging, 12*, 317–324.

Thorndike, E. L. (1923). The influence of first year Latin upon the ability to read English. *School Sociology, 17*, 165–168.

Thorndike, E. L., & Woodworth, R. S. (1901a). The influence of improvement in one mental function upon the efficiency of other functions I. *Psychological Review, 8*, 247–261.

Thorndike, E. L., & Woodworth, R. S. (1901b). The influence of improvement in one mental function upon the efficiency of other functions II: The estimation of magnitudes. *Psychological Review, 8*, 247–261.

Thorndike, E. L., & Woodworth, R. S. (1901c). The influence of improvement in one mental function upon the efficiency of other functions III: Functions involving attention, observation, and discrimination. *Psychological Review, 8*, 247–261.

van Praag, H., Kempermann, G., & Gage, F. H. (2000). Neural consequences of enrichment. *Nature Reviews Neuroscience, 1*, 191–198.

Vaynman, S., & Gomez-Pinilla, F. (2006). Revenge of the "sit": How lifestyle impacts neuronal and cognitive health though molecular systems that interface energy metabolism with neuronal plasticity. *Journal of Neuroscience Research, 84*, 699–715.

Verhaeghen, P., & Cerella, J. (2002). Aging, executive control, and attention: A review of meta-analyses. *Neuroscience & Biobehavioral Reviews, 26*(7), 849–857.

Willis, S. L., & Nesselroade, C. S. (1990). Long-term effects of fluid ability training in old-old age. *Developmental Psychology, 26*(6), 905–910.

Willis, S. L., Tennstedt, S. L., Marsiske, M., Ball, K., Elias, J., Koepke, K. M., et al. (2006). Long-term effects of cognitive training on everyday functional outcomes in older adults. *JAMA: Journal of the American Medical Association, 296*(23), 2805–2814.

Wolinsky, F. D., Mahncke, H. W., Vander Weg, M. W., Martin, R., Unverzagt, F. W., Ball, K. K., et al. (2009). The ACTIVE cognitive training interventions and the onset of and recovery from suspected clinical depression. *The Journals of Gerontology: Series B: Psychological Sciences and Social Sciences, 64B*(5), 577–585.

Wolinsky, F. D., Unverzagt, F. W., Smith, D. M., Jones, R., Stoddard, A., & Tennstedt, S. L. (2006). The ACTIVE cognitive training trial and health-related quality of life: Protection that lasts for 5 years. *The Journals of Gerontology: Series A: Biological Sciences and Medical Sciences, 61A*(12), 1324–1329.

Wolinsky, F. D., Unverzagt, F. W., Smith, D. M., Jones, R., Wright, E., & Tennstedt, S. L. (2006). The effects of the ACTIVE cognitive training trial on clinically relevant declines in health-related quality of life. *The Journals of Gerontology: Series B: Psychological Sciences and Social Sciences, 61B*(5), S281–S287.

Wolinsky, F. D., Weg, M. W. V., Martin, R., Unverzagt, F. W., Ball, K. K., Jones, R. N., et al. (2009). The effect of speed-of-processing training on depressive symptoms in ACTIVE. *The Journals of Gerontology: Series A: Biological Sciences and Medical Sciences, 64A*(4), 468–472.

Chapter 3
Consumer-Based Brain Fitness Programs

Elizabeth M. Zelinski, Sarah E. Dalton, and Glenn E. Smith

Abstract We review the evidence relating to the value of consumer-friendly cognitive training programs for older adults. We discuss the scientific foundation of research on transfer of training. Transfer implies improving not just what is trained but other cognitive or functional activities not directly trained. We describe the behavioral and neuroscience findings suggesting the role of brain plasticity processes on transfer. We detail the results of the IMPACT study, a double-blind, randomized, controlled clinical trial of a commercially available program that can be completed at home. Guidelines for selection of scientifically sound consumer-friendly programs are presented, highlighting what we consider important characteristics: input from scientific advisory panels, research testing transfer after use of the specific programs, including whether there is transfer in older adults, and where findings of tested programs are publicly disseminated. We discuss adherence issues in cognitive training, and conclude with a statement on the lack of evidence that consumer-friendly programs can delay or reverse dementia.

Introduction

Brain fitness, as conceived in the popular news media, goes beyond learning specific information or skills. The term reflects the idea that mental exercise can increase the brain's capacity to meet the cognitive demands of everyday life. The concept of brain fitness is predicated on the idea that cognitive training benefits extend to untrained cognitive processes, including memory, attention, and response speed. This indicates that *transfer* of cognitive training has occurred. Recent studies show

E.M. Zelinski (✉)
Leonard Davis School of Gerontology, University of Southern California,
Los Angeles, CA, USA
e-mail: zelinski@usc.edu

transfer effects for certain types of cognitive training in older adults (Li et al., 2008), including people well over age 80 (e.g., Buschkuehl et al., 2008; Smith et al., 2009). This suggests that advanced age is not an impediment to improvement of cognitive performance through transfer. At the same time, an industry based on cognitive training for older consumers has emerged. The growth of this industry has been rapid and impressive. In 2009, cognitive training was a $295 million industry, driven by consumers, senior communities, and insurance providers, and has been increasing at an annualized growth rate of 31% since 2005. Projections suggest that this will be a $2–8 billion industry by 2015 (SharpBrains, 2010). Yet there is considerable confusion for consumers as they try to navigate advertised claims about the effects of particular products and training approaches on cognition.

In this chapter, we examine the scientific basis of the development of computer-based cognitive training products designed for older adult users. Although products also exist for younger age groups and for patients with a variety of clinical diagnoses, we will restrict our discussion to the types of programs available for healthy older adults interested in maintaining or improving their mental abilities. We begin by reviewing the concept of transfer, how to define the extent of different transfer outcomes, the connection between findings of far transfer and models of brain plasticity, applications of brain plasticity theory to cognitive training, and a study that tested a consumer product in a randomized controlled clinical trial. A comprehensive and current review of computer-based training products is impossible, as the industry is rapidly expanding, but we will suggest some guiding principles to help consumers decide whether specific products hold promise for improving brain fitness based on the scientific research. We also discuss whether people are likely to use computer training programs for extended periods of time, and describe the most recent conclusions regarding whether these programs can actually delay or reverse dementias such as Alzheimer's disease.

Key Concepts and Principles

Transfer

The primary purpose of cognitive training of older adults is to improve or rehabilitate performance on skills that decline with age (e.g., Winocur et al., 2007). However, it has also been suggested that cognitive training could help preserve older adults' abilities, so that those who participate in training are less likely to show declines than those who receive no training (e.g., Ball, Edwards, & Ross, 2007). A third objective of training is that it not only benefits the specific skills that are trained, but should extend or *transfer* either to improvements or to maintenance of performance on different tasks that were not trained. It is generally assumed that transfer involves an overlap in processing skills from one task to another, that is, that training of the skill improves performance across different tasks requiring the skill. What is less clear is how to define the relative *amount* or distance of transfer, which has traditionally been referred to as "near," as closer to, or not very different from, the trained task, or "far," as more distantly associated with, or quite different from, the trained task (Barnett & Ceci, 2002).

Herein, we will use specific definitions of transfer of cognitive skills. We note that a major assumption of cognitive training of older adults is that the skills trained are critical to either maintaining or improving everyday functioning. Another important assumption is that because cognitive ability is a major predictor of physical function, cognitive interventions may improve physical as well as cognitive performance (e.g., Jobe et al., 2001). Age-related cognitive declines can be accompanied by functional impairments that lead to a loss of independence, increased risk of nursing home placement, and mortality (e.g., Kelmen, Thomas, Kennedy, & Cheng, 1994; St. John, Montgomery, Kristjansson, & McDowell, 2002).

However, the measurement of everyday functioning is not sensitive to many aspects of cognition that are affected by aging. For example, middle-aged adults show deficits on neuropsychological tests that predict executive function problems in planning or organizing behavior, yet have no difficulty in completing everyday tasks such as finding, selecting, and purchasing items in a shopping mall (Garden, Phillips, & MacPherson, 2001). Studies of the role of emotion in everyday decision-making in older adults show only very subtle difficulties (Mather, 2006). Furthermore, what people report about their cognitive abilities in everyday contexts is not a good indicator of everyday functioning. For example, the frequency of various memory complaints, such as difficulties remembering people's names or word-finding problems, is more strongly associated with higher depression scores and low levels of conscientiousness, a personality trait, than actual performance on memory tests (Zelinski & Gilewski, 2004), and do not consistently predict eventual diagnosis of dementia (Smith, Peterson, Ivnik, Malec, & Tangalos, 1996). Because it is difficult to show objective performance changes in everyday functioning and actual everyday cognitive functioning has not been measured in any of the studies we consider, we must restrict our discussion to changes associated with training that transfer to other cognitive tasks only.

Zelinski (2009) adapted a model categorizing near and far transfer (Barnett & Ceci, 2002) to classify transfer findings with older people. Zelinski's adapted model identifies three dimensions of context transfer; temporal, functional, and modality dimensions that bear on the when and where of transfer. *Temporal* aspects of transfer relate to the time elapsing between training and the transfer test. Obviously, it is important to show that effects last beyond the final day of training! Transfer effects observed shortly after training are identified as representing near temporal transfer, whereas effects that persist for several weeks to years after training has ended representing far temporal transfer. Far *functional* transfer is defined as a transfer of a trained skill to a function that involves a different mind-set (e.g., handicapping horses at the racetrack to handicapping stocks in the stock market; Ceci & Liker, 1986), whereas near functional transfer requires the same mind-set. Near *modality* transfer is defined as representing either the same sensory modality (near sensory modality transfer) or the same format of the transfer test (near format modality; for example, a recognition test) as the trained materials. Far modality transfer indicates

Table 3.1 Dimensions of context transfer (adapted from Zelinski, 2009)

Dimension of transfer	Near		Far	
	Description	Example	Description	Example
Temporal	Immediately after training completion	Within 3 weeks after intervention: Smith et al., (2009)	Weeks to years after training with no practice in between	Three months later after posttraining tests: Li et al., (2008)
Functional	Same mind-set for training as for transfer task	Discriminating between high and low-pitched sounds in training; discriminating between smooth and rough sounds of the same pitch at transfer: Bherer et al., (2005)	Different mind-set for training than for transfer task	Simultaneous monitoring and alphabet arithmetic in training; simultaneous paired associates recall and scheduling at transfer: Kramer et al., (1995)
Modality: sensory	Same sensory modality for training as for transfer task	Visual at training, visual at transfer: Buschkuehl et al., (2008)	Different sensory modality for transfer task than for training	Visual test at training; multiple sensory modalities test at transfer: Ball et al., (2007)
Modality: testing format	Same testing format for training as for transfer task	Recognition test at training and at transfer: Jennings, Webster, Kleykamp, and Dagenbach (2005)	Different testing format for training than for transfer	Recognition test at training; recall test at transfer: Smith et al., (2009)

a different sensory modality (far modality transfer, for example, training on visual materials with the transfer test on auditory ones) or format (far format modality transfer, for example, training of recall, whereas transfer is tested with a multiple choice recognition test). Table 3.1 shows the dimensions of context transfer observed in aging research, summarizes their descriptions, and provides examples from studies of older adults within each dimension.

Several studies have shown far transfer from dual-task training, that is, multitasking. Dual task studies require that participants perform two very simple activities at once, for example, deciding whether easy-to-discriminate tones are low- or high-pitched while deciding whether a letter shown on a computer screen is a *B* or a *C*. Though these tasks are undemanding, and produce low error rates, participants are generally slower and a bit less accurate when they perform both tasks simultaneously, producing a discrepancy known as dual task *cost*. With training, these costs are reduced, that is, people become faster and more accurate at responding. Without training or extensive practice in multitasking, older adults show larger dual task cost than younger ones. However, with several hours of training, the cost is reduced to the point where discrepancy between doing one task at a time compared to both is not any different than what young adults experience (e.g., Kramer, Larish, & Strayer, 1995). Thus, with training, older adults can multitask with about as much decrement as younger adults (we state it this way to remind our readers that there are always costs to doing two tasks simultaneously, not to suggest that older adults can successfully drive while texting, for example!).

Moreover, this reduction in cost shows transfer to completely different pairs of tasks, indicating that the skill of managing two activities simultaneously, a supervisory or executive function, translates to greater mental efficiency in older adults (Bherer et al., 2005; Kramer et al., 1995). The mental management skills observed in this research were also retained without additional practice when tested 2 months later (Kramer et al., 1995). These studies thus showed far functional transfer with application to tasks requiring a different mindset, that is, from monitoring changes of a display of six gauges while performing an alphabet-arithmetic test that used letters instead of numbers (e.g., $K - 3 = ?$) to assigning a box to the shortest of four moving lines while remembering the most recently paired letters and numbers ($D = 7$) from a continuously changing set of pairs (Kramer et al., 1995). This research demonstrates that, with training, older people can become more efficient at applying supervisory cognitive skills to different kinds of activities, an important aspect of brain fitness.

Transfer Across Multiple Dimensions

The categorization of transfer model uses the heuristic that the number of far transfer dimensions on which an effect of transfer is observed is an indicator of how much far transfer has been demonstrated (Barnett & Ceci, 2002). Some studies have demonstrated more far transfer than others with older adults. More far transfer indicates greater generality of the transferred skill, which in turn suggests that some training approaches may support brain fitness somewhat more broadly than others.

Jennings et al. (2005) trained participants to discriminate words that had been studied from words not studied but tested repeatedly. This skill was associated with better performance on other untrained tasks requiring that the context in which items were experienced be remembered, demonstrating far transfer on one dimension. Transfer on two dimensions, or further transfer, has been observed in working memory training. For example, Buschkuehl et al. (2008) found that healthy adults over the age of 80 improved on the trained tasks as well as on visual sequencing and recall tasks taken from a neuropsychology battery. A 1-year follow-up showed that the transfer improvement was retained, thus far temporal transfer was also observed. A study using a similar approach also resulted in far functional and temporal transfer (Li et al., 2008). The UFOV or speed of processing task (Ball et al., 2007, and discussed elsewhere in this book in the Chap. 15) has shown far transfer on two or all three dimensions in multiple studies for people with poor UFOV scores.

The studies reviewed here, all of which demonstrated far transfer, used extensive practice of specific cognitive skills during training. This is in contrast to studies where the primary intervention was to train strategies for improving performance (e.g., mnemonic strategies). As described elsewhere (see Zelinski, 2009), training in use of strategies does not appear as beneficial to transfer as engaging in repetitive practice of skills. This is presumably because strategies are effortful and therefore reduce efficiency in processing whereas repetition of cognitive skills increases efficiency because they have become less effortful with practice. However, it is not merely repetition that is conducive to transfer; the principles of brain plasticity suggest otherwise. Next, we examine the science behind the concept of improving cognition.

Principles of Brain Plasticity

Most of the initial research in neuroplasticity was with animals; recent work in humans uses neuroimaging to study effects of plasticity. Research in both animal and human models over the last 40 years shows that the adult brain is constantly remodeling itself based on its experiences. Human functional MRI research, for example, shows that adults experience changes in activation of specific brain regions after dual task training (e.g., Erickson et al., 2007). This is known as neuroplasticity or brain plasticity. It can be either structural or functional. That is, experience may produce changes to the physical characteristics of the brain or to its response characteristics (e.g., Draganski & May, 2008). Sensory input experiences are dynamically represented and influence perceptual functions and learning (see Xerri, 2008). The degree of change due to plasticity is related to the degree of learning (e.g., Polley, Steinberg, & Merzenich, 2006). The duration of structural plastic changes is not well understood; however, a study of changes in medical students over the course of preparing for an intensive preclinical examination indicated that increases in gray matter observed during the learning period remained 3 months later (Draganski et al., 2006). However, a parallel study that trained young adults to juggle showed structural increases after 3 months of daily practice that degraded back to pretraining levels 3 months after discontinuing the exercises (Draganski et al., 2004).

Merzenich and coworkers (e.g., Mahncke, Bronstone, & Merzenich, 2006) argue that top-down processes such as attentional focus are important mediators of sensory neuroplasticity. For example, rats trained to respond to either the frequency or the intensity of sounds that varied on both dimensions produce a plasticity response congruent with the animal's attentional focus. Thus, animals trained to respond to frequency showed a frequency-related response, and those trained to respond to intensity showed an intensity-related response, though the stimuli were the same for both groups (Polley et al., 2006).

It should be noted that neuroplasticity effects can be both positive and negative. Just as systematic stimulation is associated with gains in representation and possibly structural growth, systematic reductions of stimulation or undifferentiated stimulation are associated with less differentiated representations and less efficient processing (e.g., Wang, Merzenich, Sameshima, & Jenkins, 1995). For example, individuals who have experienced hand movement dysfunction due to repetitive stress syndrome may also have less differentiated input into specific areas of the cortex (see Draganski & May, 2008).

Merzenich and coworkers (Mahncke et al., 2006) suggest that cognitive aging deficits follow the principles of negative plasticity. Declines are the result of (1) reduced schedules of brain activity related to engaging in less cognitively demanding behaviors with age, (2) a reduced signal-to-noise ratio in information processing, that is, a decline in the brain's ability to detect signals against the spontaneous background activity of neural networks associated with declines in sensory inputs, (3) reduced neuromodulatory control of the attention and reward systems in the brain because of reduced cognitive stimulation due to (1) and (2), and (4) negative learning, that is, coping with reduced stimulation by engaging in behaviors that reduce cognitive and sensory demands even more, creating a negative spiral (Table 3.2).

However, cortical neurons are responsive to task demands, so negative plasticity effects should be reversed by undoing the activities associated with the negative spiral. Tasks, however, must follow the principles of plasticity (Mahncke et al., 2006a). These principles imply that specific brain activity can be increased by repeated engagement in specialized tasks over thousands of trials. This enhances the representation of stimuli and connections between neural networks. Signal-to-noise ratio is improved by training of sensory discrimination and processing speed. The use of adaptive methods during training keeps levels of challenge high and attention to the task intense. Reward through feedback enhances neuromodulatory control.

These principles of training were used to reverse hand movement disorders in people with dystonia generally acquired by playing musical instruments. Training of specific areas of the hand with sensory discrimination, movements, and other

Table 3.2 Principles of positive and negative brain plasticity (adapted from Mahncke et al., 2006)

Principle	Attributes Positive	Negative	Reversing negative plasticity
Schedules of engagment in cognitively challenging activities	Intense, frequent involvement	Relatively less or decreasing engagement	Increasing the frequency and intensity of engagement
Ability to detect signals and representations in memory	Strong representations leading to strong signal detection	Weakened representations that are difficult to discriminate from background neural activity	Extensive practice to strengthen representations and improve processing efficiency
Neuromodulation of attention and reward systems	Deep attention and concentration leading to strong representations	Poor attention and reward control system connectivity	Engage in rewarding activities that increase attentional capacity

motor practices was associated with more normal brain electrical responses and improved hand use (e.g., Byl, Nagarajan, & McKenzie, 2003). Merzenich and coworkers (e.g., Mahncke et al., 2006b) suggested that a gradual recovery of cognitive function should occur with cognitive task training using the same principles in healthy older adults.

Applications of Brain Plasticity Principles to Cognitive Training

The previously cited training studies implicate brain plasticity principles as necessary to reverse negative effects and to produce far transfer. First, the studies increased the schedule of engagement of brain systems. That is, all required extensive practice of the skills trained. For example, Jennings et al.'s (2005) study provided four 15-min training sessions per day, 2 days a week, for 3 weeks, with 2,160 recognition trials over 6 h. UFOV training studies involved approximately 5–10 h of training (Ball et al., 2002, Edwards et al., 2005; Roenker, Cissell, Ball, Wadley, & Edwards, 2003). The dual task studies involved varying amounts of practice: 3 h over 4 sessions (Kramer et al., 1995), 4 h over 6 sessions (Kramer, Larish, Weber, & Bardell, 1999), and 1,600 dual task trials as well as 2,000 single task trials over 5 one-hour sessions (Bherer et al., 2005). Working memory training studies included two 45-min sessions per week for 12 weeks (Buschkuehl et al., 2008), and 15 min of training per day for 45 days (Li et al., 2008).

Second, most of the previously cited studies improved the quality of information processing by improving signal-to-noise ratio. This involves improving discrimination and speed of information processing. Jennings et al. (2005) trained discrimination of context in which test items occurred. UFOV training involved improving both speed and accuracy of discriminating visual information (e.g., Ball et al., 2007), and the dual task studies the speed and accuracy of performing two tasks simultaneously (Bherer et al., 2005; Kramer et al., 1995, 1999). Processing speed was trained and improved in the two working memory studies showing transfer effects for older adults (Buschkuehl et al., 2008; Li et al., 2008). Thus, the training in the studies with far functional transfer also improved information processing efficiency.

The third principle of brain plasticity is to enhance neuromodulatory control. This may be evidenced by upregulation of metabolism and connectivity of modulatory control systems. Upregulation implies an increased number of receptors for specific sensory experiences, and increased activity of control systems. Upregulation occurs when practiced activities involve attention and reward. The UFOV studies required practice of visual attention (Ball et al., 2007), and this was also practiced in the dual-task (e.g., Kramer et al., 1995) and working memory studies (Buschkuehl et al., 2008; Li et al., 2008). Upregulation also results from the consistent increase in difficulty produced by adaptive training to maintain challenge at the individual's level of ability (e.g., Jennings et al., 2005). Accurate feedback provides reward and continued interest in the activities.

The IMPACT Study

To reverse the negative effects of plasticity, Merzenich and associates at Posit Science Corporation applied the principles of brain plasticity described here to develop a series of computer exercises. The *Brain Fitness Classic* program was developed as a product for consumers, not just as a research tool. The personal computer-based program cycles through six different exercises that range in complexity from identifying the direction of sound sweeps through answering questions about a story from memory. The exercises are as follows:

High or Low: pairs of frequency-modulated sound sweeps. Participants indicate whether the direction of the sweeps is upward (from low to more high pitched) or downward (from high to more low pitched).

Tell Us Apart: pairs of confusable syllables, such as $b\bar{o}$ and $d\bar{o}$, are presented on the screen. One syllable is spoken and participants indicate which one they heard from the pair on the screen.

Match it: a matrix of buttons is presented on the screen. Clicking a button reveals a syllable that is spoken aloud. There are two buttons with the identical syllables in the matrix. Participants find the matched pairs; as they identify them correctly, the buttons disappear until all are gone.

Sound Replay: Sets of two, three, or more confusable syllables are presented in a working memory span task. Participants listen to the syllables, then click buttons identifying the syllables in the order in which they were presented. There may be more buttons on the screen than there were syllables.

Listen and Do: A set of spoken instructions is presented. Participants see a scene with various characters and structures on it, with instructions to click particular characters or structures or to move the characters. Participants follow the instructions in the order given.

Story Teller: Participants listen to segments of stories and answer multiple-choice questions about them.

Participants complete approximately 15 min of each of four of the exercises in a 1-h training session. The exercises are rotated over sessions. The goal of the training is to complete 40 sessions, thereby strongly increasing the schedule of engagement in cognitively demanding activity. The signal-to-noise ratio is augmented through discrimination training that increases in difficulty. Difficulty is varied by the speed of item presentation (from relatively slow to more rapid) and by the duration of the items (from longer to shorter). Difficulty is also increased by the use of phonemes that are more easily confused when presented in isolation. All tasks besides *High or Low?* use natural language components (phonemes, syllables, words, discourse) with speech compression to slow down or to speed up the duration of those language units. Some of the training exercises also increase the complexity of the task by increasing the number of items that must be processed. In *Match It!* the size of the matrix increases from 8 to 30 items; in *Sound Replay*, 2–9 syllables are presented; in *Listen and Do,* the number and complexity of the instructions varies; and in *Story Teller*, the number of story segments presented at one time and the number of test questions increases.

To increase neuromodulation, all exercises are adaptive, that is, the level of difficulty is customized to increase as the participant reaches 75–85% accuracy at a given level. Feedback about correctness of responses is given on every trial. When participants achieve success at various levels of each exercise, "rewards" are shown on the screen. These may include an artistic design, travel illustrations, music, family, or pet scenarios with animation and sound.

This program was tested for far transfer in the Improvement in Memory with Plasticity-based Adaptive Cognitive Training (IMPACT) study (Smith et al., 2009). This study was the first large-scale multisite randomized controlled double-blind test of a cognitive intervention using a computer program developed for use at home by consumers. Use of *Brain Fitness Classic* was considered the experimental condition. The control condition was selected to reflect the same amount of exposure to a computer, to interaction with a trainer who installed the equipment and who was available for consultation as needed, and the amount of time spent on the activity. It involved an activity thought to reflect a more standard kind of cognitive stimulation: watching DVDs of educational television series on history, art, and literature. Participants were blinded to the hypothesized efficacy of the computer activity they engaged in, and neuropsychological testers were blinded to the specific intervention that participants received. Two of this chapter's authors served as principal investigators in two sites, EMZ at the University of Southern California and GES at the Mayo Clinic. Neither received personal compensation for their work; grants from Posit Science supported the research at each site.

The outcome measures included performance of two trained tasks, one involving discrimination of the direction of sound sweeps (*High or Low*) and the other, the temporal ordering of sets of 2–8 confusable phonemes, with the number of baseline phonemes at two, and increasing with subjects' ability to order them accurately (*Sound Replay*). Both were recognition tasks, that is, selection of the correct items from an array of possible choices.

The transfer tasks included auditory recall tasks from the Repeatable Battery for Assessment of Neuropsychological Status (RBANS; Randolph, 1998), a test that tends to be relatively insensitive to age declines before 65, and recall tasks from the more difficult and age-sensitive Rey Auditory Verbal Learning Test (Schmidt, 1996), working memory tasks from the Wechsler Memory Scale (Wechsler, 1997), visual memory asks from the RBANS, and discourse memory from the Rivermead Behavioural Memory Test (Wilson, Cockburn, Baddeley, & Hiorns, 2003).

Participants over the age of 65 were recruited from the community and invited to be part of a study to test whether cognition could be improved with specific activities. Of 1,112 volunteers, 625 were excluded with 568 not meeting inclusion criteria and 57 refusing to participate. Inclusion criteria were age, Mini-Mental State (MMSE) scores of 26 or better, fluency in English, and ability to participate in the study for 6 months. Exclusion criteria were a history of major neurological or psychiatric illness, use of acetylcholinesterase inhibitors, current substance abuse, communicative impairments, and concurrent enrollment in other studies. There were 487 subjects randomized either into the experimental treatment ($N=242$) or into the active control ($N=245$) groups.

Both groups completed 40 one-hour training sessions (5 days a week for 8 weeks) in their homes on computers provided during the training portion of the study. Trainers unblinded to the training condition set up and taught the participants how to use the equipment and programs. Access to the trainers was available if questions about operating the programs were raised. After each daily session, data were uploaded to the study database to ensure adherence. Those who did not adhere to the training program, defined as completing fewer than 10 sessions during the first month or skipping more than 10 sessions after that, were dropped from the study but their data were included in the intent-to-treat analyses. There were 19 who discontinued participation in the experimental group and 30 from the control group; one control subject died and another was lost to follow-up. The proportion of discontinuers did not differ across the two groups statistically.

Comparisons of baseline characteristics of the treatment groups revealed no differences in age, education, race, English as a first language, MMSE, estimated intelligence, hearing, tinnitus, or the use of hearing aids or glasses. However, there were more men in the active control group (53%) than the experimental treatment group (42%); gender therefore was a covariate in the analyses but did not interact with treatment group.

As would be expected, there were significant training effects, with the experimental group improving more than the control group on the trained tasks. More critically, the experimental group gained more than the active control group on the far transfer measures: RBANS auditory recall, the RAVLT tests, the working memory tests, and the participant-reported outcome. The experimental group did not gain more than the active control group, however, on the story recall task of the RBMT or on the RBANS visual memory tests (Smith et al., 2009).

The effect sizes of the significant transfer tasks ranged from Cohen's $d=0.20$–0.33, representing the proportional improvement in standard deviation units of the experimental treatment group over the active control group. This range of d's indicates a small effect. However, these effect sizes are equivalent to those of the effects of studies of cholinesterase inhibitors on cognitive scores in Alzheimer's patients and are considered clinically meaningful (Rockwood, 2004). The effect sizes in the IMPACT study are slightly larger than those of a study of the effects of modafinil on cognitive tests in young adults (Turner et al., 2003). The modafinil findings have been interpreted as showing that the drug "offers significant potential as a cognitive enhancer" (p. 268).

Using the transfer categorization model, the IMPACT study is classified as showing far functional transfer, from discrimination and memory on the computer task to paper and pencil neuropsychological tasks, and far modality transfer, from recognition tasks at training to recall at transfer. A 3-month follow-up of IMPACT participants showed that effects were still observed over time, indicating far temporal transfer. *Brain Fitness Classic* thus produced far transfer on three dimensions.

Evaluating Commercial Products

The IMPACT study is the only one of the studies showing far transfer cited herein that involves a commercially available product. However, there are numerous products that claim to help with brain fitness. Unfortunately, these products are not regulated and claims about them may be based only on the assertions of the marketing departments of the companies selling them. In order to help consumers decide whether a product will actually have far transfer effects, we provide a set of guidelines and a checklist at the same page to simplify identification of scientifically sound programs (Table 3.3).

Table 3.3 Checklist for training products

Scientific Criteria	Points Scored
Scientific advisory board	
Yes (+1)	
No (0)	
Research with the product?	
Double-blind randomized controlled (+4)	
Randomized controlled (+3)	
Controlled (+2)	
Practice on task only (+1)	
Testimonials only (0)	
Study done with a separate group of older adults?	
Yes (+1)	
No (0)	
Transfer to another task not trained in the study?	
Yes (+1)	
No (0)	
Transfer to another task in older adults?	
Yes (+1)	
No (0)	
Results published?	
In a scientific journal? (+3)	
At a scientific meeting (+2)	
Not yet, but a study is ongoing (+1)	
No publications (0)	
Total Scientific Criteria	
Practical Criteria	
How many times did you use the trial application?	
10 or more sessions over 3 weeks (+3)	
6–9 sessions over 3 weeks (+2)	
2–5 sessions over 3 weeks (+1)	
Once (0)	
Add Total Scientific + Practical Criteria	

Does the company have a scientific advisory committee to guide product development?
Because the idea of brain fitness is relatively new, and research testing the adequacy of products is relatively limited, we suggest that an important first step in evaluating products is whether they have been developed by companies that have consulted with scientific experts, and better yet, have an advisory board composed of scientists from major research universities. This information is generally available on product websites. If a careful search of the site indicates that there is no advisory committee, it suggests that the product is not necessarily scientifically sound. Consumers should be aware that websites may use the words "science" or "scientific" in the absence of a scientific advisory committee.

Has research been done on the specific training product?
Drug and medical device (e.g., cardiac pacemaker) companies must extensively test every product according to standards set by the federal Food and Drug Administration (FDA). Products cannot be sold until they are proven safe and effective. Computer training devices, however, are not currently regulated by the FDA or any other federal agency. So, a second major criterion that consumers should look for is whether a company has voluntarily evaluated and demonstrated that their *specific* product has efficacy for far transfer. For cognitive training, not enough is known about exactly which training approaches produce specific improvements. As we have noted, improvements are very specific, as they involve transfer of particular skills. The few studies we have cited use different methods and different outcomes, and most are small. Some companies have developed products that provide practice in cognitive test activities known to decline with age, (e.g., memory, attention, or working memory), but it is not clear they have followed brain plasticity principles. As we have suggested, it is the use of these principles that differentiates studies that show successful far transfer. It is possible, but we think unlikely, that other approaches would produce far transfer. Nevertheless, it is incumbent on companies offering these products to demonstrate whether they produce far transfer.

What kind of research with products?
The gold standard for research that tests the efficacy of a brain plasticity program, like a drug or other medical product, is a double-blind randomized clinical trial, that is, a study where the research participants and research staff assessing the participants do not know whether the participants are in the experimental or control group. Randomization means that participants who choose to be in the study are randomly assigned to the experimental or control condition, and have no choice about the condition to which they have been assigned. Double-blind randomized trials have the advantage of assuring that any benefit of the program is due to it, rather than to the expectation of the participant that it will be helpful, or to subtle clues from the staff that they should be benefitted, and that the characteristics of the participants, such as their gender, income, or education, do not systematically affect findings.

Having control groups allows comparisons to be made between any improvements obtained from the training and the effects of taking the outcome tests repeatedly, because people often improve on cognitive tests as they become more familiar with the procedures and more relaxed in taking the tests. This is known as a *practice* effect.

There are two major classifications of control groups: active controls and inactive, no-contact controls. An active control group may be getting a benefit from the activities in which they engaged, which could improve their outcome test scores more than just by practice, so pitting them against the training group is a strong test of the program. Inactive control groups allow for comparisons of no training against the experimental group. However, the experimental group may improve for reasons related more to experiences related to the process of being in a study: they have interacted with project staff more, learned to use a computer for the task, or felt special to be participating actively in a research project. Thus, an active control group is preferable to an inactive or no-contact control group.

Some studies simply observe differences in test performance by giving participants pretests, having them train on the product, then giving them posttests. Although this is common, it is not scientifically very useful, as it is impossible to determine whether the training provided on the product is what caused the changes or simply whether practice or other factors simply improved performance. So a no-contact control study is preferable to an uncontrolled pretest-posttest study.

Was far transfer evaluated?
Another consideration is whether the transfer of the training from the activity practiced is identified. If the study just shows that there is considerable improvement on the task trained, that is normal but probably does not have clinical significance. People with dementia or amnesia improve on tasks that they practice regularly, even if they don't remember doing the tasks. This is known as procedural or implicit memory and indicates that learning has taken place, even without the person's conscious awareness. Obviously, the practice does not even improve the person's ability to remember consciously if she can't even remember doing the task, and it is very unlikely that this kind of memory transfers to other tasks or to cognition in everyday living.

Generally, when products are touted as "showing improvement" just by practice, testimonials by users are used to support its efficacy in everyday activities. However, the relationship between what people believe about their everyday cognition and their objective test performance is modest, at the very best (e.g., Zelinski & Gilewski, 2004). Thus, even if people feel that their performance on everyday tasks is improving, it may not be.

Were older people tested on the product, separately from younger ones?
Finally, it is critical that the studies conducted include a sample of older adults and report findings for the older adults separately from the younger ones. Although older adults show neuroplasticity effects, that is, improvements in trained task performance, and effects of transfer, the older adults' performance, especially on memory or working memory tasks generally never reaches the level of younger adults' (e.g., Li et al., 2008), may still be worse that than of untrained younger adults (e.g., Dahlin, Stigsdotter-Neely, Larsson, Backman, & Nyberg, 2008) and may not show transfer even though the trained task has shown improvement (Dahlin, Nyberg, Backman, & Stigsdotter-Neely, 2008). Thus, studies with older adults are necessary to determine whether they benefit from the specific type of training and most critically, whether they show transfer as younger ones do.

Are the findings of studies published? Where?
It is also important that results of studies be disseminated through appropriate channels of communication. The most methodologically sound studies are those that have been reviewed by the peers of the researchers and published in scientific journals. This indicates that the peers have scrutinized the research and essentially approved the findings as scientifically acceptable. Peers and journal editors generally help temper interpretations of findings made by the research team.

A second means of disseminating research results is though presentations, either oral or in the form of a poster, at a scientific meeting. Presentations undergo a peer review process, but acceptance is relatively lenient, compared to publication in a scientific journal. For example, only about 10% of submissions may be rejected for a meeting, but 85% or more are rejected by prestigious journals. A paper presented at a meeting may very likely be rejected for publication in a peer-reviewed journal. Thus meeting presentations are not considered as strong an outlet for dissemination of research findings.

There are several reasons why study results might be presented at a meeting rather than being published in a journal. Some studies of cognitive training are ongoing but nearly finished, and the generally positive preliminary findings are made public in the meeting as a preview. Another reason for reporting presentations at meetings rather than in peer reviewed journals is that some studies are not as methodologically strong, with findings that are not statistically significant, or do not include a large enough sample to be considered scientifically adequate. Or they may not include a control group.

However, meeting findings are superior to company-produced white papers, which do not involve an external review process and have not been evaluated as to their scientific rigor. They are also superior to ongoing studies that do not yet have enough data to be evaluated. Nevertheless, even reporting an ongoing study is superior to making completely unfounded claims about a product.

The checklist included in this chapter follows our recommendations for selecting science-based consumer programs and uses a scoring system that weights the information for the product with respect to its basis in scientific research. This includes whether the company has a scientific advisory board, any research on the product that has been done, with more points for better-controlled studies, points for research that demonstrates transfer, for research with older adults, and whether the study has been published or presented at a meeting. This checklist can be used for one individual product or for comparing two or more products.

The checklist is designed to help consumers be able to determine for themselves what products are really science-based and are likely to produce the expected improvements in cognitive function. Higher scores indicate a greater likelihood of producing transfer.

When deciding about investing in a cognitive training product for a community center, it is important to determine whether a group license is available for use of the product. Most of the products available to consumers are for individual use, though companies do provide multiple user licenses for a fee upon request. However, many of the products are for use by individuals rather than groups, so having them available for personal use in a computer center is an option.

If you buy it, use it!
Unless the products are used regularly and frequently, the first principle of brain plasticity, increasing the scheduling of engagement in cognitively demanding activities, is not being adhered to, so even if products have strong scientific criteria scores, they may not produce the intended transfer effects. It is well known that most people begin self-improvement activities that require regular engagement in them, but they discontinue them for various reasons, even when they see the benefits. The best example is of physical exercise. Approximately, 50% of people who begin a research-based exercise program stop within the first 6 months (Dishman & Buckworth, 1996). A meta-analysis of randomized controlled exercise trials indicated that people are more likely to drop out from longer exercise interventions (Hong, Hughes, & Prohaska, 2008). This is after they agree to remain in the program and have the extra motivation provided by being in a research study! Even when older people continue to exercise, there are decreases in the amount of physical activity they report. McAuley et al. (2007) found a substantial decrease in older adults' self-reported activity 3–5 years after participating in a walking/toning trial. Thus, it would not be surprising to see that people might stop using challenging consumer friendly programs. Transfer effects do fade over time (Buschkuehl et al., 2008; Li et al., 2008), so the benefits will wane even if training was sufficient to allow for transfer.

Because people are not likely to adhere to self-improvement programs over time, we add a practical criterion to the checklist of scientific criteria for selection of consumer-friendly products: for how long will the user actually use the product? A simple experiment can be conducted: nearly all consumer cognitive training products have trial subscriptions or practice versions of the programs that can be used for a while. Many products now also have smart phone apps that are either free or inexpensive, and can be used for testing user's steadfastness in engaging in the brain fitness activity frequently and regularly. So, the user can test his or her commitment by using the product for at least 15 min in a session, and monitoring how many sessions are practiced, say, over a 3-week period, which should predict use once the novelty of the activity has worn off. The more practice sessions completed during the trial period, the greater the probability that the user will engage in the training regularly.

Commercial Entertainment Products and Cognitive Plasticity

It might be argued that user-friendly products that are entertainment-oriented, such as those developed for game platforms such as the Nintendo DS or the Wii, are more likely to encourage participation because they are fun to play and can be played by more than one user at a time, encouraging social interaction. Several studies have found that simple arcade-type video games do show some transfer to cognitive tasks (Drew & Walters, 1986; Dustman, Emmerson, Seinhous, Shearer, & Dustman, 1992). A recent study of an action video game also showed transfer to other cognitive tasks in older adults (Basak et al., 2008). In Basak's study, 23 h of play was required to show improvements; there were no statistically reliable improvements after 10 h of play. Comparisons of those who played the games in all three studies cited here were made against no-contact controls. Thus, there may be some value in playing video games, but these studies were small and require replication and there may be biases from participants being compared against no-contact controls. People may be more willing to play video games and perhaps they will be of benefit, but more research is needed to determine this.

What We Don't Know Yet

In summary, we have discussed in detail the importance of science-based approaches for development of consumer products, especially with respect to issues of transfer. Obviously, the point of training is not just to improve the trained skill, but to extend the effects of training to other outcomes, the most important one being quality of life.

Cognitive Reserve

The appeal of cognitive training products is the hope that they may increase "cognitive reserve." However, cognitive reserve research may mislead people into thinking that they can increase their reserve.

Correlational studies are those that find a relationship between two phenomena. The idea of *cognitive reserve* is based on findings that people who have more education need to experience more brain degeneration to be diagnosed with dementia, that is, they start at a higher cognitive ability level, so it takes longer for them to reach the threshold whereby the deterioration is so extensive that they cannot function independently. A recent study indicated that participation in cognitive activities is correlated with a delay in rapid memory decline in those who develop dementia (Hall et al., 2009).

However, we don't know how people acquired that cognitive reserve in the first place. It could be that they came from families that encouraged education and cognitively stimulating activities and were more stimulated from birth. Or they sought out stimulation as young, middle aged, or older adults. It could be argued that correlational studies based on comparisons of people who worked in different professions show strong evidence of developed brain plasticity. The famous study of larger regions of the brain associated with spatial navigation (the hippocampus) in London cab drivers compared to bus drivers (Maguire et al., 2003) suggested that the complex requirements of cab driving, with dynamic requirements to traverse all of London, compared to driving specific bus routes, was associated with greater development of neural pathways to represent the spatial layout of the city. However, what is not known is what selection factors exist in the brains of cab drivers vs. bus drivers. That is, with people who are better navigators and who have larger hippocampi may be more attracted to being cab rather than bus drivers, or are more likely to work as cab drivers for many years. The same argument can be made for the observation that people with different levels of intelligence show different amounts of neural connections (see Draganski & May, 2008).

There is an assumption that cognitive reserve can be increased, but the research suggesting this comes largely from animal studies where rats or mice are exposed to "complex" environments and are compared with those in ordinary cages. The animals in the ordinary cages show less brain connectivity, but if they are then exposed to the more complex environment, they develop more connections. This sounds very promising, but we need to remember that many findings observed in animal studies do not translate to humans. A 2008 article published by the senior members of the research team that showed brain changes in people learning how to juggle (Draganski et al., 2004) and medical students studying for an important examination (Draganski et al., 2006) underlines that there is a *need to understand the relationship between animal studies and training-related processes in humans*, not that they have been established:

> Brain plasticity is an inherent property not only of the developing but also of the adult human brain. Despite the promising results of longitudinal morphometric studies, we still lack a substantial amount of knowledge regarding the underlying morphological substrate, the exact time course and the relation to learning/training related functional processes in the human brain (Draganski & May, 2008).

Note also that the studies by Draganski and his colleagues do not involve assessment of transfer. We cannot replicate the experiments done with animals with humans, where we randomly assign people from birth to more or less stimulating environments. And we should acknowledge that even the study showing delayed memory decline in those with greater cognitive reserve was of people who developed dementia (Hall et al., 2009). *Cognitive reserve **did not eliminate** the risk of dementia.*

It is important to test products because at this point in time, there are more *correlational* studies about effects of cognitive activities on cognitive outcomes, including risk of Alzheimer's disease or dementia, than there are experimental studies or clinical trials of training by using principles of brain plasticity. Thus, little is known directly about general effects of training.

Buyer Beware!

Our final consideration is of the ultimate value of cognitive programs for consumers. What consumers may hope for is that practice of cognitive exercises lead to either a delay in the development of Alzheimer's or other dementias, a major reduction in risk of Alzheimer's, or even reversal of dementia. *However, none of the studies of consumer products or the experiments using principles of brain plasticity effects on cognition has evaluated any of these outcomes.* It is often suggested that older adults engage in physical, cognitive, and social activities, because at the very least, it doesn't hurt them (e.g., Valenzuela & Sachdev, 2009). However, whether these will help prevent or reverse dementia is unknown at this time. Based on our understanding of brain plasticity, it would appear that sufficient training of a wide range of cognitive abilities could ultimately increase cognitive reserve. However, we emphasize again that there is only *speculation* that training may increase cognitive reserve. A recent article on this suggests that it is possible:

> The strength of the epidemiological, clinical, basic science and neuroimaging evidence **seems (emphasis added)** to strongly support testing whether an intervention of "complex mental activity" is preventative against development of dementia (Valenzuela & Sachdev 2006).

However, it does not *yet* support prevention of dementia. The same authors conducted a review of randomized clinical trials of cognitive interventions with longitudinal follow-ups that was published in 2009. *They reported that cognitive exercise has not been shown to prevent dementia* (Valenzuela & Sachdev, 2009).

The Alzheimer's Association lists 10 myths about Alzheimer's Disease on their website (http://www.Alzheimers.org). It has this to say about treatment and cures for Alzheimer's disease:

> **Myth 8**: There are treatments available to stop the progression of Alzheimer's disease
>
> **Reality:** At this time, there is no treatment to cure, delay or stop the progression of Alzheimer's disease. FDA-approved drugs temporarily slow worsening of symptoms for about 6–12 months, on average, for about half of the individuals who take them.

The home page of the National Institutes of Health allows navigation to a website that provides consumer information for an A–Z list of diseases. Under the "Alzheimer's Disease" heading, it provides a listing of information on research sponsored by the National Institute on Aging. It currently indicates that there are suggestions that lifestyle factors may be associated with the risk of Alzheimer's disease and that there are exploratory studies on interventions for cognitive training. However, *exploratory* is the watchword here. If interventions are identified as reducing risk, delaying, or reversing Alzheimer's, they will be announced by the National Institutes of Health, it will be in the news, and otherwise made public. Until then, any product with a claim made that it delays, cures, or stops the progression of Alzheimer's, or may help prevent it is essentially unfounded. There is no watchdog organization that prevents companies from making such claims on the Web or in other media.

As a result, we think it is very important that consumers understand this, and advise them to be extremely cautious about purchasing access to a computer program making this claim. It is more prudent to select products that use research to test whether they produce far transfer, though it is seems less impressive than preventing or reversing Alzheimer's.

References

Ball, K., Berch, D. B., Helmers, K. F., Jobe, J. B., Leveck, M. D., Marsiske, M., et al. (2002). Effects of cognitive training interventions with older adults: A randomized controlled trial. *Journal of the American Medical Association, 288*, 2271–2281.

Ball, K. K., Edwards, J. D., & Ross, L. A. (2007). The impact of speed of processing training on cognitive and everyday functions. *Journal of Gerontology: Psychological Sciences, 62B*(Special Issue I), 19–31.

Barnett, S. M., & Ceci, S. J. (2002). When and where do we apply what we learn?: A taxonomy for far transfer. *Psychological Bulletin, 128*, 612–637.

Bherer, L., Kramer, A. F., Peterson, M. S., Colcombe, S., Erickson, K., & Becic, E. (2005). Training effects on dual-task performance: Are there age-related differences in plasticity of attentional control? *Psychology and Aging, 20*, 695–709.

Basak, C., Boot, W. R., Voss, M. W., & Kramer, A. F. (2008). Can training in a real-time strategy video game attenuate cognitive decline in older adults? *Psychology and Aging, 23*, 765–777.

Buschkuehl, M., Jaeggi, S. M., Hutchison, S., Perrig-Chiello, P., Däpp, C., Müller, M., et al. (2008). Impact of working memory training on memory performance in old-old adults. *Psychology and Aging, 23*, 743–753.

Byl, N. N., Nagarajan, S. S., & McKenzie, A. L. (2003). Effect of sensory discrimination training on structure and function in patients with focal hand dystonia: A case series. *Archives of Physical Medicine and Rehabilitation, 84*, 1505–1514.

Ceci, S. J., & Liker, J. (1986). A day at the races: A study of IQ, expertise, and cognitive complexity. *Journal of Experimental Psychology: General, 115*(3), 255–266.

Dahlin, E., Nyberg, L., Backman, L., & Stigsdotter-Neely, A. (2008). Plasticity of executive functioning in young and older adults: Immediate training gains, transfer, and long-term maintenance. *Psychology and Aging, 23*, 720–730.

Dahlin, E., Stigsdotter-Neely, A., Larsson, A., Backman, L., & Nyberg, L. (2008). Transfer of learning after updating mediated by the striatum. *Science, 320*, 1510–1512.

Dishman, R. K., & Buckworth, J. (1996). Increasing physical activity: A quantitative synthesis. *Medicine and Science in Sports and Exercise, 28*, 706–719.

Draganski, B., Gaser, C., Busch, V., Schuierer, G., Bogdahn, U., & Arne, M. (2004). Neuroplasticity: Changes in gray matter induced by training. *Nature, 427*, 311–312.

Draganski, B., Gaser, C., Kempermann, G., Kuhn, H. G., Winkler, J., Büschel, C., et al. (2006). Temporal and spatial dynamics of brain structure changes during extensive learning. *The Journal of Neuroscience, 26*, 6314–6317.

Draganski, B., & May, A. (2008). Training-induced structural changes in the adult human brain. *Behavioural Brain Research, 192*, 137–142.

Drew, B., & Walters, J. (1986). Video games: Utilization of a novel strategy to improve perceptual motor skills and cognitive functioning in the non-institutionalized elderly. *Cognitive Rehabilitation, 4*, 26–31.

Dustman, R. E., Emmerson, R. Y., Seinhous, L. A., Shearer, D. E., & Dustman, T. J. (1992). The effects of videogame playing on neuropsychological performance of elderly individuals. *Journal of Gerontology: Psychological Sciences, 47*, 168–171.

Edwards, J. D., Wadley, V. G., Vance, D. E., Wood, K., Roenker, D. L., & Ball, K. K. (2005). The impact of speed of processing training on cognitive and everyday performance. *Aging & Mental Health, 9*, 262–271.

Erickson, K. I., Colcombe, S. J., Wadhwa, R., Bherer, L., Peterson, M. S., Scalf, P. E., et al. (2007). Training-induced functional activation changes in dual-task processing: An fMRI study. *Cerebral Cortex, 17*, 192–204.

Garden, S. E., Phillips, L. H., & MacPherson, S. E. (2001). Midlife aging, open-ended planning, and laboratory measures of executive function. *Neuropsychology, 15*, 472–482.

Hall, C. B., Lipton, R. B., Sliwinski, M., Katz, M. J., Derby, C. A., & Verghese, J. (2009). Cognitive activities delay onset of memory decline in persons who develop dementia. *Neurology, 73*, 356–361.

Hong, S.-Y., Hughes, S., & Prohaska, T. (2008). Factors affecting exercise attendance and completion in sedentary older adults: A meta-analytic approach. *Journal of Physical Activity and Health, 5*, 385–397.

Jennings, J. M., Webster, L. M., Kleykamp, B. A., & Dagenbach, D. (2005). Recollection training and transfer effects in older adults: Successful use of a repetition-lag procedure. *Aging, Neuropsychology, and Cognition, 12*, 278–298.

Jobe, J. B., Smith, D. M., Ball, K., Tennstedt, S. L., Marsiske, M., Willis, S. L., et al. (2001). ACTIVE: A cognitive intervention trial to promote independence in older adults. *Controlled Clinical Trials, 22*, 453–479.

Kelmen, H. R., Thomas, C., Kennedy, G. J., & Cheng, J. (1994). Cognitive impairment and mortality in older community residents. *American Journal of Public Health, 84*, 1255–1260.

Kramer, A. F., Larish, J. F., & Strayer, D. L. (1995). Training for attentional control in dual task settings: A comparison of young and old adults. *Journal of Experimental Psychology: Applied, 1*, 50–76.

Kramer, A. F., Larish, J. F., Weber, T. A., & Bardell, L. (1999). Training for executive control: Task coordination strategies and aging. In D. Gopher & A. Koriat (Eds.), *Attention and performance XVII: Cognitive regulation of performance: Interaction of theory and application* (pp. 617–652). Cambridge: MIT Press.

Li, S.-C., Huxhold, O., Smith, J., Schmiedek, F., Röcke, C., & Lindenberger, U. (2008). Working memory plasticity in old age: Practice gain, transfer, and maintenance. *Psychology and Aging, 23*, 731–742.

Maguire, E. A., Spiers, H. J., Good, C. D., Hartley, T., Frackowiak, R. S. J., & Burgess, N. (2003). Navigation expertise and the human hippocampus: A structural brain imaging analysis. *Hippocampus, 13*, 250–259.

Mahncke, H. W., Bronstone, A., & Merzenich, M. M. (2006). Brain plasticity and functional losses in the aged: Scientific bases for a novel intervention. *Reprogramming the Brain, 157*, 81–109.

Mahncke, H. W., Connor, B. B., Appelman, J., Ahsanuddin, O. N., Hardy, J. L., Wood, R. A., et al. (2006). Memory enhancement in healthy older adults using a brain plasticity-based training program: A randomized, controlled study. *Proceedings of the National Academy of Sciences, 103*, 12523–12528.

Mather, M. (2006). A review of decision-making processes: Weighing the risks and benefits of aging. In L. L. Carstensen & C. R. Hartel (Eds.), *When I'm 64: Committee on aging frontiers in social psychology, personality, and adult developmental psychology* (pp. 145–173). Washington, DC: National Academies Press.

McAuley, E., Morris, K. S., Motl, R. W., Hu, L., Konopack, J. F., & Elavsky, S. (2007). Long-term follow-up of physical activity behavior in older adults. *Health Psychology, 26*, 375–380.

Polley, D. B., Steinberg, E. E., & Merzenich, M. M. (2006). Perceptual learning directs auditory cortical map reorganization through top-down influences. *Journal of Neuroscience, 26*, 4970–4982.

Randolph, C. (1998). *Repeatable battery for the assessment of neuropsychological status*. San Antonio, TX: Psychological Corporation.

Rockwood, K. (2004). Size of the treatment effect on cognition of cholinesterase inhibition in Alzheimer's disease. *Journal of Neurology and Neurosurgical Psychiatry, 75*, 677–685.

Roenker, D. L., Cissell, G. M., Ball, K. K., Wadley, V. G., & Edwards, J. D. (2003). Speed-of-processing and driving simulator training result in improved driving performance. *Human Factors, 45*, 218–233.

Schmidt, M. (1996). *Rey auditory and verbal learning test: A handbook*. Los Angeles: Western Psychological Services.

SharpBrains. (2010). *Transforming brain health with digital tools to assess, enhance, and treat cognition across the lifespan: The State of the Brain Fitness Market 2010*. San Francisco: SharpBrains.

Smith, G. E., Housen, P., Yaffe, R. R., Ruff, R., Kennison, R. F., Mahncke, H. W., et al. (2009). A cognitive training program based on principles of brain plasticity: Results from the improvement in memory with plasticity-based adaptive cognitive training (IMPACT) study. *Journal of the American Geriatrics Society, 57*, 594–603.

Smith, G. E., Peterson, R. C., Ivnik, R. J., Malec, J. F., & Tangalos, E. G. (1996). Subjective memory complaints, psychological distress, and longitudinal change in objective memory performance. *Psychology and Aging, 11*, 272–279.

St. John, P. D., Montgomery, P. R., Kristjansson, B., & McDowell, I. (2002). Cognitive scores, even within the normal range, predict death and institutionalization. *Age and Ageing, 31*, 373–378.

Turner, D. C., Robbins, T. W., Clark, L., Aron, A. R., Dowson, J., & Sahakian, B. (2003). Cognitive enhancing effects of modafinil in healthy volunteers. *Psychopharmacology, 165*, 260–269.

Valenzuela, M. J., & Sachdev, P. (2006). Brain reserve and dementia: A systematic review. *Psychological Medicine, 36*, 441–454.

Valenzuela, M., & Sachdev, P. (2009). Can cognitive exercise prevent the onset of dementia? Systematic review of randomized clinical trials with longitudinal follow-up. *American Journal of Geriatric Psychiatry, 17*, 179–187.

Wang, X., Merzenich, M. M., Sameshima, K., & Jenkins, W. M. (1995). Remodeling of hand representation in adult cortex determined by timing of tactile stimulation. *Nature, 378*, 71–75.

Wechsler, D. (1997). *Wechsler Memory Scale-III*. San Antonio: Psychological Corporation.

Wilson, B., Cockburn, J., Baddeley, A., & Hiorns, R. (2003). *The Rivermead behavioral memory test – II, supplement two*. San Antonio, TX: Harcourt Assessment.

Winocur, G., Palmer, H., Dawson, D., Binns, M. A., Bridges, K., & Stuss, D. T. (2007). Cognitive rehabilitation of the elderly: An evaluation of psychosocial factors. *Journal of the International Neuropsychological Society, 13*, 153–165.

Xerri, C. (2008). Imprinting of idiosyncratic experience in cortical sensory maps: Neural substrates of representational remodeling and correlative perceptual changes. *Behavioural Brain Research, 192*, 26–41.

Zelinski, E. M. (2009). Far transfer in cognitive training of older adults. *Restorative Neurology and Neuroscience, 27*, 455–471.

Zelinski, E. M., & Gilewski, M. J. (2004). A 10-Item Rasch modeled memory self efficacy scale. *Aging and Mental Health, 8*, 293–306.

Chapter 4
Synapse: A Clinical Trial Examining the Impact of Actively Engaging the Aging Mind*

Jennifer Lodi-Smith and Denise C. Park

Abstract A fundamental challenge and responsibility for modern science is to progress toward understanding neuroprotective factors that will support and optimize cognitive aging. The present chapter describes the scientifically driven efforts of our research group to this end. We do this in three ways beginning with a review of the latest findings regarding the neurocognitive declines that are part of the normal aging process. Next, we present the Scaffolding Theory of Aging and Cognition (STAC; Annu Rev Psychol 60:173–196, 2009), which describes a model for how the brain adapts to the neural deterioration that occurs as a natural part of the aging process. Finally, we introduce a program of research designed using the tenets of the STAC model to investigate how engaging in cognitively and socially stimulating activities may promote the neurocognitive health of seniors long term.

The Aging Mind

One of the most pervasive findings in developmental cognitive neuroscience is that there is a gradual decline in neurocognitive functioning during adulthood, even in healthy adults. However, even in the face of these changes in neurocognitive function, many faculties are maintained and protected well into old age and many seniors continue to maintain a healthy neurocognitive life. In the pages that follow, we review the normative patterns of age-related change in neurocognitive functioning. In addition, we present the Scaffolding Theory of Aging and Cognition (STAC),

---

*Chapter prepared for the *Enhancing Cognitive Fitness in Adults: A Guide for the Use and Development of Community-Based programs*.

J. Lodi-Smith (✉)
Canisius College, Department of Psychology,
2001 Main Street, Buffalo, NY 14208, USA
e-mail: lodismij@canisius.edu

a model that proposes how the brain compensates for the neurocognitive challenges that come with age, and provide empirical evidence to support this model.

Cognitive change. Behavioral findings show that cognitive decline starts in young adulthood and continues across the lifespan. In a sample of 350 normal, healthy adults, Park et al. (2002) observed reliable cross-sectional declines from age 20 to 80 and older in speed of processing, working memory, and long-term memory. By contrast, word knowledge was largely unaffected by age and may even be higher in older adults. While these findings compared people across different age groups and could, therefore, be due to cohort differences among the age groups rather than actual age differences over time, evidence from longitudinal studies that track individuals often show a similar pattern. For example, the Victoria Longitudinal Study (Hultsch, Hertzog, Dixon, & Small, 1999) tracked individuals age 60 and older across a variety of behavioral measures of cognitive performance and found results that are remarkably similar to the lifespan results found by Park et al. (2002). These two studies serve as examples of the large body of literature that delineate a pattern of normative declines in cognitive performance across the lifespan.

Structural changes in the brain. At the same time that age-related declines occur in cognitive behavior, parallel changes occur in the structure of the brain. Three primary patterns of change in brain structures occur with age (see Raz & Kennedy, 2009 for a recent comprehensive review of this topic). First, there are characteristic patterns of decline in the volume of certain brain regions such that prefrontal regions of the brain are the most subject to volumetric declines with age and regions such as the hippocampus, temporal lobe, and parietal lobe show nonlinear decreases in volume while sensory cortices remain relatively intact over the lifespan (Raz, 2000, 2004; Raz & Kennedy, 2009; Raz, Rodrigue, Head, Kennedy, & Acker, 2004). Second, there is evidence for cortical thinning in the brain with age (Fjell et al., 2009; Salat et al., 2004). Finally, some of the most important changes in the structure of the brain with age involve white matter – the areas of the brain where myelin-coated axons transfer signals between neurons. Specifically, Head et al. (2004) note significant degradation with age to white matter in the frontal regions of the brain. Additionally, abnormalities in white matter, known as white matter hyperintensities, increase with age, particularly in frontal and occipital areas of the brain (Raz & Kennedy, 2009; Wen & Sachdev, 2004). Taken together, these findings suggest reliable, age-related changes in the brain, particularly in frontal regions.

Changes in brain function. Functional magnetic resonance imaging (fMRI) measures brain activation by examining the changes in cerebral blood flow that accompany cognitive tasks completed while in the MRI scanner. Three findings related to decreased neural function are of particular note in functional imaging studies of neurocognitive changes in older adulthood. First, there is evidence for a pattern of lowered activation in mediotemporal regions of the brain including the hippocampus when comparing younger and older adults when performing long-term memory tasks (Park & Gutchess, 2005; Persson et al., 2006). Second, when presented with cognitively challenging tasks, older adults show significant impairment compared to young adults in suppressing activation in regions of the brain known as the default network – the areas of the brain that are active when the brain is not engaged in complex activities (Persson et al., 2006). Finally, many older adults show decreased specificity in patterns of activation to certain stimuli when compared to young adults, a phenomenon known as dedifferentiation. For example, a young adult viewing faces would show activation in the fusiform area of the ventral visual cortex (Kanwisher, McDermott, & Chun, 1997) while a young adult viewing pictures of places would show activation in the parahippocampus (Epstein & Kanwisher, 1998) and a young adult looking at words and numbers would have increased activation in the left fusiform gyrus and collateral sulcus (Polk et al., 2002; Puce, Allison, Asgari, Gore, & McCarthy, 1996). Older adults show significantly less specialization of these areas compared to young adults (Park et al., 2004). In addition to these age-related declines in brain function, however, there are also increases in adaptive functional activations with age as discussed below.

The Scaffolding Theory of Aging and Cognition

Despite the normative declines in cognitive and neural function described above, it is important to recognize that many older adults function at a high and optimal level, even into very old age. The STAC model proposes that, as we age, the brain responds to some of the neural declines just described by employing compensatory scaffolding – the engagement of new brain areas and pathways in response to changes in the structure and function of other brain regions (Park & Reuter-Lorenz, 2009).

Some of the best empirical evidence supporting the STAC model comes from fMRI research. As described above, functional decline is present in the aging brain in the form of lowered activation, changing patterns in default networks, and decreased neural specialization of older adults. Given these findings and the behavioral and structural declines that occur as a normative part of the aging process, one might expect corresponding declines in neural activation across the board in older adults. However, empirical evidence shows that this is not the case. Rather than holistic patterns of deactivation, the brains of older adults demonstrate more activation in key processing areas when compared to the brains of young adults on certain tasks. For example, during verbal memory tasks, young adult brains show left prefrontal activity while the brains of older adults show bilateral activation of the prefrontal cortex – activation of the same areas in both the left and the right hemispheres (Cabeza et al., 1997; Grady, McIntosh, Rajah, Beig, & Craik, 1999; Reuter-Lorenz et al., 2000).

Since these early findings indicating the presence of prefrontal bilaterality in older adults, evidence increasingly supports the hypothesis that this bilaterality is an adaptive, compensatory brain mechanism. For example, patterns of bilateral activation are linked to better task performance (Cabeza, Anderson, Locantore, & McIntosh, 2002; Cherry, Adamson, Duclos, & Hellige, 2005; Fera et al., 2005; Reuter-Lorenz et al., 2001; Reuter-Lorenz, Stanczak, & Miller, 1999; Rypma & D'Esposito, 2001) and enhanced memory in memory-based performance tasks (Gutchess et al., 2005). Even young adults show bilateral patterns of prefrontal activation when put in highly challenging situations (Banich, 1998; Hillary, Genova, Chiaravalloti, Rypma, DeLuca, & 2006; Reuter-Lorenz & Cappell, 2008) suggesting that the natural response of the brain to challenge is to recruit additional areas of processing – or scaffolds. The bilateral activation seen in older adults is thought to directly compensate for decrease in both the volume and activation of the hippocampus (Cabeza et al., 2004; Morcom, Good, Frackowiak, & Rugg, 2003; Persson et al., 2006). Whether compensation occurs in response to external forces, as in increasing the difficulty of a task for young adults, or from the internal changes that come with age, the brain is an adaptive organ that readily and automatically responds in a natural, homeostatic way by bringing scaffolds online. This is not to say that performance will be maintained at every level or that the scaffolds are as efficient as original systems. It is likely that scaffolding becomes limited with age and with the onset of Alzheimer's and other dementia-related disorders. However, for the normal, healthy older adult, the compensatory engagement of scaffolding allows for a general maintenance of everyday performance (Park & Reuter-Lorenz, 2009).

Creating Scaffolds

The research presented to this point provides evidence that the natural response of the brain to the neural challenges of aging is to create compensatory scaffolds as we age. In addition, there are a number of empirical findings suggesting that scaffolds are not just a response of the brain to aging and challenge but are also created in response to life experiences. Animal models of aging suggest that both cognitive stimulation and physical exercise can promote neurogenesis (the growth of new neurons) in keeping with the STAC model (Jessberger & Gage, 2008). For example, aged rats that had substantial degradation in their auditory cortices can be trained to have normal hearing not due to reactivation of the auditory areas of the brain but, rather, to a restructuring of the brain (Zhou & Merzenich, 2007). Additionally, animal models suggest that a lifetime spent in a stimulating environment promotes the generation of new neurons in the hippocampus of old rats (Kempermann, Kuhn, & Gage, 1998) as does physical exercise (Pereira et al., 2007). Similarly, when older rats are exposed to stimulating environments over a short period of time they show improved learning (Kobayashi, Ohashi, & Ando, 2002), a fivefold increase in the growth of new genes in the hippocampus, and decreased degradation in other parts of the brain (Kempermann, Gast, & Gage, 2002).

These findings may not be limited to nonhuman animals. There is correlational evidence that engaging in cognitively stimulating activities may be beneficial to neural health. Staying engaged in intellectually challenging work during late life relates to increased cognitive function (Bosma et al., 2003; Schooler, Mulatu, & Oates, 1999) and more highly educated individuals, who tend to spend more time in cognitively challenging activities, have a decreased risk of Alzheimer's disease even when taking into consideration other variables related to Alzheimer's disease risk (Bennett et al., 2003; Wilson & Bennett, 2003; Wilson et al., 2000).

Evidence also suggests that certain broad life experiences play a role in brain organization. For example, London cab drivers have larger brain structures related to spatial representation than normal individuals (Maguire et al., 2000) and professional musicians have larger auditory, motor, and visual–spatial regions compared to amateur and nonmusicians (Gaser & Schlaug, 2003). Similarly, while number recognition and letter recognition are relegated to separate areas of the brain, this appears not to be the case for Canadian postal workers who spend much of their time sorting mail by Canadian postal codes – which are a combination of both letters and numbers (Polk & Farah, 1998). There is also evidence that both exercise and exercise training are related to better cognitive performance, increases in brain volume, and better functional performance of frontal and parietal regions of the brain (see Boot & Blakely, Chap. 2; Potkanowicz, Chap. 15 for additional reviews linking exercise to neurocognitive health; Colcombe & Kramer, 2003).

While there is a substantial literature suggesting that targeted skill training can enhance cognitive performance on select tasks (see Lustig, Shah, Seidler, & Reuter-Lorenz, 2009 for a review), preliminary evidence from human intervention research suggests that engaging in stimulating new activities may facilitate performance on measures of cognitive processing. For example, seniors who took 4 weeks of theater classes showed better problem-solving skills and word recall relative to seniors who engaged in an art appreciation class or a no-treatment control condition. Further, the theater students retained these benefits 4 months after the intervention was terminated (Noice, Noice, & Staines, 2004). Similarly, seniors who spent 24 (nonconsecutive) hours learning to play a strategy-based video game increased in executive control relative to no-treatment controls (Basak, Boot, Voss, & Kramer, 2008) (see Boot & Blakely, 2011). In addition, older adults who participated in long-term problem-solving activities through the Senior Odyssey program showed greater speed of processing, inductive reasoning, and divergent thinking skills after 7–8 months in Senior Odyssey relative to no-treatment controls (see Stine-Morrow & Parisi, Chap. 9).

Two recent studies provide preliminary evidence that scientifically driven interventions may even be able to promote change at the neural level. Training designed to target a particular cognitive skill generally shows benefits to linked neural structure and function (for a recent comprehensive review of this literature see Lustig et al., 2009). Additionally, preliminary evidence suggests that engaging in novel, cognitively stimulating, real world activities can impact neurocognitive function in the Experience Corps model that recruited older adults who participated in literacy positions in community elementary schools (see Carlson et al, 2009; Rebok et al., Chap. 27).

In a very different type of novel activity, 25 seniors who could juggle three balls for more than 40 seconds at the end of 3 months of juggling training had increased gray matter in areas of the brain associated with vision, motion, memory, and learning relative to no-treatment controls. Unfortunately, these effects reversed such that the jugglers showed declines in gray matter in these regions when they were imaged again after 3 months without juggling (Boyke, Driemeyer, Gaser, Buchel, & May, 2008). These findings provide preliminary support for the idea that new patterns of neural activation – or scaffolds – may be generated in response to life experiences.

With this idea in mind, the *Synapse* Intervention Trial was created to provide an environment that might facilitate the development of neural scaffolding. *Synapse* provides a setting where seniors can engage in structured, cognitively stimulating activities for a sustained period of time with the hypothesis that over time the environment will stimulate the development of neural scaffolds and result in enhanced neurocognitive functioning. In the pages that follow, we discuss the details of this intervention trial in order to present the intervention to the scientific and public communities as well as provide guidance for scientists, community groups, and individuals interested in using a similar approach to promote neurocognitive health.

The Synapse Intervention Trial

The Study Design

The *Synapse* Intervention Trial takes place in Dallas, Texas. Given the size of the city, considerable effort was spent on identifying an area of the city that has a particularly dense and vibrant senior population. With this goal in mind, the White Rock Lake area of East Dallas, a historic area with many cultural draws including White Rock Lake Park, the Dallas Arboretum, and the Bath House Cultural Center, was identified as the optimal setting for *Synapse*. *Synapse* is located in two sites in this area, one in a storefront shopping center that had recently been targeted for revitalization and the other in a retirement community dedicated to fostering the involvement of community-dwelling Dallas seniors in stimulating activities.

Involvement in *Synapse* begins with a structured recruitment and screening protocol. Potential participants attend an informational meeting to learn more about the study. At this meeting, participants receive information ranging from our university affiliation and funding, to the assessments and requirements of the study, to the logistical details of the study. The goal of these meetings is to give potential participants as much information about the study as possible so that they can make an informed decision about whether *Synapse* is a good fit for them. At this point, interested individuals complete a series of screening protocols to ensure that the potential participant is a good fit for *Synapse*. Eligible participants must be over 60 years of age; spend less than 10 hours each week engaging in work and/or volunteer activities; be novice quilters and novices at the use of a sewing machine, a digital camera, and computer; demonstrate that they have functional vision and hearing; pass both a dementia and depression screening test; have no current major psychiatric disorders; and be willing to commit to the time frame of the study. Approximately, half of the participants who attend informational meetings are both interested in and eligible for *Synapse*.

Once participants are determined to be qualified for *Synapse*, they are randomly assigned to their research group based on study needs. There are eight research arms to *Synapse*. The first four research arms are the productive engagement groups. These groups spend 15 hours a week for 14 weeks learning a new activity – quilting, digital photography, a combination of the two skills, or a combination of quilting and exercise. The other four groups serve as structured controls for various components of the productive engagement groups: (1) a social control group has the same time commitment as the productive engagement groups but spends time in passive, social activities such as watching movies or going on field trips to local attractions, (2) a placebo control group gives the same time commitment as the productive engagement groups but spends this time completing passive activities at home that they are told stimulate cognitive function but likely have a less substantive impact on neurocognitive outcomes (activities include listening to classical music, reading National Geographic, and watching documentaries), (3) an exercise control group receives the same personally customized exercise intervention of 30 minutes a day for 3–4 days a week given to members of the group that both quilts and exercises, and (4) a no-treatment control group completes the assessment portions of *Synapse*.

Enrollment and retention of *Synapse* participants have been excellent. Initial advertisements in the senior section of the local newspaper drew little response for the cost of the advertisement. Targeted mailings to seniors living in the White Rock Lake area were more successful and 25 seniors enrolled the first round of *Synapse* from August to December 2008. Targeted mailers and recent local media attention have allowed us to increase enrollment to approximately 70 participants per round. To date, 255 participants have enrolled in *Synapse* with 193 fully completing all of the assessments and 62 currently engaging in their assigned activities. By the end of the study in December 2011, approximately 500 participants will have completed *Synapse*. To date, only 17 participants have had to withdraw from *Synapse* – 15 for personal reasons and 2 men (one placebo control, one no-treatment control) who did not enjoy their assigned activity after 3 weeks of engagement.

During the 2 weeks before the initiation of the new activities, each *Synapse* participant undergoes a 2½ hours cognitive assessment to measure their performance on behavioral markers of cognitive performance including processing speed, verbal fluency and ability, working memory, long-term memory, inductive reasoning, and mental control. In addition, *Synapse* participants complete a psychosocial battery during this time period to collect information about demographics, health and fitness, social networks, lifetime and daily activities, psychological health, perceptions of their cognitive life, and personality variables. Eligible participants complete a 45-minutes MRI protocol where they undergo both structural and functional neuroimaging protocols. Approximately, one third of all *Synapse* participants are eligible for the MRI portion of the study. Participants in the two arms of the intervention including an exercise component complete two 1-hour long physical health assessments. During the 12th and 13th week of the engagement period, participants complete identical cognitive, psychosocial, neuroimaging, and physical health protocols. Additionally, participants complete 30 minutes mini-assessments at weeks 3, 6, and 9 of *Synapse* to facilitate statistical modeling of change in key cognitive and psychosocial variables of interest and each *Synapse* participant completes a weekly checklist of activities throughout the study. Finally, participants complete a short questionnaire of their daily activities 3 and 6 months after the end of their time in *Synapse* and complete a final full cognitive, psychosocial, neuroimaging, and physical health assessment 1 year after they finish *Synapse*.

Productive Engagement

One of the most common questions participants and scientists alike ask about *Synapse* is "why quilting and digital photography?" Quilting and digital photography are the focal tasks of *Synapse* for a number of reasons:

1. Quilting and digital photography are productive engagement tasks that engage many cognitive processes – they are activities that require the sustained activation of working memory, long-term memory, and reasoning skills – rather than being receptive engagement tasks that have relatively low cognitive demands and rely on the use of existing knowledge structures and automatic behaviors.
2. Quilting and digital photography are skills that have a sufficient number of novices in the older adult population to allow only novices to participate in the study without unduly harming enrollment.
3. Quilting and digital photography are noncompetitive skills that foster a collaborative learning environment. It is quite common for students to help each other learn during the program and, in doing so, gain a greater understanding of the skill and develop strong interpersonal relationships.
4. Quilting and digital photography provide tangible end products for the students to take home throughout their time in the program. Quilting students complete coasters on their first day of class, finish their first quilt by the end of the fourth week of class, and have numerous additional projects that are theirs to keep by the end of the program. Digital photography students produce work ranging from standard 3×5 prints to full portfolios, digital presentations of photojournalism projects, and mounted canvas prints of their favorite photographs.
5. Both quilting and digital photography are commonly taught in the community. This provides three concrete benefits: we were able to hire an expert quilter and an expert digital photographer from the community, participants can easily continue their engagement after the study ends, and the public can readily find resources for these activities in their own communities.
6. As we describe below and as shown in Table 4.1, both quilting and digital photography are real world tasks that facilitate the development of unique skill sets that may enhance specific areas of cognitive functioning.

The skills involved in quilting require processing speed, working memory, long-term memory, inductive reasoning, and mental control. For example, simply learning how to use the sewing machine involves processing speed, visual–spatial working memory, long-term memory, and reasoning. Planning tasks such as following and

Table 4.1 Cognitive domains influenced by *Synapse* productive engagement tasks

Task	Speed	Visual–spatial working memory	Verbal working memory	Long-term memory	Reasoning	Mental control
Quilting						
Using sewing machine	x	x		x	x	
Planning		x	x	x	x	x
Preparation		x		x	x	x
Creating quilt		x		x	x	x
Photography						
Using digital camera	x	x		x	x	
Computer skills		x	x	x	x	x
Artistic skills		x	x	x	x	x
Creating final products		x	x	x	x	x

Note: x's indicate cognitive domains that are thought to be facilitated by the listed skill

designing patterns, choosing fabric, and following instructions may benefit visual–spatial and verbal working memory, long-term memory, reasoning, and mental control. The skills necessary to prepare a quilt including piecing, measuring, and cutting use visual–spatial working memory, long-term memory, reasoning, and mental control. The composition of the quilt itself through sewing, pressing, binding, and the final quilting may also help these same cognitive processes. We hypothesize that the process of learning and perfecting these important quilting skills will enhance cognitive performance in these domains.

Digital photography also requires skills that may support cognitive performance. The first skill participants in the photography group learn is simply to operate the digital camera provided for their use during the study. The use of the camera is a novel skill to many and is expected to benefit speed of processing, working memory, long-term memory, and reasoning. In addition to being new to the camera, many students are also novice computer users. From learning the basics of how to use a computer to create and download files to more advanced skills such as manipulating photographs in Adobe Photoshop and using the internet to share their photographs with others, students become experts in using modern technology as a photographic tool. Working with their photographs on the computer is only a part of what the photography students learn, however. From the first day of class, students in the digital photography module of *Synapse* also learn the art of photography through learning how to plan for factors such as lighting, composition, and layout. Finally, the creation of a final product through cropping and editing, printing, designing and creating portfolios, and enhancing photographic quality provides the students with concrete end products of their time in the class. We hypothesize that each of these areas of activity engages both visual–spatial and verbal working memory, long-term memory, reasoning, and mental control. Examples of the work of the participants in the photography group can be seen in Fig. 4.1, a compilation of photographs of participants engaging in *Synapse*.

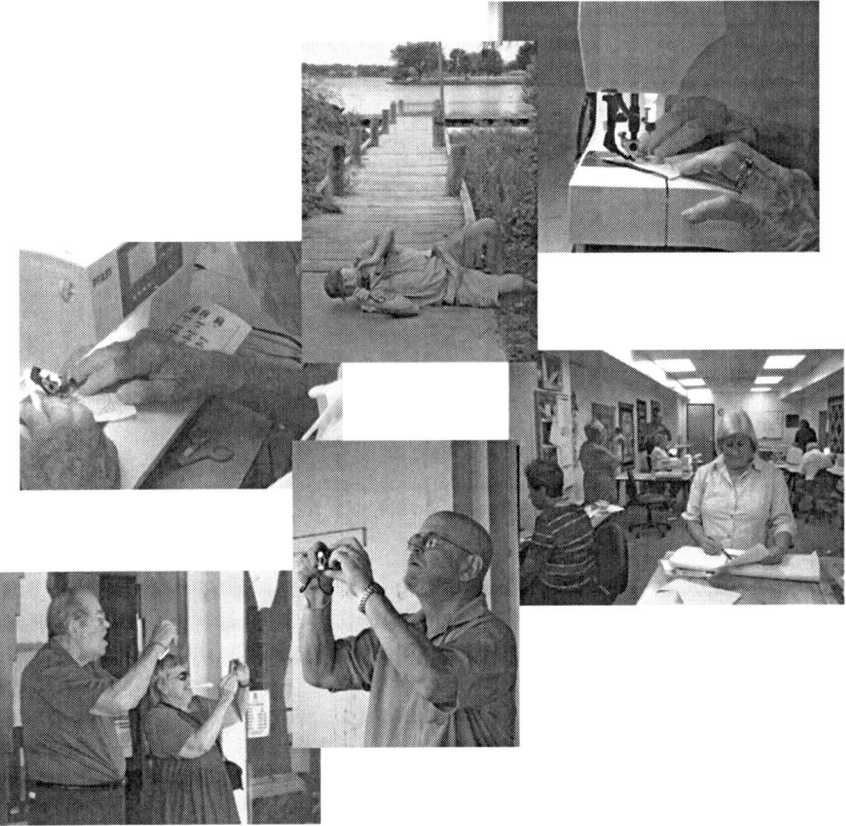

Fig. 4.1 Pictures by *Synapse* participants of the *Synapse* experience

Is Synapse Making a Difference?

All of these factors are designed to address four key hypotheses. First, we anticipate that each of the productive engagement groups will show more improvement to their neurocognitive function than any of the control groups. Specifically, we expect little to no improvement in either the no-treatment or placebo control groups and while we expect some minor improvement in neurocognitive function for the social and exercise groups, the salutatory effects of the productive engagement are expected to be more robust than those seen in any other groups. In addition, it is likely the case that the breadth of engagement experienced by the productive engagement group that spends 6 weeks learning digital photography and 6 weeks learning quilting will afford the most opportunity for scaffolding and may have the strongest effect. Second, based on the findings from pilot data described below, we anticipate that the effects of productive engagement will be even more beneficial for the "older" older adults in the study than for the "younger" older adults. Third, all participants undergo a complete cognitive and psychosocial battery and eligible participants have a third

MRI 1 year after the end of their time in *Synapse*. This will allow us to assess the effect of the scaffolding environment over the long term. Finally, we examine numerous secondary variables during *Synapse*. This allows us to investigate the impact that factors such as personality, life context, health, and social behavior may impact the individual response to *Synapse*. This information will help us isolate individual differences in response to the intervention and make preliminary suggestions on how to cater scaffolding interventions for individual needs.

Because *Synapse* is a clinical trial funded by the National Institute on Aging (NIA), we will not examine any of our hypotheses until the full complement of participants has completed the intervention period in 2011. That said, two sources of information provide us with preliminary evidence for the efficacy of *Synapse*.

First, before applying for funding from NIA, we completed a pilot study of the central interventions in *Synapse*. In the pilot study, *VIVA!*, participants spent 15 hours a week for 8 weeks learning either quilting ($N=30$) or digital photography ($N=9$) with 39 participants included in a no-treatment control group. Participants were healthy, community-dwelling older adults who ranged in age from 60 to 83 with an average age of 68. All participants were assessed before and at the end of the 8-week intervention period on cognitive variables including speed of processing, visual–spatial working memory, verbal working memory, long-term memory, and verbal fluency. Even given the relatively small number of participants and the shortened time frame, the data from *VIVA!* show that productive engagement can have a short-term impact on cognitive performance. Specifically, quilting participants increased in processing speed and visual–spatial working memory relative to no-treatment controls while participants in the digital photography intervention increased in long-term memory relative to no-treatment controls, as shown in Fig. 4.2. Treatment effects

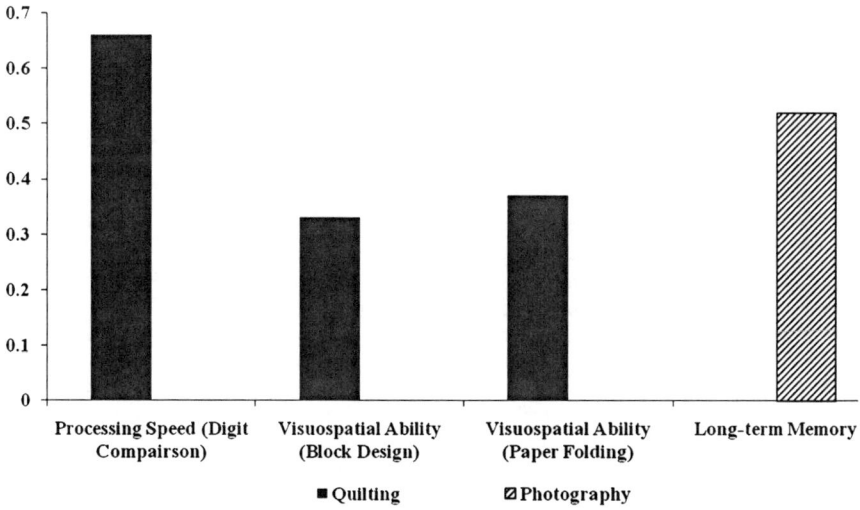

Fig. 4.2 Effect size of differences in cognitive change between experimental and control groups in *VIVA!*

sizes were moderate or larger by usual statistical standards and were most robust in participants over the age of 75.

Although verbal reports may not be reliable for assessing cognitive change, we do know that people enjoy the *Synapse* intervention and they report that it has affected their life. Given that evidence from young adults suggests that stories individuals tell of personality change during college correspond with measured changes over time (Lodi-Smith, Geise, Roberts, & Robins, 2009), the stories *Synapse* participants tell in response to the question "How do you feel you have changed as a part of your participation in the *Synapse* study?" can provide preliminary insight into the impact *Synapse* has on their lives. Participants have, to date, been positive about their time in the study. Repeated themes from these stories include enjoying life more, accomplishing goals, having greater focus, a deep sense of gratitude for the opportunity to be part of the study, and a positive outlook on the future. Table 4.2 has sample stories from participants in the productive engagement groups.

The stories of our youngest and our oldest participant to date are particularly poignant examples of the impact they report that *Synapse* is having. Our youngest participant, at 60 years of age, was a self-described "couch potato" when she was

Table 4.2 Example stories of study effects from participants in *Synapse*'s productive engagement groups

Engagement group	Story
Quilting	My concentration and focus have improved with learning a new skill. I intend to continue to learn new things. I'm going to enroll at Eastfield Community College in January for a beginner computer class. I also plan to continue quilting and improving my skills
Photography	I have become more disciplined and creative in all other aspects of my life. I notice photogenic qualities of what I see now. The overall effect of the class is mentally stimulating and life enriching. Thanks for everything!
Quilting + photography	I feel that participation in the *Synapse* program has been a very positive experience in my life. It has been beneficial in many ways – mentally through problem solving and socially by my interaction with new people
	The discipline of having more scheduling in my life, attending classes, and meeting goals has been very helpful. The instructors are informative, patient, and great motivators for my study and learning of new skills
	My initial reason for wanting to attend was the learning of digital photography, and my skills are much improved. Initially I had little interest in quilting class, but I thoroughly enjoyed learning new techniques, the creativity of design, and meeting new people. The sense of satisfaction in my completed work has given me a real feeling of accomplishment. In addition, I feel that the routine, the discipline, the learning in classes, and the social interaction have improved my mental and physical health
	I am very grateful to those who gave me this opportunity for enrichment

assigned to the group that learned both quilting and digital photography. She reported to us that *Synapse* changed her life, stating:

> The *Synapse* study has gotten me out of a rut; I looked forward to coming to classes. It's letting me know I don't have to sit around home with limited skills. The completion of projects made me feel better about myself. My family was happy for me, that I was happy and enjoying the experience of doing something new.
>
> I probably would not have ventured out of my alone space except for this opportunity.
>
> I enjoyed the interactions with everyone.
>
> I think I am going to try to find a new outlet for myself after *Synapse*.

Six months after she wrote this story, at a party to celebrate the end of one of the intervention phases, she reported that she was volunteering in the community and appeared to have lost a significant amount of weight with many people commenting on the change they could see in her.

The story of our oldest participant, an 87-year-old man, is also suggestive of a positive life impact. He shared his story with us at the end of the program during a session we held with the participants to hear their suggestions and advice for future rounds of the study. He told us that for the past 15 years he had been treated as a "has been." He described physical features that contributed to this treatment such as his hunched back, patchy skin, and clouded eye. He then went on to describe how his time learning to quilt helped him realize that he is not a has been and, instead, still has much to do and learn. He spent many months after the study recovering his old school records and is now enrolled in college completing the degree he began in his youth.

Conclusion

Synapse is an intervention program that tests whether an environment that is designed to facilitate productive engagement in cognitively stimulating activities will in fact promote cognitive performance through the development of neurocognitive scaffolding. While the primary aim of *Synapse* is to enhance neurocognitive function, as the stories of our participants illustrate, *Synapse* may have a much broader reach and is benefiting individuals across broad domains of functioning. In addition to normative changes in neurocognitive processes with age, one of the most profound challenges facing seniors today is the change they face in their social environment. Social role changes due to retirement, widowhood, loss of friends, and changes in health pose serious threats to seniors. These social roles are fundamental components of the self-concept (McCrae & Costa, 1988) and, according to the Social Investment Theory of personality development, are important determinants of a healthy and consistent identity in adulthood (Lodi-Smith & Roberts, 2007; Roberts, Wood, & Smith, 2005). By promoting active engagement in stimulating activities, *Synapse* provides the opportunity for seniors to develop new self-defining roles and, therefore, not only benefits neurocognitive health but the individual as a whole. In the words of one participant, *Synapse* provides "a new lease on life."

Acknowledgments Research supported by the National Institutes on Aging grants #R01AG026589 and 1RC1AG036003.

References

Banich, M. T. (1998). The missing link: The role of interhemispheric interaction in attentional processing. *Brain and Cognition, 36*, 128–157.

Basak, C., Boot, W. R., Voss, M. W., & Kramer, A. F. (2008). Can training in a real-time strategy video game attenuate cognitive decline in older adults? *Psychology and Aging, 23*, 765–777.

Bennett, D. A., Wilson, R. S., Schneider, J. A., Evans, D. A., Leon, C. F. M. D., Arnold, S. E., et al. (2003). Education modifies the relation of AD pathology to level of cognitive function in older persons. *Neurology, 60*, 1909–1915.

Boot, W., & Blakely, D. (2011). Mental and physical exercise as a means to reverse cognitive aging and enhance well-being. In P. E. Hartman-Stein & A. La Rue (Eds.), *Enhancing cognitive fitness in adults: A guide for use and development of community-based programs*. New York: Springer.

Bosma, H., Boxtel, M. P. V., Ponds, R. W., Houx, P. J., Burdorf, A., & Jolles, J. (2003). Mental work demands protect against cognitive impairment: MAAS prospective cohort study. *Experimental Aging Research, 29*, 33–45.

Boyke, J., Driemeyer, J., Gaser, C., Buchel, C., & May, A. (2008). Training-induced brain structure changes in the elderly. *The Journal of Neuroscience, 28*, 7031–7035.

Cabeza, R., Anderson, N. D., Locantore, J. K., & McIntosh, A. R. (2002). Aging gracefully: Compensatory brain activity in high-performing older adults. *NeuroImage, 17*, 1394–1402.

Cabeza, R., Daselaar, S. M., Dolcos, F., Prince, S. E., Budde, M., & Nyberg, L. (2004). Task-independent and task-specific age effects on brain activity during working memory, visual attention and episodic retrieval. *Cerebral Cortex, 14*, 364–375.

Cabeza, R., Grady, C. L., Nyberg, L., McIntosh, A. R., Tulving, E., Kapur, S., et al. (1997). Age-related differences in neural activity during memory encoding and retrieval: A positron emission tomography study. *The Journal of Neuroscience, 17*, 391–400.

Carlson, M. C., Erickson, K. I., Kramer, A. F., Voss, M. W., Bolea, N., Mielke, M., et al. (2009). Evidence for neurocognitive plasticity in at-risk older adults: The Experience Corps Program. *The Journals of Gerontology Series A: Biological Sciences and Medical Sciences, 64*, 1275–1282.

Cherry, B. J., Adamson, M., Duclos, A., & Hellige, J. B. (2005). Aging and individual variation in interhemispheric collaboration and hemispheric asymmetry. *Aging, Neuropsychology, and Cognition, 12*, 316–339.

Colcombe, S., & Kramer, A. F. (2003). Fitness effects on the cognitive function of older adults. *Psychological Science, 14*, 125.

Epstein, R., & Kanwisher, N. (1998). A cortical representation of the local visual environment. *Nature, 392*, 598–601.

Fera, F., Weickert, T. W., Goldberg, T. E., Tessitore, A., Hariri, A., Das, S., et al. (2005). Neural mechanisms underlying probabilistic category learning in normal aging. *The Journal of Neuroscience, 25*, 11340–11348.

Fjell, A. M., Westlye, L. T., Amlien, I., Espeseth, T., Reinvang, I., Raz, N., et al. (2009). High consistency of regional cortical thinning in aging across multiple samples. *Cerebral Cortex, 19*(9), 2001–2012.

Gaser, C., & Schlaug, G. (2003). Brain structures differ between musicians and non-musicians. *Journal of Neuroscience, 23*, 9240.

Grady, C. L., McIntosh, A. R., Rajah, M. N., Beig, S., & Craik, F. I. (1999). The effects of age on the neural correlates of episodic encoding. *Cerebral Cortex, 9*, 805–814.

Gutchess, A. H., Welsh, R. C., Hedden, T., Bangert, A., Minear, M., Liu, L. L., et al. (2005). Aging and the neural correlates of successful picture encoding: Frontal activations compensate for decreased medial-temporal activity. *Journal of Cognitive Neuroscience, 17*, 84–96.

Head, D., Buckner, R. L., Shimony, J. S., Williams, L. E., Akbudak, E., Conturo, T. E., et al. (2004). Differential vulnerability of anterior white matter in nondemented aging with minimal acceleration in dementia of the Alzheimer type: Evidence from diffusion tensor imaging. *Cerebral Cortex, 14*, 410–423.

Hillary, F. G., Genova, H. M., Chiaravalloti, N. D., Rypma, B., & DeLuca, J. (2006). Prefrontal modulation of working memory performance in brain injury and disease. *Human Brain Mapping, 27*, 837–847.

Hultsch, D. F., Hertzog, C., Dixon, R. A., & Small, B. J. (1999). *Memory changes in the aged.* Cambridge: Cambridge University Press.

Jessberger, S., & Gage, F. H. (2008). Stem-cell-associated structural and functional plasticity in the aging hippocampus. *Psychology and Aging, 23*, 684–691.

Kanwisher, N., McDermott, J., & Chun, M. M. (1997). The fusiform face area: A module in human extrastriate cortex specialized for face perception. *The Journal of Neuroscience, 17*, 4302–4311.

Kempermann, G., Gast, D., & Gage, F. H. (2002). Neuroplasticity in old age: Sustained fivefold induction of hippocampal neurogenesis by long-term environmental enrichment. *Annals of Neurology, 52*, 135–143.

Kempermann, G., Kuhn, H. G., & Gage, F. H. (1998). Experience-induced neurogenesis in the senescent dentate gyrus. *The Journal of Neuroscience, 18*, 3206–3212.

Kobayashi, S., Ohashi, Y., & Ando, S. (2002). Effects of enriched environments with different durations and starting times on learning capacity during aging in rats assessed by a refined procedure of the Hebb-Williams maze task. *Journal of Neuroscience Research, 70*, 340–346.

Lodi-Smith, J., Geise, A. C., Roberts, B. W., & Robins, R. W. (2009). Narrating personality change. *Journal of Personality and Social Psychology, 96*, 679–689.

Lodi-Smith, J., & Roberts, B. W. (2007). Social investment and personality: A meta-analysis of the relationship of personality traits to investment in work, family, religion, and volunteerism. *Personality and Social Psychology Review, 11*, 68–86.

Lustig, C., Shah, P., Seidler, R., & Reuter-Lorenz, P. A. (2009). Aging, training, and the brain: A review and future directions. *Neuropsychology Review, 19*, 504–522.

Maguire, E. A., Gadian, D. G., Johnsrude, I. S., Good, C. D., Ashburner, J., Frackowiak, R. S., et al. (2000). Navigation-related structural change in the hippocampi of taxi drivers. *Proceedings of the National Academy of Sciences of the United States of America, 97*, 4398–4403.

McCrae, R. R., & Costa, P. T. (1988). Age, personality, and the spontaneous self-concept. *Journal of Gerontology, 43*, S177–S185.

Morcom, A. M., Good, C. D., Frackowiak, R. S., & Rugg, M. D. (2003). Age effects on the neural correlates of successful memory encoding. *Brain: A Journal of Neurology, 126*, 213–229.

Noice, H., Noice, T., & Staines, G. (2004). A short-term intervention to enhance cognitive and affective functioning in older adults. *Journal of Aging and Health, 16*, 562.

Park, D. C., & Gutchess, A. H. (2005). Long-term memory and aging: A cognitive neuroscience perspective. In R. Cabeza, L. Nyberg, & D. C. Park (Eds.), *Cognitive neuroscience of aging: Linking cognitive and cerebral aging* (pp. 218–245). New York: Oxford Press.

Park, D. C., Lautenschlager, G., Hedden, T., Davidson, N. S., Smith, A. D., & Smith, P. K. (2002). Models of visuospatial and verbal memory across the adult life span. *Psychology and Aging, 17*, 299–320.

Park, D. C., Polk, T. A., Park, R., Minear, M., Savage, A., & Smith, M. R. (2004). Aging reduces neural specialization in ventral visual cortex. *Proceedings of the National Academy of Sciences of the United States of America, 101*, 13091–13095.

Park, D. C., & Reuter-Lorenz, P. A. (2009). The adaptive brain: Aging and neurocognitive scaffolding. *Annual Review of Psychology, 60*, 173–196.

Pereira, A. C., Huddleston, D. E., Brickman, A. M., Sosunov, A. A., Hen, R., McKhann, G. M., et al. (2007). An in vivo correlate of exercise-induced neurogenesis in the adult dentate gyrus. *Proceedings of the National Academy of Sciences, 104*, 5638–5643.

Persson, J., Nyberg, L., Lind, J., Larsson, A., Nilsson, L. G., Ingvar, M., et al. (2006). Structure-function correlates of cognitive decline in aging. *Cerebral Cortex, 16*, 907–915.

Polk, T. A., & Farah, M. J. (1998). The neural development and organization of letter recognition: Evidence from functional neuroimaging, computational modeling, and behavioral studies. *Proceedings of the National Academy of Sciences of the United States of America, 95*, 847–852.

Polk, T. A., Stallcup, M., Aguirre, G. K., Alsop, D. C., D'Esposito, M., Detre, J. A., et al. (2002). Neural specialization for letter recognition. *Journal of Cognitive Neuroscience, 14*, 145–159.

Potkanowicz, E. S. (2011). The role of physical activity in cognitive fitness: a general guide for community programs. In P. E. Hartman-Stein & A. La Rue (Eds.), *Enhancing cognitive fitness in adults: A guide for use and development of community-based programs*. New York: Springer.

Puce, A., Allison, T., Asgari, M., Gore, J. C., & McCarthy, G. (1996). Differential sensitivity of human visual cortex to faces, letter strings, and textures: A functional magnetic resonance imaging study. *The Journal of Neuroscience, 16*, 5205–5215.

Raz, N. (2000). Aging of the brain and its impact on cognitive performance: Integration of structural and functional findings. In F. Craik & T. A. Salthouse (Eds.), *The handbook of aging and cognition* (2nd ed., pp. 1–90). New York: Psychology Press.

Raz, N., & Kennedy, K. M. (2009). A systems approach to age-related change: Neuroanatomical changes, their modifiers, and cognitive correlates. In W. Jagust & M. D'Esposito (Eds.), *Imaging the aging brain* (pp. 151–268). New York: Oxford University Press.

Raz, N., Rodrigue, K. M., Head, D., Kennedy, K. M., & Acker, J. D. (2004). Differential aging of the medial temporal lobe: A study of a five-year change. *Neurology, 62*, 433–438.

Rebok, G. W., Carlson, M. C., Barron, J. S., Frick, K. D., McGill, S., & Parisi, J. M. (2011). Experience Corps®: A civic engagement-based public health intervention in the public schools. In P. E. Hartman-Stein & A. La Rue (Eds.), *Enhancing cognitive fitness in adults: A guide for use and development of community-based programs*. New York: Springer.

Reuter-Lorenz, P. A., & Cappell, K. (2008). Neurocognitive aging and the compensation hypothesis. *Current Directions in Psychological Science, 18*, 177–182.

Reuter-Lorenz, P. A., Jonides, J., Smith, E. E., Hartley, A., Miller, A., Marshuetz, C., et al. (2000). Age differences in the frontal lateralization of verbal and spatial working memory revealed by PET. *Journal of Cognitive Neuroscience, 12*, 174–187.

Reuter-Lorenz, P. A., Marshuetz, C., Jonides, J., Smith, E. E., Hartley, A., & Koeppe, R. (2001). Neurocognitive ageing of storage and executive processes. *The European Journal of Cognitive Psychology, 13*, 257.

Reuter-Lorenz, P. A., Stanczak, L., & Miller, A. (1999). Neural recruitment and cognitive aging: Two hemispheres are better than one especially as you age. *Psychological Science, 10*, 494–500.

Roberts, B. W., Wood, D., & Smith, J. L. (2005). Evaluating Five Factor Theory and social investment perspectives on personality trait development. *Journal of Research in Personality, 39*, 166–184.

Rypma, B., & D'Esposito, M. (2001). Age-related changes in brain–behaviour relationships: Evidence from event-related functional MRI studies. *The European Journal of Cognitive Psychology, 13*, 235.

Salat, D. H., Buckner, R. L., Snyder, A. Z., Greve, D. N., Desikan, R. S., Busa, E., et al. (2004). Thinning of the cerebral cortex in aging. *Cerebral Cortex, 14*, 721–730.

Schooler, C., Mulatu, M. S., & Oates, G. (1999). The continuing effects of substantively complex work on the intellectual functioning of older workers. *Psychology and Aging, 14*, 483–506.

Stine-Morrow, E. A. L., & Parisi, J. M. (2011). A practical guide to senior Odyssey. In P. E. Hartman-Stein & A. La Rue (Eds.), *Enhancing cognitive fitness in adults: A guide for use and development of community-based programs*. New York: Springer.

Wen, W., & Sachdev, P. (2004). The topography of white matter hyperintensities on brain MRI in healthy 60- to 64-year-old individuals. *NeuroImage, 22*, 144–154.

Wilson, R. S., & Bennett, D. A. (2003). Cognitive activity and risk of Alzheimer's disease. *Current Directions in Psychological Science, 12*, 87.

Wilson, R. S., Bennett, D. A., Gilley, D. W., Beckett, L. A., Barnes, L. L., & Evans, D. A. (2000). Premorbid reading activity and patterns of cognitive decline in Alzheimer disease. *Archives of Neurology, 57*, 1718–1723.

Zhou, X., & Merzenich, M. M. (2007). Intensive training in adults refines A1 representations degraded in an early postnatal critical period. *Proceedings of the National Academy of Sciences of the United States of America, 104*, 15935–15940.

Chapter 5
Meditation, Mindfulness, Cognition, and Emotion: Implications for Community-Based Older Adult Programs

Alfred W. Kaszniak

Abstract Meditation practices have become increasingly popular in the United States among both older and younger adults. This chapter summarizes research on the emotional and cognitive benefits of meditation practices that have been derived from Buddhist tradition and from contemporary secular mindfulness meditation. The potential for meditation-based cognitive enhancement for older adults is discussed, and special attention is paid to studies of meditation to reduce stress and improve well-being among caregivers of persons with dementia. Program planners are encouraged to consider several factors, including training requirements and the need for program evaluation, when considering the use of meditation in community-based applications.

Introduction

Over the past few decades, a growing number of people in the Western world have been engaging in the practice of meditation, including many older adults. It has been estimated that within the United States alone there are ten million meditation practitioners (Deurr, 2004). Meditation practice occurs within various spiritual traditions, and increasingly through nonsectarian approaches that have been derived from these traditions and implemented in hospitals, clinics, and other settings (Salmon, Santorelli, & Kabat-Zinn, 1998). Simultaneously, there has been a dramatic increase in behavioral and neuroscientific studies examining cognitive, emotional, and health-relevant changes associated with meditation practice, and in the funding of such studies by the U.S. National Institutes of Health (Shapiro & Carlson, 2009).

A.W. Kaszniak (✉)
Department of Psychology, University of Arizona, 1503 E. University, Tucson, AZ 85721, USA
e-mail: kaszniak@email.arizona.edu

The proliferation of popular books, magazines, and websites concerned with meditation, and the spiritual traditions in which meditation has played a central role also bears witness to the extent of contemporary interest (McMahan, 2008).

The present chapter focuses upon practical application and relevant scientific study of meditation practices that have been derived primarily from Buddhist tradition (particularly the Theravada, Chan or Zen, and Vajarayana schools) and those modern secular forms referred to as mindfulness meditation. This focus reflects four considerations: (1) An increasingly large body of practically relevant meditation research concerns practices from these traditions and training in mindfulness meditation. This research can help to guide decisions regarding whether the teaching of meditation might have potential benefit in community-based programs for older adults; (2) The term meditation has been used to describe a very wide range of practices derived from an equally wide range of spiritual and secular traditions, and even a cursory discussion of each of these practices would be far beyond the scope of a single chapter; (3) It cannot be assumed that all practices labeled as meditation have the same cognitive, affective, behavioral, and brain correlates and consequences, and it is important to be clear about what kind of practice is being considered (for discussion of this point, see Lutz, Dunne, & Davidson, 2007); (4) Another chapter in this volume, Chap. 24 authored by Khalsa and Newberg, provides information regarding meditation practice, Kirtan Kriya, derived from a different tradition, along with the results of some recent research on the correlates and consequences of this practice.

Following the present general introduction, a rationale for considering meditation among the possible choices of strategies for cognitive enrichment of older adults within community-based programs is provided. This rationale draws from traditional and contemporary claims concerning meditation and its role as a path to the alleviation of suffering and enhancement of human flourishing. Then, following a brief description of the general characteristics of the types of meditation practice derived from Buddhist tradition and conducted within mindfulness-based clinical interventions, select examples of those behavioral and neuroscientific empirical studies with the greatest relevance in regard to cognitive and emotional functioning of older adults are selectively reviewed. Following this review, recent mindfulness-based intervention studies with older adult caregivers of persons with dementia are discussed, as an illustration of the potential application of mindfulness meditation instruction in addressing the consequences of a particularly prevalent and challenging situation affecting older adults. The chapter concludes with an exploration of the implications of available research for the planning of community-based programs for older adults, as well as the utilization of established meditation teaching centers and groups.

Why Meditation?

It may initially seem incongruous to include a chapter on meditation within a book concerned with community-based cognitive enrichment programs for older adults. However, an examination of both the role of meditation within Buddhist tradition and scientific studies of meditation practices derived from this tradition illustrates why meditation is relevant. Although there were earlier Indian contemplatives, both Buddhist tradition and historical scholarship (e.g., Lopez, 2001; Rahula, 1974; Sangharakshita, 1993) identify the type of meditation of interest for the present chapter as originating with Siddhartha Guatama, born over 2,500 years ago in what is today southern Nepal. According to tradition, this person now known as the Buddha (meaning awakened one) realized the causes of suffering and a path to its alleviation, while meditating under the Bodhi tree, after several years of ascetic practices. Although the formal practice of meditation is only one component of the path of liberation that he taught (various ethical practices also being very important), it does play a critical role.

The meditation practice refined by the Buddha has been described as a training method for stabilizing and clarifying attention so that it becomes a clear and reliable introspective instrument for observing the processes of one's own mind. Within Buddhist tradition, the untrained mind is seen as dysfunctional, and training is held to be essential for a clear observing of the nature of mind. Through this trained observation, there occurs insight into, and liberation from, delusive views that are held to be the cause of mental suffering. As meditation teacher and Buddhist scholar B. Allan Wallace (2007) states:

> Without such training, it is certainly possible to direct one's attention inward, but the undisciplined mind has been found to succumb very swiftly to attentional excitation, or scattering; when it eventually calms down, it tends to drift into attentional laxity in which vividness is sacrificed. A mind that is alternatively prone to excitation and laxity is a poor instrument for examining anything... (p. 136).

In addition to emphasizing the role of attention in the mental training of meditation, Wallace's statement also hints at the inextricable component of arousal and emotion regulation in this practice. It is therefore not surprising that contemporary scientific studies of meditation have focused so heavily upon measures of attention and emotion, as will be described later in this chapter.

Why would this training of attention in meditation be relevant to an interest in cognitive enhancement for older adults? First, although not without theoretical controversy, there is a body of research evidence supporting the hypothesis that many of the cognitive changes associated with aging may reflect a reduction in that mental resource for the simultaneous processing and storage of information that cognitive psychologists call working memory (Hasher & Zacks, 1988; Salthouse, 1990; Salthouse, Atkinson, & Berish, 2003). Further, this age-related reduction in working memory may be associated with impaired attentional processes, particularly selective attention involving enhancement of task-relevant information and suppression of task-irrelevant information (Gazzaley, Cooney, Rissman, & D'Esposito, 2005). Given that attention training is a key aspect of meditation practice, it has been proposed as a potential intervention for age-related attention changes (e.g., McHugh, Simpson, & Reed, 2010). Second, chronic psychosocial stress has been shown to induce long-lasting, though reversible, impairment in attention-shifting and those prefrontal brain physiological processes that correlate with attention-shifting (Liston, McEwen, & Casey, 2009). Further, even the transient high emotional arousal that accompanies acute stress can disrupt attention control. This likely reflects the dense and reciprocal interconnection of those brain regions associated with attention control, such as the anterior cingulate cortex and the lateral prefrontal cortex, with other areas commonly linked to emotion, such as the amygdala, and to motivation, such as the nucleus accumbens (for review, see Pessoa, 2008).

On average, resilience, sense of coherence, emotion-regulation, and overall hedonic well-being appear to increase, and experienced stress to decrease, in older age (Carstensen, Pasupathi, Mayr, & Nesselroade, 2000; Nilsson, Leppert, Simonsson, & Starrin, 2010; Stone, Schwartz, Broderick, & Deaton, 2010). However, many older adults are in chronically stressful situations, such as caring for a family member with dementia. Caregiving stress is associated with a higher incidence of depression, more physical symptoms, greater medication utilization, and more hospitalizations than for similar aged persons who are not caregivers (Schultz, O'Brien, Bookwala, & Fleissner, 1995). Chronic stress exposure has also been linked to a measure of cellular aging, specifically the shortening of telomeres that are protective caps at the ends of chromosomes (for review, see Epel, Daubenmier, Moskowitz, Folkman, & Blackburn, 2009). As reviewed in the following section of the present chapter, evidence exists linking the attention training of meditation practice to enhanced emotion regulation (for more comprehensive review, see Wadlinger & Isaacowitz, 2010), and this may, in turn, reduce the experience of stress and its negative cognitive and biological consequences, including attention control and possibly even cellular aging (Epel et al., 2009).

What is Meditation?

The word meditation evokes images of someone seated in a quiet room, in a still and erect though relaxed posture, and with downcast or closed eyes. Indeed, setting and posture have traditionally been considered to be critical prerequisites for the relaxed, alert, and quietly attentive practice of meditation, and instructions in this regard can be quite specific. This is captured in the recommendations of the thirteenth century founder of the Soto School of Zen Buddhism in Japan, Eihei Dogen, instructing followers in meditation (referred to as *zazen* within this school):

> Sit straight up without leaning to the right or left and without bending forward or backward. The ears should be in line with the shoulders and the nose in line with the navel. Rest the tongue against the roof of the mouth, with lips and teeth closed… (Tanahashi, 2004, pp. 4–5).

Dogen's specificity also extends to the choice of a quiet place for meditation practice that is free of distractions. Such instructions on posture and setting are designed to facilitate remaining physically still over a period of time (typically 20–30 min or longer in a single meditation period), alert, without excessive discomfort or drowsiness, and with minimal distraction.

Having assumed such a sitting posture within an appropriate setting, what does the meditation practitioner actually do? As already noted, different spiritual traditions in which meditation has been practiced vary considerably in how this question would be answered, and there are different practices even within a particular tradition. Some practices involve maintaining mental focus on a particular visual object, sound, sensation (e.g., of the breath), visual image, or auditory image. Other practices attempt to broaden the field of attention without preferential selection of any focus, and with the gentle releasing of attention whenever it is pulled to any experience in the mental continuum. Despite this variability, it is reasonable to think of all these practices as different approaches to training in the voluntary regulation of attention.

Because there exist many popular misconceptions, it is worth noting some of the things that meditation is not. The Buddhist monk and author Matthieu Ricard (2010) provides the following helpful summary:

> Let me point out right away that meditation is not an attempt to create a blank mind by blocking out thoughts – which is impossible anyway. Nor is it engaging the mind in endless cogitation in an attempt to analyze the past or anticipate the future. Neither is it a simple process of relaxation in which inner conflicts are temporarily suspended in a vague, amorphous state of consciousness (pp. 20–21).

The Sri Lanka vipassana Buddhist meditation teacher Henepola Gunaratana (1993) adds to this list that meditation is not a form of trance or hypnosis, a way of escaping reality or "getting high," a self-centered preoccupation ("navel gazing"), a mysterious practice which cannot be understood, a procedure for becoming a psychic superbeing, something only for saints and holy people, or a panacea that will make all problems go away within a couple of weeks. Although meditation can begin to facilitate some desirable changes fairly quickly, these changes are often rather subtle, and more profound shifts appear to require longer-term regular practice that is incorporated into daily life.

Lutz, Slagter, Dunne, and Davidson (2008) provide a useful conceptual framework for understanding those forms of meditation derived from Buddhist tradition, in their broad distinction between "focused attention" vs. "open monitoring" practices. These terms capture fundamental aspects of meditation practice and help bridge to contemporary psychological constructs. According to Lutz et al., focused attention meditation involves the directing and sustaining of attention on a selected object (e.g., breath sensations), as well as detecting mind wandering (thoughts unrelated to the focus or other distractions). When mind wandering is detected, the practice then involves disengaging attention from the mental narrative, images, or other distractions and gently (without self-judgment regarding the distraction) shifting attention back to the object of focus. Focused attention meditation can thus be considered as a method for developing attention skills, and with repeated daily practice, facilitating effortless and single-pointed concentration. Such practice would also be expected to enhance the ability to monitor one's own attention and more readily notice when mind wandering occurs.

Open monitoring meditation is typically practiced once some stability of attention regulation is achieved via focused attention meditation. Open monitoring involves no explicit focus on objects, maintaining an alert nonreactive and nonjudgmental "openness" or "presence" to whatever arises in conscious experience. It also involves awareness of the conscious field itself in which mental phenomena arise, which contemporary psychology would term meta-awareness. This calm, nonreactive and nonjudgmental awareness includes all sensations, thoughts, images, and feelings, as well as automatic cognitive-emotional interpretations or associations that arise in the stream of experience. However, the practitioner does not "attach to," dwell upon, or get lost in these experiences or associations, but allows them to enter and pass out of mind while remaining alert and aware of the conscious field itself. Thus, open monitoring meditation emphasizes the self-monitoring skill developed initially through focused attention meditation practice, and cultivates moment-to-moment meta-awareness with no strong distinction between selection and deselection of phenomena to which attention is drawn.

The term mindfulness has been used as the English equivalent of the Pali word *sati* in Buddhist tradition, with connotations of awareness, retention, and discernment. The state of mindful awareness thus involves remembering to attend in a discerning way to what is in immediate experience. This sustained, present-centered, precise, nonjudging, and nonreactive awareness includes sensations, thoughts, images, and emotional experiences. Contemporary mindfulness practice derives from vipassana meditation in Buddhist tradition, and involves aspects of both focused attention and open monitoring as described above. In this practice, focused attention rests upon breath sensations, while open monitoring detects, and brings awareness to when the mind has wandered, and repeatedly, without judgment, brings it back to the breath. As skill in this open monitoring aspect develops, the practitioner learns to observe the functioning of his/her own mind in a calm and unattached manner, gaining insight into the causes and conditions of behavior (Gunaratana, 1993). As noted by Shapiro and Carlson (2009), mindfulness meditation involves intention, attention, and attitude: Intention is the personal vision for why meditation is being practiced, which may be dynamic and evolving as practice continues. Although a person might start practicing meditation with the goal of controlling stress symptoms, over time there may be an evolution to goals that include personal growth and spiritual concerns. Attention in mindfulness meditation "…is discerning and nonreactive, sustained and concentrated, so that we can see clearly what is arising in the present moment…" (Shapiro & Carlson, 2009, p. 10). Attitude refers to qualities of openness, acceptance, curiosity, and affection in the attention brought to present experience.

Kabat-Zinn (1994), the originator of mindfulness-based stress reduction (MBSR), defines mindfulness meditation as a process of paying attention on purpose, in the present moment, and nonjudgmentally. MBSR is a well-defined, 8-week, systematic training program in which the central component is mindfulness meditation. MBSR was designed to provide a secular approach to teaching people how to use their resources and abilities to respond more effectively to stress, pain, and illness (Kabat-Zinn, 1990). Within MBSR, up to 35 people meet as a group weekly for 2.5–3 h, and there is also a 6-h silent retreat that occurs on a weekend between the sixth and seventh week of classes. In addition to mindfulness meditation in a sitting posture, other mindfulness practices taught in MBSR include the body scan (a guided bodily awareness exercise in which attention is directed through various body parts, with encouragement to notice whatever arises with kindness and acceptance, and without judgment), walking meditation (with similar attention to the bodily sensations while walking), and mindful, gentle yoga. During the day-long silent retreat, loving-kindness meditation (LKM) is also taught, with feelings of kindness and compassion cultivated, through silently repeated phrases (e.g., "May you be safe. May you be healthy, May you be happy, May you live with ease."), directed toward oneself, loved ones, others in one's life, and eventually to all beings. In each week's group meeting, these practices are taught and practiced, with time allocated for discussion of participants' experience and feedback from instructors. Participants are instructed to practice at home for 45 min, 6 days/week. They are also encouraged to engage in informal mindfulness practices throughout each day, during such activities as eating, washing dishes, talking with others, etc. MBSR has been combined with cognitive-behavioral therapy (CBT), termed mindfulness-based cognitive therapy (MBCT), developed to help prevent relapse in depression (Segal, Williams, & Teasdale, 2002). In addition to a therapist manual (Segal et al.), MBCT is also now taught with a patient self-help book that includes a guided meditation CD (Williams, Teasdale, Segal, & Kabat-Zinn, 2007).

Behavioral and Neuroscientific Research on Meditation

Interest in the relationships between Buddhism and science has existed for over 100 years (Lopez, 2008; McMahan, 2008; Wallace, 2003, 2007). However, for most of this period, interest took the form of speculation concerning whether the introspection methods of Buddhist meditation qualified as a first-person science of the mind, and debate regarding the similarities between Buddhist metaphysics and theory in the physical sciences. For example, Buddhist formulations of the interdependence and insubstantiality (lack of any fundamental essence) of all phenomena were compared to relativity theory and quantum mechanics. Despite this long-standing interest, it is only during the past few decades that a vigorous field of "contemplative science" has taken form. Particularly within the most recent years, this field has been characterized by a rapid growth in publication of rigorous scientific studies of meditators, in which a sophisticated first-person appreciation of the details of meditation practice have been brought together with the third-person experimental technologies of cognitive science, affective science, and neuroscience.

Several writers (e.g., Ricard, 2010; Wallace, 2007) have attributed much of the growth and sophistication of this field to the efforts of the Mind and Life Institute (MLI: http://www.mindandlife.org/). MLI is a nonprofit organization that has sponsored conferences, research institutes, books, and grant programs that foster an integration of first person knowledge from the world's contemplative traditions with methods and findings from contemporary science. The MLI mission is to "… support rigorous, multi-disciplinary scientific investigation of the mind which will lead to the development and dissemination of practices that cultivate the mental qualities of attention, emotional balance, kindness, compassion, confidence and happiness" (http://www.mindandlife.org/about/mission/). By bringing into dialog contemplative practitioners, teachers, scholars, and scientists, MLI has had a significant influence on both the amount and quality of scientific meditation research.

Given the rapid growth and consequent size of the research literature in contemplative science, the present chapter can only briefly highlight select studies that are relevant to the focus on community-based cognitive enhancement programs for older adults. A more extensive and comprehensive review of research on mindfulness-based interventions in medical and mental health settings can be found in the recent volume by Shapiro and Carlson (2009). Their book also contains practical guidance and detail regarding specific mindfulness instructions employed in these interventions. More extensive reviews of the effects of meditation on attention and emotion regulation can be found in Lutz et al. (2008) and in Wadlinger and Isaacowitz (2010).

As already noted, it is of no surprise that behavioral and neuroscientific research on meditation has often focused on the measurement of attention, emotion, or brain structures and processes related to these psychological constructs. Experienced practitioners do appear to be maintaining greater attention focus during their mindfulness meditation practice. For example, Cahn and Polich (2009) studied 16 vipassana practitioners with an average of 20 years of meditation experience, comparing event-related brain electrical potentials to distracting sounds during meditation vs. a period in which they were instructed to let their mind wander. Meditation effects (compared to mind wandering) were found in brain responses to the distracter stimuli, with the reduction in amplitude of the distractor response found to be strongest in participants reporting more hours of daily meditation practice.

There also exist studies demonstrating an association between meditation practice and performance on laboratory attention tasks while participants are not engaged in formal meditation. Slagter et al. (2007) studied 17 participants at the beginning and end of a 3-month vipassana meditation retreat, in comparison to 23 novices who meditated 20 min daily for 1 week prior to each experimental session. The attentional blink task was administered while brain electrical activity was recorded. In the attentional blink task, participants are shown a rapid succession of letters on a computer screen, within which are embedded two numbers. When these two numbers have relatively few letters intervening between them, persons tend to be able to report seeing the first number but fail to report the second, as though their attention had "blinked." Although this attentional blink effect had previously been thought to reflect a general and fixed refractory period characteristic of the brain, Slagter et al. found that the intensive meditation retreat practitioners, compared to novices, showed a smaller attentional blink effect for the testing session after retreat, in contrast to that before. Further, this enhanced detection of the second number was associated with brain electrical response evidence for a reduction in brain-resource allocation to the first number. This is consistent with attention not "clinging" onto the processing of the first number, and therefore interfering less with processing of the second.

In another study, Jha, Krimpinger, and Baime (2007) studied 17 participants in 8-week MBSR training program, 17 meditation-experienced participants in a month-long vipassana retreat, and 17 nonmeditating control participants, administering the Attention Network Test (Fan, McCandliss, Sommer, Raz, & Posner, 2002) before and after the training and retreat. In this test, various warning and spatial cues precede sequential trials in which the participant must identify whether arrows flanking a target arrow are facing in the same or different directions as the target. By decomposing the response times for these trials, separate measures of alerting, orienting, and conflict-monitoring aspects of attention are obtained. Participants in the vipassana retreat group, who were already experienced meditators, were found to be better than those in the other groups in conflict-monitoring measured at baseline, before their retreat experience. Participants in MBSR training program showed a greater improvement than the other groups, from pre- to post-training, in their ability to orient attention to cued regions of the display. The vipassana retreat participation facilitated greater receptive attention skills, which improved alerting to visual cues, in comparison to the other groups. Thus, brief and longer-term meditation training appear to have differential impact on aspects of attention. The briefer MBSR training facilitated improved "top–down" or volitional attention control, while the longer-term and more intensive practice of the vipassana retreat group facilitated enhanced "bottom–up" or stimulus-driven aspects of attention.

In a recently published report from what has been labeled the "Shamatha Project" (MacLean et al., 2010), visual discrimination and sustained attention were assessed before and after an intensive shamatha meditation retreat involving more than 5 h/day of practice for 3 months. Shamatha is a breath-focused meditation training intended to develop attentional stability and equanimity. Participants were randomly assigned either to receive training first (30 participants) or to serve as wait-list controls and receive training during a second 3-month retreat (30 participants). The meditation group, compared to the wait-list group, showed improvements in visual discrimination that were linked to increases in perceptual sensitivity and improved vigilance during sustained visual attention task performance. In another analysis of data collected from this same project (Sahdra et al., 2011), the intensive meditation training, compared to the wait-list group, was also found to result in improved performance in a response inhibition task. This focused attention improvement predicted enhanced adaptive functioning (based on an index derived from a combination of self-report measures of emotion regulation, depression, anxiety, and psychological well-being), underscoring the relationship between attention and emotion regulation in meditation practice.

The relationship between emotional and cognitive effects of mindfulness meditation is also illustrated in a report by Ortner, Kilner, and Zelazo (2007). In one study, Ortner et al. had 28 experienced mindfulness meditation practitioners categorize tones that were presented 1 or 4 s after the onset of pictures with emotional content vs. neutral pictures. Reaction times to tones following the emotional pictures vs. the neutral pictures revealed participants with greater amounts of meditation experience to show less interference from the emotional pictures, as well as greater self-reported mindfulness and psychological well-being in their daily lives. In a second study reported in this paper, 82 participants were randomly assigned either to a 7-week mindfulness meditation training, a relaxation training, or no training (a wait-list control group). Using the same experimental procedure as described for the first study, the mindfulness meditation training group showed greater pre- to post-training reductions in interference from emotionally unpleasant pictures. In combination, these two studies support the conclusion that mindfulness meditation reduces prolonged attentional sensitivity to emotional arousal.

Other studies have also provided evidence consistent with the hypothesis that persistent meditation practice enhances emotion regulation. For example, Nielsen and Kaszniak (2006) employed an experimental procedure in which emotional scenes were exposed for very brief durations, and both preceded and followed by scrambled visual noise, termed visual masking. Masking effectively interrupts the processing of visual information at a very early stage in the brain, and those shown masked pictures are not consciously aware of what they have been shown, even though various bodily reactions to the images can be recorded. Nielsen and Kaszniak found long-term Zen and vipassana meditators with greater than 10 years of practice experience, in comparison with matched nonmeditating controls, to report higher emotional clarity in an extensive self-report inventory. Those reporting higher emotional clarity showed lower physiological (skin-conductance response) and self-reported arousal, and greater subtle positive facial expression (by facial muscle electromyography) in response to very briefly presented and masked emotional pictures. Thus, long-term meditation appears associated with enhanced regulation of emotion very early in the emotion response process.

Wadlinger and Isaacowitz (2010) have argued that while the attention training of mindfulness meditation practice may have a greater impact on the regulation of negative emotion, LKM may be more likely to increase positive emotion by bringing attention and generating positive feelings to the silently repeated phrases. In a relevant study, Fredrickson, Cohn, Coffey, Pek, and Finkel (2008) randomly assigned 139 working adults to a 7-week LKM training or a wait-list group. Using statistical procedures that allow for causal inference from a time series of correlational data, it was found that, compared to the wait-list controls, LKM practice led to greater increases over time in daily experiences of positive emotions, which in turn led to increases in a wide range of personal resources (e.g., increased mindfulness, sense of purpose in life, social support, and decreased illness symptoms). In turn, these increments in personal resources predicted increased life satisfaction and reduced depressive symptoms. Surprisingly, another study found that even a few minutes of LKM practice, compared to a closely matched control group, resulted in an increase in the experience of positive social emotions and sense of social connectedness with strangers (Hutcherson, Seppala, & Gross, 2008).

These studies on the relationships between meditation, attention, and emotion provide encouragement for the consideration of meditation training for older adults, with the expectation that they might consequently experience enhanced cognitive functioning through improved attention, emotion regulation, and emotional positivity. There are now studies in the literature suggesting that meditation practice may also impact the body's immune system and some of the biological correlates of aging.

In a study of 25 work environment participants in an 8-week MBSR training, compared to 16 wait-list controls, Davidson et al. (2003) found that meditators showed a greater decrease following training in self-reported trait anxiety, in a brain electrical measure of left anterior brain activation (previously shown to be associated with positive emotion), and increases in antibody titers to an influenza vaccine. This enhanced immune response was correlated with the measure of left frontal brain activation.

In analyses of data collected from the Shamatha Project described above, Jacobs et al. (2011), the 3-month meditation training group, in comparison to the wait-list group, showed higher levels of telomerase activity in peripheral blood mononuclear cells at the end of the intensive retreat. Telomerase is known to repair and lengthen telomeres, which, as described above, are DNA-protein complexes at the end of chromosomes that predict cell viability. As telomeres become shorter, cells age and die more quickly. It has also been found that telomere length and telomerase activity decrease with chronic psychological distress (see Epel et al., 2009). Statistical analyses from the Shamatha Project data also suggested that increases in perceived control and decreases in negative emotional experiences contributed to the increase in telomerase activity.

Recent research also suggests that meditation practice may have an effect on the actual structure of the brain. In the first study investigating such anatomical neuroplasticity, Lazar et al. (2005) found mindfulness meditators to show significantly greater brain cortical thickness (by magnetic resonance imaging) than nonmeditators in the right anterior insula, the left superior temporal gyrus, and the right middle and superior frontal sulci. As Lazar et al. describe, these are areas that previous research had associated with interoception (internal bodily awareness), somatosensory processing, and attention regulation. In the Lazar et al. and subsequent studies (for review, see Grant, Courtemanche, Duncan, & Rainville, 2010), the amount of meditation practice of participants has been significantly correlated with measures of cortical thickness or volume. There is also recent evidence that increased cortical thickness in pain-processing brain areas is related to lower pain sensitivity in meditators (Grant et al., 2010).

Of particular interest, regarding this chapter's focus on implications for older adults, is a study by Pagnoni and Cekic (2007). In this study, regular practitioners of Zen meditation (which includes focused attention and open monitoring practice aspects) did not show a significant correlation between age and performance on a sustained attention task, or between age and brain gray matter volume. Matched nonmeditator control participants did show the typical age-related decline in both attention and the brain volume measures. The authors suggest that the regular practice of meditation may thus have neuroprotective effects and reduce the cognitive decline associated with aging.

Mindfulness-Based Programs for Older Caregivers of Persons with Dementia

According to published estimates summarized by the Alzheimer's Association (2010), 5.3 million Americans of all ages (5.1 million of those over age 65) have Alzheimer's disease, the most frequent cause of the age-associated syndrome of progressive cognitive deterioration known as dementia. By the year 2030, it is predicted that 7.7 million Americans will be diagnosed with Alzheimer's disease, and by the year 2050, 11–16 million. Unpaid caregivers of persons with Alzheimer's disease are primarily family members, and caregiving can be highly stressful. More than half of caregivers are of age 50 and older. Over 40% of caregivers of persons with dementia rate the emotional stress of caregiving as high or very high, and one third of these caregivers have symptoms of depression. Caregivers are more likely than noncaregivers to have reduced immune function and slow wound healing, new hypertension, new heart disease, and a higher mortality rate (Alzheimer's Association). Contributors to caregiver distress include behavior problems, such as agitation (Duke & Kaszniak, 2000), impairment in the comprehension and facial expression of emotion (Allender & Kaszniak, 1989; Burton & Kaszniak, 2006), and impaired awareness of deficits (Kaszniak & Edmonds, 2010) manifest by the person with dementia for whom they are providing care.

Various psychosocial interventions intended to reduce the consequences of caregiver stress have, overall, had only modest impact (Brodaty, Green, & Koschera, 2003). Over recent years, evidence-based caregiver education and skills-training approaches have been developed (Gallagher-Thompson & Coon, 2007), and made more widely available. Finding ways to enhance their use of active coping strategies, such as caregiving skill development, is one of the challenges in developing interventions to help caregivers cope with their stress. Caregivers tend to rely upon characteristic individual coping strategies that remain invariant even as their family member's dementia progresses, and passive coping strategies are associated with greater caregiver depression (Powers, Gallagher-Thompson, & Kraemer, 2002). Engaging caregivers in skillful ways to help reduce some of the troublesome emotional aspects of their family member's dementia may also help reduce their own emotional distress. One example of this comes from a randomized controlled clinical trial of two active caregiver-administered behavioral interventions, one emphasizing patient-pleasant events and the other emphasizing caregiver problem-solving (Teri, Logsdon, Uomoto, & McCurry, 1997). Dyads of caregivers and their person with dementia were randomly assigned to one of these two interventions, to a typical care control group, or to a wait-list control group. The persons with dementia in both active behavioral intervention conditions showed significant improvements in depression symptoms and in the number meeting clinical diagnostic criteria for depression, compared with other two conditions. Gains were maintained at a 6-month follow-up. Interestingly, the caregivers in the active intervention groups also showed a significantly greater improvement in their depression symptoms than did those in the typical care or wait-list groups.

Of course, not all persons providing care for a family member with dementia experience severe emotional distress. It has been reported that higher levels of interdependence between spouse-caregiver dyads, and more time spent with the care receipt, are the strongest predictors of positive affect in the caregivers (Poulin et al., 2010). In describing her experience in caring for her husband who had Alzheimer's disease, Olivia Hoblitzelle (2008) exemplifies this interdependence and positive affect as she writes:

> We had gone through an initiation, as great an initiation as life can offer two people… As we were held in the fire of transformation, we were burned and burnished until the gold of love shone unobstructed between us. That was, ultimately, the blessing and gift of the journey (pp. 281–282).

It is of interest to note that both Hoblitzelle and her husband were long-term meditation practitioners and teachers. Based on several recent studies, it has been hypothesized that watching the care recipient's suffering may be what is the most stressful and health-deleterious aspect of caregiving, but that caregiver compassion, perhaps leading to greater amounts of care provided, may be health-beneficial (Schulz et al., 2007). This begs the question of how the established emotional and health benefits of engaging in compassionate action/altruism (Post, 2007) can be enhanced for caregivers, while minimizing their empathic distress.

One possibility is raised by studies of perspective taking when observing another's distress. Self-focused perspective-taking arouses more intense experience of empathic distress, perhaps because self-focused perspective-taking is more likely to evoke associations with painful events in one's own past (Batson, Early, & Salvarani, 1997). Researchers have also found that those who show greater physiological emotional response to others' distress tend to be more self-focused and less empathic (for review, see Eisenberg, 2002). Meditation practice within the Buddhist tradition has been claimed (e.g., Loy, 2008) to deconstruct the illusion of self, by directly experiencing its emptiness, that is, as without having a permanent and independent nature or essence, arising from an ever-changing flow of concepts, beliefs, images, and sensations. There is recent evidence from functional neuroimaging research (Pagnoni, Cekic, & Guo, 2008) showing that experienced Zen meditators, compared to meditation-naive persons, following stimulation with meaningful words, exhibit a faster return to baseline in brain "default network" activity associated with conceptual thought and sense of self. This more rapid "letting go" of self-relevant processing could arguably be expected to result in less self-focused perspective taking when seeing another who is suffering. These considerations, as well as those based upon studies that have evaluated emotion response and regulation in meditators, reviewed above, suggest the possibility that meditation training could be a useful adjunct in efforts to decrease the distress of those providing care for persons with dementia.

Among those questions that might be raised about teaching meditation to caregivers is whether the burden of their day-to-day responsibilities and resultant stress might simply be too severe to permit the kind of practice that would be required. McBee (2003) reported on a feasibility study of eight caregivers, aged 60–85 years, who participated in a 10-week series of MBSR classes in which they were taught mindfulness seated meditation, walking meditation, and the mindful body scan. These caregivers were able to complete the program and reported decreased stress and somatic complaints after the training. Although the lack of any control comparison group limits any conclusions regarding efficacy, this study does support the feasibility of MBSR for older adult caregivers.

In a more recent and controlled study by Oken et al. (2010), caregivers of persons with dementia (age 45–85) completed a trial in which they were randomized either into one of two 7-week active interventions – a mindfulness training based on MBSR and MBCT or the Powerful Tools for Caregivers education program (Services, 2006), or a respite-only control condition. Each of the two active intervention programs was taught for 90-min sessions each week, with at-home implementation of practices or knowledge learned. There was a high rate of caregiver completion of the study, and adherence (assessed by class attendance and a biweekly diary logbook) to the intervention programs, and comparable expectancy of improvement from, and perceived credibility of, the two active interventions. Caregivers in both of the active interventions showed greater improvement than the respite-only group on a caregiver stress self-report measure, a caregiver self-efficacy measure, and a performance-based measure of attention (Attention Network Test; Fan et al., 2002). However, there were no significant intervention effects observed on measures of mood, fatigue, mindfulness, sleep self-report, salivary cortisol (an endocrine measure sensitive to stress), and cytokines (an immune system marker).

In an ongoing study within my own laboratory (O'Donnell, Kaszniak, & Menchola, 2010), we are testing the efficacy of MBSR, compared to another active intervention, for older adult family caregivers of persons with dementia. The study design employs a randomized assignment to an 8-week Mindfulness Based Stress Reduction (MBSR) program or a Progressive Muscle Relaxation/Autogenic Imagery (PMR) program, matched for length of weekly instruction sessions (2.5 h), length of daily home practice assignments (45–60 min/day, 6 days/week), and 1 day of a silent 7-h retreat (for MBSR) or day of relaxation practice (for PMR) at week 6. Measures are taken at baseline, post-training, and at 8-weeks, 6 months, and 1-year post-training. Of the 26 caregivers (mostly spouses) who initially volunteered for the study, 24 completed the pre and postintervention data collection. Their mean age was 71 years, the mean age of their care-recipient was 78 years, and the mean length of their care-recipient's illness was nearly 8 years. Primary and secondary outcome measures include several perceived stress, perceived caregiving burden, sleep quality, and mindfulness inventories. Intervention program credibility, expectancy for benefit, compliance (by diary records of home practice), and intervention program veracity (ratings based on taped sessions from experts in the respective training approaches) were also assessed. Biological outcome measures included resting and stress-challenge blood pressure, heart rate, and salivary cortisol; weight and height for body mass index; and daily saliva samples at awakening, 30 min after awake, 4:00 p.m., and 9:00 p.m., for assays of cortisol and alpha amylase (endocrine measures associated with stress). Although all epochs of data collection have not yet been completed, and analyses of several outcome measures are ongoing, results to date show a significantly greater pre to postintervention reduction in perceived stress and depression for the MBSR compared to the PMR group. However, both groups showed a reduction in perceived caregiving burden, daily peak cortisol measures at 30 min after awakening and in systolic blood pressure both prior to and after the induced stress of recalling a difficult caregiving episode.

In summary, recent studies, although quite preliminary, support the feasibility, compliance with, and potential impact of mindfulness-based approaches for reducing caregiver distress, depression symptoms, and biological indices of stress, as well as for improving attention task performance. However, continuing research will be necessary to determine relative efficacy in comparison to other available approaches (e.g., relaxation training, caregiver education programs) and determine whether changes seen following training are maintained over time.

Implications for Planning Community-Based Programs for Older Adults

When considering whether available research encourages the consideration of implementing a meditation program within a community based setting, a few words of caution are appropriate. Despite the rapid growth of research in contemplative science, the field remains in an infant stage of development. There exist many studies providing documentation that amount of meditation practice is correlated with various cognitive, emotional, and brain measures obtained from self-selected practitioners. In assessing such research evidence, it is important to resist the automatic inference that meditation has directly caused changes in the measures of interest. Correlation is not causation, and other possibilities should be considered. For example, it could be that preexisting differences in the measures of interest influence whether and for how long one continues in meditation practice. It could also be the case that meditation practice is correlated with some other unmeasured variable that itself mediates the relationship between meditation and what was measured. Further, there exist few direct comparisons of different meditation practices to help guide decisions regarding what specific practice might be most efficacious for what desired outcome.

From a practical perspective, these considerations suggest that available research results may best be considered as conditional encouragement for teaching of meditation within community settings. Questions to consider include whether the encouraging studies are of solid design, have employed measures of relevance to the community setting in which the program would be instantiated, and recruited participants of comparable demographic characteristics to those in the setting. In addition, it is worth asking whether a community setting that is considering a meditation program has the resources to mount its own evaluation of the program being considered. Many variables can affect the success of such programs, and feedback from outcome evaluation within a particular setting plays an important role.

Caution is also necessary in interpreting published research on the practical applications of mindfulness-based programs. The quality of outcome research on mindfulness-based interventions for medical conditions (for review, see Ospina et al., 2008) and for mental health problems (for review, see Rubia, 2009) has improved over time. For example, there has been an increase in the number of clinical trials wherein persons are randomly assigned to either the mindfulness intervention or a control condition such as wait-list or some other active intervention.

However, many trials have been of poor methodological quality, and there remains the need for future trials to increase the rigor of research design, execution, analysis and reporting of results. Also, as is true for basic contemplative science research concerning relations between meditation practice and various behavioral or biological measures, only a few trials of mindfulness-based interventions have examined the relative efficacy of different types of interventions directly compared to one another (Ospina et al., 2008). Again, it is worth considering whether it is feasible to conduct an evaluation of any mindfulness-based intervention program within the community setting in which it is implemented.

Another consideration concerns the qualifications of those who teach meditation and mindfulness-based intervention programs within community settings. In regard to teachers within Buddhist traditions, it is encouraging that there have been recent efforts toward establishing organizations such as the American Zen Teachers Association http://www.americanzenteachers.org/. These organizations strive to enhance the quality of teachers by fostering dialog among teachers and providing access to information about meditation practice and teaching. However, teachers within particular spiritual traditions are generally authorized to teach individually by their own teacher, and there does not exist anything comparable to national or regional licensing or certification. Those who are considering meditation training within a particular spiritual tradition would therefore be well advised to consult available guidance for finding a teacher and evaluating their qualifications (e.g., http://buddhism.about.com/od/findingatempleandsangha/a/teacherfine.htm).

The Center for Mindfulness in Medicine, Healthcare, and Society at the University of Massachusetts Medical School provides a training program and certifies MBSR instructors (http://www.umassmed.edu/cfm/oasis/index.aspx). Qualifications that are considered in evaluating applicants for this training are personal psychological development, meditation training and regular practice, including silent retreat attendance, yoga or other bodywork training, and professional training and graduate work in a related field (e.g., psychology, education, medicine, etc.). At this point, there exists little research on the relationship between meditation teacher characteristics, qualifications, and outcome of meditation training. Until there is such research available to guide selection of a teacher, it would appear wise to consult all available resources as well as those who have been students of a particular teacher. It should not be assumed that meditation is a practice entirely without risk. Any training or intervention capable of effecting significant positive personal change is also capable of harm if taught incorrectly or by someone unskilled or with motivations that do not make the student's well-being their first priority.

On balance, the rationale for the relevance of meditation as an approach to cognitive enhancement for older adults, and the relevant research reviewed in this chapter, encourage the consideration of including meditation within community-based programs. However, there are limitations to research that has been published to date, and community program planners will need to exercise judgment, wisdom, and, wherever possible, their own on-site evaluation of meditation programs that are initiated within their settings. Mindfulness-based approaches hold promise for enhancing the cognitive and emotional functioning of older adults, including those in highly stressful ongoing situations. Future research, employing the most careful and rigorous methods, will be necessary to determine the extent to which this promise may be fulfilled.

References

Allender, J. A., & Kaszniak, A. W. (1989). Processing of emotional cues in patients with dementia of the Alzheimer type. *International Journal of Neuroscience, 46*, 147–155.

Alzheimer's Association. (2010). Alzheimer's disease facts and figures. *Alzheimer's & Dementia, 6*, 158–194.

Batson, C. D., Early, S., & Salvarani, G. (1997). Perspective taking: Imagining how another feels versus imagining how you would feel. *Personality and Social Psychology Bulletin, 23*, 751–758.

Brodaty, H., Green, A., & Koschera, A. (2003). Meta-analysis of psychosocial interventions for caregivers of people with dementia. *Journal of the American Geriatric Society, 51*, 657–664.

Burton, K., & Kaszniak, A. W. (2006). Emotional experience and facial muscle activity in Alzheimer's disease. *Aging, Neuropsychology, and Cognition, 13*, 636–651.

Cahn, B. R., & Polich, J. (2009). Meditation (Vipassana) and the P3a event-related brain potential. *International Journal of Psychophysiology, 72*, 51–60.

Carstensen, L. L., Pasupathi, M., Mayr, U., & Nesselroade, J. R. (2000). Emotional experience in everyday life across the adult life span. *Journal of Personality and Social Psychology, 79*, 644–655.

Davidson, R., Kabat-Zinn, J., Schumacher, J., Rosenkrantz, M., Muller, D., Santorelli, S. F., et al. (2003). Alterations in brain and immune function produced by mindfulness meditation. *Psychosomatic Medicine, 65*, 564–570.

Deurr, M. A. (2004). *Powerful silence: The role of meditation and other contemplative practices in American life and work*. Northampton: Center for Contemplative Mind in society.

Duke, L. M., & Kaszniak, A. W. (2000). Executive control functions in degenerative dementias: A comparative review. *Neuropsychology Review, 10*, 75–99.

Eisenberg, N. (2002). Empathy-related emotional responses, altruism, and their socialization. In R. J. Davidson & A. Harrington (Eds.), *Visions of compassion* (pp. 131–164). Oxford: Oxford University Press.

Epel, E., Daubenmier, J., Moskowitz, J. T., Folkman, S., & Blackburn, E. (2009). Can meditation slow rate of cellular aging? Cognitive stress, mindfulness, and telomeres. *Annals of the New York Academy of Science, 1172*, 34–53.

Fan, J., McCandliss, B., Sommer, T., Raz, A., & Posner, M. (2002). Testing the efficiency and independence of attentional networks. *Journal of Cognitive Neuroscience, 143*, 340–347.

Fredrickson, B. L., Cohn, M. A., Coffey, K. A., Pek, J., & Finkel, S. M. (2008). Open hearts build lives: Positive emotions, induced through loving-kindness meditation, build consequential personal resources. *Journal of Personality and Social Psychology, 5*, 1045–1062.

Gallagher-Thompson, D., & Coon, D. W. (2007). Evidence-based treatments to reduce psychological distress in family caregivers of older adults. *Psychology & Aging, 22*, 37–51.

Gazzaley, A., Cooney, J. W., Rissman, J., & D'Esposito, M. (2005). Top-down suppression deficit underlies working memory impairment in normal aging. *Nature Neuroscience, 8*, 1298–1300.

Grant, J. A., Courtemanche, J., Duncan, G. H., & Rainville, P. (2010). Cortical thickness and pain sensitivity in Zen meditators. *Emotion, 10*, 43–53.

Gunaratana, H. (1993). *Mindfulness in plain English*. Boston: Wisdom Publications.

Hasher, L., & Zacks, R. T. (1988). Working memory, comprehension, and aging: A review and new view. In G. H. Bower (Ed.), *The psychology of learning and motivation* (Vol. 22, pp. 193–225). New York: Academic Press.

Hoblitzelle, O. A. (2008). *The majesty of your loving: A couple's journey through Alzheimer's*. Cambridge: Green Mountain Books.

Hutcherson, C. A., Seppala, E. M., & Gross, J. J. (2008). Loving-kindness meditation increases social connectedness. *Emotion, 8*, 720–724.

Jacobs, T. L., Epel, E. S., Lin, J., Blackburn, E. H., Wolkowitz, O. M., Bridwell, D. A., et al. (2011). Intensive meditation training, immune cell telomerase activity, and psychological mediators. *Psychoneuroendocrinology, 36*, 664–681.

Jha, A., Krimpinger, J., & Baime, M. J. (2007). Mindfulness training modifies subsystems of attention. *Cognitive, Affective, and Behavioral Neuroscience, 7*, 109–119.

Kabat-Zinn, J. (1990). *Full catastrophe living: Using the wisdom of your body and mind to face stress, pain and illness*. New York: Delacorte.

Kabat-Zinn, J. (1994). *Wherever you go, there you are: Mindfulness meditation in everyday life*. New York: Hyperion.

Kaszniak, A. W., & Edmonds, E. (2010). Anosognosia and Alzheimer's disease: Behavioral studies. In G. Prigatano (Ed.), *The study of anosognosia* (pp. 189–228). New York: Oxford University Press.

Lazar, S. W., Kerr, C. E., Wasserman, R. H., Gray, J. R., Greve, D. N., Treadway, M. T., et al. (2005). Meditation experience is associated with increased cortical thickness. *Neuroreport, 16*, 1893–1897.

Liston, C., McEwen, B. S., & Casey, B. J. (2009). Psychosocial stress reversibly disrupts prefrontal processing and attentional control. *Proceedings of the National Academy of Sciences, U.S.A, 106*, 912–917.

Lopez, D. S. (2001). *The story of Buddhism: A concise guide to its history and teachings*. San Francisco: Harper.

Lopez, D. S. (2008). *Buddhism and science: A guide for the perplexed*. Chicago: University of Chicago Press.

Loy, D. (2008). *Money, sex, war, karma: Notes for a Buddhist revolution*. Boston: Wisdom Publications.

Lutz, A., Dunne, J., & Davidson, R. (2007). Meditation and the neuroscience of consciousness. In P. Zelazo, M. Moscovitch, & E. Thompson (Eds.), *The Cambridge handbook of consciousness* (pp. 497–549). Cambridge: Cambridge University Press.

Lutz, A., Slagter, H. A., Dunne, J. D., & Davidson, R. J. (2008). Attention regulation and monitoring in meditation. *Trends in Cognitive Sciences, 12*, 163–169.

MacLean, K. A., Ferrer, E., Aichele, S. R., Bridwell, D. A., Zanesco, A. P., Jacobs, T. L., et al. (2010). Intensive meditation training improves perceptual discrimination and sustained attention. *Psychological Science, 21*, 829–839.

McBee, L. (2003). Mindfulness practice with the frail elderly and their caregivers. *Topics in Geriatric Rehabilitation, 19*, 257–264.

McHugh, L., Simpson, A., & Reed, P. (2010). Mindfulness as a potential intervention for stimulus over-selectivity in older adults. *Research in Developmental Disabilities, 31*, 178–184.

McMahan, D. L. (2008). *The making of Buddhist modernism*. New York: Oxford University Press.

Nielsen, L., & Kaszniak, A. W. (2006). Awareness of subtle emotional feelings: A comparison of long-term meditators and non-meditators. *Emotion, 6*, 392–405.

Nilsson, K. W., Leppert, J., Simonsson, B., & Starrin, B. (2010). Sense of coherence and psychological well-being: Improvement with age. *Journal of Epidemiology and Community Health, 64*, 347–352.

O'Donnell, R., Kaszniak, A. W., & Menchola, M. (2010). *Evaluating mindfulness-based stress reduction for older family caregivers of persons with neurocognitive disorders*. Poster presented at the annual Mind and Life Summer Research Institute, Garrison, NY.

Oken, B. S., Fonareva, I., Haas, M., Wahbeh, H., Lane, J. B., Zajdel, D., et al. (2010). Pilot controlled trial of mindfulness meditation and education for dementia caregivers. *The Journal of Alternative and Complementary Medicine, 16*, 1031–1038.

Ortner, C. N. M., Kilner, S. J., & Zelazo, P. D. (2007). Mindfulness meditation and reduced emotional interference on a cognitive task. *Motivation and Emotion, 31*, 271–283.

Ospina, M. B., Bond, K., Karkhaneh, M., Buscemi, N., Dryden, D. M., Barnes, V., et al. (2008). Clinical trials of meditation practices in health care: Characteristics and quality. *The Journal of Alternative and Complementary Medicine, 14*, 1199–1213.

Pagnoni, G., & Cekic, M. (2007). Age effects on gray matter volume and attentional performance in Zen meditation. *Neurobiology of Aging, 28*, 1623–1627.

Pagnoni, G., Cekic, M., & Guo, Y. (2008). "Thinking about not-thinking": Neural correlates of conceptual processing during Zen meditation. *PLoS One, 3*(9), e3083. doi:10.1371/journal_pone.00-3083.

Pessoa, L. (2008). On the relationship between emotion and cognition. *Nature Reviews Neuroscience, 9*, 148–158.

Post, S. (Ed.). (2007). *Altruism and health: Perspectives from empirical research*. New York: Oxford University Press.

Poulin, M., Brown, S., Ubel, P. A., Smith, D., Jankovic, A., & Langa, K. (2010). Does a helping hand mean a heavy heart? Helping behavior and well-being among spouse caregivers. *Psychology and Aging, 25*, 108–117.

Powers, D. V., Gallagher-Thompson, D., & Kraemer, H. C. (2002). Coping and depression in Alzheimer's caregivers: Longitudinal evidence of stability. *Journal of Gerontology: Psychological Sciences, 57B*, P205–P211.

Rahula, W. (1974). *What the Buddha taught* (2nd ed.). New York: Grove Weidenfeld.

Ricard, M. (2010). *Why meditate?* Carlsbad: Hay House.

Rubia, K. (2009). The neurobiology of meditation and its clinical effectiveness in psychiatric disorders. *Biological Psychology, 82*, 1–11.

Sahdra, B. K., MacLean, K. A., Ferrer, E., Shaver, P. R., Rosenberg, E. L., Jacobs, T. L., et al. (2011). Enhanced inhibition during meditation training predicts improvement in self-reported adaptive social-emotional functioning. *Emotion, 11*, 299–312.

Salmon, P. G., Santorelli, S. F., & Kabat-Zinn, J. (1998). Intervention elements promoting adherence in mindfulness-based stress reduction programs in the clinical behavioral medicine setting. In S. A. Shumaker, E. B. Schron, & J. K. Okene (Eds.), *The handbook of health behavior change* (2nd ed., pp. 239–268). New York: Springer.

Salthouse, T. A. (1990). Working memory as a processing resource in cognitive aging. *Developmental Review, 10*, 101–124.

Salthouse, T. A., Atkinson, T. M., & Berish, D. E. (2003). Executive functioning as a potential mediator of age-related cognitive decline in normal adults. *Journal of Experimental Psychology General, 132*, 566–594.

Sangharakshita. (1993). *A survey of Buddhism: Its doctrines and methods through the ages* (7th ed.). Glasgow: Windhorse Publications.

Schultz, R., O'Brien, A., Bookwala, J., & Fleissner, K. (1995). Psychiatric and physical morbidity effects of dementia caregiving: Prevalence, correlates, and causes. *Gerontologist, 35*, 771–791.

Schulz, R., Hebert, R. S., Dew, M. A., Brown, S. L., Scheier, M. F., Beach, S. R., et al. (2007). Patient suffering and caregiver compassion: New opportunities for research, practice, and policy. *The Gerontologist, 47*, 4–13.

Segal, Z. V., Williams, M. G., & Teasdale, J. D. (2002). *Mindfulness-based cognitive therapy for depression: A new approach to preventing relapse*. New York: Guilford Press.

Services, L.C. (2006). *The caregiver handbook: Powerful tools for caregivers*. Portland: Legacy Health Systems.

Shapiro, S. L., & Carlson, L. E. (2009). *The art and science of mindfulness: Integrating mindfulness into psychology and the helping professions*. Washington: American Psychological Association.

Slagter, H. A., Lutz, A., Greischar, L. L., Francis, A., Nieuwenhuis, S., Davis, J. M., et al. (2007). Mental training affects distribution of limited brain resources. *PLoS Biology, 5*(6), e138. doi:10.1317/journal.pbio.0050138.

Stone, A. A., Schwartz, J. E., Broderick, J. E., & Deaton, A. (2010). A snapshot of the age distribution of psychological well-being in the United States. *Proceedings of the National Academy of Sciences, U.S.A, 107*, 16489–16493.

Tanahashi, K. (Ed.). (2004). *Beyond thinking: A guide to Zen meditation – Zen master Dogen.* Boston: Shambhala Press.

Teri, L., Logsdon, R. G., Uomoto, J., & McCurry, S. M. (1997). Behavioral treatment of depression in dementia patients: A controlled clinical trial. *Journals of Gerontology: Psychological Sciences, 52B*, P159–P166.

Wadlinger, H. A., & Isaacowitz, D. M. (2010). Fixing our focus: Training attention to regulate emotion. *Personality and Social Psychology Review.* Retrieved April 30, 2010, doi:10.1177/1088868310365565.

Wallace, B. A. (Ed.). (2003). *Buddhism and science: Breaking new ground.* New York: Columbia University Press.

Wallace, B. A. (2007). *Contemplative science: Where Buddhism and neuroscience converge.* New York: Columbia University Press.

Williams, J. M., Teasdale, J. D., Segal, Z., & Kabat-Zinn, J. (2007). *The mindful way through depression: Freeing yourself from chronic unhappiness.* New York: Guilford Press.

Part II
Community-Based Programs to Enhance and Sustain Healthy Aging

Chapter 6
Keys to a Sharp Mind: Providing Choice and Quality Programming in a Retirement Community

Jeanette S. Biermann and Paula E. Hartman-Stein

Abstract Keys to a Sharp Mind (K2SM) was a pilot project designed to change the way intellectual programming was produced for residents of the independent living section of a continuing care retirement community (CCRC). The intention was to apply current research in cognitive science that suggests age-related mental decline may be delayed or at least slowed by engaging in cognitively stimulating activities within a social context. The program was built on the idea that independent living residents will have greater motivation to participate in lifelong learning if they are given the opportunity to create and choose course offerings. In this chapter we delineate defining principles and program evaluation methodology along with lessons learned and the impact the project had on participants and subsequent programming at the facility. A list of the programs and suggestions for future implementations in similar retirement communities are provided.

Introduction

Mrs. Jones, a 77-year-old widow who was a retired consultant to the Library of Congress, thoroughly enjoyed participating in a lifelong learning program that had courses on a wide variety of topics such as the frescoes of the Sistine Chapel, the operation of the U.S. Supreme Court, creative writing, and techniques to enhance memory. Her active participation went beyond note taking and class discussions. She also had a role in choosing the courses and the instructors. An added benefit was that she was able to participate without leaving the retirement center.

J.S. Biermann (✉)
Center for Healthy Aging, 265 W. Main Street, Suite 102, Kent, OH 44240, USA

Counseling Psychology, University of Akron, Akron, OH, USA
e-mail: jsb37@zips.uakron.edu

However, when she had first moved into the continuing care retirement community (CCRC) 2 years earlier, she had been disappointed with the programs that were then being offered to the residents in the independent living (IL) section. "They have very good programs for the residents with dementia, but few intellectually stimulating programs for those of us who still have good memory capacity. We need to be challenged too," she had said to the second author of this chapter (G. Jones, personal communication, August 25, 2005).

Dr. Jeanette Reuter, professor emeritus from Kent State University, resided in the same retirement community as Mrs. Jones and had observed the same void in programming for older adults who wanted intellectually challenging courses. An active and outspoken member of the retirement center's Wellness Committee, Dr. Reuter said, "The decisions about which opportunities are offered to us are made by staff who are decades younger than we are. What do they know about what we'd like to do with our time?" (J.M. Reuter, personal communication, December 17, 2005).

Encouraged by Dr. Reuter to change the intellectual offerings of the retirement community, the second author of this chapter approached the administration with a proposal for a program to evaluate the impact of a 3-year series of courses, Keys to a Sharp Mind (K2SM), which the residents would help to design and which would be professionally evaluated for its impact. The administration was receptive, identified a potential funding source, and offered in-kind staff support of the project. The second author of this chapter wrote the grant which a local private foundation funded for $90,000 over 3 years.

Mrs. Jones and other residents seeking similar challenges and choices in their intellectual lives embraced the project. To these residents and others like them, offerings of bingo, bridge, and cruise ship theme nights represent the dinosaur days of retirement activities. Administrators are becoming aware of expanded expectations of incoming retirees. Growing numbers of healthier older adults choose CCRCs based on their offerings of entertainment, exercise as well as intellectually challenging programs.

Activity directors of many of the institutions where older adults live out their lives are responsible for designing quality programs to meet the needs of the residents and have the additional task of attracting residents to participate. This is true at all levels of care, from IL, to assisted living, to dementia and long-term nursing care units. At many such institutions, the activity director is evaluated on the basis of participation levels (Hall & Bocksnick, 1995).

Robertson (1988) referred to the "intervention continuum" of staff behaviors for accomplishing that second task of getting residents to participate in programs: "inform, encourage, coax, coerce, require" (p. 62, both quotes). One can assume that there is a matching continuum of responses from the resident, from free choice (if the person readily agrees to participate and does not feel pressured to do so), to giving in, to not needing to respond at all when the resident has no control at the end of Robertson's continuum. Robertson made the case that if the recreation therapist or activity director believed it was in the resident's best interest, it was "legitimate" (p. 68) for staff in nursing home settings to coerce and even to require attendance at a leisure activity.

However, Hall and Bocksnick (1995) concluded from their interviews of nursing home staff and residents that residents' needs for self-determination, control, and autonomy were being undermined. Whereas the residents reported attending activities merely to avoid boredom, administrators and activity professionals – perhaps naively – assumed residents enjoyed and benefited from them. Further, while the staff believed that residents would make any suggestions they might have about the design of the programs, the residents felt they had no say in evaluating or modifying programs.

Four decades ago, Langer and her colleagues had demonstrated "the power of making choices" (Langer, 2009, p. 4). In a randomized controlled experiment, Langer and Rodin (1976) found that when nursing home residents were given choices, such as choosing a houseplant, so that they had control over aspects of their lives for which they were the sole decision-maker (such as deciding where to place the plant and when to water it), they improved in mental alertness and active participation and felt happier. Control group participants who were not offered those choices nor given that responsibility had an increase in debilitation during the same time frame. The researchers concluded that if the right to make decisions and a feeling of competence were retained by (or returned to) older adults living in an institutional setting, then some negative aspects of aging would be prevented or at least delayed.

In a subsequent paper, Rodin and Langer (1980) called for "social change that provides opportunities for real control, not simply strategies that increase perceived control while options for actual control remain unavailable" (p. 27) for all older adults, not just those in nursing homes. Rodin (1986) reviewed a number of studies on the relation between health and a sense of control in old age, noting that results showed detrimental impact on health when individual control in the environment was restricted and health promotion when options for control were enhanced. However, she also cautioned that with increasing age, some studies found the possibility of self-blame, stress, and worry with greater control. Kasser and Ryan's (1999) study of higher functioning nursing home residents found that it was important for the older adult to not only have autonomy but also to feel supported in that autonomy by his/her family and the staff. When autonomy support was present, vitality, well-being, and physical health were facilitated at greater levels.

Although the studies cited here were primarily conducted on nursing home residents, the generalized finding that autonomy is a necessary ingredient of well-being has been widely validated in all age groups, children and adult, and in many settings, under the rubric of Deci and Ryan's Self-Determination Theory[1] (Deci & Ryan, 2008; Ryan & Deci, 2000).

---

[1] Self-determination theory has identified three general motivational orientations that refer to the way people orient to their environment and the extent to which they want to and feel that they do have control. The orientations are also conceptually related to mindfulness vs. mindlessness, which has also been associated with positive psychological outcomes (Deci & Ryan, 2008). "Making choices leads to mindfulness" (Langer, 2009, p. 5). Such individual differences may explain the negative aspects of control reported in Rodin's (1986) review.

In summary, it is important for the physical and psychological health and well-being of older adults that they have autonomy and control over aspects of their lives, whether they are able to live in the community or have entered an institution such as a CCRC. This is especially important for residents in a CCRC because the institutionalization has necessarily taken control over some aspects of their lives, most obviously at the highest level of care (skilled nursing) but also in assisted living and even IL.

The remainder of this chapter describes K2SM, a pilot project designed to change the way intellectual programming was done at a 150-acre CCRC campus that offers multiple levels of care to approximately 500 residents. Funded by a grant from a private foundation for $90,000 over 3-years (2007–2009), the second author served as Project Director, and the first author assisted in the research aspects of the project. On average, the 370 residents in IL at the start of K2SM were 80.7 years old (ranging from 70 to 92 years) and had been in residence for 4 years, 8 months (range of 8 months to 17 years); virtually all had college degrees and many had graduate degrees.

The Essence of Keys to a Sharp Mind

K2SM was defined by two principles: (1) that the residents themselves should not only decide whether they will participate in a program but also share in the decision-making regarding the topics and content of the programming; (2) the programming needed to be intellectually challenging, not merely entertaining. The intent of K2SM was not to offer more "leisure activities," done for the sake of the activity per se (Robertson, 1988). Rather, it was motivated by the recent neuroscience findings that brains have a lifelong ability to grow new neurons and that brain plasticity (the responsiveness of the brain to the ways it is used) can continue throughout life (Bruel-Jungerman, Rampon, & Laroche, 2007). That is, K2SM was undertaken with the intention of applying current research in cognitive science that suggests age-related mental decline may be delayed or at least slowed by engaging in cognitively stimulating activities within a social context. We differentiated K2SM activities from leisure activities by referring to them as "pursuits" that were both enjoyable and produced "cognitive sweat." The residents embraced our use of these terms and understood the distinction.

The K2SM programming differed from some of the previous programming provided at the CCRC in several ways in addition to the two defining principles described above.

- The program was targeted to the independent, high-functioning residents. However, residents from any of the levels of care at the CCRC were welcome to participate, and some programs were open to the outside community.
- Rather than rely upon facility staff or volunteer instructors from the experienced and well-educated residents, the Project Director recruited outside instructors who had experience teaching adult learners.

- Instructors were provided continuous feedback from formal class evaluations in order to continuously improve the course structure and style of teaching.
- Each of the class offerings was intended to elicit active cognitive effort from the attendees.
- Participants were periodically asked to self-evaluate mood, perceived memory functioning, and quality of life in order to evaluate the program's impact.

Making the Case for K2SM

The first tangible product of K2SM was a report on the science behind the project (Hartman-Stein & Biermann, 2007), that is, a review of the literature suggesting that:

1. Older adults may increase the "cognitive reserve" that protects them against decline.
2. Neurogenesis can be promoted in older adult brains.
3. Cognitive fitness has a variety of positive outcomes for older adults.

(see especially Gould, Beylin, Tanapat, Reeves, & Shors, 1999; Kempermann, Kuhn, & Gage, 1997; Olson, Eadie, Ernst, & Christie, 2006; Scarmeas & Stern, 2003; Stern, 2007).

The report formed the basis of a widely attended presentation that the Project Director made to the residents, administrators, and staff to enable them to understand how the new program would differ from the previous programming offered. The essence of the difference was a greater role for residents, and the success of the program would be dependent on their acceptance of this new role offered to them. In essence, K2SM set out to change the culture of the facility for both staff and residents. The presentation also introduced the term "pursuit" to provide the language with which to talk about K2SM in contrast to the other activities that were available. This initial presentation turned out to be the first of a series of presentations to residents and staff throughout the 3-year grant period in which the Project Director communicated the state of the project and its accomplishments in an effort to maintain ongoing support for the programs.

Focus Groups and Surveys to Select Pursuits

At the outset of the project and again at the beginning of the second programming year, focus groups of residents were conducted to determine where the residents' interests lay. A program evaluation firm, Luther Consulting LLC, was contracted for this task, part of the program evaluation (described below). The consultant facilitated the focus groups of 10–12 residents who brainstormed topics and activities that interested them. Over 60 different topics were generated during the focus groups. Subsequently, the ideas spawned in the focus groups were organized into a

Table 6.1 Top "Pursuits" based on planning survey results

2007 (154 respondents)	2008 (173 respondents)
Basic computer skills	American politics/American history
American history	World affairs
Music appreciation	Health
Art appreciation	Science and the environment
Creative writing	Music appreciation
World affairs	Art appreciation
Health	World religions
Best-seller discussion groups	Computer skills
Flower arranging	American education system
Painting, drawing	Best-seller discussion groups
Movement pursuits: walking club	Creative writing

planning survey that was distributed to every IL resident via the in-house mail boxes. The survey asked the respondents to choose the ten pursuits of most interest to them.

One hundred fifty four (154) respondents completed the 2007 survey, and 173 respondents completed the 2008 survey (42% and 47% of the IL residents). The research team tallied and analyzed the results to determine the pursuits of greatest interest to the residents. Table 6.1 provides the ranked results.

Within the first month of the grant, the Project Director convened an ad hoc group of residents who had shown a high level of interest in the project. These individuals became members of The Resident Advisory Committee for Keys (TRACK). Throughout the project they provided a channel of communication between other residents and the Project Director and an ongoing source of consultation and support. TRACK's initial contribution was to recruit residents to participate in focus groups. Subsequently, they took attendance at classes and distributed and collected planning surveys, class evaluations, informed consent forms, and initial self-assessments. They also interviewed, assessed, and checked references of some instructors. The work of these volunteers was more extensive and essential for measuring outcomes than initially anticipated at the outset of the grant. The final format and delivery of K2SM would not have been feasible without their continued involvement and dedication to the success of the project.

Implementing Residents' Selection of Pursuits

The residents' top ranked pursuits framed the selection of classes and courses. The Project Director sought out potential instructors with strong reputations in their respective fields. Candidate instructors were interviewed, reference-checked, and assessed for the appropriateness of their teaching style to an audience of adult learners. The Project Director made an effort to attend candidates' lectures/programs in the community when possible as part of the vetting process. Candidates were briefed on the essence of K2SM, that is, that the participants had a role in choosing the class topics, and that the intention was to offer cognitively challenging programs not mere leisure activities. Therefore, class material was to be intellectually stimulating and suitable for college or graduate level courses. The Project Director encouraged the instructors to use an interactive style of teaching whenever possible, and she provided instructors with regular feedback from the residents based upon data from questionnaires taken at the end of each course.

Instructors had a range of backgrounds and experience including current and retired university professors and award winning high school teachers, the curator of a regional art museum, a retired geriatric social worker, a former school superintendent, a geriatric neurologist, an advanced graduate student of medical anthropology, research scientists specializing in dementia, an environmental attorney, local poets, a musician, and a photo journalist. The Project Director identified many of the instructors from contacts she had throughout the community, and she also requested suggestions from members of the resident committee.

For this pilot program, instructors were paid a modest honorarium that ranged from $100 to 250 per class session, averaging $150 per 90 min class plus mileage costs. One instructor donated his fee to the retirement community's Foundation. One resident of the retirement community, who also served on TRACK, took an active role in voluntarily teaching the computer classes. She had been a tutor for several residents in the past, and her participation as an instructor was invaluable to the program. In addition to the classes chosen by the residents, during each year of the grant the Project Director, a clinical geropsychologist, taught multi-part basic courses in memory enhancement techniques and relaxation/meditation strategies in order to offer to evidence-based programming to improve memory efficiency and overall cognition.

Classes Offered

Over a period of 33 months, a total of 60 different courses were offered via K2SM. Classes met on-site at the CCRC (except for one that was held at a local university that is a 20-min drive away; Fig. 6.1). There were no attendance fees for any of the programs. Residents and members of the community enrolled in the class ahead of time and for the most part there was compliance with this request. However, classes also witnessed some hallway-word-of-mouth effect by which residents would join in at the spur of the moment. Courses had varying numbers of sessions, ranging from 1 to 20. Class periods generally were 60–90 min. Class size varied from 8 to over 300 as determined by room size or instructor preference (e.g., the writing instructor preferred a limit of 12 students). Over the 33 months during which courses were offered, the average number of class sessions offered per month was 4.6. Course titles and number of sessions are listed in the Appendix.

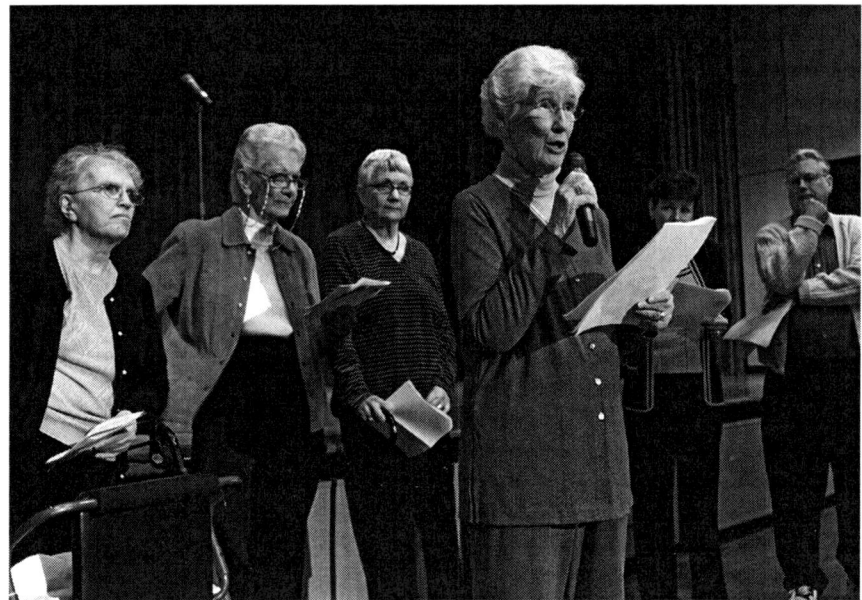

Fig. 6.1 Intergenerational creative writing class performs at Kent State University's *Giving Voice* program to the community

Class Satisfaction and Quality Indications

Satisfaction with the classes was measured in two ways: by attendance levels and by formal surveys. Attendance is an especially good indicator of satisfaction when neither cost nor distance is a barrier to participation and where there is a total absence of coercion to attend. In a small community like a CCRC, it is also an indicator of the word-of-mouth reputation of the class instructor.

Overall attendance at the K2SM offerings was excellent, from which it can be inferred that the program was very well received by residents. At no time was there pressure to participate from any staff. On average, each IL resident attended at least eight different K2SM classes or courses (a course is a multiple-class series). Considering that the usual, traditional activity programming at the CCRC ran in parallel during the entire grant period with a full menu of other on-site entertainment activities, support groups, religious programs, occasional guest lectures, field trips, resident-led discussions or peer-led autobiography classes, for residents to choose so many from the K2SM offerings speaks well of the quality. Attendance data indicated that interest in K2SM programming among IL residents increased over the 3 years with no evidence of decreasing enthusiasm.

During the second and third years of the grant, classes held in the auditorium-community room were widely advertised to the public by the CCRC. A number of the non-residents who attended a program also enrolled for subsequent programs when advertised, and we interpret this as a sign of satisfaction with what they experienced.

Table 6.2 Attendance

Number of residents in independent living (rough census)	370
Number of residents attending at least one class	313
Number of community members attending at least one class	206
Total number of individuals who attended at least one class	519
Average number of courses attended by a resident	8.35

Table 6.3 Top attended classes

American politics: presidential campaign of 2008	153
Art appreciation: architecture, prehistoric, and Egyptian art, Sistine frescoes	151
Health: myth of Alzheimer's disease, current diagnosis and treatment ideas	122
World religions: Hinduism, Buddhism, Islam	119
American history: presidential courage	119
Art appreciation: The Parthenon, classical Christmas art	119
Art appreciation/history: statue of liberty, art of the nativity	112
Music appreciation: Broadway musicals	102

Attendance counts are in Table 6.2. These are enrollee counts and do not necessarily include walk-ins (for large classes held in the auditorium, it was often difficult to capture the attendance of those who had not previously enrolled).

Table 6.3 identifies the eight classes for which attendance exceeded 100. All these were held in the auditorium. Certainly attendance at this level is a tribute to the speaker and his topic; however, classes with a lower attendance cannot be inferred to have a lower level of satisfaction because there were size limits, as explained above.

An informal analysis of the attendance data promotes several conclusions. A great many of the IL residents at this facility preferred the lecture-and-discussion format. The extent of group discussion and interaction varied with both timing of the courses in the 3-year program as well as the instructor. The Project Director observed that by the final six months of classes, the liveliness of group discussions and frequency of questions in classes had increased in comparison to the start of K2SM. One speculation is that the older adults in this particular community were formal in their style of learning, and as they became more comfortable with the K2SM program, they became more animated and interactive. Two sets of focus group data indicated that the majority did not prefer learning through performance-based skills such as classes in painting, acting, or learning to play musical instruments.

In addition to inferring satisfaction from participation levels, satisfaction with instructor and content was formally assessed via evaluation at the end of each class or course. Attendees evaluated five criteria on a Likert scale: engaging presentation, interesting content, mentally stimulating and challenging, enjoyable, and rewarding. The evaluation instrument also had three open questions that solicited the following: (1) comments on how the class had affected perceptions of their mental clarity, ability to concentrate, and memory; (2) general comments and suggestions for class improvement; and (3) for multi-session courses the number of sessions they had attended.

Table 6.4 The best courses, as rated by at least 90% of the attendees who completed an evaluation

Highest ratings for "engaging instructor"	Creative writing workshop Best sellers II Environmental science
Highest ratings for "stimulating instructor"	Memory enhancement The Christmas series The election
Highest ratings for "engaging and challenging content"	Supreme court Presidents Creative writing workshop
Highest ratings for "enjoyable"	Presidents Supreme court Best sellers II
Highest ratings for "personally rewarding"	Presidents (92.6%) Creative writing workshop (100%) Best sellers II

Participation in the class evaluations was high: 1,162 satisfaction surveys were turned in. Overall, classes were well received by participants. The courses getting the highest ratings from at least 90% of those completing that survey are shown in Table 6.4.

The following are representative responses to the open question on a course's impact on the participant's cognition: "Intellectually stimulating," "I exercised my brain today," "Extremely effective delivery to enhance concentration and memory." Responses on the satisfaction surveys strongly suggest that participants perceived a high level of benefit from the courses.

Results of the evaluations were provided to the teacher and to the project director to aid planning future class offerings. Returning instructors found the survey data to be helpful in adjusting the curriculum of upcoming offerings or to improve aspects of the teaching style. For example, the instructor of Best Sellers modified her selection of books based on feedback.

Impact of K2SM on Participants' Cognition and Well-Being

A significant aspect of the K2SM project was its expectation that it would have a benefit to the participants' cognition, especially memory skills, mood, and social connectedness. To gather evidence of the effects upon participants, the Project Director selected several established and psychometrically valid instruments to create what we called the Thinking Survey. The Multi-factorial Memory Questionnaire (Troyer & Rich, 2002) measured respondent's perception of his/her memory and cognitive functioning. This instrument comprises three scales: Feelings about Memory, whose items refer to self-evaluations of memory ability; Everyday Memory Situations, whose items refer to incidents of poor memory; and Memory Aids &

Strategies, whose items refer to strategies one could use. The UCLA Loneliness Scale (Russell, 1996) measures social contentment and sense of isolation. A three-item version of the geriatric depression scale (GDS) measured mood (Bank, MacNeill, & Lichtenberg, 2000). The first two instruments are self-assessments with Likert-type responses, which were subsequently numerically coded from 1 to 5. The GDS had yes/no responses, coded as 1 or 5. The resulting Thinking Survey comprised 80 questions.

Participants completed the Thinking Survey before they attended their first class. This initial measurement set a baseline for that individual against which any change could be measured. The initial survey was completed at different times by different participants, depending on when they first attended a class. Each person who completed an initial survey was subsequently mailed another copy six months later by the program evaluation firm (Luther Consulting, LLC), and then sent another identical survey every six months during the 3-year program period, to complete and mail back to the contractor.

These repeated surveys were associated to the individual by means of an identity number assigned by the consulting firm but unknown to CCRC staff and K2SM personnel. Hence, any changes could be measured at the individual level, and not merely on a group level. Because the surveys could not be completely anonymous, participants in the Thinking Survey research signed an informed consent document before completing the initial survey. Attending a class was not dependent on participation in the survey research, although very few participants declined to fill out serial surveys. TRACK's efforts to identify first-time K2SM attendees and invite their participation in the program evaluation were very important. An exception to recruitment of research participants was made for the classes held in the large auditorium-like community room, especially in the second and third years when such programs were open to the public.

Response to the request to complete an initial Thinking Surveys was very good. All 48 attendees of the first class on memory in April 2007 complied with the request. By the end of the year, a total of 111 individuals had done so. A remarkable number of these 111 continued to complete and mail back the additional surveys every 6 months. Seventy nine people (71%) completed at least three, and 55 (50%) of the 111 completed at least four in total. This is an excellent response rate for a repetitive survey for which respondents were not being paid.

On the initial survey, people generally responded above the mid-point in the positive direction, and subsequent phases saw little change, on average, from that baseline. Hence, this population did not view themselves as having immediate difficulty with their memory or lacking in social connections at the start of K2SM. See Table 6.5 for the descriptive measurement at baseline.

The biggest change in the means across all five scales and the five phases of measurement occurred at 18 months in the "Feelings about Memory" scale, for which the change was approximately one fifth of a point. Positive improvement from baseline for the "Feelings about Memory" scale reached statistical significance at 6, 12, 18, and 24 months. Improvement in the responses on the Everyday Memory Situations scale, compared to baseline, also reached significance at the 6-month

Table 6.5 Descriptive statistics at baseline

	N	Minimum	Maximum	Mean	Std. deviation
Feelings about memory	116	2	5	3.65	0.608
Everyday memory situations	118	3	4	3.49	0.406
Memory aids and strategies[a]	117	2	5	3.06	0.475
UCLA loneliness scale	116	2	4	3.61	0.429
Three-item GDS	118	1	5	4.80	0.594

[a]A lower score is better

Table 6.6 Statistically significant differences from baseline

	Mean difference	t	df	Significance (two-tailed)
Feelings about memory				
At 6 months	0.14847	2.682	71	0.009
At 12 months	0.12952	3.072	83	0.003
At 18 months	0.19344	3.958	63	0.000
At 24 months	0.15900	1.730	19	0.100
Everyday memory situations				
At 6 months	0.07736	2.133	71	0.036
Memory aids and strategies[a]				
At 18 months	−0.11541	−1.892	60	0.063

[a]Lower score is better

phase, and those for the Memory Aids and Strategies scale at 18 months. Note that these are not cumulative differences. Table 6.6 lists those changes that were significant. All other phases and scales are interpreted as "no change." It is noteworthy that there were no declines over the measurement period for this older adult population.

Overall, the results of the Thinking Survey are supportive of the notion that participation in K2SM was a factor in increasing individuals' contentment with their memory functioning. This finding is noteworthy because studies generally indicate that older adults commonly perceive deterioration in their cognitive function over time (e.g., Cavanaugh, 1996). One hypothesis is that participating in cognitively challenging programs triggers memory recall about facts the individuals once knew. For example, historical, scientific, or autobiographical information may have been retrieved by engagement in the class, thus raising participants' contentment with their memory skills.

A limitation of the program evaluation data is that participants who dropped out of the evaluation process could not be tracked as to the reason for dropping. Thus, those whose cognition declined may have been among the drop-outs, skewing the remaining sample toward cognitive maintenance or improvement. It is also possible that some individuals who were concerned about their cognitive functioning may have self-selected out of the evaluation process.

This project was not conceived as nor funded as empirical or experimental research, although theoretically, statistically stronger results on the variables measured may have been obtained had there been a comparison group of nonparticipants who also completed Thinking Surveys every 6 months. Experimental research with its requirement for randomized groups was not considered realistic for the CCRC setting because it would have required prohibiting some residents from attending classes of interest to them in order to create the comparison group.

Lessons Learned

If a retirement facility is interested in replicating this program, developers need to be aware that activity staff members may view the insistence on a shift for residents to be actively involved at the programming level to be a criticism of the status quo. Early buy-in from the activity staff is essential to success. Explaining the research findings on autonomy, support, and self-determination, reviewed in the first part of this chapter, to the activity staff, marketing personnel, and upper level administrators is a step in the process that must not be skipped. The change we are advocating should be appealing to administration because it is the sort of improvement that successful businesses are constantly looking for, one that can be expected to result in a better customer response, i.e., more participation and improved customer (resident) satisfaction.

Buy-in is also more likely if the activity coordinator meets regularly with the Project Director and is actively involved in brainstorming and planning sessions for the purpose of developing a good working relationship. In order to publicly show the activity director's level of professional involvement, the Project Director included her as an author of a poster of the preliminary findings of K2SM presented at a professional conference (Hartman-Stein, Luther, Biermann, & Busko, 2007). Perhaps most importantly, the Chief Executive Officer of the retirement community must understand the benefits of increased involvement from residents. If the CEO is wholeheartedly behind the project and committed to the culture change, then success of the program is much more likely.

A small group of enthusiastic residents such as those participating in TRACK, who have a large social network within the CCRC, provides an important element in the support structure for implementation and execution. For K2SM, TRACK was able to identify people whose communication skills were appropriate for the focus groups, solicit opinions about solving problems that are bound to arise, and be identified by residents as point of contact for new ideas. Furthermore, from our experience it is important that this was a self-determined group, independent from staff or other administrative influence.

The level of funding obtained to execute K2SM required a high level of volunteer involvement, much more than anticipated. This led to some "burn out" of several volunteers. Our recommendation is to earmark funds to hire additional help such as students or interns from local universities to be involved in data collection and clerical support functions.

Offering high-quality programs brings a marketing advantage for the administration of the CCRC. Opening classes to the community, if space allows, provides a major marketing opportunity.

We think it is important to plan at the start to measure program impact. Participants demonstrated a prolonged willingness to complete several different types of evaluative surveys: (1) topics to be addressed in classes; (2) the quality of the classes; and (3) the impact on mood, social connections, and perceptions about memory functioning.

The changes that were expected as a result of K2SM participation were difficult to measure, and other characteristics have since come to light as likely and perhaps more easily measured outcomes. The baseline levels of the Thinking Survey were higher than expected, and subsequent changes were perhaps not captured due to ceiling effects. We suggest that projects stemming from the principles underlying K2SM look for increased mindfulness in the participants. Mindfulness is increased attention to and interest in one's surroundings, an open awareness, and it has been linked to improved well-being. "Making choices leads to mindfulness" (Langer, 2009, p. 5). The four-item measure of subjective vitality used by Kasser and Ryan (1999) is suggested as an instrument that could capture important changes. Subjective vitality (Ryan & Frederick, 1997) is the feeling of aliveness and energy. Kasser and Ryan found that it varies systematically with anxiety, depression, well-being, and life satisfaction, as well as physical health.

Conclusion

The stimulus for the K2SM grant was the expressed wisdom of a resident who predicted that independent, high-functioning residents of a retirement community would respond enthusiastically to self-determination in their intellectual programming. This is a stark contrast to the usual approach, program design by staff, supplemented with self-programming by residents that has minimal staff support. It is important to keep in mind that the people who work at a CCRC are, by definition, younger than the residents, who have retired from full-time work up to 30 years earlier. By providing an opportunity for the residents to select their own topics of interest to pursue and study on the CCRC site with professional instructors, K2SM assured that the classes offered were age-appropriate for the IL residents (mean age 81). Consistent with the findings and recommendations of Hall and Bocksnick (1995), Kasser and Ryan (1999), Langer and Rodin (1976), and Rodin and Langer (1980), this pilot project and the on-going changes it stimulated in that CCRC's programming for IL residents demonstrate that when choice and autonomy are returned to older adults, they perceive a high level of personal benefit and an increase in well-being.

The second principle on which K2SM was based is that age-related mental decline may be delayed or at least slowed by engaging in cognitively stimulating activities within a social context. The data collected in periodic surveys of participants suggest that participants increased their contentment with their memory functioning, but measures of change in other variables proved difficult to capture.

As described in the introduction, the inspiration for the change in culture regarding the intellectual programming for this CCRC stemmed from the wisdom and insight of Dr. Jeanette Reuter who sadly passed away three months before the funding of

K2SM began. However, the spirit of her influence continues, even nearly two years since the initial grant ended. A second grant at a much lower amount was obtained in 2010 to pay for distance learning programs sponsored by a local museum that offers periodic high-quality lectures on a variety of topics in the arts and sciences. Besides offering intellectually challenging programming in this new format, one major change is that the activity department now uses questionnaires to gain feedback from the residents about the topics of most interest to them.

We began the chapter with the case presentation of Gerry Jones. The following are her comments about the impact of K2SM a year after the grant ended.

> Without a doubt K2SM had a positive effect on subsequent programming. K2SM made us aware of the large number of very qualified people available as experts in fields that were identified as of "high interest" on the resident questionnaires. Contacts are everything and the Project Director's wide range of experience in this geographic area, both professional and personal, made it possible to obtain highly regarded individuals who probably never would have crossed our radar. I think of the museum curator, a truly renaissance man in the arts, the dynamic political science teacher who had audiences on the edge of their seats, the creative writing instructor who thought to combine her college-age students in the same class with the CCRC residents. But it's a lot of work to delve into these resources… At least, now, residents' consciousness has been aroused to the possibilities out there.

Appendix: Classes and Courses Offered

One Session Classes and Multi-Part Courses

American politics and American history (25 sessions):

1. Rating and debating the presidents
2. The supreme court
3. Parties, presidential campaigns, platforms, propaganda, and polls
4. Presidential courage: past and present
5. The history of Walt Disney, American entrepreneur

Enhancing memory and healthy aging (18 sessions):

1. Maximum memory fitness
2. Alzheimer disease current theories and treatment
3. A group discussion of presentation on dementia
4. Relaxation and mindful meditation
5. Exercise strategies for the over 50 crowd
6. Boost your memory skills
7. Memory impairment in late life: what's normal, what's not
8. Enhancing quality of life for memory impaired adults
9. Enhancing quality of life for memory impaired adults: an up close and personal perspective
10. Meditation for memory enhancement

Art history and appreciation

1. Art of the statue of liberty
2. Art of the nativity
3. Intro to architecture
4. Prehistoric art
5. Egyptian art
6. Sistine frescoes of Michelangelo
7. Love in art
8. Jesus in the film media
9. The Parthenon
10. Classical Christmas art
11. Kimono as art
12. Art of Leonardo Da Vinci
13. Celebrating watercolor
14. Celebrating ceramics
15. Clyde singer's America
16. Photo journalism: *The Growing Season*, a story of migrant workers in Ohio

Note:

1. A week after the class on Kimonos (number 11), residents went to a local museum to view a traveling exhibition of Japanese kimonos.
2. As an offshoot of the class on DaVinci's Art (number 12), the CCRC's foundation provided funding for a one act play, *The Incredible Life of Leonardo DaVinci*, staged and performed on-site by a local acting company at the retirement community.

Computer skills training (48 small group sessions)

1. Intro session, internet, email
2. Creating documents
3. Managing directories of documents each of the 16 sessions was offered 3 times on the same day in groups of 8–12

Note: Money from the grant was used to purchase four additional computers that remain available to the residents.

Best-seller discussion groups and literary classics (21 sessions)

1. Literature of Christmas
2. Best-seller discussion group
3. Best-seller discussion group

Music history and appreciation (12 sessions)

1. The music of Christmas
2. Roaring twenties
3. Classical curios, musical oddities

4. Opera: exploring opera (23 sessions: 19 for writing, 4 for poetry reading) Berlioz, Puccini, Tchaikovsky, Madame Butterfly (5 sessions)
   5. Broadway musicals

Creative writing/recitation/readings (23 sessions: 19 writing & 4 poetry reading)

   1. Introductory creative writing workshop series
   2. Writing for health and healing
   3. Advanced creative writing/poetry
   4. Guided reminiscence series
   5. Poetry reading by class participants to the retirement community residents
   6. Intergenerational readings by residents and college students
   7. *Creative voices*, performed by class participants for the community of Kent
   8. Frost, Sandburg, and Keats poetry recitation by local older adult poet

Religions of the World (6 sessions)

Two sessions about each of the following religions: Hinduism, Buddhism, and Islam.

Science (6 sessions)

   1. Environmental issues: Can the U.S. build a green city? Must the U.S. make the world green?
   2. Energy series
   3. Physics made simple: our place in the universe
   4. Physics made simple: the universe within

World affairs (5 sessions)

   1. Politics of the Middle East
   2. Afghanistan and Pakistan
   3. Colombia: a culture of violence
   4. Politics of Russia
   5. Politics of China

The American education system (3 sessions)

   1. The history and future of American education: an intergenerational program.
   2. The Intergenerational School: example of an award winning charter school in Cleveland.

References

Bank, A. L., MacNeill, S. E., & Lichtenberg, P. A. (2000). Cross validation of the MacNeill-Lichtenberg decision tree: Triaging mental health problems in geriatric rehabilitation patients. *Rehabilitation Psychology, 45*, 193–204.

Bruel-Jungerman, E., Rampon, C., & Laroche, S. (2007). Adult hippocampal neurogenesis, synaptic plasticity and memory: Facts and hypotheses. *Review of Neuroscience, 18*, 93–114.

Cavanaugh, J. C. (1996). Memory self-efficacy as a moderator of memory change. In F. Blanchard-Fields & T. M. Hess (Eds.), *Perspectives on cognitive change in adulthood and aging* (pp. 488–507). New York: McGraw-Hill.
Deci, E. L., & Ryan, R. M. (2008). Self-determination theory: A macrotheory of human motivation, development, and health. *Canadian Psychology, 49*, 182–185.
Gould, E., Beylin, A., Tanapat, P., Reeves, A., & Shors, T. J. (1999). Learning enhances adult neurogenesis in the hippocampal formation. *Nature Neuroscience, 2*, 260–265.
Hall, B. L., & Bocksnick, J. G. (1995). Therapeutic recreation for the institutionalized elderly: Choice or abuse? *Journal of Elder Abuse and Neglect, 7*, 49–60.
Hartman-Stein, P., & Biermann, J. S. (2007). *Literature review for Keys to a Sharp Mind*, unpublished manuscript.
Hartman-Stein, P. E., Luther, J. L., Biermann, J., & Busko, S. (2007) *Determining preferences and feasibility for instituting "brain healthy" lifestyle programs for older adults in a continuing care retirement community.* Poster presentation at the Alzheimer's Association International Conference on Prevention of Dementia, Washington.
Kasser, V. G., & Ryan, R. M. (1999). The relation of psychological needs for autonomy and relatedness to vitality, well-being, and mortality in a nursing home. *Journal of Applied Social Psychology, 29*, 935–954.
Kempermann, G., Kuhn, H. G., & Gage, F. H. (1997). More hippocampal neurons in adult mice living in an enriched environment. *Nature, 386*, 493–495.
Langer, E. J. (2009). *Counterclockwise: Mindful health and the power of possibility*. New York: Ballantine.
Langer, E. J., & Rodin, J. (1976). The effects of choice and enhanced personal responsibility for the aged: A field experiment in an institutional setting. *Journal of Personality and Social Psychology, 34*, 191–198.
Olson, A. K., Eadie, B. D., Ernst, C., & Christie, B. R. (2006). Environmental enrichment and voluntary exercise massively increase neurogenesis in the adult hippocampus via dissociable pathways. *Hippocampus, 16*, 250–260.
Robertson, R. D. (1988). Recreation and the institutionalized elderly: Conceptualization of the free choice and intervention continuums. *Activities, Adaptation and Aging, 11*, 61–73.
Rodin, J. (1986). Aging and health: Effects of the sense of control. *Science, 233*, 1271–1276.
Rodin, J., & Langer, E. J. (1980). Aging labels: The decline of control and the fall of self-esteem. *Journal of Social Issues, 36*, 12–29.
Russell, D. (1996). The UCLA loneliness scale (version 3): Reliability, validity, and factor structure. *Journal of Personality Assessment, 66*, 20–40.
Ryan, R. M., & Deci, E. L. (2000). Self-determination theory and the facilitation of intrinsic motivation, social development, and well-being. *American Psychologist, 55*, 68–78.
Ryan, R. M., & Frederick, C. M. (1997). On energy, personality, and health: Subjective vitality as a dynamic reflection of well-being. *Journal of Personality, 65*, 529–565.
Scarmeas, N., & Stern, Y. (2003). Cognitive reserve and lifestyle. *Journal of Clinical and Experimental Neuropsychology, 25*, 625–633.
Stern, Y. (Ed.). (2007). *Cognitive reserve: Theory and applications*. Philadelphia: Taylor and Francis.
Troyer, A. K., & Rich, J. B. (2002). Psychometric properties of a new metamemory questionnaire for older adults. *Journal of Gerontology: Psychological Sciences, 57B*, P19–P27.

Chapter 7
Osher Lifelong Learning Institute at the University of Montana: A Model of Successful University and Community Partnerships

Sharon Alexander, Cynthia Aten, Dannette Fadness, and Kali Lightfoot

Abstract This chapter provides the history of the Osher Lifelong Learning Institutes (OLLIs), university-based programs designed to promote personal growth and provide intellectually stimulating programs for those age 50 and older. The recent experience of the program at the University of Montana in Missoula is featured.

Introduction

As the aging landscape changes, many different demands are placed on communities and the services they provide. While fewer communities are offering physical wellness programs or those that provide intellectual stimulation for the population over age 50, recognition of the need to positively impact aspects of aging is definitely on the rise. Current research findings draw a direct correlation between healthy aging and keeping the brain engaged through a variety of pursuits, as highlighted throughout this volume. Among the programs in the US that provide intellectually stimulating courses and workshops for those over 50 years of age are the Osher Lifelong Learning Institutes (OLLIs). In 2001 Bernard Osher, a magnanimous supporter of lifelong learning for "seasoned" adults, funded the first OLLI that led to a network of institutes spread throughout the country.

To date, the Bernard Osher Foundation has provided significant funding for 117 OLLIs at colleges and universities in all 50 states.

S. Alexander (✉)
Osher Lifelong Learning Institute, University of Montana,
32 Campus Drive, Missoula, MT 59812, USA
e-mail: molli@umontana.edu

History of the OLLI

Mr. Osher was born and raised in Biddeford, Maine, son of Russian and Polish immigrants. He graduated from Bowdoin College and soon after followed his sister Marion to California, settling in the Bay Area, where he established himself over the years as a respected businessman and community leader. Mr. Osher was successful in a number of ventures, including the purchase, with his sister, of a small savings and loan bank which grew to be World Savings, the largest of its kind in California.

In 1977, Mr. Osher created the Bernard Osher Foundation which *seeks to improve quality of life through support for higher education and the arts. The Foundation provides post-secondary scholarship funding to colleges and universities across the nation, with special attention to reentry students. It also benefits programs in integrative medicine in the United States and Sweden, including centers at the University of California, San Francisco; Harvard Medical School and Brigham and Women's Hospital in Boston; and the Karolinska Institute in Stockholm. In addition, the Foundation supports a growing national lifelong learning network for seasoned adults… . An array of performing arts organizations, museums, and selected educational programs in Northern California and in Mr. Osher's native state of Maine receive Foundation grants* (http://www.osherfoundation.org/index.php?foundation).

Mr. Osher's earliest ideas of supporting lifelong learning activities came from his association with Alfred Fromm, who, together with his wife, underwrote a lifelong learning program at the University of San Francisco (USF). During a trip to Maine, he heard various people speak of the University of Southern Maine (USM) Senior College and, after talking with officials of the university and senior college leaders, he decided to fund the operation. He was impressed with the Senior College as an organization and thought it had growth potential. The local leadership changed the name Senior College to OLLI to reflect the generosity of its new donor. The Osher Foundation adopted the name for its new program and went on to fund more OLLIs at other universities, starting with Sonoma State University.

By 2004 there were some 40 Osher Institutes, primarily in California and along the Eastern seaboard. It became clear that there was a need for some sort of organizing body to think about the Osher Institutes as more than just individual programs. The staff at the OLLI at USM had gained valuable experience coordinating the Maine Senior College Network, a loose confederation of 18 independently managed lifelong learning programs located at a variety of sites around the state of Maine. That experience gave the staff the confidence to propose a similar kind of resource network to the Osher Foundation. Deemed the National Resource Center (NRC), the original vision was of a central hub with no fiduciary or policy responsibilities that would exist to create opportunities for the leaders of the various Osher Institutes to communicate with each other through face-to-face conferences and online tools and share news and information about successful and not-so-successful programs and initiatives. A tour through the NRC website (http://www.osher.net) will give the reader a sense of the depth and breadth of issues OLLI leaders confront, as well as the joy with which they approach their work. The Osher Foundation found this to be an attractive enough proposal to support it with a $2 million endowment, as well as matching support for a new building that houses the NRC and the local OLLI at the USM.

All lifelong learning institutes for older adults spring from an initial program that was founded at the New School for Social Research in New York City in 1962. The Institute for Retired Professionals (IRP) began when a group of retired New York City public school teachers approached the New School with a request for a set of courses that would be something more intellectually stimulating than the usual fare offered at senior centers at that time. The New School operated with a particular collaborative philosophy about adult students:

> The New School does not set any limits to its programs in regard to subject matter. Whatever seriously interests persons of mature intelligence properly falls within the province of the school. History and philosophy, the social and behavioral sciences, literature and art, the natural and biological sciences, education, and ethics naturally take up a significant part of The New School curriculum, since these are the fields in which The forces of culture and change are most significantly active, and in which human beings, their institutions, and their products are directly studied. The centrality of the liberal arts is maintained and strengthened in every possible way, but not to the exclusion of other educational programs that serve a legitimate need for mature adults in a mature community (http://www.nsu.newschool.edu/01b_history.htm).

In fact, this could be considered a blueprint for the curriculum at the 450 or so lifelong learning institutes and OLLIs that have come into existence since the IRP opened its doors in 1962. Further, the IRP website includes the following statement: *The IRP encourages students to challenge themselves by taking part in study groups, and by assuming academic and administrative leadership roles.* The IRP philosophy of shared leadership and volunteer participation in the inner workings of the institute, to a greater or lesser degree, is a hallmark of the national network of OLLIs, not because the Osher Foundation demands it, but because we have discovered it to be the best way to run a program for empowered, experienced, "seasoned" adults and make it financially accessible to the widest range of participants.

The Foundation is remarkably non-prescriptive about the use of its funds. In the early years, it funded startups as well as established institutes, using a formula based on membership benchmarks. As it has gained more experience, it has concentrated on funding institutes with strong membership and a good management track record. The initial two institutes funded in 2001 were the heavily volunteer-driven Senior College at USM, and a startup program with very few volunteers at Sonoma State University in California. The two programs had vastly different administrative structures and were the first indication that the network of OLLIs was going to include a variety of approaches to the delivery of courses and activities.

It has become clear that the only common core vision that the OLLIs share is a belief in the joy of learning for its own sake within a community of learners. This is a radical vision in our very utilitarian world, but an important one. In her recent book, *The Third Chapter: Passion, Risk and Adventure in the 25 years after 50*, Sarah Lawrence Lightfoot (2009, p. 246) writes about the need for "organization innovations, and creative invention of other scenarios and arenas of learning that support a more fluid and frequent movement across boundaries, allowing for shifts in our routines and rhythms across time, and offer us multiple opportunities to recalibrate the balance between work and love, between work, family and community, and between work and play – all of which may help us revise and expand our definitions of a meaningful, purposeful life."

Far from being about earning credits, or certificates and degrees, the learning that takes place in OLLI is aimed at creating opportunities for sampling new thoughts and ideas, trying out a different way of being purposeful, changing the rhythm and routine of life, and looking at identity in a new way. In the larger society, old age is thought of as the end, the time of winding down. The OLLI population thinks as well about new beginnings: "what will I learn, whom will I meet, what will that learning and that person bring to my life?"

As of 2011, the Osher Foundation is not funding new institutes. The network will continue to mature, hopefully with 117 successful programs in 50 states. There is no other foundation or grantmaking entity that is currently funding lifelong learning institutes on a national scale although small local grants may be available to groups that want to start an institute. Most lifelong learning institutes (including many that are now OLLIs) have begun with very small grants (up to $5,000) from local sources, magnified by a lot of elbow grease on the part of passionate prospective students over the age of 50. The more than 300 institutes that exist in the US today without Osher funding are living proof that successful, inspiring programs can grow on their own with no outside funding sources.

Information and technical assistance are available on the NRC website (http://www.osher.net) to anyone wanting to start an institute, and the staff members of the NRC are available for phone or email consultation (check the website for contact information). Prospective institutes can also find startup information and technical assistance, though not funding, on the Elderhostel/Road Scholar Institute Network website http://www.roadscholar.org/ein/intro.asp

One of the newest OLLIs is at the University of Montana (UM). Launched late in 2005 with free "appetizer" lectures given by two of UM's most respected faculty members, the OLLI at UM (MOLLI) has provided significant outreach to the community and been highly successful in creating exciting learning opportunities for its members. Indeed, MOLLI has taken on a vibrant life of her own!

Courses are dynamic and highly interactive, designed to stimulate the intellectual interests of members. Care is given to structuring the program to ensure a balance between and among the arts, humanities, sciences, and current affairs. Motivation for attending courses includes interest in a course topic, the joy of learning more about oneself, one's community, and the world in a challenging, intellectually rigorous and supportive environment, and social interaction with like-minded people.

Given the program's location in the heart of the Rockies and the relatively small population, its ability to succeed might have been doubted. However, the community of Missoula, in partnership with the university, has a strong reputation for not only being "one of the best mountain towns in the nation" (Koeppel, 2007) but also being considered a "destination point" conveniently situated between Glacier and Yellowstone National Parks. The university has produced 28 Rhodes Scholars and eight Pulitzer Prize winning journalists. One of MOLLI's faculty members, Steve Running, was part of the team who won a Nobel Peace Prize in 2008 for their work on global warming.

Many MOLLI members are newcomers to Missoula and are delighted to find the Institute's programs. One member wrote:

> My husband and I moved to Missoula four and a half years ago... . We knew we needed to get involved in the community to begin to make a place for ourselves here, and we set out to do just that ... . It's hard to express the depth of my delight in finding MOLLI classes. I began taking classes like a mad woman: politics of the Middle East, world cuisine, medicinal plants, the latest in bird research, medical anthropology, memoir writing, piano literature of the Romantic, Classical and Baroque eras, the "Axial Age," determining one's spiritual type, the Civil War, staging to Kill a Mockingbird, "Yes, You Can Draw" (and suddenly, yes, I could!), Islamic Art and Architecture, and I could go on. Suddenly I was planning my life around the six-week fall, winter and spring terms, scheduling our visits with our son and his family in Virginia so that I could fit in all of my MOLLI classes ...

Not only does the MOLLI program enhance the cultural and educational environment of Missoula, it is also of great importance to the University, as it brings hundreds of new people to campus each year.

The mission of MOLLI is to "promote lifelong learning and personal growth for adults plus 50. Older adults are a valuable resource for society, and through the Institute we will speak to their continuing intellectual needs." We accomplish this through a diverse collection of non-credit short courses primarily offered in three 6-week terms. Our courses are taught by university professors, both active and emeritus, as well as experts from the community. By creating an accessible and innovative learning environment, we ensure that older adults from all backgrounds and levels of education can pursue learning without concern for grades or exams, with accountability for attendance and completion of any homework assignments only to themselves. For newcomers to the community, MOLLI provides an excellent opportunity to learn and meet new like-minded friends. For long-time residents, we offer new educational opportunities at a reasonable cost. For everyone, MOLLI creates an increased awareness of the vital role the University of Montana plays as a valuable and vibrant community resource.

Our institute began in 2005 as the Montana Lifelong Learning Institute. Upon recognition by the Bernard Osher Foundation, it officially became the OLLI at the University of Montana, although we retain the familiar MOLLI moniker locally. We also lowered the age limit from 55 to 50 to be congruent with other Osher institutes around the country. Over time, we have learned that those members in the 50–65-year-old group are often still working; thus those taking courses are often 65 or older. As a result, we are exploring options that will help us meet the needs of this younger audience; for instance, we offer brown-bag lunches in the downtown area, evening courses, and recently we have begun to develop online courses which will provide access to learning at any time or place regardless of employment or mobility.

Originally, the program was self-funded. In 2006, we were invited to apply for a grant from the Bernard Osher Foundation. This funding proved to be "life-changing," as it provided a solid financial base upon which to plan and grow program, instruction and marketing, all of which culminated in dramatic growth in participation. This success was recognized by the Osher Foundation, and we were funded for 2 additional years, culminating in a $1,000,000 endowment grant. At this writing, we have over 1,200 members with annual individual course enrollments of over 2,500.

Organizationally, MOLLI is a program of the University of Montana and is administered by Continuing Education; however, its strength comes from the leadership of a volunteer Council comprised of university representatives and community members with a variety of backgrounds. The Council is a key component of the organization, having oversight of programs and marketing as well as playing a major role in the development of policies and procedures. This group is guided by a set of by-laws and assisted by an active committee structure including Executive, Program, Marketing and Membership, and Nominating Committees. This core group of volunteers, supported by Continuing Education personnel, has attained remarkable success, as both membership and attendance at courses and special programs attest. The partnership between volunteers and professional staff has provided a strong foundation that addresses all aspects of effectively running a large institute including program logistics, financial operations and contractual obligations.

From the outset, the decision was made that MOLLI courses would focus primarily on academic topics. We avoided "how to" courses, such as use of computers and digital cameras or those with purely social intent. Because of the rich resources available through the university and a highly accomplished community, this decision fit our community of learners well. Volunteer members of the Program Committee are responsible both for identifying what is taught and by whom as well as recruitment of faculty. Without the tireless efforts of this dedicated group, we would not be as successful as we are, and without excellent programming, there would be no reason to become a member of MOLLI.

In planning, the Program Committee balances the mix of large and small courses as well as offerings in the arts, humanities, sciences, social sciences and current events. Offerings range from *Iran between Two Revolutions*, which drew 150 students, to *Fist Fights to First Kisses: Rites of Passage in Literature,* which attracted 15. Having both large and small class sizes enables individuals to select learning activities that meet their particular needs and styles.

We have also offered several unique opportunities, such as going behind the scenes of *Hamlet* and *To Kill a Mockingbird*, each produced by university-affiliated companies; taking an historical walking tour of Missoula; or day-long bus tours to historical sites in Butte and Helena. Our participants enjoy these alternative programs. One person noted about the latest bus tour: *Super day – can't wait until another is offered…This is a fun way to learn about my new home [Montana].*

Another highly successful collaboration has been with the University of Montana's President's Lecture Series. Through this lecture series, national and international experts are invited to speak on a wide variety of topics, and MOLLI has offered courses designed to enhance the lectures. For example, Dr. Marcia Angell, former Editor-in-Chief of the *New England Journal of Medicine* and Senior Lecturer, Department of Social Medicine at Harvard Medical School, gave a presentation entitled: *Discoveries, Discoveries, What You Should Know about the Drugs*

You Take. The accompanying MOLLI course, presented by a panel of pharmaceutical and medical experts from UM and the community, met with our students three times before the lecture and once after, to discuss local views and applications while stimulating audience participation on a very relevant topic.

Keeping the program diverse is essential in meeting the needs of our 1,200 members, whose ages range from 50 to over 90 years. When the program was first initiated, the Program Committee had to actively recruit faculty. Now we are finding that many faculty members want to teach again and again. We are also receiving unsolicited course proposals for consideration. Guided by course evaluations from participants at the end of each term, Program Committee members ask previous faculty to teach again, follow up with those who have submitted course proposals or seek out faculty for newly proposed topics. On the MOLLI website, www.umt.edu/molli, prospective instructors can find directions for submitting course proposals, all of which are considered by the committee.

We are pleased to offer an honorarium which acknowledges our instructors for their support of lifelong learning. The instructors receive a $1,200 honorarium for a 6-week term. Co-instructors may decide how to split the honorarium accordingly. Other OLLIs reduce operating costs by offering peer-led courses, eliminating the need for professor honoraria. Although MOLLI is not presently considering peer-led courses, we note that some of our courses have led to the creation of peer-led groups continuing to explore writing, drawing and painting.

It is worth mentioning that faculty members who teach in the program thoroughly enjoy working with students who are engaged, read course materials and who actively participate in class discussion. One of our favorite art historians has noted: *These students engage me and help me formulate new ideas…they help me see things in a new way, a way I don't normally see things…*[teaching in MOLLI] *is a marvelous experience!*

If the Council and the Program Committee, are two legs of the MOLLI "stool," then the Membership and Marketing Committee is the third leg. Their work to both market the program and increase membership is essential to our continued success. This committee has become increasingly adept at identifying potential participants and reaching out to them through a combination of advertising in print media and on billboards, and strategic distribution of printed informational materials before each term at senior centers, assisted living facilities, libraries, churches, lecture series and the like. Committee members are available to speak about MOLLI to organizations such as local service clubs. We have also found that incentive promotions, e.g., offering $10 off a course fee for each new member recruited during a recent membership drive, have been very popular. We also distribute attractive cards that can be used to gift a MOLLI membership or course. It must be said, however, that we have found that our most powerful recruitment tool remains enthusiastic members; "word of mouth" has brought us the most new participants.

A strong working partnership with the Dean of Continuing Education and the MOLLI Coordinator, supervised by the dean, support the functionality of the "stool." The coordinator works closely with faculty, volunteers and members to ensure satisfactory experiences.

One of the major goals of MOLLI has been to build partnerships with other community organizations and programs. These range from sharing advertising in each other's newsletters and concert programs to co-sponsoring events. As a result, our members can enjoy many benefits at little or no cost. In our partnership with the Missoula Symphony Orchestra, our members are treated to two interactive lectures by the orchestra's dynamic music director and are then invited to the dress rehearsal for the spring concert. Another partnership has been with The Springs Retirement Community where courses are offered, on site, for individuals with physical limitations who are unlikely to be able to attend one of our regular on-campus sessions. MOLLI benefits from the outreach opportunity while the Springs reciprocates by opening their facility to non-residents.

MOLLI has another unique partnership with the Montana Museum of Art and Culture, on the UM campus. Our collaboration has included art lectures (plus wine and cheese) associated with current exhibits. One of the most powerful collaborations was a 6-week course in conjunction with the exhibit *Capture the Moment: Pulitzer Prize Photographs*. One member noted: *The history of photography, the technical aspects of photos and the composition (I'll never again look at a photo with the same eyes), a new view of the race issue and news photography…both the exhibit and the class have blown me away!*

Missoula is home to the *International Wildlife Film Festival*, which gave us the opportunity to have Michele and Howard Hall, internationally known oceanographers, give a presentation related to their work. This spring we joined with the IWFF to sponsor a talk on wildlife trade issues in Southeast Asia.

First Night Missoula, an alcohol free celebration for the New Year is another Missoula community collaboration. This has been a great success, with over 500 individuals of all ages participating thus far.

During the lifetime of MOLLI, the leadership has made a concerted effort to engage older learners in science, knowing that many over 50 are intimidated by the topic. We began with a 2-day summer intergenerational science camp for grandparents and their grandchildren 8–12 years of age. The camp, *MOLLI Grandparents and Grandkids: Connecting the Circle,* brought together the generations to engage in shared scientific exploration. Topics included: *The Buzz about Bees, Fun with Stars*, and *The Magic of Chemistry.* In each case pairs were able to participate in hands-on learning, with science experiments that were both challenging and entertaining. One of the young students in the "Bee" course was visually impaired and the instructor placed a male bee (which has no stinger) in the student's hand, enabling him to feel what he could not see. This experience was significant not only for the child, but also for the professor, as he learned how best to engage visually impaired students. Participants in the camp noted: *An absolutely terrific experience to share with the kids…Great idea to connect the generations…Yes, yes, yes, [I would attend again] quality time with a grandchild, plus it will keep the old brain alive and tingling!* The camp was so successful in its first summer (2009) that it was held again in 2010. The age range was expanded to include children of 6–8, and participation doubled. Catchy titles surely played a part, with *Incredible Edible Bugs,*

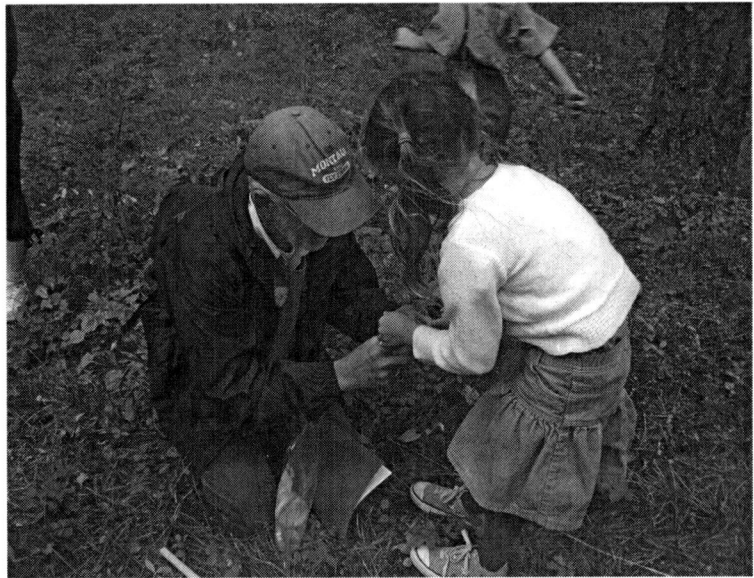

Grandparents and Grandchildren summer camp from the *Incredible Edible Bugs* course

Bones and Stones, and Wild Weather Wonders among the offerings. The summer camp was sponsored in part through a grant from Montana EPSCoR and the National Science Foundation through the spectrUM Discovery Area, UM's interactive applied science museum.

This led to a second science project, one which is associated with the NRC for OLLIs that received a planning grant from the National Science Foundation to encourage more effective ways to connect informal science learning and older adults. The Montana institute was one of six OLLI's selected to receive funding to support development of a partnership with local informal science educators to conduct pilot projects; in our case, we once again worked with spectrUM. Two courses were presented, *Wonder Wheels* which focused on the physics of bicycling and *Classic Mediterranean Cuisine: Chemistry in the Culinary Laboratory*. The latter brought together a master chef and a UM chemistry professor for an evening of food, wine and the chemistry of each. The goal was to increase the participants' knowledge of science through a multimodal learning experience. A full evaluation of the project indicated that the 30 older adults not only thoroughly enjoyed the experience, but also, based on pre- and post-tests, actually learned a great deal about the chemistry of cooking. One participant indicated, *Best class ever; really enjoyed combining science and cooking…[It] had everything from sensory pleasure to cultural cuisine* [and] *science.*

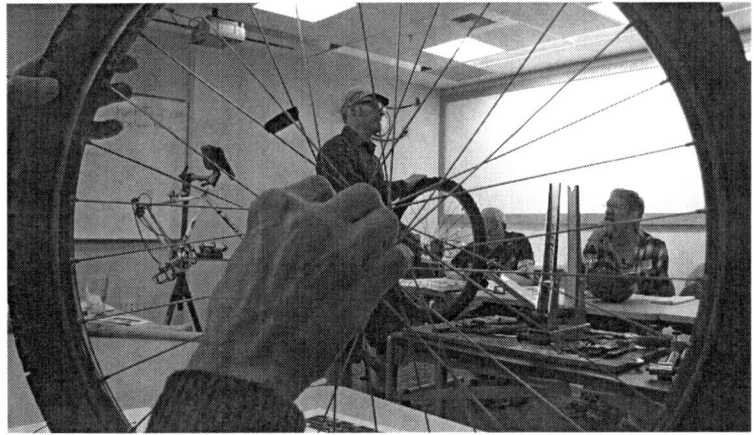

National Science Foundation Grant course *Wonder Wheels* bike physics course

The importance of planning, as it relates to sustainability, cannot be overemphasized for organizations such as MOLLI. In the long run, it is as important as program content and marketing. According to Collins (2005), "A great organization is one that delivers superior performance and makes a distinctive impact over a long period of time…Performance must be assessed relative to mission, not financial returns …" The critical question is not "How much money do we make?" but "How effectively do we deliver on our mission and make a distinctive impact, relative to our resources?" Measured by that yardstick, MOLLI is meeting the objectives of its mission. As one member noted, *I'm living my life differently because of this course*, which vividly describes the power of an organization devoted to elder learning.

Support from a university for an OLLI is required by the Osher Foundation, creating an invaluable partnership that allows the institute to utilize the university's resources such as staff and location as well as its image and brand for excellence. Meeting the needs of the university is important as well, so a partnership was formed with the UM Staff Senate granting staff members a 20% discount on MOLLI courses.

The OLLI at the University of Montana has several strengths:

1. It was initiated at the suggestion of the president of the university, and continues to enjoy his enthusiastic support, along with that of the provost and faculty members.
2. It is an approved institute of the University of Montana under the direction of the Dean of Continuing Education.
3. It has a passionate, dedicated advisory council and committee members who work hard to achieve sustainability.
4. It has over 1,200 passionate members.

MOLLI is a strong organization and, through good leadership, it will continue to achieve its mission to address the intellectual needs of individuals 50-plus who are excited about learning. To ensure that the program will continue well into the future, fundraising initiatives must be created to add to our established revenue streams. Thus, to supplement endowment income and membership and course revenues, we anticipate establishing a planned giving program as well as strategically directed giving. Already we receive donations from members, and faculty members often donate part or all of their honoraria. These donations go into a fund to provide tuition waivers for students who cannot afford to attend courses. We acknowledge that continuing to investigate other fundraising and grant opportunities is necessary to sustain the program over time.

The Culture of a Responsive Organization

According to Collins (2001), the road to greatness is paved with discipline: disciplined people, thought and action. Passion, though a great resource, doesn't always result in greatness. While MOLLI Council, committees, and staff members do admit to being very passionate about MOLLI, we also act on the knowledge that a balanced and forward-looking budget, continued recruitment of dynamic faculty, development of varied program formats, and cultivation of new members are all important to ensure a great organization.

Viewing MOLLI from the outset, there was no single defining action that created the program. Ours was a cumulative process that developed one step at a time. With strong community response coupled with dynamic volunteer participation and supported by university capabilities, we have achieved results well beyond our original vision. If we maintain all of this while sustaining our enthusiasm and commitment, we will continue to influence positively the lives of older adults in our community.

Sharon Alexander was the Dean of Continuing Education at the University of Montana (retired) and the former director of the Osher Lifelong Learning Institute at UM. A founding member of the Institute, Dean Alexander has guided its development from the outset and has participated actively as a MOLLI member. She has degrees from University of Toronto, University of Victoria and a doctorate from Brigham Young University.

Cynthia B. Aten, MD is a graduate of Yale School of Medicine, Goddard College and Duke University. She practiced pediatrics and adolescent medicine in New Haven, Connecticut prior to serving as Chief of Undergraduate Medicine at Yale University. In 2004 she moved to Missoula, Montana, to be near one set of grandchildren. She has served on the Osher Lifelong Learning Institute at the University of Montana's Council and Membership and Marketing Committee.

Dannette Fadness is the Coordinator of MOLLI. She earned undergraduate degrees in art and counseling psychology from the University of Great Falls and graduated, with distinction, with an MS in Science of Managing Organizations and Human Development. She recently received a Public Anthropology Award for Excellence in Writing on Public Issues. In 2007, she moved back to her home state of Montana after her husband retired from 22 years in the U.S. Air Force to be closer to family, including their six grandsons.

Kali Lightfoot is the Executive Director of the National Resource Center for the Osher Lifelong Learning Institutes.

References

Collins, J. (2001). *Why some companies make the leap ... and others don't: good-to-great*. New York: Harperbusiness.
Collins, J. (2005). *Why business thinking is not the answer: good to great and the social sector: A monograph to accompany good to great*. Boulder, CO: Jim Collins.
Koeppel, D. (2007, August). Best places to live + play: Mountain towns. *National GeographicAdventure*. Retrieved February 7, 2010, from http://www.nationalgeographic.com/adventure/relocating/best-places-to-live-2007/mountains/mountains.html
Lawrence-Lightfoot, S. (2009). *The third chapter: Passion, risk and adventure in the 25 years after 50*. New York: Farrar, Straus and Giroux.

Chapter 8
Closing the Generation Gap: Using Discussion Groups to Benefit Older Adults and College Students

Kelly E. Cichy and Gregory C. Smith

Abstract Designing class activities that enable students to interact with older adults in meaningful ways is one of the most powerful tools of undergraduate gerontological education. This chapter describes the benefits of participating in intergenerational discussion groups for undergraduate students and older adults. Throughout the semester, older adults attended four to five *Introduction to Gerontology* class sessions, where together with the undergraduate students they participated in thought provoking dialogs about current gerontological issues. The goal was for older adults and college students alike to gain knowledge, improve problem solving skills, and question their own belief systems. After participating in the discussion groups, the undergraduate students indicated that they had an increased understanding of older adults. Further, older adults' self-report questionnaires and focus group participation indicated that attending the groups helped them feel mentally sharp and more knowledgeable about aging. Benefits for both generations will be discussed.

Introduction

Baby Boomers expect more from retirement than previous generations and tend to view retirement as an opportunity for pursuing lifelong learning, civic engagement, and volunteerism (Putnam, 2000; Wilson & Simson, 2003). Volunteerism and lifelong learning have grown internationally due to such worldwide trends as the aging of the population, an emphasis on information and knowledge, and rising levels of formal and informal education (Hori & Cusack, 2006). Both of these endeavors

K.E. Cichy (✉)
Department of Human Development and Family Studies, College of Education, Health, and Human Services, Kent State University, PO Box 5190, Kent, OH, USA
e-mail: kcichy@kent.edu

promote positive health and well-being of older adults by offering opportunities to maintain and enhance their cognitive functioning and by availing them of meaningful and valued social roles (Hinterlong & Williamson, 2006; Simone & Scuilli, 2006).

Universities and colleges are consequently defining their missions in broader terms as centers for lifelong learning, thereby positioning them to support aging boomers who transition to late maturity. Intergenerational service and learning opportunities developed within educational settings deserve special attention in this regard because they have been shown to yield positive outcomes for older and younger participants alike (Public Health, 2004).

Gerontological education represents an ideal context for bringing together undergraduate students and older adult volunteers within an intergenerational context. While studying gerontology, students are encouraged to explore their feelings about being members of an aging society and to think more deeply about their own aging (Alpeter & Marshall, 2003; Whitbourne, 1977). Additional goals of gerontological education are to challenge myths and stereotypes held by students about aging as well as to increase their understanding of the realities of the aging process and their awareness of the diverse experiences of older adults (Stanberry & Azria-Evans, 2001). These are critical goals because ageist beliefs contribute to a host of negative outcomes for older adults, including, but not limited to: isolation from the community, unnecessary institutionalization, and untreated physical and mental illnesses (Nussbaum, Pitts, Huber, Raup Krieger, & Ohs, 2005; Sanders, Fitzgerald, & Bratteli, 2008). Thus, ideal programming should simultaneously confront ageism and provide concrete benefits to both generations.

Here, we report on an innovative intergenerational group discussion activity that was included within an introductory gerontology course at a public research university. In addition to describing the goals, content, and format of this intergenerational activity, we also consider its benefits as perceived by college students and the community-dwelling older adults who participated. Our description of this unique classroom activity is also used to illustrate several key points from the growing literature on civic engagement and volunteerism in the later years.

The Intergenerational Discussion Group Program

An underlying principle behind the intergenerational discussion groups was that class activities which enable students to interact with older adults in meaningfully ways are powerful tools within undergraduate gerontological education (Anderson-Hanley, 1999; Lohman, Griffiths, Coppard, & Cota, 2003). Since educationally-based interactions between college students and older adults typically involve service-learning arrangements in residential care settings where older adults have significant cognitive or physical impairments (Blieszner & Artale, 2001; Shapiro, 2002), our goal was to create an intergenerational learning environment where younger and older adults were equals. This encouraged an atmosphere in which all persons, regardless of age, had their opinions heard and valued (Stanberry & Azria-Evans, 2001). In contrast, interactions with older patients in care settings (e.g., nursing homes) often lead to one-sided discussions that inadvertently reinforce students' ageist beliefs (Shapiro, 2002).

Our program addressed these issues by inviting community-dwelling older adults into the college classroom to participate in intergenerational discussion groups with college-aged adults.

The older adult guests were recruited through the University alumni office, from existing university programs for older adults, through articles in the local newspaper, and later through word of mouth from previous older adult guests. The newspaper articles appeared to be the most fruitful recruitment approach. The intergenerational discussion groups occurred across several semesters and involved a total of 35 older guests, many who participated during multiple semesters. The older adult guests ranged in age from their early 60s to early 90s, and each semester the group of older adult guests included equal numbers of men and women. The majority of our participants had some college and many completed a Bachelor's degree.

Each group discussion included at least two older adults and five to eight students. The groups were designed so that both generations had equal status within the discussions to ensure that all participants, regardless of age, could have their opinions expressed and valued (Stanberry & Azria-Evans, 2001). Equal status among participants was demonstrated by various group roles (e.g., timekeeper, moderator, recorder, and reporter) that were shared equally among the students and older adult members of each group. Additionally, the older adults were purposely referred to as "guests," which is in stark contrast to the "patient" or "client" labels typically assigned to older adults involved with intergenerational service-learning activities.

To further reinforce the equal status of both generations, students and older adults rated each others' contributions to the discussion sessions.

Prior to each session, the students and guests read articles on the specific topic to be discussed, and received a series of discussion questions to address during that session. These materials were selected and distributed in advance by the course instructor. The overarching goals of this intergenerational learning activity, from a liberal education perspective, were for both the older "guests" and students to explore jointly issues of high societal importance, gain knowledge, improve problem solving skills, question their own beliefs, hear the views of others, and to examine the consequences of their beliefs. After each intergenerational discussion session, students completed a one page written reflection requiring them to relate their intergenerational discussion group experiences to course content as well as to their personal views on aging.

Each session included a 45-min intergenerational group discussion period where six different groups met in separate locations to discuss thought provoking topics related to aging (e.g., healthcare rationing; radical life extension; gender and ageism; the future of retirement). This was followed by a 30-min "plenary" session where each group reported on the major points raised by its members, and all participants were encouraged to further express their views in this larger forum. The plenary sessions typically involved anywhere between 50 and 60 students and "guests." Table 8.1 provides a description of program highlights.

Table 8.1 Program highlights for the intergenerational discussion groups

Students and older adults received readings and discussion questions to read and review prior to meeting in their discussion groups

Two older adult guests were assigned to each discussion group. Each week older adult guests were assigned to different student discussion groups to provide both generations with optimal exposure to a diverse group

Discussion groups met in separate, semiprivate locations throughout a university building to engage in the intergenerational discussion groups

Members divided responsibilities and assigned roles (i.e., timekeeper, moderator, recorder, and reporter) for group members

5-Min break

Each group returned to classroom for a Plenary session with the entire class, where a reporter from each group presented the main points of their group's discussion to the larger audience

Discussion was opened up to the entire class

Both students and older adult guests evaluated each others' preparation and group participation

Expected Outcomes

We believed that participation in the intergenerational discussion groups would be of mutual benefit to the older guests and college students alike in view of considerable evidence that learning activities which involve intergenerational experiences provide benefits for both generations (Hinterlong & Williamson, 2006; Rebok et al., 2004). For example, older adult volunteers for the school-based program, Experience Corps achieved improved health and well-being while at the same time academic achievement improved for the elementary school students who worked with the older adult mentors (Rebok et al., 2004; Chapter 27 this volume).

Benefits to Older Guests

We anticipated positive outcomes for the older "guests" because the intergenerational discussion group activity combined lifelong learning with volunteerism. In fact, the goals of lifelong learning mirror the motivations for volunteerism in later life given that both can provide older adults with meaningful, valued, and productive social roles (Bradley, 1999; Hinterlong & Williamson, 2006; Simone & Scuilli, 2006). In turn, productive roles give older adults an enhanced sense of purpose by allowing them to give back to society (Bradley, 1999). In fact, a review of the literature on older volunteers suggests that they are motivated by altruistic concerns and esteem values, such as the desire to be useful, to feel productive, to fulfill moral obligations, and to a lesser extent by factors such as the opportunity to learn new skills or the opportunity for social interaction (Grano, Lucidi, Zelli, & Violani, 2008). There is even speculation that younger volunteers may not experience the same benefits because their volunteering is usually obligatory (e.g., tied to other duties, such as parenting), whereas volunteering by older persons is more likely to be discretionary and thus provides them with purposeful roles in their community (Grim, Spring, & Dietz, 2007).

There is also evidence that some older adults are motivated to volunteer in order to learn more about a particular issue and to expand their knowledge (Guterbock & Fries, 1997). Similarly, the majority of older adult learners appear to be motivated by expressive goals that emphasize learning and knowledge for its own sake (Kim & Merriam, 2004; Leung, Lui, & Chi, 2005). Older adults perceive learning experiences to be most effective and interesting when the experience is deeply engaging and focuses on familiar or relevant topics (Duay & Bryan, 2008). Older adults have also been found to express deep interest in volunteering as mentors or tutors to young people or to help elderly adults live independently (Moore, 2008). To a large extent, the intergenerational discussion groups satisfied the above motives by directly involving the older adult volunteers in discussions with undergraduate students. Further, the focus of the discussions was on gerontological topics that they were quite familiar with due to their own aging and where they believed that the students would benefit from hearing their personal experiences first hand.

Evaluating Outcomes from the Older Adult Guests' Perspective

Method

Procedure and measure. We employed a multi-method approach to evaluate the benefits of participating in the intergenerational discussion groups for the older guests. First, the perceived benefits of participating in the intergenerational discussion groups were assessed through a self-report questionnaire. Participants answered a series of questions about their experiences by indicating how much they agreed with each statement using a 4-point scale ranging from 1 (*strongly disagree*) to 4 (*strongly agree*). Examples of the items include: *I felt like I was giving back to the younger generation as a result of participating in the intergenerational discussion groups* and *I found that participating in the intergenerational group discussions helped to keep me mentally sharp.* This questionnaire was mailed to the older adult guests, and was subsequently completed by 11 older adult guests.

After completing the self-report questionnaires, the older adult guests were invited to participate in a focus group held on-campus. A subsample of the older guests attended the focus group ($n=7$, 2 males, 5 females), where they answered a series of open-ended questions about their experiences participating in the intergenerational discussion groups. The questions asked during the focus group focused on obtaining more open-ended descriptions of reasons for volunteering to participate in the groups (e.g., *What did you expect the groups to be like when you first expressed interest in participating?*), the perceived benefits of participating in the intergenerational discussion groups (e.g., *How did your view of your own aging change as a result of participating?*), and suggestions for improving the quality of this program in the future.

Results: Older Adult Guests' Perspective

Self-Report Questionnaire Findings. The results from the self-report questionnaires indicated that the majority of older guests perceived participating in the intergenerational groups as a positive experience. All said that they would encourage other people their age to participate and that participating made them feel like they were giving back to the younger generation (Table 8.2). As expected, the majority also agreed that after participating in the groups they had a more positive view of college-aged adults. The questionnaire results also revealed that most respondents felt that participating in the groups made them feel better about themselves, made them feel more self-confident and capable, helped to keep them mentally sharp, helped them to realize strengths in themselves they never knew existed or had forgotten about, and helped them to become more knowledgeable about aging in general.

Table 8.2 Means and standard deviations for older adult guests' self-questionnaires

Self-report questionnaire items	Mean (SD)
I would encourage other people my age to participate in intergenerational discussion groups	3.92 (0.29)
I have a more positive view of college-aged adults after participating in the intergenerational discussions	3.45 (0.69)
I have a more positive view of other adults my own age after participating in the discussions	3.00 (0.45)
Participating in the discussions made me feel older	1.42 (0.52)
Participating in the intergenerational discussions is a good way to make new friends	3.00 (0.60)
I have a more negative view of other adults my own age after participating in the discussions	1.55 (0.52)
I felt better about myself after participating in the intergenerational discussion groups	3.09 (0.94)
My participation in the intergenerational discussion groups was a waste of my time	1.08 (0.29)
I felt like I was giving back to the younger generation as a result of participating in the intergenerational discussions	3.58 (0.52)
Participating in the intergenerational discussion groups was an important social outlet for me	3.08 (0.52)
At times, participating in the intergenerational discussion groups made me feel younger than I actually am	2.83 (0.58)
Participating in the discussions made me feel more self-confident and capable	2.91 (0.94)
I found that participating in the intergenerational group discussions helped to keep me mentally sharp	3.17 (0.58)
Participating in the intergenerational discussion groups helped me to keep my mind off some problems in my life right now	2.55 (1.04)
Participating in the intergenerational discussion groups helped me to realize strengths in myself that I never knew existed or had forgotten about	2.92 (0.90)
I have a more negative view of college-aged adults after participating in the intergenerational discussions	1.45 (0.69)
I feel as though I have become more knowledgeable about aging in general as a result of participating in the intergenerational discussion groups	3.27 (0.79)

Note. Response scale: 1 (*strongly disagree*), 2 (*disagree*), 3 (*agree*), and 4 (*strongly agree*)

Table 8.3 Thematic codes for focus group responses

Thematic Code	Examples	Kappa
Interest in college-aged adults	Interest in understanding college-aged grandchildren; interest in working with a student population	1.00
Opportunity for productive roles	Productive role in retirement; lifelong volunteerism	0.53
Share aging experience with students	Share experiences with aging with the younger generation	1.00
Change in perspective	Change view of college-aged adults; broaden mind; exposure to new ideas	1.00
Receive advice from students/faculty	Generate ideas for coping with late adulthood	1.00
Understanding of generational/cohort differences	Cohort differences in education, family life, employment opportunities, technology, etc.	1.00
Increased knowledge/interest in study of aging	New ideas about aging; increased knowledge of aging/aging process; beliefs on controversial issues	1.00
Ability to compromise	Ability to compromise; clearly articulate and explain point of view	1.00

Focus Group Findings. The focus group session was audio recorded and then transcribed to categorize responses and identify transcendent themes. The first author identified thematic codes. Then, the second author independently coded the transcribed responses using the identified thematic codes. Table 8.3 provides the inter-rater reliabilities and a description for each code. In addition to the specific codes, we also discuss a number of transcendent themes that emerged.

Motivation for participating emerged as one obvious theme. One primary motive for attending the groups involved an interest in college-aged adults, including the desire to better understand one's own college-aged grandchildren. A second motive focused on the opportunity for productive and meaningful roles in retirement or in response to lifelong volunteerism. As one guest who participated with her husband explained, *We've always been involved in volunteer work, even more so since we retired.* There was also consensus among the guests that it was important to give college-aged adults hands on experience with older people. Everyone endorsed the idea that participating in the intergenerational discussion groups made them feel as if they were giving back to the younger generation. Specifically, they all emphasized the importance of helping today's students understand differences between generations, such as how things have changed from when they themselves were in young adulthood, especially in terms of career opportunities and expectations for family life. These observations are consistent with prior survey findings where adults aged 44–79 expressed a deep interest in volunteering as mentors or tutors to young people (Moore, 2008).

A second theme had to do with the older guests' positive perceptions of the experience. They unanimously said that they would encourage other people their age to participate in the intergenerational discussion groups. They expressed that volunteering for the intergenerational discussion groups gave them an opportunity to share the aging experience with students and to change their own perspectives by changing their view of college-aged students and broadening their mind. The majority agreed that by participating in the discussion groups, they realized that college-aged students are motivated, prepared, and genuinely interested in trying to relate to older adults. As one female said, *You hear so much about the younger generation, and I don't think we have anything to worry about if these young people are an example of what to look forward to.* Her spouse (also a guest) added, *We thoroughly enjoyed it. Really it was, as [she] indicated, very enlightening, that these children, these young people were so sensitive to the needs of the aged and to their family matters over the years.*

The older guests also mentioned they would encourage others to participate to receive advice from students and faculty. For example, one 70-year-old female said, *I got a lot of good ideas about coping with my senior years. The students helped me adjust to that, and I learned a lot from them, just listening to them.* As noted earlier, like these focus group participants, the majority of older adult learners appear to be motivated by expressive goals that emphasize learning and knowledge for its own sake (Kim & Merriam, 2004; Leung et al., 2005).

A third theme concerned social and cognitive benefits derived from the experience. The older guests unanimously agreed that participating in the groups helped to keep them mentally sharp by requiring them to think. Despite their already positive attitudes toward aging, many believed that participating in the groups increased their knowledge and interest in gerontology by offering new ideas about aging, increasing their knowledge of the aging process, and encouraging them to explore their beliefs on controversial issues, such as radical life extension. After participating in the groups, one male shared, *Reading the resource material given to us on the subject matter opened some doors. If I came across a subject in a paper or magazine on the subject, then I was more interested in reading it to get a different opinion.* Another social benefit mentioned was that participating in the groups helped with the ability to compromise, particularly when the groups were required to reach some kind of consensus on a controversial issue. A female guest noted, *I think when you had to make a choice either for or against the program, it took compromise, and you had to explain your point of view. Sometimes it meant changing someone's mind, and I think it was good for the students and the seniors.*

Although not deliberately included as part of the focus group interview protocol, several transcending themes also emerged that are particularly noteworthy because they reinforce several of the key findings and recommendations found in the literature on older volunteers. One transcending theme echoed by the majority of participants was how their involvement was associated with the close ties they had to the university. With very few exceptions, most indicated that they had children or grandchildren who had graduated from or were currently enrolled at the university. One male guest explained that, *Generations have gone through as a result of the University being here. Two sons have graduated from here, three daughters-in-law, and three grandchildren; they paid our dues.* The discussions further revealed that the guests sought additional ways to remain actively involved with the University community.

A female guest said, *I'm scheduled to take a trip to Ireland this August with the [University] group, and I'm delighted to be going.* Although not mentioned during the focus group, many of the guests had been former students or faculty themselves at the University.

These findings are very much in line with the literature on volunteerism where it has been reported that volunteering often serves as a way to maintain connectedness to organizations that have been important to one either currently or in the past. In fact, it is claimed that the biggest single inducement to volunteer is being asked by someone with whom one has an established relationship such that volunteering becomes an extension of one's family, work, and social life, rather than something apart from it (Public Health, 2004). In this regard, colleges and universities may serve as an ideal site for older volunteers who wish to remain connected to the educational institution that has provided a vast reservoir of happy memories and friends (Bradley, 1999). For example, one male guest graduated from the University as a young man and remained active with its Alumni Organization for over 50 years until his recent death.

Another transcending theme was that most of the guests had heard about the groups via the local newspaper or through friends who were already participating. For example, one male guest explained that *We heard from a friend of ours that was in the first session, and he was very enthused, so we joined, and we're very happy that we did.*

Although this finding is not particularly striking by itself, it does speak to the general observation that older adults do not volunteer more frequently simply because they have not been asked to do so. For example, Moore (2008) reported survey findings of 1,000 Americans aged 44–79 where almost half of the respondents said there was a lack of available information about volunteer opportunities, and 68% of those who did not *volunteer* in the past year said they had not been invited to do so. These findings, along with the high interest in the program, imply that more older adults would assume volunteer roles if they were simply asked to do so.

It was also clear from the focus group that although our participants had positive attitudes toward aging, many of them still felt that they had encountered ageism in one form or another in the real world. As one 81-year-old female proclaimed, *If you're a professional person, you don't walk around saying I'm 80. You keep your mouth shut because the stereotype takes over and you're dead in the water.* An older male summed it up by saying, *I had a doctor's appointment last evening and this nurse is beyond a teenager, and whenever she sees me she says, "Hi Sweetie, how you doing?" That really bugs an older person to be treated that way. It's almost like we're childish and we need to be fed.*

These comments took on further significance as the guests went on to mention their belief that interacting with them was a step toward changing students' attitudes toward aging. As one guest said, *I think we've educated them about what being old means. It doesn't mean put them on a shelf, no, they are still functioning people*, said one 70-year-old woman. In fact, another transcending theme was that the guests felt that the students would benefit from increased exposure to the older adults. Not only are these findings consistent with the fundamental goal of gerontology education to reduce ageism among students (Hulicka, 1979), they also reinforce the belief that volunteerism by older adults can be a significant way to replace the negative image of the frail, dependent elder with a view that emphasizes the value of elders and the meaning and purpose of one's later years (Public Health, 2004).

Evaluating Outcomes from the Student Perspective

Methods

Procedure and measures. We also used multiple methods to evaluate the outcomes for the students. These assessments were collected over multiple semesters from varying groups of students. First, we assessed the students' perceived benefits of participating in the intergenerational discussion groups using a self-report questionnaire. Participants answered a series of close-ended items using a 5-point response scale that ranged from 1 *(strongly disagree)* to 5 *(strongly agree)*. Example items included: *My understanding of others has increased* and *I would encourage others my age to participate*. Students also provided open-ended responses evaluating what they liked best about participating in the groups, what they disliked, and what they felt could be improved in the future. The open-ended responses were then reviewed to identify the three most common responses to each question.

We also conducted a separate study to examine whether participating in the intergenerational discussion groups changed undergraduate students' ageist attitudes toward aging. The students who participated in the discussion group during one semester ($n=40$) were compared to a control group of undergraduate students from another introductory gerontology course during the same semester that did not include the intergenerational discussion groups ($n=37$). Although different instructors taught each course, both groups of students were exposed to similar subject matter regarding key concepts, including age-related changes in biological systems, social relationships, social roles (e.g., retirement), cognitive abilities, and health and well-being as well as the implications of the aging of the population. The main difference between the groups was that one group also participated in intergenerational discussion groups as part of the course curriculum and the other group did not.

At the beginning of the semester and again at the end of the semester, both groups completed the Fraboni Scale of Ageism (FSA; Fraboni, Saltstone, & Hughes, 1990). The FSA assesses three components of ageism: (a) antilocution (i.e., expressions of antagonism, antipathy based on misconceptions, misinformation, and/or myths about elderly people); (b) discrimination (i.e., active prejudice regarding political rights, segregation, and intervention into the activities of the elderly); and (c) avoidance (i.e., respondent's withdrawal from social contact with the elderly).

Results: Students' Perspective

Self-Report Questionnaire Findings. The results from the students' self-report questionnaires indicated that nearly all of the students said they would encourage other people their age to participate (91.7%). The majority of students also believed that participating in the groups increased their understanding of others (84.8%) and helped them to grow as a person (61.1%).

Students' open-ended responses revealed that the single thing that the majority (66%) of the students liked best about the intergenerational discussion groups was the ability to interact with the older adults. This finding further supports the value of providing students with opportunities to interact meaningfully with older adults (Anderson-Hanley, 1999; Lohman et al., 2003). Students also indicated that they enjoyed hearing the views of others/meeting new people (37%) and the interesting topics/discussions (~7%). There was very little that the students did not like about participating in the intergenerational discussion groups. In fact, nearly 20% of students said there was nothing they disliked about the groups. About 25% of students disliked that there was not enough time for lengthier discussions. Similarly, 35% of students thought that the groups could be improved with more sessions and longer lasting sessions. This same suggestion was also offered by the older adult guests, suggesting that both generations valued the groups so much that they would appreciate more time for the discussions.

Findings for the Ageism Measure. We examined statistically how attitudinal ageism scores changed from the beginning of the semester to the end of the semester as well as differences in ageism scores between the student groups that did and did not participate in the intergenerational discussion groups. Unexpectedly, participating in the intergenerational discussion groups did not appear to change students' scores on any of the ageism subscales. In other words, participating in the intergenerational discussion groups did not significantly alter students' ageist attitudes toward aging.

Implications and Future Directions

Overall, our findings revealed benefits of participating in the intergenerational discussion groups for both generations. Both generations agreed that they would encourage other people their age to participate in the groups. After participating in the discussion groups, undergraduate students reported an increased understanding of others and personal growth, and the older adult guests indicated that they held more positive attitudes toward college-aged adults. In particular, the majority of older adult guests volunteered because of their desire to better understand their college-aged grandchildren. This increased the understanding that is likely to have implications for individuals, families, and society by improving the quality of intergenerational relationships (e.g., grandparent-grandchild relationships) and increasing support and advocacy for public policies for the aged and the younger generation alike (Hulicka, 1979). Taken together, our findings imply that both generations perceived participating in these intergenerational discussion groups to be a worthwhile educational experience.

Unexpectedly, our findings did not provide support for incorporating these intergenerational discussion groups into college courses as a strategy for improving college-aged adults' attitudes toward aging per se. Participating in the intergenerational discussion groups may not have significantly changed students' attitudes toward aging because their scores on the ageism measure were relatively low at the beginning of the semester, and so there was little room for improvement. On the other hand, our quantitative and qualitative results clearly suggested that the students appreciated the opportunity to interact with the older adults. This provides further support for the value of incorporating meaningful social interactions between older adults and students into undergraduate gerontology courses (Anderson-Hanley, 1999; Lohman et al., 2003).

Participating in the intergenerational discussion groups also offered the older adult guests a chance to share their experiences with the younger generation. This desire is consistent with prior research that suggests older adults express deep interest in volunteer opportunities that offer them the chance to mentor younger individuals (Moore, 2008). These intergenerational discussion groups offered the older adults an experience that combines elements of volunteerism with opportunities for lifelong learning. These groups are unique from other service-learning opportunities because they bring the older adult guests into the university classroom to learn alongside the undergraduate students. Both generations had equal status within the groups, providing a means for them to learn from each other (Stanberry & Azria-Evans, 2001). In particular, the older adult guests felt that they helped the students understand generational differences in education, career opportunities, and family life. At the same time, however, the older adult guests believed that they also learned a great deal from the undergraduate students.

Consistent with prior research on volunteering and lifelong learning, the older adult guests unanimously endorsed the idea that participating in the intergenerational discussion groups helped to keep them mentally sharp. Countless studies emphasize the importance of engaging in cognitively stimulating activities as a key to successful aging (e.g., Hultsch, Hertzog, Small, & Dixon, 1999; Jung, Gruenewald, Seeman, & Sarkisian, 2010; Schooler, & Mulatu, 2001). Our findings suggest that participating in these intergenerational discussion groups may represent a strategy for maintaining cognitive functioning in late life. Specifically, participation in the groups encouraged the older adults to pursue cognitively stimulating activities, such as reading articles, engaging in lively discussions, and defending their positions on controversial topics.

The older adults also revealed during the focus group that they believed that participating in the groups helped to increase their knowledge and interest in the study of aging. Indeed, older adults are often motivated to volunteer in order to expand their knowledge (Guterbock & Fries, 1997). To this end, it was clear that the older adult guests used the knowledge acquired in class to help them evaluate the quality of the information on aging they encountered in newspapers and magazines. In other words, there was qualitative evidence suggesting that the older adults used their experience as a means of becoming more informed consumers of research on aging.

The quantitative results also showed that the majority of older adults perceived other benefits to participating in the groups, including effects on their self-image, self-confidence, and attitudes toward their own aging. It is important to point out that these social and cognitive benefits were perceived as a result of participating only a few hours each month. Thus, the present findings are consistent with prior research suggesting that older adults can benefit from just a small amount of volunteering without having to make a labor or time intensive commitment (Rozario & Tang, 2003). It has been reported, for example that benefits can be obtained with a small amount of volunteering, even as little as 3 h per month (Morrow-Howell, Hinterlong, Rozario, & Tang, 2003; Musick & Wilson, 2003).

It has also been noted in the literature that older adults who volunteer too many hours may experience role strain that limits the positive benefits of volunteering (Lum & Lightfoot, 2005). Since such strain is most likely to occur among very old adults, it is noteworthy that many of the older guests in our intergenerational groups were in their late 80s and early 90s. In fact, several of them attended repeatedly despite considerable health limitations such as broken limbs, mobility difficulties, and respiratory problems requiring a portable oxygen tank. Thus, the discussion groups exemplify a much needed type of volunteerism that even very old and frail individuals can meaningfully participate in (Bradley, 1999; Guterbock & Fries, 1997).

Finding new ways, such as the intergenerational discussion groups, to involve frail older adults with volunteering is significant because numerous studies suggest that rates of both volunteerism and lifelong learning drop off after age 75 due to chronic health conditions that limit older adults' capacity to participate in such activities (Bradley, 1999; Guterbock & Fries, 1997). Still, research consistently shows that volunteering and lifelong learning benefits health and well-being, particularly at older ages (Greenfield & Marks, 2004; Hinterlong & Williamson, 2006; Lum & Lightfoot, 2005; Rozario & Tang, 2003; Van Willigen, 2000).

Intergenerational discussion groups also provide an opportunity for older adults to engage in lifelong learning beyond enrolling in noncredit college-level courses. The type of learning activity described here offers a self-structured experience characterized by less evaluation and less potential for failure than more traditional classroom experiences. As stated earlier, participation in the intergenerational discussion groups involved a relatively small time commitment that seemed to be manageable for our older adult guests.

Limitations

It is important, to acknowledge the potential limitations of our approach. The current findings are based on a relatively small sample of older adult guests. Further, research on both volunteerism and lifelong learning in later adulthood are biased toward highly educated, healthy, young old adults (Bradley, 1999; Guterbock & Fries, 1997;

Kim & Merriam, 2004). The current study also included primarily well-educated older adults, although we did have more diversity in terms of age and health status.

We also failed to examine potential physical health benefits of participating in the intergenerational discussion groups even though numerous past studies have repeatedly shown volunteering by older adults to be related to reduced mortality, increased physical function, increased levels of self-rated health, muscular strength, reduced depression, and reduced pain (see for review, Lum & Lightfoot, 2005; Tang, Choi, & Morrow-Howell, 2010). However, this particular limitation within our work is somewhat diminished by the recent conclusion that it is actually the social integration and meaningful engagement aspects of volunteer activity that best explain the positive health effects found among older volunteers (Tang et al., 2010).

It is also noteworthy that the benefits of the intergenerational discussion group activity do not end with those identified above for the student and older guest participants. For example, although guests' exposure to any particular group of students ends when the semester is over, many of the guests have developed on ongoing relationship with the instructor. Such interactions have involved email-greetings sent by guests, newspaper articles and other materials related to course content mailed to the instructor, and occasional updates from guests on their significant life events (e.g., birthdays, great-grandchildren, vacation, and personal illnesses). The benefits of the intergenerational discussion groups also extend to the University by providing a concrete demonstration of its desire to engage with and serve the larger community.

Lessons Learned

Still, our experiences with the discussion groups taught us a number of important and unanticipated lessons. First, because the older adults proved to be accurate judges of their own physical and cognitive ability to participate, there was no need for a formal screening procedure. In fact, we would caution against using physical health as a rigid inclusion criterion. For example, there were times when older guests were unable to participate in a few sessions due to injuries (e.g., broken foot) or unexpected illnesses. Rather than dropping out, these older adult guests returned to the groups as soon as they were able. Additionally, some guests attended regularly despite having substantial physical needs and limitations (e.g., portable oxygen tank) that one might reasonably expect to restrict participation. Not only did these experiences highlight the older adult guests' commitment to the groups, they also taught us the importance of being flexible and prepared for these issues to arise. To compensate for unexpected health issues, we recruited more older adult guests than needed to ensure there were always at least two older adults available for each group.

As stated earlier, the majority of our older adult guests were highly educated and had ties to the university. A second lesson is that less educated older adults are sometimes intimidated about attending college courses. For example, one female guest without a college degree expressed concerns about her ability to participate. The instructor encouraged her to attend the sessions, and she made meaningful contributions and ultimately enjoyed the experience. Thus, it is important to deliberately reach out to those with lower levels of formal education.

We also discovered that both generations preferred to have the older adult guests change discussion groups each week. Although this requires more effort on the part of the instructor, it provides both generations with increased exposure to diverse perspectives. We also found that some topics, particularly timely issues, such as radical life extension, generated the liveliest discussions. Therefore, it is important to be selective about the topics to most effectively stimulate discussion. Frequently, the older adult guests would bring newspaper articles to class related to the discussion topics. Instructors could make this spontaneous activity a more formal procedure to encourage students and older adults to actively look for examples of gerontology in the news to further inform the intergenerational discussions.

Both the students and the older adult guests also indicated that they would have appreciated more discussion sessions throughout the semester. More frequent discussions would increase students' exposure to the older adult guests, however, more frequent sessions would also take time away from the more traditional lecture format. Obviously, the instructor needs to establish a balance between traditional instruction and the intergenerational activity that fits best with his/her goals for the course.

There are a number of logistical considerations when it comes to implementing these discussion groups in the college classroom. First, this activity is best suited for a moderate class size (e.g., 50 students) to keep the groups manageable. This is important because of the inevitable space constraints and time considerations. In order to ensure the groups had privacy for their discussions, we made every effort to provide each group with a semiprivate location within a campus building. This often meant commandeering multiple classrooms and conference rooms for the intergenerational discussion groups. We were able to do this because the course met in the evening when there were fewer other classes in session. It may be more challenging to conduct these groups during the day when numerous courses are competing for space.

Similarly, because the class met once a week for 2 h, we had time for the groups to meet individually and then to come together for the plenary session. This approach would certainly be more challenging to implement in a typical 50-min class session. We were fortunate to have the optimal conditions for the intergenerational discussion groups. Adjustments would need to be made to the format to accommodate a different set of classroom conditions.

Finally, we realized that it is important to facilitate parking for the older adult guests. Parking spaces are at a premium at most universities, yet we found that this small issue made a great deal of difference for the older adult guests. Fortunately, we were able to provide the older adult guests with permits for a nearby parking lot to make it easier for them to attend the sessions. This alleviated some of the issues, but even this arrangement presented challenges during periods of inclement weather and for older adults with mobility issues. In an ideal situation, the older adult guests would be able to park as close to the building as possible.

In the future, we believe a similar approach could be adopted to develop other intergenerational programs to serve underrepresented groups of older adults (e.g., lower socioeconomic status, those with chronic health conditions). For example, a number of service-learning programs in colleges and universities involve teaching older adults how to improve their health and well-being. We believe that even these intergenerational programs focused on health promotion for older adults could be framed in terms of the older adults serving as "mentors" for the college students. In addition to the service being provided to older adults, such as exercise programs and wellness training, the older adult participants are likely to provide the students with new perspectives on aging.

In the same way, we believe these intergenerational discussion groups could also be constructive for other disciplines outside of gerontology, particularly any context where there may be different generational perspectives. For example, students in a Political Science or Sociology course are likely to benefit from considering not only their own views, but also the views of another generation of adults.

Summary and Conclusions

In conclusion, these intergenerational discussion groups bring together components of volunteerism and lifelong learning to mutually benefit two generations, college-aged students and older adult guests. Opportunities, such as these intergenerational discussion groups, simultaneously satisfy the preferences and desires of both generations by providing older adults with the opportunity to mentor young people (Moore, 2008) and enabling undergraduate students to interact with older adults in meaningful ways (Anderson-Hanley, 1999; Lohman et al., 2003). All members had equal status within the groups, and participating improved students' understanding of others and older adults' perceptions of college-aged young adults.

The older adult guests, however, also perceived a host of other social and cognitive benefits, where they believed that participating in the groups helped keep them mentally sharp, made them feel more knowledgeable about aging, and allowed them to give back in a meaningful way to the younger generation. These benefits were perceived by bringing community-dwelling older adults into the university classroom for only a few hours each month. Often older adults do not volunteer because they are not invited (Moore, 2008). In the current program, not only were they invited to participate, but they were actively recruited because of the unique perspective they could bring to the experience. Our findings remind us of the value of taking advantage of enduring ties between communities and universities forged through the generations. Finally, the overall benefits of the intergenerational discussion groups were summed up best by one of our male respondents, *I would say if you don't want to change and grow and be challenged, then stay away. You'll have all of those things.*

References

Alpeter, M., & Marshall, V. M. (2003). Making aging "real" for undergraduates. *Educational Gerontology, 29*, 739–7556.

Anderson-Hanley, C. (1999). Experiential activities for teaching psychology of aging. *Educational Gerontology, 25*, 449–456.

Blieszner, R., & Artale, L. M. (2001). Benefits of intergenerational service-learning to human services majors. *Educational Gerontology, 27*, 71–87.

Bradley, D. B. (1999). A reason to rise each morning: The meaning of volunteering in the lives of older adults. *Generations, 23*, 45–50.

Duay, D. L., & Bryan, V. C. (2008). Learning in later life: What seniors want in a learning experience. *Educational Gerontology, 34*, 1070–1086.

Fraboni, M., Saltstone, R., & Hughes, S. (1990). The Fraboni scale of ageism (FSA): An attempt at a more precise measure of ageism. *Canadian Journal on Aging, 9*, 56–66.

Grano, C., Lucidi, F., Zelli, A., & Violani, C. (2008). Motives and determinants of volunteering in older adults: An integrated model. *International Journal of Aging & Human Development, 67*, 305–326.

Greenfield, E. A., & Marks, N. F. (2004). Formal volunteering as a protective factor for older adults' psychological well-being. *The Journals of Gerontology, Social Sciences, 59B*, S258–S264.

Grim, R., & Spring, K. (2007). & Dietz, N. The health benefits of volunteering: A review of recent research. Corporation for National and Community Service.

Guterbock, T. M., & Fries, J. C. (1997). *Maintaining American's social fabric: The AARP survey of civic involvement.* American Association of Retired Persons: Washington, DC.

Hinterlong, J. E., & Williamson, A. (2006, Winter). The effects of civic engagement of current and future cohorts of older adults. *Generations*, 10–17.

Hori, S., & Cusack, S. (2006). Third-age education in Canada and Japan: Attitudes toward aging and participation in learning. *Educational Gerontology, 32*, 463–481.

Hulicka, I. (1979). *Teaching undergraduate courses in adult development and aging.* Mt. Desert, ME: Beech Hill Enterprises.

Hultsch, D. F., Hertzog, C., Small, B. J., & Dixon, R. A. (1999). Use or lose it: Engaged lifestyle as a buffer of cognitive decline in aging? *Psychology and Aging, 14*, 245–263.

Jung, Y. Y., Gruenewald, T. L., Seeman, T. E., & Sarkisian, C. A. (2010). Productive activities and development of frailty in older adults. *Journals of Gerontology, Psychological Sciences and Social Sciences, 65*, 256–261.

Kim, A., & Merriam, S. B. (2004). Motivations for learning among older adults in a learning in retirement institute. *Educational Gerontology, 30*, 441–455.

Leung, A., Lui, Y., & Chi, I. (2005). Later life learning experience among Chinese elderly in Hong Kong. *Gerontology & Geriatrics Education, 26*, 1–15.

Lohman, H., Griffiths, Y., Coppard, B., & Cota, C. (2003). The power of book discussion groups in intergenerational learning. *Educational Gerontology, 29*, 103–115.

Lum, T. Y., & Lightfoot, E. (2005). The effects of volunteering on the physical and mental health of older people. *Research on Aging, 27*, 31–55.

Moore, C. J. (2008). 73% of older Americans volunteer, survey finds. *Chronicle of Philanthropy*, 20.

Morrow-Howell, N., Hinterlong, J., Rozario, P. A., & Tang, F. (2003). Effects of volunteering on the well-being of older adults. *The Journals of Gerontology, Social Sciences, 58B*, S137–145.

Musick, M., & Wilson, J. (2003). Volunteering and depression: The role of psychological and social resources in different age groups. *Social Science and Medicine, 56*, 259–269.

Nussbaum, J. F., Pitts, M. J., Huber, F. N., Raup Krieger, J. L., & Ohs, J. E. (2005). Ageism and ageist language across the life span: Intimate relationships and non-intimate interactions. *Journal of Social Issues, 61*, 287–305.

Health, P. (2004). *Reinventing aging: Baby boomers and civic engagement.* Boston, MA: Harvard School of Public Health.

Putnam, R. (2000). *Bowling Alone*. New York: Simon and Schuster.

Rebok, G. W., Carlson, M. C., Glass, T. A., McGill, S., Hill, J., Wasik, B. A., et al. (2004). Short-term impact of Experience Corps participation on children and schools: Results from a pilot randomized trial. *Journal of Urban Health, 81*, 79–93.

Rozario, P. A., & Tang, F. (2003). Effects of volunteering on the well-being of older adults. *Journal of Gerontology, 58B*, S137–S145.

Sanders, G. F., Fitzgerald, M. A., & Bratteli, M. (2008). Mental health services for older adults in rural areas: An ecological systems approach. *Journal of Applied Gerontology, 27*, 252–266.

Schooler, C., & Mulatu, M. S. (2001). The reciprocal effects of leisure time activities and intellectual functioning in older people: A longitudinal analysis. *Psychology and Aging, 16*, 466–482.

Shapiro, A. (2002). A service-learning approach to teaching gerontology: A case study of a first-year undergraduate seminar. *Gerontology and Geriatrics Education, 23*, 25–36.

Simone, R., & Scuilli, M. (2006, Fall). Cognitive benefits of participation in lifelong learning institutes. In *The LLI Review* (Vol. 1, pp. 44–51). Portland, ME: University of Southern Maine: Osher Lifelong Learning Institute.

Stanberry, A., & Azria-Evans, M. (2001). Perspectives in teaching gerontology: Matching strategies with purpose and content. *Educational Gerontology, 27*, 639–656.

Tang, F., Choi, E., & Morrow-Howell, N. (2010). *Organization support and volunteering benefits for older adults* (pp. 1–10). Special Issue: The Gerontologist.

Van Willigen, M. (2000). Differential benefits of volunteering across the life course. *Journals of Gerontology, Psychological Sciences and Social Sciences, 55*, S308–S318.

Wilson, L. B., & Simson, S. (2003). Combining lifelong learning with civic engagement: A university-based model. *Gerontology & Geriatrics Education, 24*, 47–61.

Whitbourne, S. K. (1977). Goals of undergraduate education in gerontology. *Educational Gerontology, 2*, 131–139.

Chapter 9
A Practical Guide to Senior Odyssey

Elizabeth A.L. Stine-Morrow and Jeanine M. Parisi

Abstract This chapter describes Senior Odyssey, a program of activity engagement which offers opportunities for intellectual challenge in a social context. Core elements include ill-defined problem-solving, team-based collaboration, competition, and play. We provide the history of the Senior Odyssey, a description of program logistics, and an overview of outcomes.

Introduction

Much has been written in recent years about the swift change in global demographics over the last century. While 100 years ago, it was a relatively rare occurrence to encounter an adult past the age of 65, the number of older adults will soon outnumber children for the first time in history (e.g., Kinsella & He, 2009). We are getting older, with some recent projections suggesting that individuals born in developed countries in the twenty-first century will be as likely as not to reach their 100th birthday (Christensen, Doblhammer, Rau, & Vaupel, 2009). Old age is young!

Cultural and social models that define the sorts of activities and roles that are available to individuals during the first half of the life span are well articulated (e.g., education, work roles, parenting, civic leadership), but we are still learning how to be old. First, few social institutions are now in place that offer meaningful

---

E.A.L. Stine-Morrow (✉)
Psychology, and the Beckman Institute, University of Illinois at Urbana-Champaign, Champaign, IL, USA
e-mail: eals@illinois.edu

roles later in life, particularly those that engage cognitive and intellectual capacities in a significant way (Riley & Riley, 2000). To the extent that mind, brain, and behavior are sculpted through the life span through the activities to which we allocate our time and effort (Hertzog, Kramer, Wilson, & Lindenberger, 2008; Kramer & Willis, 2002; Li, 2003), the dearth of such roles create a cultural context that would not be expected to normatively engender lifelong cognitive vitality. Second, to some extent we learn how to be old from those who have grown old before us, and limitations in health care and medicine for older cohorts may provide successive generations with more limited conceptions of different forms of successful aging. In fact, there is some evidence that those who have been exposed in youth to older adults with more vitality age better themselves (Langer, 1997). Not surprisingly, there is a rich history and literature on cognitive interventions for older adults (Stine-Morrow & Basak, 2011; Willis, 2001). The chapters in this volume attest to the broad-based efforts to craft a new vision of what adulthood can look like if we live longer and embrace the challenge of living every day of every year to maximum potential.

The Senior Odyssey project is one model for social and intellectual engagement. The general idea for the program was derived from longitudinal findings from Schooler and colleagues (Schooler & Mulatu, 2001; Schooler, Mulatu, & Oates, 1999, 2004) showing a relationship between what they called "substantive complexity" of activities and mental flexibility. For example, these researchers observed that adults involved in complex work of the sort that demanded self-direction and frequent decisions in the face of uncertainty (e.g., lawyers who develop arguments for innocence or guilt in the face of ambiguous evidence; teachers who must develop lesson plans and actively engage students in learning activities) fare better in certain cognitive tests relative to adults who work in routinized jobs that required repetition of activities in predictable circumstances. They also noted an advantage for individuals who engaged in complex leisure activities (see also Verghese et al., 2003). They argued that the habitual engagement in environments that require an individual to consider situations from different perspectives, and take multiple viewpoints into account in making decisions and taking action, was a form of mental exercise integrated into the fabric of everyday life that enhanced mental ability. In the Senior Odyssey program, participants are thrown into what is designed to be a substantively complex environment, which also happens to be a lot of fun. At the same time, Senior Odyssey is also a research venue to test the hypothesis that such engagement can act as a form of cognitive enhancement, even though it does not involve explicit training in any of the cognitive abilities tested (Willis et al., 2006). In subsequent pages, we provide an introduction to the history of the Senior Odyssey, a description of program logistics, and an overview of outcomes. Our intent is to present this in sufficient detail to enable program coordinators and individuals working with community groups to create a program in their own communities.

A Short History of the Senior Odyssey

The story of Senior Odyssey begins with Odyssey of the Mind (OOTM; www.odysseyofthemind.org). OOTM was started over 30 years ago as an enrichment activity for children and young adults enrolled in educational programs. It is now a large international program (e.g., the 2010 World Finals tournament, a high-level competition for top performers from state tournaments and national tournaments outside the US, hosted over 5,000 students from 24 countries). OOTM was founded on the assumption that classroom instruction often involves skill training and knowledge acquisition in highly constrained contexts that may not always encourage students to creatively apply what they have learned in novel situations. The idea was to present students with "ill-defined" problems, for which there was no one perfect solution, but rather a range of solutions that could be developed with different types of personal resources. Thus, rather than the traditional teach–test rhythm, in which the students' goal is to learn what the teacher has to teach, the program encourages self-reliance in conceptualizing what the problem is and how to solve it.

OOTM teams (which fall into age-graded divisions ranging from primary grades through university level) are formed in the fall and work together through the academic year to prepare for tournament competition in the spring. So at its core, OOTM is a collaborative activity in which teams prepare themselves to face a series of challenges in the context of a community who values their performance. There are two components for the spring tournaments. Each team prepares a solution to a selected "long-term problem," and also practices working as a group to solve novel "spontaneous problems."

Long-term problems are relatively complex open-ended challenges that require cycles of reflection, attempts at implementation, evaluation, and revision. Each year, the OOTM staff develop a new set of long-term problems that form the basis for team activity through the year. The particulars of the problems are different each year but they are always of five different types: classics and history, vehicle design, science and technology, civil engineering, and humorous performance. For example, in the civil engineering problem, teams build structures of balsa wood and glue within certain parameters designed so as to maximize the weight it will bear, but in one year a constraint of the problem might be that the structure has to span a distance, and in another year a constraint might be that the structure has to withstand an impact; the classics problem generally involves elaborating on or retelling a classic tale or historical event (e.g., invent an explanation for how the Egyptian wonders came to be, or create a story involving inspiration by the Muses, one of whom is original and was not among those from classic Greek mythology). These long-term problems can be characterized in terms of the "spirit of the problem," the most important elements central to the problem, as well as more minor constraints that contribute to the multidimensional complexity of the problem (e.g., the inclusion of certain original artifacts that have to be created by the team, or a specific challenge that one character will have to face). Tournament competition of the long-term problem requires the presentation of the solution in an 8-min theatrical performance including sets, props, and costumes developed by the team. These performances are scored by trained judges who assign points for innovation according to a detailed rubric, with multiple judges scoring to assure good reliability.

Thus, participants are presented with a goal that may be effectively achieved in an infinite number of ways by people of widely varying abilities. Indeed, most OOTM problems can be solved by both third graders and by college students – and as we will describe, older adults. Individuals at different stages of development bring different skills to bear, and the nature of the solutions will vary by division, but the important point is that all age groups can solve the problem in some way. The flip side is that there is no perfect solution, so that any solution is, by its nature, subject to revision. Preparing a solution for tournament competition exercises multiple cognitive abilities in a socially meaningful context. Along the way, alternative solutions must be developed (divergent thinking) and evaluated (reasoning); a plan must be developed for how the work will be accomplished and tasks must be coordinated (executive functioning, prospective memory); sets, costumes, and structures must be built (visual–spatial processing); a short script must be written (language processing) and learned for performance (memory).

In contrast to the generate-test-revise process engendered by long-term problems, spontaneous problems encourage the fluent generation of, as the name implies, spontaneous ideas ("thinking on your feet"). They may be verbal (e.g., "name a type of water," with more points awarded for creative responses like "water lily" or "water color," in contrast to common responses like "tap water"; given a starting sentence, each team member generates a sentence that continues the story so that it is coherent and resolves a mystery, a game called "The Exquisite Corpse"); hands-on (e.g., given a mailing label, six straws, a piece of paper, and a rubber band, protect a light bulb so that it can be tossed without breaking); or verbal/hands-on (e.g., given a pair of chopsticks, suggest a novel use and enact; given a pile of marshmallows and toothpicks, the first member will create something and describe it and on each successive turn it is altered and described by adding either a toothpick or a marshmallow). These activities encourage fast-paced generation of ideas (divergent thinking, verbal and ideational fluency) in a collaborative context in which participants often have to consider and build on what others in the group have done (working memory). Thus, inherent in this program is not only the exercise of basic cognitive processes but also decision-making, creativity, evaluation of ideas, competition, and engagement in a community in which effective performance is rewarded and honored. As an established program, OOTM occurs within a well-structured social system so that roles and expectations are well defined and transmitted across generations of participants. The idea for OOTM as a cognitive intervention began to germinate in the Cognitive Aging Lab at the University of New Hampshire, where I (the first author) was on the faculty. Research volunteers from the community, who were asked to perform fairly routine cognitive lab tasks (e.g., speeded judgments, list and text memory), would often enthusiastically return to do other experiments, telling us that the sessions were fun and that they thought that the activities helped to keep them mentally sharp. At the same time, I was learning about OOTM as a coach for my son's middle school OOTM balsa wood team, and it struck me as odd that (as evidenced by my chauffeuring duties and the mess in my dining room) my son had so many opportunities for involvement in activities, but that our lab volunteers were resorting to pattern comparison and sentence span tasks as forms of mental exercise! Life was otherwise busy, so the idea of OOTM as a cognitive enrichment program for older adults had to be tucked away for another day.

There were a number of factors that led to pulling this idea out after my arrival at University of Illinois. First, there was expanding concern in the psychological literature with the question of whether engagement in mental exercise could actually alter cognitive capacity, or alternatively, whether it was simply a consequence of maintained ability (Hultsch, Hertzog, Small, & Dixon, 1999). In spite of the very strong (and probably adaptive) belief in popular culture that "using it" will keep one from "losing it" (Chabris & Simons, 2010), and the utmost urgency of the issue (Hertzog, et al., 2008; Stine-Morrow & Basak, 2011), empirical evidence for this notion is strikingly thin. Also in the air was the "structural lag" idea from sociology (Riley & Riley, 1994, 2000) that meaningful and appropriate roles for later adulthood were lagging behind the swift change in the demographic profile toward an older society. In a nutshell, the argument is that social institutions are traditionally built on the assumption that education is afforded in youth, work is expected from young to middle age, and leisure (retirement) is available in old age (collectively, an "age-segregated" social structure); longer life (and working) spans imply that the frontloading of education to early in the life span is no longer tenable (e.g., it is impossible to be educated for a job 30–50 years hence). Of course, if educational activities are normatively unavailable in later life and mental exercise can maintain and/or augment cognitive capacities, the implication is that structural lag may be a contributor to age-related declines in certain abilities in late life. Thus, "age-integration," in which meaningful roles that afford cognitive stimulation through the life span, may have broad-based potential to offset cognitive declines with aging that are often assumed to be largely grounded in biology. Ultimately, this is an empirical question, and so Senior Odyssey was developed quite deliberately as a cognitive intervention piggybacked onto OOTM so as to be embedded within existing social structures.

In fact, senior teams have participated in OOTM over the years, presenting their solutions noncompetitively at World Finals (e.g., the OOTM in Maine has organized senior teams through a community college course and sent teams to World Finals from time to time). What is unique about the Senior Odyssey project in Illinois is its dual function as (a) a venue for authentic participation in an intellectually challenging program that is not traditional for older adults, and as (b) a research project in which effects on cognition are measured.

As noted earlier, the more specific theory behind Odyssey as a cognitive intervention was that it offered a very nice operational paradigm for Schooler's notion of engagement in a "substantively complex environment." Participants are randomly assigned to participate in Odyssey or a nonengagement control, and administered a comprehensive cognitive battery at pretest and posttest. Consistent with the requirements of a complex environment (e.g., diverse stimuli, multiple decisions, ill-defined problems), we adopted the long-term problems from the existing program, taking them right off the OOTM shelf, and carefully orchestrated the types and administration of spontaneous problems so that they would provide mental exercise of a range of cognitive abilities. Working in a university context afforded the opportunity to involve undergraduate students as coaches. To standardize activities somewhat across teams, we created PowerPoint presentations that would provide coaches with a structure for weekly meetings and ensure that the quality of the visual presentation (e.g., large print) was appropriate for seniors.

Developing the Senior Odyssey

The Senior Odyssey program at Illinois was developed incrementally, incorporating both quantitative and qualitative assessments at each stage. This approach allowed us to evaluate feasibility of the program, the appropriateness of the problems chosen with an older age group, and the integration of authentic programming and controlled research; and to make revisions as needed (Stine-Morrow, Parisi, Morrow, Greene, & Park, 2007). Pilot activities included first conducting single 2-h sessions of spontaneous problems with small numbers of participants, and then a small scale 4-week spontaneous program with four groups administered brief pretest and posttest assessments of cognition (processing speed, working memory, inductive reasoning, visual–spatial processing, divergent thinking). All of these sessions were conducted by the second author, so that we started slowly with a very hands-on approach allowing us to think through logistics. Having established proof of concept, we then moved to the field experiment with small grant funding from the National Institute on Aging. During this period (two program years, 2004–2005 and 2005–2006), we registered our teams with the national organization and took advantage of OOTM resources for program materials and coaches' training. We recruited undergraduates to coach the teams and selected them in part based on an audition, in which they role-played presenting a couple of spontaneous problems to a group of unruly participants (role-played by lab staff). We developed our program to be in synch with the national program and enjoyed close collaboration with the state organization. At the end of each season, we hosted a local Senior Odyssey tournament in the community (one in a park district community center and another in a local school), and trained judges from the state organization scored long-term and spontaneous performances at the Senior Odyssey tournaments, based on the same criteria used in other OOTM tournaments running concurrently elsewhere, and prizes were awarded in closing ceremonies. Each tournament was an event with food, silly hats, and other customs of the traditional program (e.g., the award of a safety pin with one bolt for every year attended), and was well attended by family and friends of the participants. At the beginning of the season, participants were randomized to Odyssey or a retest control, so that Odyssey participants were compared with controls on change in cognitive performance.

After a 1-year hiatus, we continued on a larger scale, both in terms of the scientific aims (e.g., an additional comparison group, expanded cognitive and dispositional battery, activity logs to monitor weekly engagement in program activities) and the size and complexity of the program. Currently, the program is more embedded in the community, with project space conveniently located in a local shopping mall, where groups hold their weekly meetings, store materials, and gather for other program activities. Participants are required to engage in some form of Odyssey activity for at least 10 h per week aside from regular 90-min meetings (including a wide range of choice in games, selected by our research team based on a task analysis of exercising particular cognitive components). Participants keep point trackers for their activities and receive prizes for completion of program activities (e.g., mugs, totebags, pins with the Senior Odyssey logo).

Each year, participants are randomly assigned to the Odyssey program, a training control, or to a waitlist. Once assigned to the program, participants are invited to return to the program in subsequent years as alums who are integrated into teams of novices; alums become an important part of program context as experts who know the explicit rules (e.g., different types of problems, how points are scored, no outside assistance) and have tacit knowledge (e.g., strategies for brainstorming or adhering to cost limits). (At this point, participants are no longer in the experimental group but become part of the intervention.)

Each year, we have received an invitation to compete in the Illinois state tournament (in fact, there is currently an open invitation for any senior team to present at World Finals). We have had a couple of teams elect to do this, both of whom were keen to see how they scored in this competition. Traditional school teams carry the names of their educational institutions into the competition. Part of the culture of the Senior Odyssey teams has been the custom of coming up with their own names; some of our favorites include the Sea-Nior Odd-ta-See Players, who presented a humorous performance in 2005 on a nautical theme, and the Balsa Buster team in 2008. A particular success story was the Shockin' Seniors team, a 2009 balsa wood team. The balsa problem that year included the constraint that the structure had to withstand shockwaves created by weights dropping onto the structure at particular points during the test. Prior to the Senior Odyssey competition in Champaign, the team travelled to Belleville, IL, for the State Tournament to compete as a Division 4 (college-level) team from University of Illinois. Their structure held over 700 lb and they received the coveted OMer Award for exceptional creativity (no, there were no retired engineers on the team). From there, they went to World Finals at Iowa State. Much to their horror (when they were announced, it meant that they had to walk from the high bleachers down to the tiny little stage on the arena floor to receive their trophy), they won third place, beating out two college teams. Their structure actually did not hold nearly the amount of weight it did at state (drier wood? faulty joint?), but their spontaneous score was at the top in this university level division (Figs. 9.1 and 9.2).

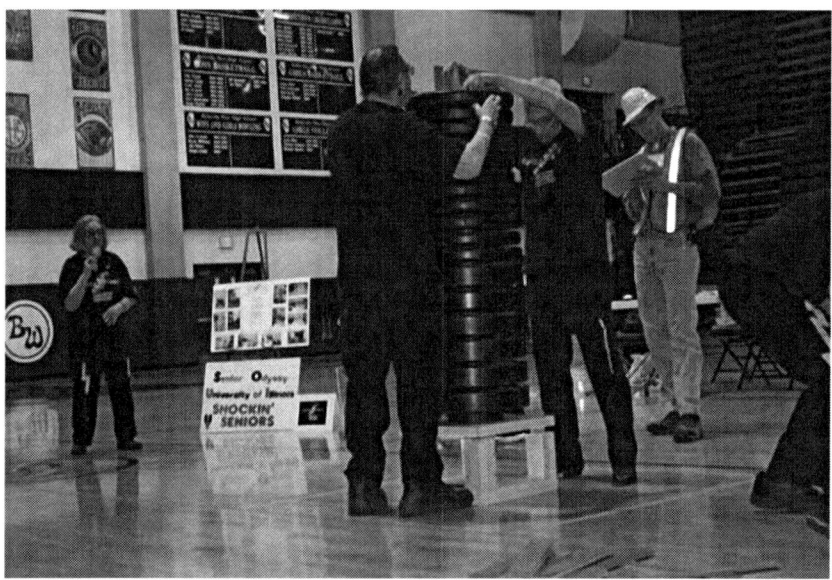

Fig. 9.1 The Shockin' Senior team performs their long-term problem (Shockwave) at the Illinois State Tournament in Belleville, IL, in 2009. The balsa structure is placed around a pipe running through the middle of the crusher, and the crusher board (weighing 9 lb) is placed on top of it. Weights are then laid over the pipe onto the crusher board until the structure breaks. Shockwaves were created by placing two boards of specified widths (just visible in the lower right corner) on top of a weight, laying another weight on the board, and then removing the boards suddenly

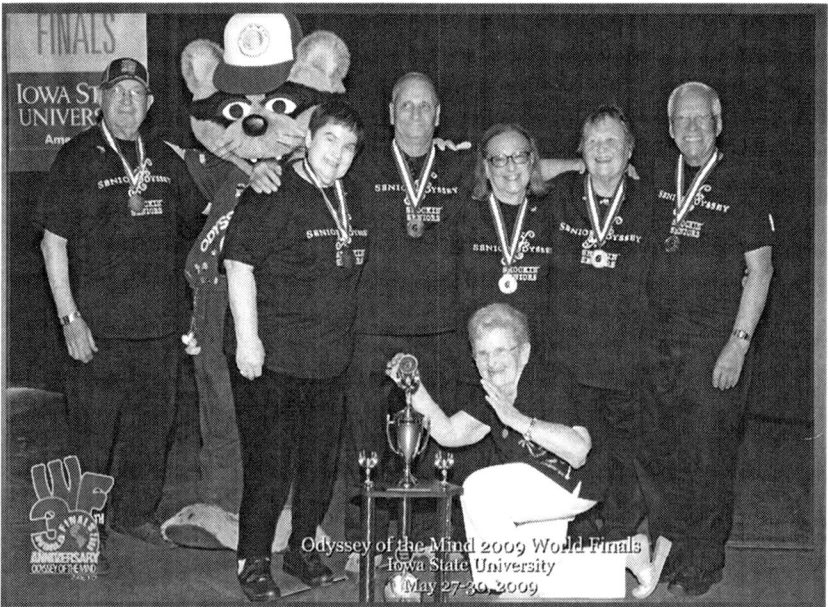

Fig. 9.2 The Shockin' Seniors received the third place trophy for the Division IV balsa problem. Team members are Bob Lewis, Charlene McQueen, Steve Palmer, Helen Miron, Peggy Yeazel, and Ken Schuele. In front is Joanne Rompel, not a team member, but Illinois OOTM Association Director

An Evidence-Based Approach to Cognitive Optimization

Given the focus of this volume, we will not go into detail about the assessment of outcomes or the evidence for beneficial effects of engagement in Odyssey activities; we sketch out our findings briefly. Suffice it to say that there is a lot of snake oil out there for consumers looking for ways to maintain cognitive health with age. In spite of the intuitive appeal of the "use it or lose it" notion, empirical evidence to define principles guiding how to allocate the precious hours of one's days to as to optimize cognitive potential is hard to find. By contrast, there are many suggestions in the popular press that activities, such as doing crossword puzzles, learning a second language, and/or generally being exposed to novel situations, will keep us sharp (with one popular book going so far as to suggest alternating the hand with which one brushes teeth, and taking a shower with one's eyes closed as cognitive interventions). Ever mindful that Senior Odyssey has the potential to become another bandwagon, we have tightly interwoven empirical assessment of its effects on cognition and other psychological functions with the development of an authentic community-based program. Findings from our 2-year pilot suggested that, relative to the control group, Odyssey participants showed modest increases in processing speed, inductive reasoning, and divergent thinking, as well as in a composite measure of fluid ability. Odyssey participants as a group did not show differential increase in predispositions toward intellectual activity, but change in the fluid composite in this group was correlated with change in both mindfulness and need for cognition (Stine-Morrow, Parisi, Morrow, & Park, 2008). This is interesting since such dispositions are predictive of cognition even controlling for their relationship with activity (Parisi, Stine-Morrow, Noh, & Morrow, 2009).

Individual Experiences

Individual and group interviews have been conducted with Senior Odyssey participants, and with the undergraduate coaches in an attempt to understand how some individuals view their experiences with the program (e.g., Parisi, Greene, Morrow, & Stine-Morrow, 2007). Although participants often mention enjoying the cognitive stimulation afforded by both spontaneous and long-term components of the program, they seem to place equal (if not greater) value on the opportunity to maintain and expand social networks. For some, the program appeared to create a broader support system in which team members helped each other through losses or adversities in life outside of the program. Those interviewed also talked about the social interactions as providing a context for personal growth and development, in particular as helping to build confidence.

Coaches typically get to know their team members quite well over a season, and occasionally bring us anecdotes of personal impact. For example, one coach told the story of a participant who seemed to use the program as an anchor in a personally difficult time: "[Alan] was a retired man with a wife and a 9-year old son. ... [He] is a naturally curious and intelligent man. It was obvious that he enjoyed the ...

puzzles and was very vocal with his guesses and reasoning. [At week 13 of the program, Alan] was floored when his wife decided to divorce him and took their child with her. The news took a very heavy toll on [him], and during the first couple weeks ... he was noticeably more quiet and reserved. ... Even with all the commotion ... in his personal life, [Alan] continued to come to the weekly Senior Odyssey meetings. ... Throughout the weeks he had grown closer to the other participants. Senior Odyssey was a time for him to momentarily forget about the troubles in his personal life and have fun. He gradually became his normal self again, joking around and voicing his answers and ideas. For Alan, Senior Odyssey has been a very stable environment that allows him to be himself, have fun, and participate in activities that are enjoyable to him" (Coach Observation).

Another participant had been forced into retirement some years before from a job in which he had funneled much of his energy. With retirement, he had become rather sedentary, plagued with joint and knee pain. His strained relationships with his children were also a factor contributing to feelings of isolation. Throughout the season, this participant was especially articulate about his enjoyment of the Odyssey experience. His coach believed that the long-term problem "sparked [his] creative and competitive drive." The participant invested a lot of his energy into the competition, focusing less on his pain. He also developed strong ties with his team members. During the season, he repaired relationships with his children and started babysitting his grandchildren.

Some participants and coaches reflect on what they learn about individual abilities, strengths, and weaknesses, and the importance of collaboration to success in the final solution. For example, "[Ruth] had chosen the long-term problem so she could be in the same group as her husband ... He was extremely into the problem and had ideas as soon as the guidelines were given [but Ruth was not engaged by the problem]. She then had her time to shine [with] the script... Once the group had decided on a theme for their performance she went home and wrote an outline for it. Then every week she would bring in a script that everyone had helped edit .... She was very modest about her work and never thought she had done that much, but she had written a great script and took in everyone's input. ... She had found her little niche in the problem and shined" (Coach Observation).

Of course, these are anecdotes about individual experiences that are certainly not necessarily representative of the typical experience. We have selected these for presentation because they illustrate how meaningful the experience is for some people.

A Step-By-Step How-To Guide to Developing a Senior Odyssey Program

An important practical advantage of this community-embedded approach to cognitive intervention is that it piggybacks onto an existing system so that much of the spadework of program development is done. Therefore, getting started is relatively easy; we outline logistics based on our experience.

1. *Familiarize yourself with the details of Odyssey of the Mind (www.odysseyofthemind.org), and register with the national program.* Take time to understand what you are getting into. There is a small fee (currently, $135/year for a community organization) for registering with the national OOTM program. Your membership provides coaches training materials, access to coaches training sessions, detailed descriptions of the long-term problems for the year, some resources for spontaneous problems, and access to web-based resources for problem clarifications.
2. *Consider whether you should seek out sponsors.* Odyssey does not have to be expensive (the registration fee covers all the long-term problems and will allow one team for each problem (5 teams × 7 members = 35 individuals) to compete at the state tournament; all long-term problems have cost limits so garage-sale savvy is more important than cash on hand). However, depending on the clients served by the program and the number of teams, some funding for registration fees, recruitment costs, program materials, and venue fees could be helpful. Odyssey does require a strong investment of human capital (e.g., one coach for every seven team members), and it may be advantageous to have a stipend (or payment for release time within an organization) to attract and maintain the most talented coaches. Because our program is a research project, we hired and trained university undergraduates to be coaches who could implement a program in a standardized fashion; also because we are in a university context, we were interested in the educational opportunity this role afforded undergraduates. The traditional OOTM program most typically runs on volunteers, which is certainly possible for the senior version. Also, once the adult Odyssey program is established, experienced participants can serve as coaches.
3. *Cultivate connections with your local, regional, and/or state OOTM association.* These are great resources for training (coaches and judges) and for materials. You might be surprised at the excitement you generate by saying you are organizing senior teams.
4. *Start small and grow slowly as you develop your local coaching talent.* Being a good coach is an acquired skill. The main role of the coach is to lead the team through selected problems and activities, without providing assistance in actually solving the problems. Instead, the coach acts as a "guide on the side," facilitating the group sessions, offering encouragement, and helping the team prepare for competition. This requires a deep understanding of the program and the development of skilled facilitation while promoting independence.
5. *Recruit participants.* Teams are typically composed of five to seven individuals. Arranging for multiple teams probably means multiple long-term problems. Again, starting small to gain confidence with program logistics before juggling too many things is wise. At the same time, if you decide you want to host your own tournament (see below), you will need at least two teams performing the same long-term problem.
6. *Set a regular schedule and keep the momentum going.* Once you have your team(s) in place, select a weekly time and location for meetings. Preparing the

long-term problem takes both work time and incubation time. A reasonable attempt will require a minimum of 14–20 weekly meetings (an hour or so each is typical). Timed with the state tournaments in March, and allowing for weeks off for holidays and bad weather, it is optimal for teams to start meeting in September or October. Teams often prefer to meet more frequently when it gets closer to the final tournament.

7. *Develop a pool of resources for spontaneous problems.* Spontaneous problems can be generated through online resources, including state OOTM websites, as well as on other web-based brainteasers and creativity problem sites. Problems and activities can also be found in books, such as those published by Creative Competitions, Inc. However, you may also want to exercise your creativity and develop your own spontaneous activities. In developing the program as a research-based cognitive intervention, we were very interested in keeping the exposure of different teams to spontaneous problems somewhat consistent, so we developed computer-based presentations (e.g., PowerPoint) of spontaneous problems for each program week in advance. This is helpful with senior teams for enhancing accessibility (e.g., large font printed presentations for problems that might be presented only aurally for younger teams).

8. *Learn the long-term problems that your teams will tackle.* Official descriptions of the long-term problem are several pages long, and at times, read like legal documents (Odyssey folks are pretty serious about the constraints of the problem ... the level playing field and all that). This can be daunting at first, but one thing coaches learn over the years is the problem schema (e.g., range of elements in an 8-min performance, cost limitations, distinguishing core elements of the problem from elements of style that are scored separately).

9. *Develop a routine for individual sessions – that is not too routinized.* Over the season, team members will practice solutions to various spontaneous problems and work on developing, evaluating, and refining solutions to their chosen long-term problem. Because the long-term problem is involved, it is not a bad idea to introduce it gradually. An emphasis on spontaneous problems early on is a good ice-breaker and can help the team learn to work together with some immediate gratification ("we solved it!"). As it gets closer to tournament time, and specific goals to ready the long-term performance have become defined, effort on the long-term problem typically accelerates. It is important to keep practicing spontaneous problems for competition; however, they are also good ways to warm up at the beginning of the session – and to relax at the end.

10. *Decide how you will arrange the competition.* An important part of the Odyssey experience is the opportunity for competition. If you have the minimum of two teams presenting one long-term performance, you may want to consider holding a local tournament (connections with local OOTM are important here since you will need judges). States with larger organizations have regional tournaments in addition to the state tournaments. Another option is to work with these groups to enter the Senior teams as Division IV participants.

Conclusion

As of this writing, we continue the Senior Odyssey program on the calendar with the international program, collecting data pretest and posttest on a wide range of cognitive and dispositional measures and tracking weekly activities with individual logs. The extent to which engagement with Odyssey activity impacts cognition in specific or broad-based ways remains to be seen. Our preliminary data (Stine-Morrow et al., 2008) were promising in showing small but reliable effects on fluid ability; we look forward to a more fine-grained examination of effects (as well as mediators and moderators of effects) with the data set from our current expanded project that is underway.

Culture shapes development, in part, by providing opportunities for activities and behaviors on a small scale ("microgenesis"; Li, 2003). Our goal with the Senior Odyssey project has been both (a) to test the engagement hypothesis, that a cognitive stimulating context requiring active construction of goals and coordination of activities to meet those goals (i.e., ill-defined problem solving) is beneficial for cognition, and (b) to develop a translational model that can be sustained. Clearly, even if one has identified a program that provides strong evidence of cognitive enrichment, it is worthless if it cannot be disseminated. Like diet and physical exercise, there is large gap between knowing what makes for healthy lifestyle and actually living that way. The strong advantage to this community-embedded research strategy for a cognitive intervention, especially one of demonstrated longevity, is that it is there even when the participants are not. It is available when the individual is ready. There is community involvement in retaining members. In relying on an existing cultural institution, it insinuates change in individual lives in subtle ways that in the long run have the potential to make a big difference.

Acknowledgments We are grateful for support from the National Institute on Aging (Grants R03 AG024551 and R01 AG029475). We also wish to thank Joanne Rompel and Sammy Micklus for their support in helping us develop the Senior version of their Odyssey; Donna Whitehill, MT Campbell, Jennifer Kapolnek, and all of the Illinois Senior Odyssey coaches for keeping the program running so smoothly; and Donna Whitehill for thoughtful comments on an earlier version. For updates on published reports and photos of Senior Odyssey events, go to www.seniorodyssey.org.

References

Chabris, C., & Simons, D. (2010). *The invisible gorilla: And other ways our intuitions deceive us*. New York: Crown.

Christensen, K., Doblhammer, G., Rau, R., & Vaupel, J. W. (2009). Ageing populations: The challenges ahead. *The Lancet, 374*, 1196–1208.

Hertzog, C., Kramer, A. F., Wilson, R. S., & Lindenberger, U. (2008). Enrichment effects on adult cognitive development: Can the functional capacity of older adults be preserved and enhanced? *Psychological Science in the Public Interest, 9*, 1–65.

Hultsch, D. F., Hertzog, C., Small, B. J., & Dixon, R. A. (1999). Use it or lose it: Engaged lifestyle as a buffer of cognitive decline in aging? *Psychology and Aging, 14*, 245–263.

Kinsellla, K., & He, W. (2009). *International Population Reports, P95/09-1, An Aging World: 2008.* Washington, DC: U.S. Government Printing Office.

Kramer, A. F., & Willis, S. L. (2002). Enhancing the cognitive vitality of older adults. *Current Directions in Psychological Science, 11*, 173–177.

Langer, E. (1997). *The power of mindful learning.* Boston, MA: Addison-Wesley.

Li, S.-C. (2003). Biocultural orchestration of developmental plasticity across levels: The interplay of biology and culture in shaping the mind and behavior across the life span. *Psychological Bulletin, 129*, 171–194.

Parisi, J. M., Greene, J. C., Morrow, D. G., & Stine-Morrow, E. A. L. (2007). The Senior Odyssey: Participant experiences of a program of social and intellectual engagement. *Activities, Adaptation, and Aging, 31*, 31–49.

Parisi, J. M., Stine-Morrow, E. A. L., Noh, S. R., & Morrow, D. G. (2009). Predispositional engagement, activity engagement, and cognition among older adults. *Aging, Neuropsychology, and Cognition, 16*, 485–504.

Riley, M. W., & Riley, J. W., Jr. (1994). Age integration and the lives of older people. *The Gerontologist, 34*, 110–115.

Riley, M. W., & Riley, J. W., Jr. (2000). Age integration: Conceptual and historical background. *The Gerontologist, 40*, 266–270.

Schooler, C., & Mulatu, M. S. (2001). The reciprocal effects of leisure time activities and intellectual functioning in older people: A longitudinal analysis. *Psychology and Aging, 16*, 466–482.

Schooler, C., Mulatu, M. S., & Oates, G. (1999). The continuing effects of substantively complex work on the intellectual functioning of older workers. *Psychology and Aging, 14*, 483–506.

Schooler, C., Mulatu, M. S., & Oates, G. (2004). Occupational self-direction intellectual functioning, and self-directed orientation in older workers: Findings and implications for individuals and society. *American Journal of Sociology, 110*, 161–197.

Stine-Morrow, E. A. L., & Basak, C. (2011). Cognitive interventions. In K. W. Schaie & S. L. Willis (Eds.), *Handbook of the psychology of aging* (7th ed.). New York: Elsevier (in press).

Stine-Morrow, E. A. L., Parisi, J. M., Morrow, D. G., Greene, J. C., & Park, D. C. (2007). An engagement model of cognitive optimization through adulthood. *Journal of Gerontology: Psychological Sciences, 62*, 62–69.

Stine-Morrow, E. A. L., Parisi, J. M., Morrow, D. G., & Park, D. C. (2008). The effects of an engaged lifestyle on cognitive vitality: A field experiment. *Psychology and Aging, 23*, 778–786.

Verghese, J., Lipton, R. B., Katz, M. J., Hall, C. B., Derby, C. A., Kuslansky, G., et al. (2003). Leisure activities and risk of dementia in the elderly. *New England Journal of Medicine, 348*, 2508–2516.

Willis, S. L. (2001). Methodological issues in behavioral intervention research with the elderly. In J. E. Birren & K. W. Schaie (Eds.), *Handbook of the psychology of aging* (5th ed., pp. 78–108). N.Y.: Academic Press.

Willis, S. L., Tennstedt, S. L., Marsiske, M., Ball, K., Elias, J., Koepke, K. M., et al. (2006). Long-term effects of cognitive training on everyday functional outcomes in older adults. *JAMA, 296*, 2805–2814.

Chapter 10
Spelling Clubs and Competitions for Older Adults: Language Boosting Within a Social Context

Paula E. Hartman-Stein and Mary DeForest

Abstract This chapter describes how a community-based spelling/language club and spelling competition for adults can provide opportunities for cognitive exercise and strengthening social connections. We also present insights into the experience of competing at an adult national spelling competition, summarize age-related spelling and language errors, describe strategies that enhance spelling skills in adults, and suggest ideas for future research about the link between spelling skills, attention, and working memory.

Introduction

In 1773 Noah Webster is credited with saying, "Spelling is the foundation of reading and the greatest ornament of writing." Webster is correct as research studies show that the relationship between English reading and spelling skills of children range from 0.66 to 0.90 (Joshi, Treiman, Carreker, & Moats, 2008–2009). In normal cognitive aging, a consistent pattern of changes in language emerges with some skills preserved and others impaired. For example, the components of reading such as comprehension of the meaning of words and sentences and the perception of the letters and speech sounds that make up words remain stable in older age, but language production, specifically spelling skills and word finding exhibit significant age-related declines (Burke & MacKay, 1997).

In this chapter, we describe ways to support adults' interests in language as a basis for cognitive exercise by creating a community-based spelling/language

P.E. Hartman-Stein (✉)
Clinical Geropsychologist, Center for Healthy Aging, 265 W. Main Street,
Ohio 44240; Adjunct Faculty, Department of Human Development and Family Studies,
College of Education, Health and Human Services, Kent State University, Kent, OH, USA
e-mail: paula@centerforhealthyaging.com

club and regional spelling bee for adults that was linked to a national adult spelling competition. The second author of this chapter, who competed in the national bee for adults age 50 plus, provides insights about her experience. The chapter also describes adult spelling strategies, summarizes the research evidence for spelling and language errors that occur more frequently with age, and suggests ideas for future studies that can shed light on the link between spelling skills, working memory, and other aspects of attention.

Spelling Competitions for Children and Adults

Thousands of children in grades 6 through 8 demonstrate their spelling acumen in local contests around the United States and other countries each year in local and regional bees. From those winners a subset of about 265 verbally precocious children compete in the Scripps National Spelling Bee (formerly the Scripps Howard National Spelling Bee and commonly called the National Spelling Bee). It is a highly competitive annual competition in the United States with participants from other countries as well. Since 1994, the television network, ESPN, has broadcast the later rounds of the bee, and since 2006 the championship rounds have been aired in primetime on ABC television. In his book, *The American Bee: the National Spelling Bee and the Culture of Word Nerds*, Maguire (2006) described the competition as nothing short of pure Americana, part Norman Rockwell and part Horatio Alger, an egalitarian event in which children from every social class can and do compete.

Maguire describes the children as obsessive etymologists or language detectives who explore linguistic patterns because good spelling requires more than rote memorization skills. Educators agree that spelling is a linguistic task that requires knowledge of sound and letter patterns, root words, word origins, and awareness of a word's internal structure, including its oddities (Joshi et al., 2008–2009).

The National Spelling Bee for children is more than an academic competition. It is a gathering of like-minded young souls, word nerds, who share a subculture. They have similar interests and idiosyncrasies, and the regional and national contests provide a structure for supporting one another. *Akeelah and the Bee*, the 2006 major motion picture with Laurence Fishburne and Angela Bassett, showcases the social context of the competition and how it can help to create positive social connections in a community and enhance confidence and emotional well-being for the participants.

In 1996 a group of members of the American Association of Retired Persons (AARP) in Cheyenne, Wyoming decided that spelling bees are not just for children by hosting the first national spelling contest for adults age 50 plus. Over the years the contest that is supported by AARP's Educator Community and the *Staying Sharp program* has grown into an event that attracts adult spellers from all over the country and Canada. In June each year approximately 50–75 adults pay a small admission fee to compete fiercely in the challenging competition, with the winner appearing the following Monday on a nationally televised morning news show.

The following is a description of the second author's AARP Spelling Bee experience:

Greek scientists explained atomic theory by saying that the physical universe is made of atoms just as words are made up of letters. English words have 26 atoms, into which we fit everything we know about the universe. Like atoms, letters combine to make pieces of words whose edges can be unscrewed and fitted onto other pieces. Sometimes, you need to smash some of the edges, to get it to fit, as when the com of companion (one you share bread with) hits an L as in collect (gather together).

I teach Greek and Latin, which is a huge help in a spelling bee because I personally know many words that show up in spelling bees and can recognize their pieces as well. I also created a spelling program, *StellarSpeller*, specifically to help those wishing to compete in spelling bees and improve their language skills in general. I collected information on about 5700 English words derived from different languages (about half Latin and Greek) for the StellarSpeller program, and had gone through the program enough times to be somewhat familiar with what happens in Spanish, for instance with Latin command. It drops the extra m in the word comandancia. I never thought of myself as a good speller—pretty good, but not great. I identified with the Ian Holm, the trainer in Chariots of Fire: I could give a speller four feet.

I certainly had no intention of competing in the AARP Bee until urged by the first author of this chapter. Of course I had to do so then, but after I saw the kinds of words they used in previous bees, I whined, "Why are we getting harder words than the ones in the Nationals? It's not fair! We're old!" But I had already registered.

I did not think I'd enjoy being exposed as a poor speller, but it was great!

A spelling bee can be a lonely place. It's you vs. the English language. The gate opens and a word flies out. Sometimes, this word lopes out like Bugs Bunny, chewing a carrot. There were quite a few of those. There are the words you know, the words you should know, and the words you might be able to guess. Amongst these were about twenty special words. These words are the ones that weed us out. These words test you, teach you, cleanse you. If you think you can spell, wait until you get your corrected test. (One word I missed was profiteroles, cream puffs that had been served to the spellers at the opening reception, and served to us again during the written test.) I thought I'd maybe missed as many as 6. Instead of 6, I missed 13. Then, I knew I would not win. Still, I squeaked onto the podium for the spell-off.

There is nothing more thrilling than facing a word as it rushes from the gate and thunders down at you. It calls up everything you have, everything you are, to meet it full charge and nail it.

On the podium, there were words I could spell, and the words I couldn't mostly went to other people, mostly: like reseaux (nets) and quaalude. I got a big one, weltanschauung, world-view, but I knew that word, and got to know it later. The biggest word I spelled right was archaeopteryx. I mention it not to boast, but because something can take over in a spelling bee, that has to do with the moment, not what you know, or have learned.

That's how it was with me and archaeopteryx. The oPTERYx ending did not bother me—I saw the feather. Where I hesitated was whether to spell the first part archae- or arche-. The former is more common: archeology, archeozoic, but for some reason, I went with the less common, archae- and it saved me for a round. How did I know? I am not a good speller. Once while doing a crossword, I spelled argyle with an I, to avoid ending a cross-word in -yd. I have a poor visual memory. I work on rules. I don't know if I'd ever seen this word, perhaps I had. It was mystical.

We got two strikes before going out, and I missed two words I should have gotten. One was "my word," zori, straw sandals, which is part of the Japanese section of my program, but I had not studied the Japanese words before coming to the spelling bee, and it served me right. Then I missed nimiety. I was so glad to recognize the stem (Latin nimis, too much), that I rushed past the suffix, which I spelled –iaty. (There are no words in English ending in –iaty.) Strike 2, and served me right.

My strike three was so delightful that it was worth being eliminated to meet: wappenschawing, "a parade of weapons." I knew the German word schau, because I had gotten it right earlier. I somehow knew that Scottish words would not end in –ung, as weltanschauung, so I got the –ing ending right. I didn't like schau, but I couldn't think of how to get out of it. If I had thought a couple of hours, I might have gotten it—go two letters down, and you have it: wappenschawing, a German word with English trousers! It is like seeing a fossil of some creature that was part of a transitional life form on its way to a form still extant.

I tell people it was worth being eliminated to glean that particular gem from the English language. Most people don't believe me, but it's true. And, even when you lose, you get to go on spelling, and the words kept coming, harder ones, words I had no idea how to spell, coming so fast, that the spellers spelled them more quickly than I could write them down.

I may have implied that lonely is the speller. That is not altogether true. At the moment of truth facing the unknown word, you are alone. But outside the contests, you get to meet other spellers, all obsessed with language, all in love with words, all—and this surprised me—eager to share our lists. I collect -aa- words (mostly Dutch), another collects birds, and trees; another, names of winds. The day spent with these people was one of the happiest of my life.

I came away impressed with the power of the AARP, the host of the bee. This organization demonstrated in the lavish banquets and tours of Cheyenne. This includes a tour of Cheyenne's public library, which should be visited by everyone who has ever loved a book.

Dr. DeForest has since competed in her second national bee and performed well enough to once again place among the top spellers, tying for tenth place in 2010. The word that was her downfall was diesis, a double dagger.

In the next section, we describe spelling competitions and spelling clubs that can be introduced in community settings.

The Northeast Ohio Senior Spelling Bee

The first author of this chapter was a competitive speller as a child, winning two county-wide competitions as a sixth and eighth grader, but not making the cut to the level of competing in the national bee. She thought her spelling bee days were over, until at age 50 she learned of an opportunity to participate in a three person team, adult spelling bee that was a fund raiser for the county Literacy Coalition. Local businesses or organizations entered the contest for marketing purposes and to show support of a charitable cause. The contest had the potential to showcase her private practice, the Center for Healthy Aging, in the community where she had recently relocated. By the time the team learned of the competition, there were only a few weeks to prepare. With healthy doses of luck and skill, the team of the Center for Healthy Aging won the bee and was rewarded by a quarter page newspaper story about the new business in town.

The following year the team decided to compete again, but this time with some serious preparation beforehand. We obtained word lists from multiple sources such as *Readers' Digest and Valerie's Spelling Bee Supplement* (Browning, 2002), and studied the origin of words and used memorization strategies based on cognitive research such as chunking, visualization techniques, and self-testing (see Dunlosky, Bailey, & Hertzog, 2011, Chap. 1). During the 3–4 months of rigorous preparation, it appeared that our speed of mental processing increased and working memory skills improved. After competing for 4 years (and placing first in 3 of the 4 years), the first author of this chapter decided to stop competing and instead teach other adults her spelling strategies and create a regional spelling competition for adults age 60 plus. Many clients and friends sought enjoyable ways to be cognitively challenged. The senior bee and preparation classes appealed to individuals who wanted to improve their knowledge of word meanings and spelling of uncommon English words. In the spring of 2005, the first author of this chapter moderated the first Northeast Ohio Senior Spelling Bee after finding a sponsoring organization that provided financial support and lent legitimacy to the community event.

A large healthcare organization showed initial interest, but it was the CEO of a local community mental center who recognized the potential advantages of hosting such a program and made a commitment to the project. The bee was held in the new building that housed their adult day program to bring community attention to their expanded program for frail older adults. The mental health center's Foundation paid approximately $5,000 for consulting costs, advertising, spelling classes for the community, prizes for participants, food and beverages for onlookers during the event, as well as round trip transportation and all expenses for the winner of the bee to participate in the AARP national spelling bee in Cheyenne, Wyoming.

Staff from the Foundation and adult day program formed a committee that met on a regular basis for 4 months with the creator of the bee to plan and execute every detail. In order to get buy-in from community leaders, we asked prominent business and educational leaders to participate as judges.

The first year the event brought a crowd of about 50 spectators who were encouraged to participate by writing down the spelling of each word to see how they may have fared in the actual competition. Thirteen intrepid spellers ranging in age from about 60 to 90 participated in the competition. Similar to the format of the AARP bee, there was a combination of written and oral rounds, with only the top ten spellers eligible to compete in the oral rounds.

One of the judges, the newspaper publisher, David Dix, wrote the following excerpt that appeared in his column on the editorial page the following Sunday in the local paper, *the Record Courier*:

> Other than the humiliation of discovering how poor a speller I truly am, serving as a judge at Thursday evening's Northeast Ohio Senior Spelling Bee at the impressive facilities of Portage Area Senior services was a blast…Mistakenly believing I would be a judge for seniors being treated for problems we encounter as we grow older, I found myself along with the other judges, confronting 13 livewires who had cheerfully volunteered to be contestants….Do you know how to spell "collywobbles," a word that means a mild intestinal disorder? How about "contumacy," a stubborn resistance to authority? How about guillotine, the French instrument for beheading? And how about trousseau, the personal possessions of a bride?

Not only did I misspell these four words. Out of 40 words Paula gave us, I failed to correctly spell a total of 23 words, some of them much easier than the four examples I've given you...Dick Schellenberger, a history teacher in his 70s, nearly backed out of the competition, but must be glad he did not. He made the cut in the written bee and then in the oral finals came in first.

There's a difference between spelling answers in writing and spelling answers orally, Dr. Paula Hartman-Stein said, 'because pronouncing the answers in front of people requires greater concentration and mental tracking skills.'

...It's no different than our muscle and bones we are all warned to take care of and use. Become a couch potato addicted to fast food and you're buying a ticket to cardiac failure. Quit using the cognitive portion of your brain by which you take in information, process it and make decisions, and you could find yourself headed for what I once heard mistakenly called, 'Old Timer's Disease.'

Their confidence growing, the spellers battled away Thursday evening and those of us watching applauded their answers, some of us realizing full well we could not come close to doing as well.

The staff and administration of the community mental health center were very pleased to receive the positive publicity. The Foundation of the mental health center funded three additional annual contests. In order to spice up the event and provide hints as to the nature of the words used in the bees, we created themes such as Cinco de Mayo, Derby Day, and Earth Day. The national publication, *Mature Living magazine* (Laird, 2008), published a two page story about the annual event and following the publication, over 40 senior centers from across the country requested information about the nuts and bolts of conducting community-wide senior spelling competitions.

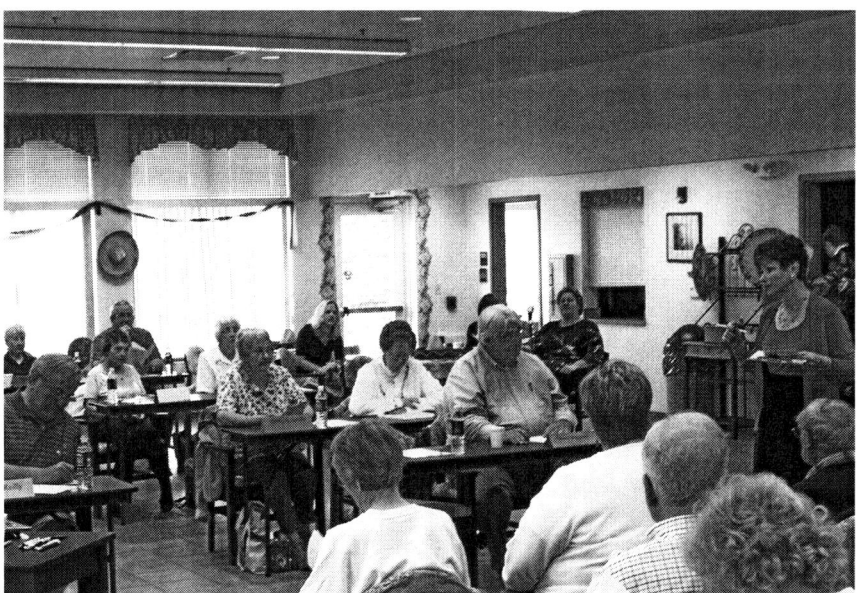

Spelling Bee with Cinco de Mayo theme

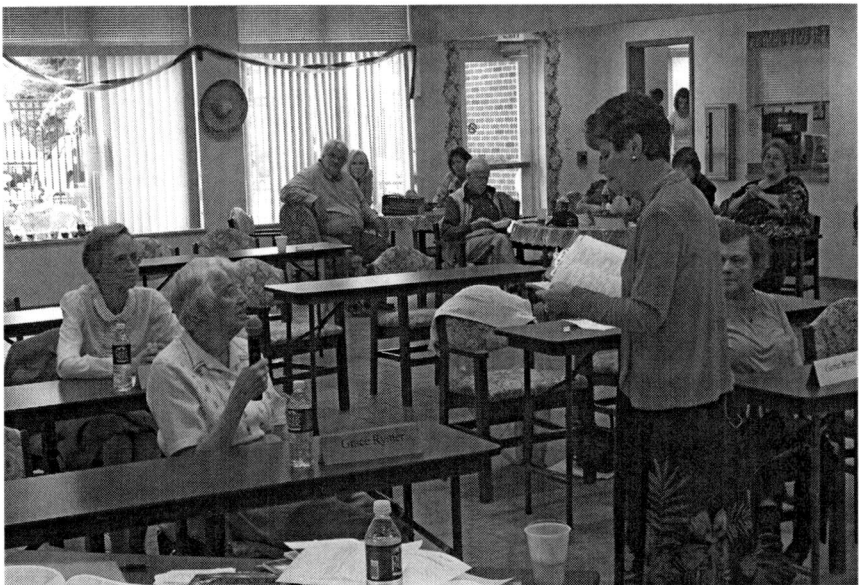

Spelling Bee with Cinco de Mayo theme

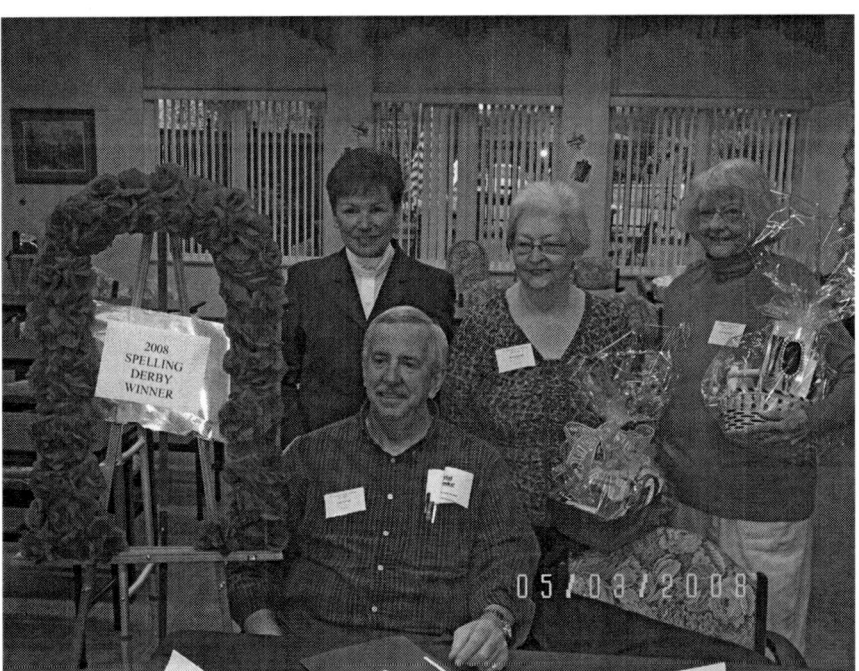

Spelling Bee with Derby Day theme

During the fifth year of the contest, a local retirement center sponsored the senior bee. As a result, the activity coordinator of the retirement center formed a spelling club, the Verbomaniacs, for residents in independent and assistant living, who meet regularly to study the meanings and practice the spelling of obscure words. The Northeast Ohio Senior Spelling Bee had a fun 5-year run. Smaller, low budget adult bees sponsored by local libraries in our area occur each year. From the experience of organizing this type of community programming for older adults who love language, the merit of such an event is clear: cognitive fitness is supported and social connections are created. Organizations such as senior centers, associations of retired professionals, churches, retirement communities, and universities are appropriate venues for similar endeavors. All that is needed is a passionate leader and a team of committed volunteers to begin such a program. Word lists from the AARP Bee are available online as well as Valerie's Spelling Supplement (Browning, 2011).

Adult Spelling Clubs

Demonstrating spelling prowess in front of an audience is not everyone's sport. Spelling/language clubs provide a framework that can fit into any community to provide a low stress, intellectually challenging pursuit with opportunities to create and strengthen social connections. Below is an account of the beginning of a typical meeting of such a group.

The atmosphere of the public library classroom was noisy, an air of energy and enthusiasm brewing around the table where eight adults, ranging in age from the early 60s to middle 80s, sat and chatted with one another. The leader, a petite, lively 70 year-old woman brought the meeting to order. "Welcome to KAOS everyone. Let's get started. We have a lot to do today," she announced. We have two new guests, and our club founder is here to interview us about why we are in this club. We must decide our holiday celebration plans also. Plus Betty will be quizzing us. Remember, we have a test today of 50 words taken from the online list from the AARP bee. "That's too many words," shouted one of the women. "It will take too much time. Let's do half of that." "Yes," said several of the women in unison. "Twenty-five is enough," said the youngest woman in the group. "Chaos is the name of this group?" asked one woman with a clipped British accent. The leader said, "Oh, I forgot to tell you. Yes, the name of our group sounds like chaos, but we spell it K-A-O-S, the Kent Area Orthography Society."

That was the beginning of the KAOS meeting in November 2010 attended by the first author of this chapter who had founded the club 4 years earlier. The club meets once a month at the local library, and several club members participate in local contests during "bee season" in the spring. During monthly meetings, every member brings a list of words along with the etymology of each word and its definition accompanied by a sentence using the word properly.

The current president of the spelling club, Garnet Byrne, wrote the following to explain her reasons for participating in a spelling club:

> (KAOS) was the perfect group for us. Consisting of seniors, 60-90+ years of age with a wide variety of backgrounds, the class reviews words from our reading, our foreign language experience and our hobbies as well as other sources. At one session, my friend, Grace, and I both focused on bird and plant life, learning that we are kindred spirits in our appreciation of nature and the environment. Through KAOS, we, like others in our group, have become very close friends, visiting each other frequently, sharing jokes and stories, and reviewing spelling words.
>
> Preparing for local bees involves class mini-bees plus individual practice sessions. Grace and I spend a couple of hours each week, researching words and pronouncing them to each other. We have concentrated on words related to a regional bee's theme, such as Cinco de Mayo and Earth Day. This method has proved successful. Grace, age 80, won second, third and fourth place in her bees; I won second place in one bee and helped in other ways, such as displaying green products from local companies and reading Chief Seattle's Native American earth prayer for our Earth Day bee.
>
> Grace and I entered the regional senior spelling bees because we want to keep our minds active and to test our ability to memorize and retain words in our senior years. We knew that bees require long hours of study, for we remember the hard work we put into school bees. Grace had participated in county bees in elementary school, and her high school spelling team took second place at the county level. I won seventh and eighth grade school and county bees and placed third in the state bees. We also both have very competitive spirits and thrive on new challenges. We seniors feel like celebrities at the bees. We and our audience are feted with delicious food, drink and live music. Competition is keen, with the bees sometimes lasting for 20–25 rounds. The audience is mesmerized by the difficulty of the words. We love the applause that follows and the generous gifts: a coveted all-expense trip to the AARP senior spelling bee in Wyoming, certificates to regional book stores, and tickets one year to the Tony award-winning play, THE PUTNAM COUNTY SPELLING BEE, among others. No one loses in these bees, for all gain just by entering and being treated in a very special way.

The following are additional responses from club members:

> I like the social aspects of the club and although I learn the words I participate in the club because it is mostly a stress reliever. It is also a way for me to overcome shyness. By being the contact person for our participation in various bees I take a leadership role….I have a high school education, and I find that spelling is a great leveler. People who went to college are just as apt to miss a letter as I am. In one of the bees I came in 6th place, and I was the person there with the least formal education. Dotty, age 60.

> I compete in spelling bees because it is a challenge… I am a storyteller and used to being out in front of the public. I am just a show off in a healthy way… I am not competitive. I don't study enough… Guenveur, age 80+

> I compete because I am very competitive in general, anything from selling cookies for the Girl Scouts or playing racquet ball. Garnet, age 72.

> It is fun to look at a word and take it apart and figure out where it came from. I am a ferocious reader, and so it helps to know what you are reading. We have a lot of fun doing this. We laugh. We are almost afraid the library will kick us out. It is a social thing but also a way to get us to focus and learn. Betty, age 70.

The club's focus is not exclusively on practicing spelling. Periodically it hosts guest speakers on word etymology and other aspects of the English language. For example, Victoria Pagán, Ph.D., a visiting professor in the Department of

Classics at the University of Florida (and daughter of one of the older adult spellers) described how the English language evolved over the past 2,000 years. Dr. Pagán said, "English is living, breathing and organic. It's a resilient language that keeps expanding with room for more contributions. That's the dynamic nature of the language."

Spelling Strategies for Adults

In the next section of this chapter, we review strategies reported to improve spelling skills of adult English spellers. There is relatively little systematic research on strategies used by adult spellers, and no research is available on techniques that improve spelling of older adult spellers. Qualitative data from asking a group of children who were finalists in the National Spelling bee revealed the major strategies of repetition, concentration on letter sequence, and visual memory (Logan, Olson, & Lindsey, 1989).

Holmes and Malone (2004) conducted an experiment using college students between the ages of 17 and 26 years to determine the strategies they used to improve their spelling and pinpoint the success of each strategy for both better and weaker spellers. Examples of the types of strategies reported include the following:

1. Rote learning through the rehearsal of letters was both the favorite strategy and highly successful in learning words that had been misspelled. This involves repeating the letters of the word aloud. Example: truculence has one c in the first syllable and no k.
2. Overpronunciation is a strategy useful for words with nonstandard pronunciations. It requires the speller to isolate different segments of the spelling, code each segment, and assemble them into a pronunciation. This is a complex sequence of operations and was more successful for the better spellers. For example, the word fuchsia lends itself to this strategy. An illustrative utterance is to divide the word into the sounds, "fuch," rhyming with such, then "si" with a long i sound, and ending with the sound "uh."
3. Morphological analysis was used when the speller distinguished the separate forms of the syllables of the word. For example, the word avgolemono (a soup made of lemons and eggs) can be chunked into "avgo," meaning egg in Greek, followed by lemon, and ending with the letter o.
4. Comparison is a strategy when the spellers compared the memory of their incorrect spelling with the correct spelling. In the Holmes and Malone (2004) study, the comparison technique worked successfully only if it also included rehearsal of the correct letters in the word, and it worked better for spellers with superior visual memory skills.
5. Visualization was reported as the least frequently used strategy but when it was used it was moderately effective for both skilled and unskilled spellers. Holmes and Malone (2004) questioned whether visualization is independent of other spelling strategies and concluded that more investigation is needed to determine the degree of importance of visual memory skills for spelling.

Additional strategies used by the first author of this chapter but not empirically tested include finding a rhythm when spelling each word and using this same rhythm or cadence each time the speller practices saying that particular word aloud. Other techniques include using visual memory strategies such as "air writing" words on an imaginary board and making a recording of word lists that can be listened to while driving or doing mundane household tasks. When recording the word, the person says the correct spelling, followed by saying aloud strategies used to remember the word, similar to those described, including letter rehearsal, overpronunciation, and morphological analysis.

In addition, when working with adult spellers using techniques such as spaced retrieval and frequent self-testing may prove helpful (see Dunlosky et al., 2011, Chap. 1). For example, if a speller records a list of unfamiliar words, he/she can use the recording as a way to self-test by stopping the recording prior to hearing the correct spelling and seeing whether he/she can spell the word correctly.

Not all older adults retain their spelling skills from their youth. In the next section, we summarize some of the research on age-related changes in language and describe two theoretical models that help to explain these age-related changes; for example, the transmission-deficit model and the graphemic buffer. Both underscore the value of spelling/language clubs and spelling competitions as promising methods for preserving language skills in late life.

Research Results of Age-Related Changes in Language and Spelling Ability

A growing number of studies have demonstrated that specific age-related changes occur in language production such as the inability to produce a well-known word, the tip of the tongue (TOT) experience. The majority of TOTs are proper nouns, especially proper nouns for names of people or TOT words that have a low frequency of occurrence generally in language (see review by Burke & Shafto, 2004).

As noted earlier in this chapter, spelling skills decline with age. Even accomplished spellers experience deterioration of spelling skills, not in the ability to recognize a misspelling but in the ability to produce the correct spelling of words from memory (MacKay & Abrams, 1998). In one study a dictation task was used to test the ability of young and older adults to spell words with uncommon spellings for their speech sounds (e.g., colonel), and older adults made more errors. In addition, older adults made more errors on words that occur with less frequency in English compared to high frequency words. This age-linked decline in correct spelling was unrelated to prior training on spelling skills and time spent per week in other language-based activities such as reading, writing, and solving crossword puzzles (MacKay & Abrams, 1998).

Language functions that comprise the input side of language, including knowledge of words and word meanings and the perception of the letters and speech sounds, are preserved in normal aging (Burke & Mackay, 1997; Madden, 1988). One theoretical framework for this pattern of age-related language change is the transmission-deficit model (Burke & Shafto, 2004). This hypothetical framework explains that language production deficits are caused by weak connections in the phonological (sound) and orthographic (spelling) systems. Activation through practice appears to strengthen connections among memory representations of language which increases the ability to subsequently retrieve words. According to the transmission-deficit model, practicing irregularly spelled words should reduce age declines in spelling. Burke and MacKay (1997) reviewed theoretical and empirical research that point to the importance of practicing language skills in older age and concluded that older adults can offset effects of cognitive aging by focusing on areas of intellectual expertise that they have developed over their lifetimes. Participation in spelling/language clubs and spelling competitions fits with this idea of preserving skills through practice. This is the same idea of supporting cognitive strengths described throughout this volume (e.g., see Camp, Zeisel, and Antenucci, Chap. 23; Caulfield, Chap. 19; Hartman-Stein, Chap. 12; La Rue, Chap. 21).

The Role of Attention in Spelling

Studies of spelling errors made by individuals with early stage dementia of the Alzheimer's type (DAT) provide insight into the role of attention in spelling skills. In comparing spelling skills of individuals with DAT to young adults and healthy older adults, semantic skills (word meaning) remain relatively intact in early stage DAT, but a breakdown in attentional control appears to be a factor in deficits in the spelling and reading of inconsistent words. Individuals with DAT have difficulty inhibiting inappropriate responses; for example, when asked to spell the word plaid, subjects with DAT had difficulty inhibiting incorrect spellings such as plad (Cortese, Balota, Sergent-Marshall, & Buckner, 2003).

In a study of 23 individuals with DAT compared to 27 intact older adults of a mean age of 72 and 70 respectively who wrote to dictation of different real words and pronounceable pseudowords, the DAT patients spelled less accurately compared to the controls, but the quality of error types suggested that their errors were due to impairment outside of the language system. The researchers concluded that the nonlinguistic functions of attention, executive control, and praxis were the underlying causes of the differences between the groups (Glosser, Kohn, Sands, Grugan, & Friedman, 1999).

Spelling data indicate age-linked declines occur also in retrieving frequently used words, not just words used rarely or infrequently, as in TOTs (see review in Burke, MacKay, Worthley, & Wade, 1991). For example, a cognitively intact older adult may make the error of spelling broom as "brum" but may immediately recognize the error upon seeing it in written form. One likely explanation for the spelling error is a deficit in attention explained by an informational processing model known as the graphemic buffer. This model can be generalized to normal individuals and to neurologically impaired populations (Neils, Roeltgen, & Greer, 1995).

The graphemic buffer is the stage in which an individual selects a spelling of a word and stores it while motor processes are activated to spell the word orally or in writing. This stage occurs after the individual generates the spelling by the lexical system or through sounding it out by the phonological system. In their review, Neils et al. (1995) explained that the main feature of the graphemic buffer is a fast decay of words that results in nonlinguistic errors. Misspellings that are unlikely by their sounds (that is, phonologically implausible) are generated by impairment in the graphemic buffer because the stored spelling degrades in the buffer. Letters are omitted, substituted, transposed, or added. For example, in one team spelling competition in which the first author participated, her teammate had the word parabrake. In such competitions members can coach their teammates. The first author whispered the correct spelling to her 25-year-old teammate who immediately spelled it incorrectly as "parabreak." This error appears to be an example of graphemic buffer impairment triggered by anxiety. In addition, the correct spelling of long words from dictation stresses the role of attention and working memory capacity of the graphemic buffer.

Neils et al. (1995) found that visual attention tests were better predictors of the number of spelling errors than a sensitive measure of language in individuals diagnosed with mild-stage Alzheimer's dementia. Normal control subjects did not misspell as many words as the AD subjects but they showed some of the same trends such as making the same types of errors in the same word position. Also, normal subjects made more errors in longer words, suggesting inattention plays a role in the error pattern of both impaired and nonimpaired older adults. This intriguing finding has implications in future directions for research.

Directions for Future Research

In reviewing existing published research to date, no studies were found that examined whether attempts to improve working memory also have an effect on spelling skills or whether interventions to improve spelling skills in middle age or late life have any effect on working memory or other aspects of attention. Hence, important questions for future research are first, whether older adults can improve their spelling and if so, how much can they be improved, and second, if spelling can be improved, is there a concomitant transfer effect to improvements in working memory efficiency?

In addition, research on the most effective strategies to improve English language spelling skills in older adults has not been published to date. With the interest adults are showing throughout the country to compete in spelling bees, this area is an area ripe for research.

Concluding Remarks

Spelling competitions for adults appear to be a growing phenomenon as increasing numbers of Baby Boomers who were spellers as children want another chance to compete, sharpen their language skills, or simply be supported and surrounded by a community of like-minded older word nerds. On their T shirts the following phrase is appropriate: "Spelling…improving the mind one word at a time."

References

Browning, V. (2002). *Valerie's 2002 Spelling Bee Supplement*. Hunt: Hexco Academic.
Browning, V. (2011). *Valerie's Spelling Bee Supplement*. Hunt: Hexco Academic.
Burke, D. M., MacKay, D. G., Worthley, J. S., & Wade, E. (1991). On the tip of the tongue: What causes word finding failures in young and old adults. *Journal of Memory and Language, 30*, 542–579.
Burke, D. M., & MacKay, D. M. (1997). Memory, language, and ageing. *Philosophical Transactions of the Royal Society of London, 352*, 1845–1856.
Burke, D. M., & Shafto, M. A. (2004). Aging and language production. *Current Directions in Psychological Science, 13*, 21–24.
Cortese, M. J., Balota, D. A., Sergent-Marshall, S. D., & Buckner, R. L. (2003). Sublexical, lexical and semantic influences in spelling: Exploring the effects of age, Alzheimer's disease and primary semantic impairment. *Neuropsychologia, 41*, 952–967.
Dix, D. (2005, June 12). Along the way. *The Record Courier*, p. 4.
Dunlosky, J., Bailey, H., & Hertzog, C. (2011). Memory enhancement strategies: What works best for obtaining memory goals. In P. E. Hartman-Stein & A. La Rue (Eds.), *Enhancing cognitive fitness in adults: A guide for use and development of community-based programs*. New York: Springer.
Glosser, G., Kohn, S. E., Sands, L., Grugan, P., & Friedman, R. B. (1999). Impaired spelling in Alzheimer's disease: A linguistic deficit? *Neuropsychologia, 37*, 807–815.
Holmes, V. M., & Malone, N. (2004). Adult spelling strategies. *Reading and Writing: An Interdisciplinary Journal, 17*, 537–566.
Joshi, R. M., Treiman, R., Carreker, S., & Moats, L. C. (2008–2009). How words cast their spell: Spelling is an integral part of learning the language, not a matter of memorization. *American Educator, 32*, 6–16.
Laird, J. (2008). Spelling bees aren't just for kids. *Mature Living, 32*, 36–37.
Logan, J. W., Olson, M. W., & Lindsey, T. P. (1989). Lessons from champion spellers. *Journal of the Education of the Gifted, 13*, 89–96.
MacKay, D. G., & Abrams, L. (1998). Age-linked declines in retrieving orthographic knowledge: Empirical, practical, and theoretical implications. *Psychology and Aging, 13*, 647–662.
Madden, D. J. (1988). Adult age differences in the effects of sentence contexts and stimulus degradation during visual word recognition. *Psychology and Aging, 3*, 167–172.
Maguire, J. (2006). *American bee: The national spelling bee and the culture of word nerds*. New York: Rodale Books.
Neils, J., Roeltgen, D. P., & Greer, A. (1995). Spelling and attention in early Alzheimer's disease: Evidence for impairment of the graphemic buffer. *Brain and Language, 49*, 241–262.

Chapter 11
Oral Life Review in Older Adults: Principles for the Social Service Professional

Thomas M. Meuser

Abstract The opportunity to tell one's life story, share personal wisdom, and leave a spoken legacy for the future can be a powerful intervention for the well-being of just about any older adult. Social service professionals hear many stories from older clients, yet few take the time to pursue these to the level of a life review. Facilitation of the life review process is not "rocket science" but there is an art to it and important ground rules to follow. This chapter reviews the theoretical basis for "life review in aging" and introduces key concepts for professionals interested in incorporating a "life review sensibility" into their daily practice with older clients.

Introduction

Tell me your story – a simple yet powerful request. To ask this of another, one must be willing to listen. Such listening takes time, commitment, intention, and care. A bond of trust is involved. For the teller, there's a risk of vulnerability and judgment. Will I be heard and how? What might I gain (or lose) from telling my story?

Reminiscence is core to our nature as human beings. It is a function of our memory system and our insatiable desire for growth. We look back and recall the past for many reasons, but most always we reminisce with an eye to the present and future. For the young, reminiscence builds a continuous sense of identity and purpose in life. For the old, it provides a source of comfort, closeness to others, and an opportunity for legacy.

Most reminiscence is automatic and occurs in the midst of daily life. We reminisce with friends from school, war buddies, when talking to an acquaintance at the bus

---

T.M. Meuser (✉)
Gerontology Graduate Program, University of Missouri – St. Louis, MO 63121, USA
e-mail: meusert@umsl.edu

stop, when getting a haircut, etc. These moments of reminiscence are typically brief, focused on one time or place, and experienced as communal and enjoyable.

Reminiscence can also be intentional and inclusive of a whole life story; in other words, a *life review*. In his seminal article on this subject, famed Gerontologist, Robert Butler, wrote:

> "I conceive of life review as a naturally occurring, universal mental process characterized by the progressive return to consciousness of past experiences, and, particularly, the resurgence of unresolved conflicts; simultaneously, and normally, these revived experiences and conflicts can be surveyed and reintegrated ... "
>
> "The life review, as a looking-back process that has been set in motion by looking forward to death, potentially proceeds toward personality reorganization. Thus, life review is not synonymous with, but includes reminiscence ... "
>
> (Butler, 1963: 65–66).

As Butler was writing this in 1963, the dominant view in psychiatry and, to some degree, medicine in general, was that reminiscence was a sign of weakness – *an unhealthy living in the past*, so to speak. Why dwell on the past when life must be lived in the present and with an eye to the future? Butler challenged this view and, in doing so, laid the foundation for the life review movement of today (Gibson, 2004; Kunz & Soltys, 2007).

For Butler, life review is natural, universal, and often transformative. We all do it and benefit in different ways and at different times. The prospect of death is a common motivator. Looking back from the vantage point of the present, and possibly decades of intervening experiences, we can frame our past selves anew and move forward with greater integrity of self and purpose. As will be discussed later, the transformative power of life review lays in the acts of telling and listening, as well as in our choice of words and how we are heard.

A number of excellent publications establish the theoretical, evidentiary and practical bases of life review and related forms of guided autobiography (Birren & Deutchman, 1996; Gibson, 2004; Haight & Haight, 2007; Kunz & Soltys, 2007; Webster & Haight, 2002), and concepts from these primary sources will be discussed throughout this chapter.

Electronic media, especially video sharing and social networking websites, are the new frontier for narrative expression. Options for personal storytelling abound today. In my view, the best combination of traditional reminiscence and life review with modern technology is StoryCorps, a partnership effort of the Library of Congress and National Public Radio.[1] StoryCorps allows individuals from all walks of life to record stories of personal, local, national and, even, global significance. Audio recordings are posted in the thousands to the StoryCorps website – a treasure trove of content and ideas for anyone interested in narrative gerontology (i.e., the study of aging through life stories).

---

[1] See http://storycorps.org/. In addition to clips from various interviews from around the US, the StoryCorps website includes excellent written and video "how to" guides for conducting life story interviews.

Life review interventions can focus on the level of the individual, couple, group of family members or friends, or even a group of strangers. Robert Butler conceptualized the process within a framework of individual discovery and growth. In contrast, James Birren, the founder of group-based Guided Autobiography (GAB), focused as much on the interpersonal power of life review for socialization and personal self-esteem. For Birren, recall of the past is most impactful when embedded in a communal process:

> The group process of priming memories works through bringing to light similarities and differences in the recalled memories of participants. In guided autobiography classes, I often hear such comments as 'Oh, I remember something like that happening to me when I started school' or 'I also broke my leg on a playground.' Differences can also evoke memories. A comment such as 'I was a healthy child and was rarely sick' can bring forth a contrasting memory: 'I had polio when I was a child, and it left its mark on me'
>
> (Birren, 2006: 7).

The communal aspect of life review enriches individual experience, as more varied and detailed memories may be evoked from the interaction of group members. Plus, the group format provides a meaningful forum for self-expression and interpersonal acceptance that's different from a 1:1 encounter. The power of positive regard in a group cannot be underestimated. Both introvert and extrovert can and do benefit.

The choice of whether to pursue an individual or group intervention often depends on the setting. Life review has its fullest expression, I believe, in the hospice movement. Individual interventions prevail here. Persons aware of impending death often feel an extra motivation to tell their story, speak their truths and wisdom, and leave a personal legacy. The book *Tuesdays with Morrie* (Albom, 1997) is a wonderful example of this genre. Retired professor, Morrie Schwartz, dying gradually from ALS, tells a story of a life, love, and wisdom to his former student, Mitch Albom. Mr. Albom wrote the book, of course, but the story is all Morrie – his values, his legacy.

Both men were enriched by their many conversations – deep and lighthearted in tone – and Morrie's personhood lives on in the pages of Albom's book, as well as through a number of fascinating interviews with ABC News' Ted Koppel.[2] Many hospice programs now offer services for the telling and recording of life stories. The *Lumina Program*, for example, offered through BJC Hospice in St. Louis, Missouri, trains community volunteers to visit hospice patients in their homes and hospital or nursing home rooms to record personal stories for reasons of personal integration and legacy.[3]

Long-term care facilities and retirement communities are fertile ground for such interventions. While most people would prefer to live independently, those who live long enough will often need extra help in managing daily tasks as a consequence of declining health. Nursing homes today are striving to be more person-centered (i.e., aware of and responsive to individual preferences and differences), emphasizing the "home" aspect as much as medical care. An important aspect of any home environment is an opportunity to share and be heard.

---

[2] See http://abcnews.go.com/video/playerIndex?id=9084429.
[3] See http://www.bjchospice.org/

Biographical interventions allow staff to know those they care for, not just as "the woman in Room 205 with the broken hip", but as "Doris, the former dancer and teacher, wife and mother, etc." Such interventions bridge the gap between staff and resident, thereby reducing loneliness and bringing meaning to an often painful reality of individual decline. The Apartment Community at The Shrine of Our Lady of the Snows in Belleville, IL, for example, is one such facility to embrace life review as an enjoyable, "value-added" intervention for residents at all levels of care.[4] Residents schedule time in the on-site studio to tell their stories, and often these are screened for others to enjoy, too. Such screenings encourage interpersonal interaction and community, drawing even the most reclusive into the dialog.

Families benefit from life review interventions as well, and not always immediately. I interviewed my grandmother about her life story in the summer of 2003. Then in her early 80s, my grandmother was becoming frail, and it occurred to me how little I knew of her history. What would be lost if she died tomorrow? I asked to interview her about her life story, suggesting that we talk about her birth, family and working lives, important memories, present values, etc. She accepted quite readily, and we met a few days later for a 2 hours tape recorded session at her kitchen table.

We covered a surprising amount of material in this short time. While the facts of her story were of interest, we spent as much time talking about lessons learned and values. She seemed pleased when finished, but not all that interested in keeping any documentation of this interview. She declined a copy of the cassette tape, suggesting that others might appreciate it in the future. This *potential legacy* was enough for her. Whatever she gained in telling her story to me was her private affair. I gained a great deal, much of which would not become apparent to me until years later.

My grandmother died peacefully in 2009. I volunteered to give the eulogy at her funeral. The cassette of her life story was a rich and comforting resource. Her voice was ever-present in my mind as I prepared and later delivered the eulogy, and her story was reflected very much in my words that day. Much as Mitch Albom gave voice to Morrie's personhood and legacy in his book, I gave voice to my grandmother in her eulogy. It was *her* story, *her* legacy. A recorded life review can be a source of learning and inspiration for years to come.

Teaching Life Review

Life review is an intentional looking back on one's life story to bring understanding and meaning to the present (see Table 11.1). This definition includes reminiscence, as suggested by Butler, but also implies a degree of purpose that incidental storytelling (i.e., what we might share at the bus stop or a breakfast with friends) often lacks.

---

[4] See http://www.apartmentcommunity.org/

Table 11.1 Definitions

Oral history	A retelling of specific events (e.g., World War II, 9/11/01) so as to leave a record for future generations
Reminiscence	Recalling past events in one's life to promote meaning, understanding and/or pleasure in present discourse with others
Life review	Typically an organized, intentional effort to recall one's life story and retell critical events and present interpretations
Guided autobiography	Typically an organized, intentional effort to recall one's life story and *write down* critical events and present interpretations

Those engaged in a form of life review interpret and reframe the past based on a lifetime of experiences and wisdom. The reviewer views him or herself differently as a result – more positively in most instances. It is this interpretive aspect that separates life review and guided autobiography from simple reminiscence.

The oral history interview is even further removed, as this approach emphasizes event-specific, chronological recall. What happened and when? The interviewee recalls events and experiences from some critical juncture in the past. The usual goal is to create a record of important events in the life of a family, community, or larger group. While some interpretation may occur in this process, the purpose of the interaction is not to promote personal well-being and self-understanding. Believe it or not, it is possible to conduct an oral history interview and never touch on personal emotions and values! The personal, felt aspects of the story are at the heart of life review.

I strive to model a humanistic, psycho-educational approach to life review with broad applicability across individuals, situations, and practice settings. Life review is not rocket science, but there is an art to doing it well. It is also important to recognize boundaries between supportive care and clinical intervention, especially for unlicensed professionals.

A challenge in teaching life review is its multiplicity of forms and functions. No two life review interventions are alike, as theoretical approaches vary and all people are essentially unique. We may share certain events in common, like graduation from high school or marriage, yet our interpretations are quite personal. While the ultimate goals may be to build self-esteem in the reviewer and leave a legacy for family, the path to these goals is as individual as a fingerprint. This does not mean to say that there is not a structure and rules of thumb to follow, however. Knowledge and preparation are keys to success in life review.

What you will learn in the coming pages is my framing life review as a semi-structured, interpersonal intervention, bookmarked by consent and planning on one side and a final product (written, audio or video) at the other. This is what I teach my graduate students. What happens in between is a function of the person reviewing his or her life story, the goals negotiated and renegotiated during the narrative process, and the journey that reviewer and interviewer share over their time together.

There are always detours and surprises along the way, but it is just as important to keep an eye on the final desired outcome. The person who wishes to leave an upbeat explication of personal values and advice for grandchildren may not wish to touch on past losses or trials, for example. Likewise, the person who wishes to put his or her whole life into honest context may desire (and even need) to hit the highs and lows, even if painful memories surface in the process. Special care must be taken when past traumas surface, however, as life review *is not psychotherapy*.

Since I teach students to conduct life review interviews within the confines of a compressed summer term, my approach emphasizes 1–2 interview/review sessions totaling no more than 2 hours of interaction. Volunteer participants prepare ahead of time by reviewing a detailed Interview Guide (see Appendix). We video record these sessions using a basic digital camcorder, and we then edit the footage on a PC into a unified "keepsake video" for the reviewer and family to have and enjoy in the future.

Other models of life review are not as restrictive in time as this approach, and often encourage six or more sessions to delve more deeply into a life story; whether brief or longer term, however, the basic principles and core values are the same.

To Tell is Human

Stories have been told around the campfire, at the dinner table, in the workplace, at places of worship, etc., since the dawn of human community and society. We teach our children through stories, share our important experiences and truths about life in what we tell each other, and leave a legacy in the tangible and intangible evidence of our existence. Stories define us on individual and collective levels simultaneously:

> … the stories that adults make and tell to provide their lives with unity and purpose are not mere psychological musings, but instead influence deeply the stories and the lives that other people make, for better or for ill. And those stories give rise still to others, in a continuous process of individual and cultural evolution. From one generation to the next, people find meaning and connection within the web of story-making, storytelling, and story-living. Through life stories, human beings help to create the world they live in at the same time that it is creating them.
>
> (McAdams, 1996: 148).

The power of story lies in the act of telling and the human interaction that surrounds it. It has been suggested that we know and even define ourselves as individuals, as unique persons, by what we say and demonstrate to others – the *narrative self*.

Some have argued, also, that our technology-driven society has damaged our ability to tell and listen to personal stories. I disagree. I hear the value placed on the "narrative self" in the older adults who volunteer for the University of Missouri – St. Louis Life Review Project.[5] I hear it every Friday morning when the StoryCorps segment is played on my local public radio station. On the contrary, I would suggest there is more storytelling today than ever before. The kitchen table may be less active of a location, but the electronic world most surely is. It just takes a teller and a listener.

---

[5] See http://www.umsl.edu/~meusert/LifeReview/

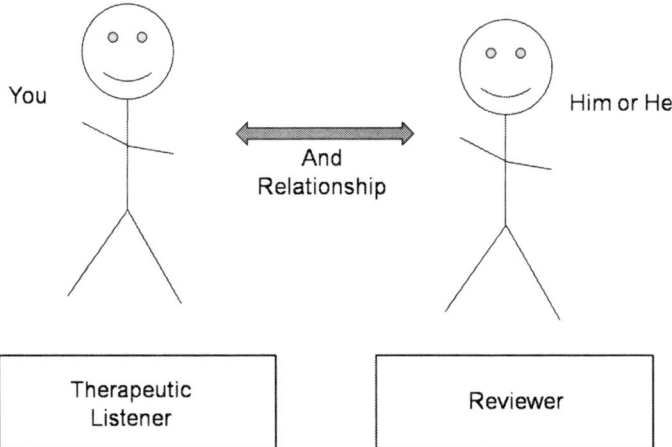

Fig. 11.1 Interpersonal communication

Life review occurs in the context of an interaction between two (or more) persons (see Fig. 11.1). Ideally, this interaction involves a relationship characterized by openness, mutuality, and trust. The *reviewer* is the person telling his or her story. Many call the other participant in this encounter the *interviewer*. While this term is perfectly acceptable and I use it, I prefer the phrase that Barbara Haight recommends: *therapeutic listener* (Haight & Haight, 2007).

The reviewer tells while the other listens. This listening is not passive, however, but empathetic, caring, and even strategic. The therapeutic listener wants the process to be a positive, integrative experience for the reviewer, and so asks questions and shapes the interaction to meet this and other goals. It is helpful for the therapeutic listener to have some background in aging, human development, and interviewing. A friendly manner, an honest interest, and willingness to follow the reviewer's lead are really the only true prerequisites, however.

Therapeutic but not Therapy

In speaking about his version of life review, Guided Autobiography, James Birren is quick to point out that reviewing one's life is not therapy, but it is often therapeutic. The Merriam Webster Dictionary defines therapeutic in this way: "(1) of or relating to the treatment of disease or disorders by remedial agents or methods; (2) providing or assisting in a cure." The person reviewing his or her life story is not diseased or in need of a cure. If this were the case, a form of therapy might well be necessary and helpful. Life review activities are *therapeutic* in the sense that all human beings need affiliation, acceptance, and love. We experience these when in the presence of caring others. The act of telling one's story and being heard is enriching and healing in itself.

Table 11.2 Key differences in clinical versus life review interviewing

Clinical interview	LR interview
Emphasis on *present* (to future)	Emphasis on *past* (to present)
Symptom/problem focus	Understanding/integration focus
Purposeful Therapeutic intent	*Incidental* Therapeutic intent
Power differential (TL >R)[a]	Power differential (TL <R)
Self-narrative is secondary	Self-narrative is primary
Involves one-sided filtering and interpretation	Involves storytelling and interested conversation
Results in recommendations and intervention	Results in an autobiographical product and enhanced self-understanding

[a] *TL* therapeutic listener/interviewer; *R* reviewer/interviewee

A supportive or psycho-educational life review intervention does just this. A PhD or clinical license is not required to conduct in life review work. I teach graduate students in the fields of Gerontology and Social Work. Most do not plan to become counselors or therapists, but rather social service professionals involved in various programmatic and supportive care activities. As clinical psychologist, I am very aware of the importance of defining professional roles and boundaries. While I may choose to incorporate life review techniques in a psychotherapeutic intervention, this usage is not an appropriate option for most of my students; and that's OK.

Awareness of professional boundaries is critical. An invisible, but quite tangible, line separates *clinical* from *supportive* (or psycho-educational) interventions. It is important for all practitioners of reminiscence and life review to be aware of their role and location relative to this boundary. The basic differences between clinical and supportive interventions, and so where to draw this line, are summarized in Table 11.2.

On the clinical side, clients or patients usually seek clinical care because of a problem or illness. Something is wrong that needs diagnosis and treatment. The clinician offers assistance, first by assessing past history and present coping, and then by working to treat the identified malady, encourage more effective coping, promote a healthier approach to daily living, etc. In such interactions, the clinician is the *expert* (i.e., authority figure) and holds the *power* to direct this encounter. The client or patient listens as the expert frames the important issues (including diagnoses) and makes recommendations for care and future benefit.

The supportive life review encounter is very different. First, the *power to* direct the encounter resides with the reviewer. It is his or her life, after all. The reviewer enters into the life review dialog with specific purposes in mind and chooses what will be discussed. The therapeutic listener may ask questions and make comments (it is important that he or she to so, in fact), but the power to choose how to respond remains with the reviewer. The past is viewed as a source of knowledge and inspiration to enrich the present and future.

Both clinical and supportive interventions may be *therapeutic* in that person's present life is enriched, but the motivators and methods are distinct.

Core Values

Most fields of professional practice have codes of ethics or norms for right behavior. I am unaware of a specific code for life review professionals, but I believe in a set of core principles that guide my efforts in this area. These relate to how we view and treat older adults, respect personal boundaries, and manage the vagaries of human memory.

Principle 1 – Older adults can handle the tough stuff.

A common ageist stereotype is that older adults become frail in body, mind, and emotion, and so need to be "protected" from undue distress and burden. If you live seven or eight decades, you have learned to manage life's ups and downs. Certainly, some older adults, such as those with advancing dementia, are vulnerable and do need reasonable protection. Most that choose to participate in a life review interview, however, are not in this situation. An important "job" of the therapeutic listener is to accept what the reviewer wishes to discuss and follow the threads, even when painful and troubling at times.

A life review that is all about pain, however, is not really a life review. There needs to be balance and a present focus. Imagine, for example, that you are interviewing a 92-year-old woman about her life story. You have developed a strong rapport – she really feels comfortable with you – and at some point she reveals that she was raped as a child. Past traumas can and do surface in the context of a life review. As the therapeutic listener, your role is not only to hear her out, but also to bring balance to the discussion. The specific details of the assault may be discussed, but what's central from a life review perspective is how this early experience shaped her life story the person she is today. You might say in response: "I recognize that this was a very painful event in your early life and I am glad you shared it. Painful events sometimes bring learning and growth, too. How did this event make you the person you are today?" This response honors the memory, but emphasizes that all life events occur in the larger context of a full life story. Few persons who have lived through and overcome a trauma like this would not find some meaning and even value for self-definition.

It can happen, also, that a trauma is discussed and the wound is still fresh. In this case, the therapeutic listener needs to do more than just honor the memory and discuss present integration. Evidence of distress should be discussed and documented, and a referral made for professional assistance.

Principle 2 – Telling the story is the most important part.

While many of those who volunteer to be interviewed by my students wish to leave a video-based record for future generations, this goal is secondary to the act of telling their stories. The deeper benefit for most participants occurs during the interview itself, as they tell of past events and frame themselves anew in a structured, insight-oriented process. The DVD or written biography that follows is a nice capstone, but nothing more. The foundation has already been laid and fulfilled the core mission.

This was my grandmother's experience. She didn't want a copy of her life story on audiotape. "I know what I went through," she remarked, "I did this for you." I would go so far as to say that when the final product becomes the primary motivator, then the life review intervention has lost essential focus.

Principle 3 – Truth as fact is secondary in life review.

The human memory system is not like a camcorder; it does not record events as they occurred for later playback. It is, rather, a distributed system of memory traces that are constructed and reconstructed over a lifetime (see a detailed review in Gibson, 2004). What and how we remember something is based as much on our attention and emotions at the time of the event, as the quality of our memory in general. Maybe with the exception of a handful of savants, most of us forget something each day, each hour. We remember what we need to for success in our family and work lives, but we often forget the finer details of events and routine aspects of our daily lives. What did you have for breakfast a week ago last Monday? Many could not answer this question and for good reason. This level of recall is not adaptive; as such memories would clutter and confuse what's most important for success in living months and years hence.

Recall of any past event or experience is always a reconstruction. Our brains draw on memory traces that are stored in visual, auditory, and association cortex, for example, and pull the key material into working memory for it to be processed and discussed. While certain powerful memories (e.g., Where were you when you learned that President Kennedy was shot? What were you doing when you heard the news of the 9/11/01 Terrorist Attacks?) may be recalled in essentially the same way each time, most memories are not of this "flash bulb" type. We remember bits and pieces, and then put these together as best we can in the moment. Intervening experiences and present interpretation often intrude and may change the content or organization somewhat.

This is not to say that memories shared in life review are not truthful – they are for that person in most instances – but they may not be completely factual (i.e., as a camcorder would record them). It is important for the practitioner to recognize this limitation of memory and respect it. *Facts are not as important in life review as are personal understandings and interpretations.*

I take this one step further with a World War II story I tell in my life review class. Imagine that you are interviewing a veteran in his living room, and his wife is preparing a meal in the kitchen nearby. He tells you about his service during the war, and he relays a detailed story of serving on the front lines during the Battle of the Bulge.[6] You listen intently and are captivated by his story. Then, moments later, his wife yells "Honey, you were State-side the whole war! What are you talking about?"

---

[6] Knowledge of important historical events can be very helpful when conducting a life review intervention. The Battle of the Bulge was the final major offensive of the German Army towards the end of World War II. It was an especially fierce and bloody campaign, leaving thousands dead on both sides. The memories of this and similar war-related experiences remain vivid in the minds of the veterans who were there.

The veteran in this case was sharing *his truth* with you. Do you pick up on the wife's comment and correct him? Maybe you would in therapy, but not in a life review encounter. What's important in this story is what he's saying *between the lines*. Some veterans who served outside the theater of combat may regret, even to this day, not having been more involved and even at personal risk. You may respond: "I sense that you are very proud of your service to your country; that your contribution was important and remains a source of strength today." He will likely agree and share more, and his wife's comment need not be addressed.

Consent and Negotiation

How is a life review encounter or intervention initiated? In the case of my Life Review Project, I distribute a simple flyer via e-mail and when I speak in the community. Prospective volunteers learn the basics of what's involved from the flyer, and those interested in proceeding will send in the interest form or call my office. Since student education is a part of my effort, volunteers must be willing to allow 2–5 min clips from their interviews to be used in a Gerontology Video Library. This library is accessible to faculty at my institution to enrich classroom instruction. There is no cost for the interview, but there's "payment" in the volunteer's support for the video library effort. The going rate for a professional life review interview and video is $300–500. A consent form is involved, and we take extra care in editing video clips so that names, other identifiers, and especially sensitive topics are excluded.

I'm often asked about the video library by faculty at other institutions and social service professionals. Most want access to use the clips for their own education and outreach. While I appreciate many aspects of our current electronic world, the integrity of our life review work is most important to me. Once video is shared on-line, even with the best of intentions, it can be captured and misused. I owe it to my volunteers to protect their self-expressions as much as I reasonably can. This is an important issue for the practitioner, and one to keep in mind whenever electronic media are utilized.

Two recent publications (Gibson, 2004; Haight & Haight, 2007) discuss the consent process for life review in great detail, including templates for the new practitioner to review and adopt.

Once consent is obtained, an interview plan must be negotiated. This can be done through a face-to-face orientation meeting (preferable) or by telephone. Why does the individual wish to review his or her life at this time? What aspects are especially important to cover? Is one sitting planned; or two, three, four? Is a chronological approach most appropriate or are there important events or themes that may guide the interview experience? Some reviewers will not have specific answers to such questions, at least when asked in such a direct way. The important thing is for the practitioner to get to know the person and the broad brush strokes of his or her life before sitting down formally. The rest is negotiated as the process unfolds.

Themes, Metaphors, and Questions

How should the life review process unfold? Barbara Haight recommends a chronological-developmental approach that touches on early childhood, childhood, etc., with emphasis on important milestones (see Haight & Haight, 2007). Haight's approach is appealing because of its strong theoretical basis (i.e., the work of Erik Erikson) and its promotion of personal integration. I draw from Haight's work, but I do not teach her specific approach to my students. It is a bit too close to the clinical boundary line discussed earlier. Those with a background in counseling can benefit greatly from learning and practicing this approach. Haight and Haight (2007) provides a helpful list of life review questions that any practitioner can use.

James Birren emphasizes the use of important life themes and metaphors to guide the review process (see Table 11.3). Participants in GAB participate in a series of group meetings each organized around a different life theme. I prefer this approach, myself, as it is understandable and accessible to just about anyone. My Interview Guide (see Appendix) combines such themes with specific questions and probes to promote self-reflection prior to the live, video recorded interview. Most participants come prepared with notes, or at least tell of having thought through what's most important to them. The themes listed in the guide are a useful starting point for negotiating how the interview will proceed; what is most important to cover and what may be less applicable or desired.

I teach my students to capture the *gist* of a persons' life story, touching on birth, family of origin, education, career, family, etc. We want the reviewer's "keepsake video" to reflect a full life story, but we can't cover everything of consequence in 1–2 hours. We hit the high points. Particular emphasis is placed on exploring personal values, considering the final years of life, and touching on beliefs about death. This latter topic may sound morbid, but not so to many older adults who consider it often. Honoring a reviewer's beliefs and hopes about death are critical tasks in any life review interview.

Table 11.3 Themes and resources for life review

Birren's themes	On-line resources
Branching points	American Folklife Center http://www.loc.gov/folklife
Your family	
Role of money	The Birren Center for Autobiography and Life Review http://www.guidedautobiography.com
Major life's work	International Institute for Reminiscence and Life Review
Health history	http://www.uwsuper.edu/cee/lll/reminiscence/index.cfm
Death and dying	USC Shoah Foundation Institute http://college.usc.edu/vhi/
Sexual identity	
Spirituality, philosophy of living	StoryCorps http://www.storycorps.net
Goals and aspirations	UMSL Life Review Project http://www.umsl.edu/~meusert/LifeReview/

I told the story of my grandmother earlier in this chapter. In addition to telling me her life story, she also spoke of how death touched her life in the past and her own eventual death. She shared that she did not fear death; her faith was a great source of strength and comfort in this regard. "We all must die someday," she commented, "that's how we were created and must accept it." This perspective added much to my eulogy and served to heal the wounds of grief.

What questions to ask in a life review encounter will depend on the reviewer, how vocal he or she may be, and the flow of chosen topics. Simple yes–no questions should be avoided. While fact-based questions (e.g., Where did you go to high school?) have their place, open-ended questions are preferable, even some that might seem a bit odd. I conducted a life review with my father last year. I asked him to recall a favorite food from his childhood. Why should a favorite food be important in life review? Well, in his case, this question yielded a flood of memories and opened multiple lines of discussion, eventually culminating in his thoughts and feelings around his mother's early death from cancer. His favorite food was spiced meatballs that his mother made on special occasions. I could see in the expression on his face that he tasted those meatballs anew in that moment. A dual reflection on the joys and the tough stuff of his early life ensued. It was a powerful moment.

Ripples in Time and Legacy

I hope that reading this chapter has given you a sense for what life review is and/or can be in your own personal or professional life. It is often said at funerals "If only (name) could be here to see how he (she) impacted so many others." We all leave a legacy – our own ripples in time – whether aware of it or not. The life review process is an intentional effort at legacy that allows the reviewer to feel the impact and know the meaning of these ripples while still alive and engaged. It empowers the reviewer, too, to learn, grow, and make changes for a better tomorrow. While the prospect of death may motivate participation, life review is not about dying, but about living. Morrie Schwartz expressed his passion for life in his many meetings with Mitch Albom. Will you support someone else in doing this, too?

Appendix

Life Review Interview Guide

A life review interview can be both an enjoyable and a challenging experience. Many questions may be considered, but rarely would all be answered in a single sitting. Your comfort is of utmost importance. You don't have to answer any question or delve into any area which causes you discomfort. You can expect your interview to last about 1–2 h.

As you prepare for the interview, consider how you have grown over the course of your life and the many things you have learned. This interview is an opportunity to learn about yourself, share your perspectives and values, and teach others at the same time.

The interview begins with three standard items (in italics below) that appear early in the edited Keepsake DVD:

- Looking at the camera, please say your *first name* (My name is_____), where you were *born/year* (I was born in_____ in 19_____), your *age* (I am _____ years old), and where you *live now* (and I live in an apartment (house, etc.) in _____).
- What 3–5 characteristics or adjectives describe you the best? (e*xample: I like to think of myself as honest, hard-working, caring, and inquisitive*).
- Why did you volunteer to participate in this interview today? What do you hope to gain from this experience?

The remainder of the interview is loosely structured around the themes and questions listed below. Over the course of the interview, we *do* want to capture the general story of your life (birth, early life, school, work, etc.), and the interviewer will help structure this. The rest will depend on you and what's important to you.

Most interviewees cover many/all of the themes below, but some in more depth than others. It is sometimes helpful to come prepared to your interview with notes (on this page is fine) or a listing of topics. The interviewer will ask you about important topics to cover (or not cover) at the start of the interview process. Since the interview is being video recorded, you can stop at any time and negotiate how to proceed.

- *Your current life*
  - Tell me about your current life and activities.
    – Who are the 2–3 *most important* people in your life now?
    – What is your daily routine like? What brings you joy?
    – What are the most challenging aspects of your life today?

- *About you/past life*
  – Tell me about your family of origin – parents, siblings.
  – What stands out in your memory about growing up?
  – Who were the 2–3 *most important* people in your life when you were young?
  – (If married or widowed) How did you and your spouse meet? What was your early relationship like?
  – What joys and/or challenges occurred during your married life?
  – (If you had children) Tell me about your child or children. What stands out in your memory about their growing up? What is your relationship(s) like today?
  – (If applicable) What did it mean for you personally to become a parent? How did parenthood mold you as a person?

- We all experience losses in our life. Looking back at the first half of your life, what losses (deaths, other losses) stand out in your memory? What has grief meant in your life?

- *Career and service*
  - What paying jobs did you hold in the past?
  - Did you consider any as a career or vocation?
  - Was volunteerism a part of your experience, then or now? How so?
  - Did you serve in the military? If so, what branch and position? What was your experience like? Hold did it mold you as a person?
  - (If applicable) What impact did retirement have on your sense of yourself and personal security?

- *Health*
  - How would you describe your health today? Do you function in handling daily life tasks much as in the past, or are there limitations now?
  - Have health problems been challenges at other times during your life?
  - Have you ever experienced a period of significant anxiety or depression? If so, would you be willing to share a bit about this experience? What helped you through it?

- *Caregiving*
  - Have you served as a caregiver, now or in the past?
  - For whom did you provide care? For what reasons?
  - How does/did serving as a caregiver enrich your life?
  - What challenges do/did you face as a caregiver? What is/was the hardest part for you?

- *Spirituality*
  - What role has faith played in your life?
  - What are the roots of your faith? Has your faith changed over time.
  - What values do you hold especially dear or meaningful?
  - Has your faith helped you to overcome challenges and/or get through some difficult times?

- *Death and end of life*
  - How as death impacted the second half of your life?
  - What losses stand out as particularly meaningful or challenging?
  - What do you believe about death and what may come after?
  - Does death frighten you?

- *Life review*
  - On balance, are you satisfied with how you have lived your life?
  - Are there any significant regrets?
  - What 2–3 accomplishments are you most proud of? Why?

- *Looking to the future*
    - What do you expect the next 5–10 years to bring in your life?
    - What are your hopes for yourself and those closest to you?
    - If you could share just one piece of advice to enrich the life of a young person, what would it be?
- *Other thoughts and comments*

References

Albom, M. (1997). *Tuesdays with Morrie: an old man, a young man, and life's greatest lesson.* New York, NY: Random House.

Birren, J.E. (2006). Benefits of memory priming: Effects of guided autobiography and reminiscence. *MindAlert 2006*, San Francisco, CA: American Society on Aging. Retrieved from http://www.asaging.org/asav2/mindalert/pdfs/booklet_2006.pdf.

Birren, J. E., & Deutchman, D. E. (1996). *Guiding autobiography groups for older adults: Exploring the fabric of life.* Baltimore, MD: Johns Hopkins University Press.

Butler, R. N. (1963). The life review: An interpretation of reminiscence in old age. *Psychiatry Journal for the study of Interpersonal Processes, 26*, 65–76.

Gibson, F. (2004). *The past in the present: Using reminiscence in health and social care.* Baltimore, MD: Health Professions.

Haight, B. K., & Haight, B. S. (2007). *The handbook of structured life review.* Baltimore, MD: Health Professions.

Kunz, J. A., & Soltys, F. G. (2007). *Transformational reminiscence: Life story work.* New York, NY: Springer.

McAdams, D. P. (1996). Narrating the self in adulthood. In J. E. Birren, G. M. Kenyon, J. E. Ruth, J. J. F. Schroots, & T. Svenson (Eds.), *Aging and biography: Explorations in adult development* (pp. 131–148). New York, NY: Springer.

Webster, J. D., & Haight, B. K. (2002). *Critical advances in reminiscence work: From theory to application.* New York, NY: Springer.

Chapter 12
Creative Writing Groups: A Promising Avenue for Enhancing Working Memory and Emotional Well-Being

Paula E. Hartman-Stein

Abstract Creative writing groups are cognitive enhancement programs that can be offered easily, with minimal expense, and are adaptable to many community settings. Healthy older adults as well as those living with cognitive impairment can benefit from them if they desire an intellectually challenging activity with a social component. This chapter presents case studies, reviews research evidence of the health and cognitive benefits of creative writing, and illustrates the value of a "building on existing strengths approach" to cognitive support and stimulation.

Case Study: Peter

Peter, a 78-year-old married, retired high school teacher, sought intellectually stimulating activities within his community. I invited him to participate in a creative writing workshop series open to residents at a nearby retirement facility and members of the community where he lived (Biermann & Hartman-Stein, Chapter 6). The following is an unedited excerpt of his writing in response to the prompt given at the first session to write about life-defining moments:

> There are times when I feel compelled to examine my character. Am I selfishly concentrating on doing only what I want to do or do I try to bend to the wishes of others, even if I don't find these suggestions pleasant? When I consider these attitudes I think of my family and I am led to concentrate on my parents since I was an only child. I would always turn to my mother because she was gentle and loving. She enjoyed providing me with delights and was always quite proud of my successes.

P.E. Hartman-Stein (✉)
Clinical Geropsychologist, Center for Healthy Aging, 265 W. Main Street,
Kent, Ohio 44240; Adjunct Faculty, Department of Human Development and Family Studies,
College of Education, Health and Human Services, Kent State University, Kent, OH, USA
e-mail: paula@centerforhealthyaging.com

My mother was sometimes demanding but rarely sharp with me. My father, on the other hand, was of a different nature. Though he was never violent, I was generally afraid of his reactions to my behavior. As I grew up, however, we began to share the same interests.

He was a journalist at the Wolverhampton Express and essentially spent his entire working life on the newspaper. He worked his way up to the Chief Sub-Editor…. He was under great pressure because of strict deadlines and quick decisions at the newspaper. Like the majority of workers, the stressful day would end with pints of beer at a local pub. He came home to a late supper, and I was careful not to engage in arguments or venture toward anything that might irritate as I never felt comfortable with him in my younger days.

The war broke out with Hitler's Germany, and a new era dawned. I clearly remember listening to the radio as Prime Minister Chamberlain announced the declaration of war. I was nine years old on that day. My father persuaded my mother to take me to Shrewsbury since it was a small market town and less likely to be a target of the expected bombardments.

We had arranged to have our coal cellar fortified as a bomb shelter furnished with cots and kerosene lamps. We recognized the characteristic drone of the German planes as they flew over, heralded by warning sirens…

The end of the war marked a great improvement in my relationship with my father as he became more relaxed…. We began to take long walks together in the countryside; he helped me learn how to play cricket and showed me how to take the correct strokes; meanwhile I had started to take piano lessons, and he and I sometimes played duets although my capacities in music soon outshone his own. At the local grammar school I found interesting teachers who put me on the path to scholarship. I was able to enter Pembroke College, Cambridge, where I became a serious student of foreign language…

Several years later I had joined the faculty at a private academy when I received a call telling me that my father was seriously ill. I flew over immediately and found him too weak to talk. He remained weak but was impressively light-hearted about the situation. This put me in a quandary when I started to wonder if he was really as harsh as I had remembered him being as a child. At one point he lay back just as the nurse arrived and announced, "he's gone." My mother wept but I could only feel a sense of relief that he had had a peaceful end.

Peter had been diagnosed with Alzheimer's disease over 2 years before he composed this piece. At the time he wrote it, he was dependent upon his wife for most instrumental activities of daily living such as food preparation, shopping, driving, and management of medications and finances. Each week of the 11 session program he was unable to find the classroom location within the retirement facility without assistance. Results of his neuropsychological evaluation conducted 6 months earlier revealed significant impairment in verbal recall and retention, executive functioning, and visual spatial organization. However, he performed in the nonimpaired, intact range on tests of language such as verbal fluency, language comprehension, common sense reasoning, and judgment.

Peter had been alarmed about his diagnosis of early dementia, so he had embarked on a self-designed program of cognitive enrichment and physical exercise. He walked each day for at least an hour and worked out a local gym three to four times a week with weight bearing exercises. He practiced foreign languages, including Russian, recited poetry in multiple languages, and practiced musical instruments, the piano and recorder. Peter had a supportive wife and family, often traveling to visit his adult children, but he recognized that his social network of friends was shrinking. Peter was determined to take few, if any, medications. He and his wife believed in life style modifications whenever possible when faced with health or emotional problems that may be ameliorated through nonpharmacological interventions. He had sought my consultation for assistance to help him cope better with his declining cognitive skills. At the time of his consultation, I was able to offer him a new program in his community that would meet his needs and support his existing strengths.

I was currently serving as project director of a lifelong learning program, *Keys to a Sharp Mind*, at a local retirement community and was about to lead one of the workshop series, "Creative Writing for Health and Healing" (Biermann & Hartman-Stein, Chapter 6). The entire programming was geared to the older adult who had minimal, if any, cognitive impairment, but individuals with early dementia were not turned away from attending if they showed interest in any of the courses.

The selected writing prompts selected for this course helped to elicit written expression of meaningful past life events. I had designed the course based on the fairly extensive body of research that suggests writing about deep thoughts and feeling on emotional issues and upsetting past life events in a way that results in "meaning-making" can produce long-term improvements in mood and health (Stuckey & Nobel, 2010). I had not geared the program in any specific way to helping individuals with mild cognitive impairment or early onset dementia syndromes.

Although Peter lived with significant cognitive impairment, I encouraged him to participate because of the potential benefit from the socialization aspect of the writing program that encouraged feedback and support from the other writers, a small group of 6–10 people. Because his remote autobiographical memory and his expressive language skills were intact, it was likely he could participate in a meaningful, appropriate way.

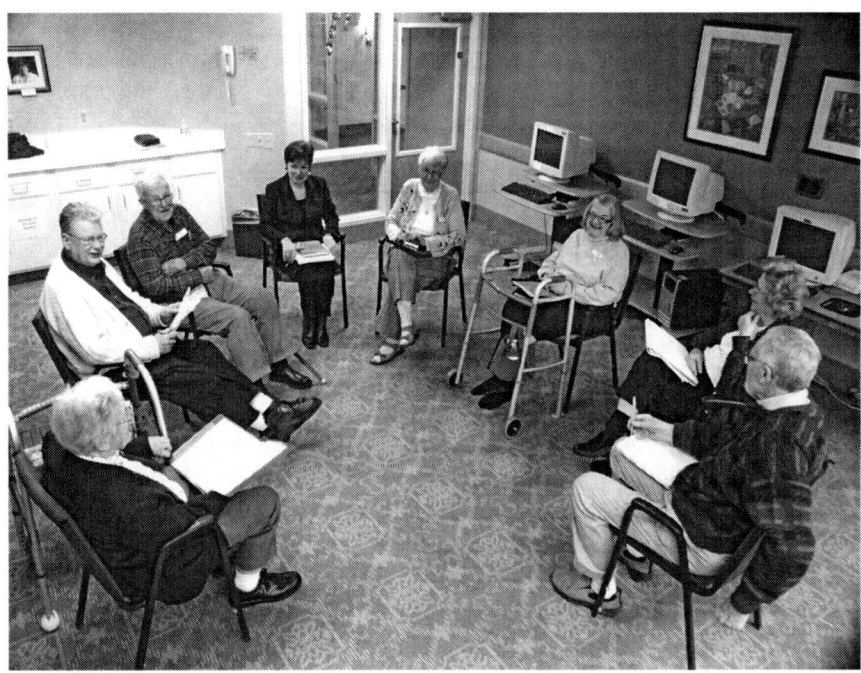

Immediately after the first day of the class, one of the other participants questioned why I had allowed Peter in the program because she was aware of his diagnosis of Alzheimer's dementia. I told her that he was interested in participating, and I believed he would be an asset to the group. As his excerpt illustrates, Peter had the ability to write with great clarity about his distant memories. He also read his pieces with theatrical eloquence, demonstrating impressive oratorical skills beyond those of anyone in the writing group. After his first reading, no one questioned the appropriateness of his presence in the program. Peter attended the majority of the sessions and reported that he looked forward to them. His mood appeared to improve in general, and his wife was pleased that he could participate in the writing program. The other members of the writing workshop appeared to enjoy listening to him read the accounts of his life in the past and his philosophical notions that came out in his work.

Peter was the first person with cognitive impairment who had participated in my writing workshops. By observing his participation and the response of others to his writing, I learned firsthand that creative writing through guided autobiography has potential benefit not only for individuals with intact memory functioning but also for some individuals who live with cognitive impairment, particularly if writing skills had been a strength and continue to be a potential interest to revive.

The rest of the chapter describes different types of therapeutic writing, reviews available research evidence of the benefits of creative writing on well-being and working memory, incorporates two additional case studies, and provides suggestions for the implementation of therapeutic writing groups in community settings.

Throughout this chapter, there is no distinction between therapeutic and creative writing. According to Gillie Bolton, a British consultant for therapeutic writing groups who has worked with populations as varied as hospice patients, prisoners, and healthcare professionals, creative and therapeutic writing would lose their power if there was a major difference (Bolton, 1999). Therapeutic writing includes journaling, memoir writing, guided autobiography, poetry, and creative nonfiction, to name a few genres (Birren & Cochran, 2001; Bolton, 1999; Carroll, 2005; Kominars, 2007).

The genre of autobiographical writing is credited as far back as St. Augustine, the fourth century theologian, who wrote about his growth in Christian spirituality (Brady & Sky, 2003). The tradition of writing one's story through journals and diaries has been found in both Eastern and Western traditions throughout the ages. In recent years, journal writing has gained popularity in American culture and has been connected with enhancing spiritual awareness and overall creativity (Cameron, 1992).

The gerontologist, James E. Birren, has conducted guided autobiographical writing group programs for older adults for more than 3 decades. In the book, *Telling the Stories of Life through Guided Autobiography Groups*, Birren and Cochran (2001) describe a structured method of guiding the writer to prepare a personal history using a series of life themes over a 10-week course. Themes include major branching points in life, family, the role of money, major life work and career, health and body, sexual identity, experiences with and ideas about death, spiritual life and values, and goals and aspirations.

Guided autobiography groups provide opportunities for introspection and sharing within groups to help leave behind old wounds, gain personal insights, reaffirm personal needs, leave behind a legacy for family members, and help people cope with life transitions (Birren & Cochran, 2001).

Research on Benefits of Expressive Writing

Writing about stressful life events has received much attention in the medical and psychological literature although there are relatively few published studies with older adults. In a qualitative study of perceived benefits of journal writing among 15 older adults (average age 69.2 years), Brady and Sky (2003) reported perceived improvements in the following areas: coping with conflicts in relationships, decision-making skills, and as an aid to memory. Regular journal writers in the study identified additional benefits of improving daily problem-solving skills, enabling personal discoveries, contemplating the meaning of one's life, and developing a new level of consciousness or spirituality.

Pennebaker and Beall (1986) published the first randomized control trial showing the health benefits of writing about traumatic events compared to superficial topics. Writing about traumatic events for as few as three 20-min sessions resulted in improvements in physical and psychological health compared to writing about trivial topics. Since that first publication, over 200 studies on expressive writing have surfaced, with a large number showing positive effects on health. In a recent review, Stuckey and Nobel (2010) summarized research that demonstrated the positive impact of expressive writing on health measured by frequency of physician visits, stress hormones, immune function, blood pressure, pain severity, depressed mood, and working memory.

Relatively few studies have specifically examined the impact of creative writing on memory functioning except for research that investigates its effect on working memory, the ability to hold information in mind while performing a mental operation such as repeating a list of digits backward (Lezak, Howieson, & Loring, 2004). Working memory is a limited capacity system that requires simultaneous storage and processing of information. Klein and Boals (2001) investigated the impact of expressive writing on working memory based on the rationale that cognitions about ongoing stressful events are among the irrelevant demands that interfere with working memory capacity, and expressive writing about these events may reduce their draw on working memory resources.

One study done with American college freshmen (35 students in the experimental group and 34 assigned to the control group) found that those assigned to write about their thoughts and feelings about beginning college compared to a group of writers assigned a trivial topic demonstrated larger working memory gains 7 weeks later (Klein & Boals, 2001). In a subsequent study, they found that students who wrote about a negative personal experience showed greater working memory improvement and reported less intrusive thoughts compared to students asked to write about a positive experience or a trivial topic.

Yogo and Fujihara (2008) obtained similar results in a study of 104 Japanese undergraduates. Those students assigned to write about traumatic experiences improved their working memory capacity after 5 weeks of writing, but writing about positive topics had no effect.

In another study of first semester college students, an expressive writing intervention about a stressful or traumatic event done in three 20 min sessions reduced depression symptoms in participants who engaged in brooding or ruminative thinking. Expressive writing appeared to help individuals restructure maladaptive cognitions and facilitate active problem-solving by actively analyzing and processing past stressful experiences (Sloan, Marx, Epstein, & Dobbs, 2008).

Klein and Boals (2001) suggested that improvements in available working memory may be responsible in part for the evidence that expressive writing benefits health and promotes a sense of well-being. Unwanted thoughts can impair problem-solving and reduce proactive coping and appropriate responses to stressors. Consequently, more stress is produced, resulting in decreases in psychological and physical well-being. Additional studies are needed to determine whether writing about stressful experiences lessens the stress-illness cycle by its effect on working memory.

Whether the positive impact writing interventions appear to have on the working memory of younger adults generalizes to older adults is another area for future research.

Case Study: Frances

The following is a case study of an individual who participated in creative writing groups as a complementary treatment of depression and to improve expressive language skills.

Frances was an 85-year-old widowed woman with a suspected diagnosis of primary progressive aphasia, a gradually progressive syndrome of loss of ability to use or understand language that occurs without memory impairment early in the disease (Lezak et al., 2004). During the 6 months prior to her consultation, her family noted she increasingly spoke in a halting, hesitant manner and engaged in conversation less often. She had been withdrawing from her usual social activities and became less physically active. Her neuropsychological test results showed intact functioning in verbal recall and retention, naming skills, construction, and reasoning. She performed poorly on a verbal fluency task involving generating words that began with specific letters in contrast to her performance on a category naming task in which she generated examples of animals. On a task of divided attention with a motor component, she scored in the mildly impaired range due to slow response time, but her visual deficits due to macular degeneration likely contributed to her slowness in responding to visual stimuli.

Frances acknowledged feeling depressed and lacking enjoyment in her life. She reported fears of death and feelings of inadequacy due to slowness in her verbal expressive skills. As a child she had a severe stuttering problem, and in the last few years since her husband's death her speech pattern reverted to a similar halting, hesitant pattern. Her neurologist suggested she exercise more, learn Tai Chi, and practice speaking more often by reading books aloud to her dog because she lived alone and had relatively few social contacts during the day.

I recommended that she participate in individual and group psychotherapy to mitigate her depressive it with thoughts and have opportunities for interacting with other older adults as well as engage in regular aerobic exercise at a community health club that offered a "Silver Sneakers" program geared to older adults. Because of her expressive language difficulties, I offered her a therapeutic guided autobiographical group to provide structure and encouragement for self-expression, both written and oral. A high school graduate and former bookkeeper, Frances agreed to try the program.

The group members readily accepted Frances despite the fact that she rarely initiated conversational remarks to others during the group; however, she used a magnifier during the writing portion of the program and responded to each writing prompt. A visible change occurred in her mood and speech pattern after she wrote the following excerpt based on the prompt, "Describe your thoughts and experiences with the death of a family member or friend":

> The day my husband died, I knew he was going to die…I got him ready for bed and gave him insulin and cleaned him up. I regret that I could not stay awake but I was so exhausted from trying to keep him in his chair that I fell asleep. When I woke up, I looked over at him; he looked so peaceful that I knew he had passed into heaven. I took the dog for a walk, for I knew she needed to go out. Then I called the paramedics and the family. The sheriff came down to take pictures; it seems they had to take pictures to make sure he died of natural causes…I asked my doctor what would make feet cold and icy and turn blue, and he said it was a blood clot.
>
> I secretly wished he would die because he took my freedom away from me, but yet I don't regret taking care of him…I cannot complain as there are people worse off than he was…When he was talking to a visitor once, he said I was an angel for taking care of him. He never told me that.

Almost immediately after Frances composed the above piece and read it aloud with the group of writers, her speech became less halting, less dysfluent. She smiled more frequently in the writing group, and during individual therapy she agreed to begin the exercise program because she had more energy. Two months of previous therapy had been unsuccessful in achieving the same profound effect. During therapy she had not mentioned ambivalent thoughts about the death of her husband or the guilt she secretly harbored. She rarely spoke of him or the extent of her past caregiving responsibilities.

Following unsuccessful exploration of possible triggers of her depressive mood and behavioral withdrawal, I used a behavioral activation approach, encouraging her to increase the frequency of pleasant activities and engaging in problem-solving with the goal of decreasing her isolated lifestyle. It appeared that the writing prompts helped to increase her insight and acknowledgement of her ambivalent feelings regarding her husband's death. In addition, listening to others read about deaths of children and parents modeled a manner of expression within a group that offered acceptance and emotional safety.

However, the improvement in her fluency lasted about 6–8 months. One possibility is that when Frances had felt stressed, she resorted back to ruminative thinking, and her speech deteriorated. She continued to write therapeutic homework assignments within the context of individual therapy. During the first half of each psychotherapy session, Frances' speech had been dysfluent as it had been previously, but as she gained confidence in self-expression, her speech improved during the second half of the therapy sessions. Psychotherapeutic treatment included a combination of problem-solving to reduce isolation, cognitive restructuring, and insight-oriented techniques.

Nuts and Bolts of a Therapeutic Writing Workshop

For the past 3 years, therapeutic writing workshops have been part of the services offered to many of my clients. Because these programs are complementary treatment to psychotherapy for my clients and open to the public for self-development, they are not group psychotherapy. No insurance claims are accepted. The participants pay an out-of-pocket fee, similar to the customary rates charged for writing workshops in our locality. I advertise the programs through churches, local writers' groups, and my website, www.centerforhealthyaging.com. The themes of the workshops vary and have included intergenerational programs on topics such as connections between the mind and body, guided autobiography, spiritual autobiography, coping with caregiving and connecting with nature, an eco-therapeutic approach.

Case Study: James

I invite select clients to participate, including those who live with mild cognitive impairment or dementia syndromes, for the purpose of supporting their needs for cognitive stimulation within a social context. James' story is such an example. A 92-year-old retired psychotherapist, James had vascular dementia with depression. I invited him to participate in writing sessions because of his complaints about the lack of cognitively stimulating activities offered at the assisted living facility where he lived. James had a major stroke 5 years earlier. He was unable to walk independently. He had an indwelling catheter and could not manage any instrumental activities of daily living independently. He often became disoriented to time and place. He had a devoted caregiver, Greta, who had been his lover for many years prior to his stroke. She brought him to my office for psychotherapy for his depressive symptoms as well as the writing workshop. Because James' right arm was paralyzed, he dictated his thoughts to Greta who transcribed them. James was able to read his pieces aloud to the group. The following is an excerpt of his writing from the prompt to describe thoughts and experiences about death.

> My one time love and former assistant, Pat, had gone down to the basement and sat on a bench with a bunch of pills in front of her. She was serious about ending her life. I felt very keenly that she wanted to die as I knew she had taken steps to bring about her death. I don't remember many details about my efforts to change her mind. I believe I helped her think more about this frightful decision, and in the end she decided not to commit suicide. I remember talking to her about the impact of such a decision on her family, friends, and the people she loved…

> Another time when Pat and I no longer lived together, she called me about 2.00 a.m. and told me she was going to commit suicide. I felt she was a precious person, and I didn't want to see her suffer. I remember using every effort I could to convince her not to take her life. … There didn't seem to be any particular event or events going on in the life at the time to warrant her feelings of desperation. …I convinced her to go with me to the hospital. She remained at the hospital for several weeks. Over time her attitude about life became more positive. I saw her frequently and remained a close friend. Her concerns with dying seemed to become less and less important in her life. Her situation provoked constant concern on my part because I felt personally threatened that I might lose her. She was so very important to my life at that time.

James reported a sense of relief after recalling the above life experience and reading it to others. Group participants praised the former psychotherapist for his willingness to talk about preventing a suicidal death. He clearly enjoyed the attention and support from the group.

James was able to participate in the group for only a few sessions because of his fragile health status and increasing difficulty to travel outside the facility. However, his caregiver requested a list of all of the themes of the guided autobiography group. For several months he dictated his memories while she transcribed them, creating a written legacy for his daughters. Greta reported that the activity was a meaningful one for her as well.

The possible benefit of creative writing for individuals living with moderate cognitive impairment may be the enhancement of mood through processing life experiences and engaging in "meaning making" rather than by impacting working memory. Future research is needed to clarify the effects of expressive writing and participation in writing groups upon individuals who live with memory impairment.

Structure of the Groups

Sessions last 2 to 2½ h and vary in scheduled number of sessions, from 2 to 12, depending upon the topic and interest of the group members. Group size has ranged from 7 to 12 individuals, and I have had occasional intergenerational groups with members ranging in age from early 30s to early 90s. Larger groups are possible, but all members may not have time to read their submissions aloud. Dividing larger groups into several smaller, more intimate size ones so that everyone can read aloud and have an opportunity to receive reactions from others can work as well.

Positive connections between generations can occur in intergenerational writing groups. I have witnessed younger participants express amazement to learn about aspects of life unfamiliar to them such as the impact of polio on family members or the effect of the 1970 Kent State shootings on the community (Hartman-Stein, 2010). Anecdotally, the older writers reported that they found the writing of the younger group members to be surprisingly direct and open about topics such as money, relationships, and sexuality.

Michael, a 34-year-old builder and designer, wrote the following to a prompt about the impact of money in his life, entitled *Depression Blood*:

My grandparents filled my summer calendar every year with tasks around the farm, but every task finished with a lesson.

I spent the whole summer of 1987 painstakingly tearing down an old barn that wasn't even fit for the wild animals that lived in it. I couldn't understand why, at the time, we stacked each piece of this 80 year old barn with great care…It was rewarding to see the big piles of wood all nicely stacked at the end of my summer vacation, but still quite pointless in my eyes.

Then came the summer of 1988. I spent the first 3 weeks pulling nails out of the old barn wood, every day filling my hands with splinters from the rough timbers. Another wasted summer of pointless work – until it was finished. Grandpa laid out the plan for the new 16' by 32' barn that was going to house the evaporator for making maple syrup that I tore apart four summers ago. I couldn't believe it; my brother and I had been given the task to build the new barn by ourselves. Grandpa handed us the coffee can full of old, bent, rusty nails that we pulled from the old barn wood. I asked Grandpa why we were using this stuff instead of buying new. He answered, "It's called depression blood; we use what we can. There will be nothing new needed for this barn. We need to save the money for equipment, and every dollar counts." I was 12 years old, and I only truly understood what he meant now. He would often tell us that money was a good servant but a bad master.

His poignant story sparked a lively discussion about the Great Depression and what it had meant in the lives of the families of the older writers in the group.

Ingredients of an Effective Group

To promote a sense of calm and focused concentration before writing, I begin each session with a brief deep breathing or meditative exercise followed by reading of an inspirational poem from a source such as *Love Poems from God: Twelve Sacred Voices from the East and the West* (Ladinsky, 2002) or a humorous piece from *Good Poems for Hard Times* (Keillor, 2005). I also recommend that participants read *Writing down the bones: Freeing the writer within*, as an inspirational writing guide (Goldberg, 2005).

In order for writing groups to be effective, a sense of security and trust needs to develop. "Groups don't happen, they have to be created and nurtured" (Bolton, 1999, p. 130). One issue is confidentiality. Although writing workshops are not psychotherapy, a frank discussion about confidentiality helps to set the stage for trust to develop among participants.

Emotional reactions such as bursting into tears while writing or reading occur during writing groups. I prepare the group at the onset, suggesting that it is a normative response. The most stalwart looking participants may have unexpectedly intense emotional responses. Baikie and McIlwain (2008) found that expressive writing has particular benefits for individuals scoring high on alexithymia, i.e., difficulty identifying and labeling their emotions.

In guided autobiography groups, I have used the nine writing prompts that give structure to the program (Birren & Cochran, 2001). I have also created writing prompts with broad, emotionally evocative themes such as meaningful gifts, deeply prized objects, anger, forgiveness, guilt, coping with adversity and partings.

A 78-year-old woman who had been estranged from her adult daughter wrote this piece, entitled, *The Gift of Joy*, from the prompt, "meaningful gifts":

This day may be one I'll always remember. Nan wrote a note about celebrating "Christmas." She did not even mention her celebrating "Solstice," as in years past. The note was included in a box of homemade cookies, chocolate ones, shortbread cut-outs, pecan, and ginger. I feel that Nan is ready to have a relationship with us as she also sent us a donation card made in honor to Heifer Project International which she knows is our favorite charity. What joy after 10 years of estrangement!

During mind–body connection workshops, I have asked participants to write about a symptom of their own or that of a family member that may be triggered by emotional stress. Topics covered by recent groups included jaw pain, tinnitus, back pain, seizures, and neurological symptoms initially thought to be from multiple sclerosis. A 72-year-old woman wrote about her parents' headaches. She reported that she gained great insight about the stress and pressures they likely experienced that she had not realized until she wrote the piece.

Also part of the mind–body workshop, I have asked participants to write from the "voice" of a symptom. One 64-year-old man wrote about his hemorrhoids. When they pop out, he said, he knows he is pushing too hard in many aspects of his life.

In each workshop session, participants spend 30–35 min writing within the confines of the workshop. Occasionally they have additional writing assignments outside the session to bring in and read during the subsequent group. Many participants edit their writings outside of the workshop although that is not required. The purpose of these workshops is not to fine-tune the craft of writing, but rather to stimulate old memories and gain insight about coping strategies, conflicts, and physical symptoms. The expectation is for each participant to read aloud two pages of his/her work, followed by time for brief reactions from other participants.

In order to ensure a powerfully therapeutic group experience, I recommend that group facilitators have experience leading groups or arrange for professional consultation or supervision. It is useful to record a brief summary following each group session to reflect what occurred in order to help plan the next session. Although writing groups are not therapy, they are highly therapeutic if conducted well (Birren & Cochran, 2001).

Role of the Group Leader

My decision to take on two roles, that of writer-participant, in addition to facilitator, turned out to be an unexpectedly powerful element of the writing workshops. Acutely aware of therapist–client boundary issues, I made a deliberate decision to write during the group session along with the participants and self-disclose memories and insights aloud after others have had the opportunity to read their stories. This is different from that of the typical teacher–therapist (for an in-depth discussion of boundary issues when leading groups, see Meuser, Chap. 11). By modeling a willingness to disclose insights about my life, deeper levels of insight and greater willingness to self-disclose are fostered more quickly, compared to when the facilitator reveals little of a personal nature. In reviewing available research literature, I have found no studies to date that examined the impact of differences in outcome based upon the role of the facilitator during writing workshops, but it is an intriguing topic to pursue from a research perspective.

Examples of topics I have self-disclosed are my reaction to the auction of my parents' house after their deaths, cherished objects, resilience modeled by my coal miner father, and stress-induced physical symptoms.

Compilation of Excerpts from the Writing Groups

The creation of a collection of excerpts of the writing produced during the workshops is a meaningful, cherished product for many participants. Although it is a time-consuming, labor intensive task, many writers find it meaningful to have a collective "chapbook" of select writing from their fellow workshop participants. When a workshop has produced outstanding insights, I have compiled selected works, dividing them thematically, and choosing a cover that exemplifies a theme of the workshop. One such chapbook is the *Tour of the Writers' Garden: Reflections for Health and Healing through Guided Autobiography*.

As a surprise, at the last session one writer had read aloud a metaphorical description of each participant using the theme, the tour of gardens. An excerpt follows:

> Sherry: A garden of SOLOMON'S SEAL—which prefers to rest in a shaded area and is one that many are not familiar with. Their flowers are often hidden by foliage—they are adaptable and not invasive.
>
> Carla—A garden brimming with BLACK-EYED SUSANS—They are hardy, loved by all and are dependable by readily reseeding themselves with more and more blooms.
>
> Frances—A garden of beautiful WISTERIA—Upon nearing the plant, the fragrance puts all into a good mood. A plant of patience—the longer its years, the more amazing the growth. It is a forgiving plant that can transform the ordinary into a regal estate…

Anecdotal Evidence of Benefits from Therapeutic Writing Groups

A retired school teacher in her early 70s, Carla had bouts of clinical depression since childhood. She was concerned about her memory functioning because of a history of small strokes. The following is a description of how the writing programs were beneficial to her:

> A major benefit was that I was able to put into sequence events that have emotionally impacted my life. One of the things I find interesting is that as I remember the incidents and write them down sequentially, I am able to "remember" the details much more clearly.

There have been times when the writing itself has been very emotional, lots of tears. But there have been other times when the impact of what I wrote really didn't 'hit home' until I read it orally.

A major benefit in having all this in writing is the ability to go back and reread it. There are some that I have reread repeatedly.

The power of the group cannot be over emphasized. They gave me support, helped me to clarify things, and gave me a sense of direction on areas that were still somewhat 'fuzzy' and came across that way in the writing. At times they saw things I didn't see but when I heard it, it made total sense. Very helpful!

In summary, there is an extensive body of research evidence that suggests a linkage between expressive writing and health/psychological benefits for a variety of medical and psychological conditions. Few studies have focused specifically on the impact on the well-being of older adults, a potentially rich avenue of future research. In addition, an area of future investigation is the potential added value of therapeutic writing within small groups. The available research showing the positive impact of expressive writing on working memory is intriguing and presents an exciting new direction for research with both cognitively intact older adults as well as those living with impaired memory functioning.

In regard to research methodology, qualitative studies that document individual and unique results are needed in addition to the use of quantitative methods to understand creative engagement and its impact on health and well-being (Stuckey & Nobel, 2010). In her ground-breaking book, *Counterclockwise*, Ellen Langer (2009) challenges researchers to adopt the empowering pursuit of what she calls "the psychology of possibility," i.e., that exceptional cases should not be disregarded as unwanted noise in the data but rather become focal points of an investigation.

Creative writing groups are rich sources of cognitive stimulation, with the potential of boosting memory, emotional resilience, and enhancement of physical well-being at a relatively low cost. They can be offered to older adults encompassing many themes including coping with caregiver stress (Mackenzie, Wiprzycka, Hasher & Goldstein, 2008). They can occur in a variety of settings including behavioral health practices, primary care clinics, senior centers, retirement communities, and assisted living facilities. Writing workshops specifically geared to adults living with memory impairment are a promising venue especially if participants consider writing a skill they had developed earlier in their lives or if the individuals are motivated to develop writing as a cognitive pursuit.

References

Baikie, K. A., & McIlwain, D. (2008). Who does expressive writing work for: Examination of alexithymia, splitting, and repressive coping styles as moderators of the expressive writing paradigm. *British Journal of Health Psychology, 13*, 61–66.

Biermann, J., & Hartman-Stein, P. E. (2011). Keys to a sharp mind –providing choice and quality programming in a retirement community. In P. E. Hartman-Stein & A. La Rue (Eds.), *Enhancing Cognitive Fitness in Adults: A guide for use and development of community-based programs*. New York: Springer.

Birren, J. E., & Cochran, K. N. (2001). *Telling the stories of life through guided autobiography groups*. Baltimore: The Johns Hopkins University Press.
Bolton, G. (1999). *The therapeutic potential of creative writing*. London: Jessica Kinglsey.
Brady, E. M., & Sky, H. Z. (2003). Journal writing among older learners. *Educational Gerontology, 29*, 151–163.
Cameron, J. (1992). *The artist's way*. New York: G.P. Putnam's Sons.
Carroll, R. (2005). Finding the words to say it: the healing power of poetry. *Evidence-based Complementary and Alternative Medicine, 2*, 161–172.
Goldberg, N. (2005). *Writing down the bones: Freeing the writer within*. Boston: Shambhala.
Hartman-Stein, P. E. (2010). Expressive writing groups: A powerful modality to promote health and wellness in older adults. *Psychologists in Long Term Care Newsletter, 24*, 13–16.
Keillor, G. (2005). *Good poems for hard times*. New York: Viking Penguin.
Klein, K., & Boals, A. (2001). Expressive writing can increase working memory capacity. *Journal of Experimental Psychology: General, 130*, 520–533.
Kominars, S. B. (2007). *Write for life: Healing body, mind, and spirit through journal writing*. Cleveland: Cleveland Clinic Press.
Ladinsky, D. (2002). *Love poems from God: Twelve sacred voices from the east and the west*. New York: Penguin.
Langer, E. (2009). *Counterclockwise: Mindful health and the power of possibility*. New York: Ballantine Books.
Lezak, M. D., Howieson, D. B., & Loring, D. W. (2004). *Neuropsychological assessment* (4th ed.). New York: Oxford University Press.
Mackenzie, C. S., Wiprzycka, U. J., Hasher, L., & Goldstein, D. (2008). Seeing the glass half full: Optimistic expressive writing improves mental health among chronically stressed caregivers. *British Journal of Health Psychology, 13*, 73–76.
Meuser, T. (2011). Oral life review in older adults: Principles for the social service professional. In P. E. Hartman-Stein & A. La Rue (Eds.), *Enhancing Cognitive Fitness in Adults: A guide for use and development of community-based programs*. New York: Springer.
Pennebaker, J. W., & Beall, S. K. (1986). Confronting a traumatic event: Toward an understanding of inhibition and disease. *Journal of Abnormal Psychology, 95*(3), 274–281.
Sloan, D. M., Marx, B. P., Epstein, E. M., & Dobbs, J. L. (2008). Expressive writing buffers against maladaptive rumination. *Emotion, 8*, 302–306.
Stuckey, H. L., & Nobel, J. (2010). The connection between art, healing, and public health: A Review of the current literature. *American Journal of Public Health, 100*, 254–263.
Yogo, M., & Fujihara, S. (2008). Working memory capacity can be improved by expressive writing: A randomized experiment in a Japanese sample. *British Journal of Health Psychology, 13*, 77–80.

Chapter 13
Peer-Led Memory Training Programs to Support Brain Fitness

Linda M. Ercoli, Paul A. Cernin, and Gary W. Small

Abstract Despite evidence supporting the effectiveness of cognitive enhancement interventions in older adults with age-related changes, few if any cognitive enhancement programs are available in the community that can be administered with ease and high quality, and reach a large number of persons. Just as peer-led programs are widely used to promote health awareness, health self-maintenance, and wellness, peers can promote memory awareness and education in community-residing older adults with mild age-related memory concerns. Overall, there has been a gap between the development of effective cognitive intervention programs to help offset the daily minor challenges associated with mild age-related memory loss, and convenient availability to the general population. Given this need, in association with the University of California, Los Angeles (UCLA) Longevity Center our group developed a unique 5-week, peer-led community education/intervention program to improve memory functioning in older adults. In this chapter, we detail the development and implementation, and present preliminary data regarding the effects on memory of this MTP program. We discuss the benefits and challenges associated with administering this kind of peer-led memory enhancement strategy. Given the many older adults experiencing age-related memory decline and the potential benefits of the intervention, the potential impact of peer-led memory training programs could be considerable.

Introduction

Successful aging has been defined as maintaining both cognitive and physical health throughout life (Rowe & Kahn, 1998). As people age, however, they often experience cognitive and physical challenges.

L.M. Ercoli (✉)
University of California, Los Angeles, CA, USA
e-mail: lercoli@mednet.ucla.edu

The influence of age-related physical and cognitive decline on society is projected to grow as the proportion of the population older than age 60 years increases over the next decades. The mildest form of such cognitive decline known as age-associated memory impairment (AAMI) (Crook et al., 1986; Larrabee & Crook, 1994) is characterized by self-perception of memory loss and a standardized memory test score indicating a decline in objective memory performance compared with younger adults. In people 65 years of age or older, its estimated prevalence is 40% in the United States. The condition is often referred to as normal aging, and it tends to remain stable in most cases. However, as people continue to age, their risk increases for becoming more cognitively impaired and developing mild cognitive impairment (MCI) (Winblad et al., 2004), a condition defined by more severe memory deficits without functional impairments. Although MCI patients are able to continue to live independently, they show objective memory impairments similar to those seen in people with very mild Alzheimer's disease (AD). Approximately, 10% of people 65 years or older suffer from MCI, and nearly 15% of them develop AD each year. Cognitive problems in aging are of concern not only because they may predict the development of dementia but also because of their immediate impact on quality of life.

Some studies suggest that mentally stimulating activities may protect against age-related declines in cognition and lower the risk for dementia; however, definitive evidence proving a causal relationship between mental stimulation and lower dementia risk is lacking. Several lines of evidence indicate that learning and mental activities are associated with improved cognitive functioning and/or lower dementia risk. People with advanced education and professional accomplishments tend to have greater density of neuronal connections in brain areas involved in complex reasoning (Del Ser, Hachinskim, Merskey, & Munoz, 1999). Epidemiological studies indicate that increased frequency of engaging in everyday mental or leisure activities is associated with significantly reduced risk for developing dementia or cognitive decline (Akbaraly et al., 2009; Desai, Grossberg, & Chibnall, 2010; Fillit et al., 2002; Fritsch, Smyth, Debanne, Petot, & Friedland, 2005; Paillard-Borg, Fratiglioni, Winblad, & Wang, 2009; Verghese et al., 2003; Wilson, Barnes, & Bennett, 2003; Wilson et al., 2002). In randomized clinical trials, cognitive training improves memory, reasoning, and mental speed in persons with normal aging or mild memory declines (Ball et al., 2002; Cavallini, Pagnin, & Vecchi, 2003; Craik et al., 2007; O'Hara et al., 2007; Stuss et al., 2007; Valentijn et al., 2005; Verhaeghen, Marcoen, & Goossens, 1992; Willis et al., 2006). A major hurdle that most programs have not overcome is in transferring such cognitive gains to improvement in everyday memory challenges.

Despite evidence supporting the effectiveness of cognitive enhancement interventions in older adults with age-related changes, few if any programs are available that can be administered with ease and high quality, and reach a large number of people in their own communities. Overall, there has been a gap between the development of effective cognitive intervention programs to help offset the daily minor challenges associated with mild age-related memory loss, and convenient availability to the general population. Given this need, in association with the University of California, Los Angeles (UCLA) Longevity Center our group developed a unique

5-week, peer-led community education/intervention program to improve memory functioning in older adults (Ercoli, Hedberg, & Johnson, 2006). This memory training peer (MTP) program includes memory improvement techniques, such as association and visual imagery, which other clinical trials have found to augment memory ability in older adults. This MTP program is innovative in that it trains lay volunteers to use a scripted, standardized curriculum to teach memory strategies to community-residing older adults; thus, the MTP program can be readily adopted in a variety of settings where seniors congregate. One of the most novel aspects of this program is its portability and ability to reach large numbers of older adults. Since its inception in 2003, more than 3,000 individuals have taken the course, which has been taught in seven US states (California, Iowa, Pennsylvania, Texas, Illinois, Florida, and Maryland) in a variety of venues (e.g., senior and community centers, hospitals and other healthcare provider organizations, and academic institutions). Approximately 500 volunteers have been trained to administer the program. In this chapter, we detail the development and implementation of this MTP program and discuss the benefits and challenges associated with administering this kind of peer-led memory enhancement strategy.

Development

Peer-led educational programs are implemented worldwide to promote adaptive health behaviors and wellness. They have been administered in developed and underdeveloped countries and to people of all ages and socioeconomic backgrounds (Alcock et al., 2009). There are several advantages to peers providing educational interventions. For instance, compared to non-peer health professionals, peer leaders may be more approachable, may have more credibility than health professionals, and often can relate better to the experiences and concerns of the participants (Gammonley & Luken, 2001; Nettles & Belton, 2010; Rogers, 1983). As examples, peer-led programs have targeted alcohol awareness, breast cancer awareness, sexual health, tobacco cessation, prevention of functional decline in older adults, successful aging, chronic mental illness self-management, and self-management of chronic physical diseases, such as diabetes and arthritis (Chodosh et al., 2005; Fabacher et al., 1994; Kim & Sarna, 2004; Kocken & Voorham, 1998; Lawn et al., 2007; Lorig et al., 1999; Maticka-Tyndale & Barnett, 2010).

While peer-led education programs have been widely disseminated for health self-management and raising awareness, memory function is one area that has received relatively little attention. Our main goal was to devise a portable, empirically based, and engaging entertaining memory training program that could raise awareness in older adults about memory health and train memory enhancement skills. We chose a peer-led education program model in order to increase accessibility to the community.

In developing the MTP program, we used approaches and content from research, educational, and popular resources. The intervention itself is modeled after a multifactorial memory training program (Stigsdotter, 2000). Multifactorial memory training programs address both cognitive and noncognitive factors that contribute to memory function including (1) Education about memory; (2) Preliminary instruction in the basic elements of memory improvement strategies prior to the teaching of specific techniques (i.e., "pretraining"); (3) Instruction in specific memory strategies; (4) Home practice; (5) Discussion of noncognitive factors such as self-confidence, anxiety, and negative expectations; (6) Group-based training; and (7) Sessions of relatively brief duration. The UCLA MTP program includes all of those components.

The MTP program teaches specific techniques drawn from empirical studies that have demonstrated the effectiveness of memory training strategies in older adults with age-related cognitive changes (Cavallini et al., 2003; Craik et al., 2007; McCarthy, 1980; O'Hara et al., 2007; Stuss et al., 2007; Valentijn et al., 2005; Verhaeghen et al., 1992; Willis et al., 2006; Yesavage, 1983; Yesavage, Rose, & Bower, 1983). A meta-analysis of 33 memory training clinical trials of over 1,500 adults 60 years and over showed that gains due to use of memory training techniques are large – on average, effect sizes of 0.73-standardized difference, posttest mean minus pretest mean – compared to control (0.37) and placebo (0.38) conditions (Verhaeghen et al., 1992). Benefits from memory and other cognitive training interventions are robust, and may last from 6 months up to 5 years (Anschutz, Camp, Markley, & Kramer, 1987; O'Hara et al., 2007; Scogin & Bienias, 1988; Stigsdotter & Backman, 1993; Willis et al., 2006). Techniques and education material also were based upon a popular book about memory health and memory improvement techniques (Small, 2003).

In addition to empirically supported methods for memory enhancement, the MTP program also incorporates basic principles of memory function, behavior modification, learning theory, and cognitive-behavioral approaches. The MTP program targets functions that are primarily subserved by the declarative memory system, which involves the conscious recollection of information, such as facts (semantic memory) and experienced events linked to time and place (episodic memory) (Tulving, 1983). Daily life examples of declarative memory include autobiographical information and remembering people, object placement (e.g., keys, purses, reading glasses), appointments, errands, shopping lists, and more. Forgetting in these daily life situations reflects the kinds of challenges experienced by older adults with minor memory difficulties (Craik & Rabinowitz, 1984; Hill, Backman, & Stigsdotter, 2000; Olofsson & Bäckman, 1996; Schai & Wills, 1991). Elements of behavior modification are incorporated into the program and in the training of the peer-trainers, who are taught the importance of *positive reinforcement* and *shaping*. Trainers reinforce correct or even partially correct execution of the memory strategies to gradually shape effective use and mastery of a technique. They provide encouragement, feedback, and praise to maintain the participants' motivation. The curriculum emphasizes *chaining and shaping* by breaking down a memory technique into steps and teaching each step sequentially to facilitate learning the complete technique. Finally, participants are encouraged to use *distributed practice* to space learning and practice trials over time in short sessions (Baddeley & Longman, 1978), rather than attempting to acquire the same information though "cramming." Home practice assignments are distributed weekly to reinforce learning.

From learning theory, *the levels of processing* approach (Craik & Lockhart, 1972) makes an important contribution to the MTP program. Levels of processing posits that memory is a function of the degree to which a new or to-be-learned piece of information is analyzed – the deeper and more meaningful the analysis, the better the stimulus is remembered. During learning, "deep" analysis that focuses on meaning is associated with higher levels of retention than "shallower" processing that focuses on physical or sensory aspects of a stimulus. Therefore, peer-trainers encourage deep analysis by having participants make associations to information in ways to make it more personally meaningful and distinctive, and help integrate that new information with a framework of preexisting knowledge that provides cues for later retrieval.

Finally, from cognitive-behavioral approaches, the MTP program includes exercises for *cognitive restructuring* to help shape more positive attitudes about memory and aging for participants. As described in Section "Specifics of the Curriculum," participants learn cognitive restructuring techniques to counter negative self-statements that may hinder learning the techniques.

Our group initially developed and piloted a multifactorial memory training intervention in older adults (Ercoli et al., 2005) that was instrumental in developing the MTP program. The pilot memory training program was a 7-week intervention taught by psychologists. We evaluated the pilot program in 63 older adults and found that the subjects who received training in associative memory enhancement techniques improved significantly on objective memory tests, with a medium effect size (ES = 0.63), compared to a health education control condition. We then shortened the pilot program to 5 weeks, which better accommodated participants' busy schedules. We also edited the pilot program to include techniques that were most easily taught in 15–20 min and added other educational material about lifestyle factors that affect memory (Small, 2003).

After shortening the curriculum, the final step was to manualize, script, and stage it so that trained peer volunteers could administer it. The manual includes everything that peer-trainers need. A professional educator developed the initial scripting, which was then revised extensively by a geriatric psychiatrist and psychologist. In developing the script, we paid special attention to terminology so that jargon and complexity were minimized. We also avoided the use of emotionally charged words that might increase the participants' anxiety. For example, the term "skill-builder" is used instead of "homework," and the word "memory check" is used instead of "memory quiz" or "test". The script also has a Flesch-Kinkaid Grade Level rating of 5.4; thus, the program is accessible to a broad range of reading-level abilities. Volunteers use the manual to present all of the material and examples, but they may adjust the discourse as needed to ensure that the participants fully understand the concepts and memory techniques.

Given the barriers to mobility and expenses that some seniors face for transportation, an additional important step was to develop a portable program that could be presented in locations where seniors congregate. We therefore purposefully made the MTP program "low tech" using readily available and inexpensive materials (e.g., paper and pencil, handouts) and decided not to use expensive, technical, or less available methods for dissemination (e.g., computers and LCD projectors).

Specifics of the Curriculum

The MTP program includes specific memory enhancement strategies, often called "mnemonics" that involve the use of verbal associations, visual imagery, and organizational strategies to remember information relevant to daily life, such as book and movie titles, dates, pin-codes, phone numbers, addresses, a shopping or to-do list; and, faces and names. The curriculum is divided into five sessions; each session is structured in the same way and includes instruction in two to three mnemonic techniques, class examples, group- and pair-wise exercises, and assignment of the "skill-builder" home practice exercises, which are initially easy to facilitate participants' confidence and provide mastery experiences. Skill builders become increasingly challenging and include reviews of previous material. Skill builders are reviewed weekly to reinforce the concepts. Over half of each session is devoted to practicing techniques through exercises. Class exercises are interactive, instructive, and fun. We have found that participants very much enjoy partnering with a classmate for the exercises. A team of two trainers presents the program. They teach and model the memory enhancement techniques and help participants with in-class exercises. Trainers also acknowledge individual differences and praise effort as well as excellence. We have found that this positive approach, along with pairing classmates for exercises, encourages participation and makes people feel comfortable.

At the start of the course, each participant receives materials including a pencil and a folder for keeping blank paper and handouts. Course content for each week is outlined in Table 13.1. Following the model of multifactorial memory training programs, in the first session, trainers discuss the rationale for the course, the importance of practice and regular attendance, and the benefits of memory training and basic education on memory functions, such as how memories are formed and how memory abilities change with aging. Trainers also discuss noncognitive factors that also can interfere with optimal memory functioning. For example, participants learn about how to identify negative expectations and thoughts (e.g., "I'll never be able to do this.") and how to use basic cognitive restructuring techniques to promote more positive thinking. Participants also engage in self-exploratory exercises to discover if they are visual or auditory learners, which helps to raise their awareness and focus their practice to enhance abilities that they may use less. In the first session, participants also complete a self-report questionnaire about their memory complaints, as well as a memory check (i.e., quiz). Participants take two additional memory checks and another self-report questionnaire at subsequent sessions and track their complaints and memory check scores throughout the 5 weeks.

In the first session, following the educational component, the next step is "pretraining" or the introduction of basic memory enhancement concepts. Research has shown that pretraining in the basic techniques of association and imagery facilitates the learning of specific mnemonic techniques (Verhaeghen et al., 1992; Yesavage, 1983). Attention pretraining involves studying a photograph and recalling the details. Association pretraining involves forming associations or thinking of jingles for products and names. For visualization pretraining, trainers talk participants through guided imagery exercises.

Table 13.1 Peer-led memory training program content

Session	Techniques and topics	Other activities
1	Introduction/Course Rationale Education on Memory Function Learning Styles Assessment Countering Negative Thinking Pretraining: Association and Imagery	Distribute Course Materials Take Memory Check #1 Complete Subjective Memory Questionnaire #1 Assign Skill Builder #1
2	Chunking Method Look-Snap-Connect	Review Skill Builder #1 Assign Skill Builder #2
3	Sentence and Link Methods Remembering Faces and Names	Review Skill Builder #2 Take Memory Check #2 Assign Skill Builder #3
4	Remembering Numbers, Addresses, and Dates Expanding Vocabulary Versatility Training	Review Skill Builder #3 Assign Skill Builder #4
5	Organizational Strategies Other Factors Affecting Memory Staying Mentally Fit Review of Techniques	Take Memory Check #3 Complete Subjective Memory Questionnaire #2 Review Skill Builder #4 Complete Course Evaluation Collect Course Evaluation, Memory Check, and Subjective Memory Questionnaire Scores

Instruction in specific techniques continues in subsequent sessions. The categorization or "chunking" method, the easiest technique, is placed first in the curriculum to instill confidence and provide a successful experience for participants. Categorization involves breaking down or categorizing a list of items into smaller subgroups of items that have something in common. Words can be grouped under category headings, and the headings then act as cues to retrieve the items. Participants perform in-class exercises, one of which involves categorizing a list of 12 items into three groups – tools, sports equipment, and vegetables – and the use of category headings to cue their memories for the words. Look-Snap-Connect (Small, 2003) is an attention, visualization, and association technique, wherein multiple items can be visualized in a single scene or image. For instance, participants use Look-Snap-Connect to remember parking a car on level 3B in a parking structure. One way to do this is to form an image of three bumble bees hovering over a car. Participants learn the Sentence and Link methods; and how to remember names and faces. The Sentence and Link methods, respectively, involve creating sentences to remember short lists and creating stories to remember longer lists. Visualizing the sentences or stories is also helpful. For example, participants will create a sentence to remember three things on a to-do list: Buy a cooked chicken, bring flowers to a sick friend; RSVP to a nephew's wedding. A possible result would be "the chicken brought a bouquet of flowers to the wedding." Remembering faces and names requires first paying attention to a face, forming an association with a name or changing the name slightly to sound like something familiar, and then linking the face and name using an image. This technique is based on McCarthy's (McCarthy, 1980) three-step method (1) identify a prominent facial feature, (2) change the name to sound familiar or meaningful, and then (3) associate the face and the transformed name using an image. Exercises focus on learning how to form associations to names (e.g., Terry sounds like merry) and how to pick out an outstanding facial feature to focus attention on a face (e.g., teeth), and link the face with the person's name using imagery (e.g., Terry has a merry smile). The face-name class exercises and skill builder exercises reflect ethnic diversity. For instance, we include photographs of Asian, African-American, and Caucasian individuals, and name association exercises provide tips for learning ethnic names (e.g., "Frank Soto," "Bob Castini").

Participants learn associations for remembering numbers and months. For example, the number 10 is associated with a dime; 747 is associated with a jet. The month of November can be associated with a Thanksgiving turkey. In one exercise, participants will remember a doctor appointment on November 5th. November can be associated with a turkey; the number 5 can be associated with a nickel, and participants can visualize a turkey with a nickel on its chest, wearing a stethoscope. Association and imagery can be applied to expand vocabulary. For instance, participants use association and imagery to learn the word "silage." Trainers will associate the word with a sound (e.g., "silage" as rhyming with "mileage"), meaning (animal feed made by fermenting grain in a silo), spelling (contains the word "silo"), and with an image (e.g., visualize cows eating grain near a silo). Versatility training involves being flexible in using techniques. Trainers lead exercises to interchange using sentences/stories, imagery, and Look-Snap-Connect to remember the same information. The topic of organizational strategies includes tips and class discussion for using practical memory aids, such as written and auditory reminders, and having special places for important things like keys. Participants learn about multiple factors affecting memory, including lifestyle and health-related variables, such as distraction, multitasking, stress, and anxiety. Participants apply the various memory techniques learned over the 5 weeks to new material as a final review. At the end of the course, trainers distribute a handout with resources (e.g., books, websites) where people can learn more about memory enhancement. Participants also are asked to complete an anonymous evaluation of the MTP program.

The MTP program manual includes information to help peer-trainers pace the class. For instance, the manual suggests how many participants the trainers should call on during an exercise or provides approximate time limits for exercises (e.g., "call on two participants" or "allow three minutes") to help keep the course on track and ensure adequate time to practice the various exercises. Possible examples and answers to class exercises are provided in italics to help trainers if participants need additional assistance or have questions about examples. The curriculum is paced at a rate comfortable for most adults over 60 years of age. Each trainer is fully self-contained for training in the community. They are equipped with a file with all materials needed to present the course.

Implementing the Program

Characteristics for MTP Program Participants

The MTP program targets people 60 years of age or older with mild, age-related memory concerns or changes. Patients with dementia will find the program too difficult and will become frustrated and generally unable to implement or learn the memory training strategies (Cahn-Weiner, Malloy, Rebok, & Ott, 2003; Yesavage, 1982). Memory training studies yielded mixed results for effectiveness in persons with MCI (Belleville, 2008; Rapp, Brenes, & Marsh, 2002; Unverzagt et al., 2007; Wenisch et al., 2007); therefore, some persons with MCI may not be optimal candidates for the program.

Participants typically can have a range of visual and auditory acuity for participation in the program. During screening, staff inform people who report sensory deficits that the MTP program requires reading and listening. Participants then make the choice whether or not to enroll. The material and environment in the course is sufficient for individuals with mild age-related hearing or visual deficits. For instance, most visual materials are printed in larger (size 14) font, and trainers are taught to present auditory information clearly and at a reasonable pace. Participants with sensory deficits are encouraged to position themselves closer to the trainers. At times, some participants with severe sensory deficits who started the course have self-selected out, mainly due to hearing difficulties.

Participants come from various sources in the community. Some respond to advertisements or learn of the MTP program through word of mouth. Others are relatives of patients from memory disorder clinics, or are patients who were originally referred for cognitive assessments who were found to have no significant memory impairment. MTP program staff do not perform cognitive screenings on potential participants. Instead, staff members inform interested callers that the MTP program is an educational course for persons with mild memory complaints. Addressing upfront that the MTP program is not a cognitive rehabilitation program for persons with brain injury, dementia or MCI has been generally effective in recruiting appropriate participants. In organizations that have different programs for people with varying degrees of cognitive ability, persons ineligible for the MTP program may be directed to a different course or activity. There have been occasions where persons with more severe cognitive impairment have taken the course, and in those cases, the individuals sometimes drop out, or may enjoy the course but not necessarily benefit from it. In the event that someone with more significant cognitive difficulties enrolls in the MTP program, peer-trainers will work individually with that person so the progress of other participants who are not cognitively impaired is not affected.

Recruitment, Training, and Retention of Peer-Trainers

As indicated in Table 13.2, there are several core factors relevant to the recruitment, training, and retention of successful peer-trainers for the MTP program. Trainers are initially recruited via newspaper advertisements and word of mouth. Potential trainers responding to the advertisements call administrative staff who then describe the MT program and the role of trainers in detail. Typically, after 15–25 potential volunteers are recruited, a psychologist with expertise in neuropsychology and aging conducts a 2-day training seminar to orient the volunteer memory trainers.

During the 2-day seminar, potential trainers learn about the rationale behind the program, memory systems, functions, and changes with age. Potential trainers learn the techniques and review the curriculum in detail. The psychologist models how to present the techniques, provides examples, and demonstrates class exercises using the manual. Each potential trainer then reads sections of the script aloud and role plays teaching portions of the course to the group. At the end of the training, the staff determines which potential trainees appear to be a good match for the program. Once the trainers are selected, they undergo further training and certification. New trainers are required to learn the script thoroughly and then return for mock presentations which are reviewed by peer and staff. Trainers that meet the standards of the Longevity Center at the mock presentations are then considered to be "certified". Those who do not meet the standards undergo additional training. New trainers are typically paired with and mentored by an

Table 13.2 Factors for successful recruitment, training, and retention of memory training peer (MTP) program trainers

Recruitment
Advertise in local papers, newsletters, word of mouth
Liaison with community groups
Recruit from MTP courses
Characteristics of successful MTP peer trainers
"People persons" with strong social and communication skills
Comfortable with public speaking
Confidence in and ability to understand and implement the mnemonic methods
Sensitive to diversity of participants
Quality control
Require peer-trainer applicants to take the MTP course
Conduct 2-day training seminar
Conduct certification of trainers, consisting of mock teaching of MTP material with peer-review/feedback
Experienced peer-trainers mentor new trainers
Retention of trainers
Meet needs of trainers for supplies and materials
Provide trainer appreciation days and continuing education
Require a minimum commitment to MTP program
Retain larger volunteer pool to prevent burn-out
Minimize time between recruitment and teaching first MTP course
Consider stipends for peer-trainers

experienced trainer for approximately two courses. The UCLA Longevity Center also collects anonymous reviews from participants at the end of each course, which are used to monitor quality of the training experiences. In addition, the Center holds trainer meetings twice yearly for continuing education on related or supplementary topics.

The Longevity Center has recruited volunteer trainers from all walks of life and of all ages (20s to 80s). Successful trainers usually have strong social skills, relate well to peers, and are comfortable with public speaking. They also have confidence in their ability to learn and use the memory techniques. Successful trainers are dedicated to fostering an understanding of the techniques, are sensitive to individual differences in learning ability and style. They are also sensitive to the diversity of participants with respect to age, gender, culture, ethnicity and race, sexual orientation, socio-economic status, and disability. Many of the trainers have backgrounds in education, business, or social work, but the most important quality is being a "people person." Many trainers have had a family member with dementia, which led to their interest in age-related memory loss and memory training.

National and Local Venues

The MTP program has been administered locally in the Greater Los Angeles area and nationally. Locally, the program is presented at UCLA or hosted by venues that provide activities or services for older adults, such as senior centers, churches, synagogues, adult education and cultural centers, and museums. The local venues pay a fee to cover program expenses. Venues are responsible for recruiting participants, and then the peer-trainers from UCLA present the course at the venue. The MTP program has also been licensed to venues who then independently host the program for an entire year in a designated geographical catchment area. The licensees receive the manual and templates for administrative and promotional materials. Licensees are responsible for recruiting their own peer-trainers and participants and for providing all supportive functions and materials for the program. Licensees have included nonprofit healthcare organizations, memory disorders clinics, senior centers, and businesses. The MPT program psychologist from UCLA travels to the licensee site and trains their peer-trainers in the same 2-day seminar used for training local peer volunteers. Organizations that license the program are required to present it in its current form; however, adjustments can be made depending on the community of participants. For instance, the MTP program has been licensed to a Japanese-American nonprofit healthcare provider and also to a healthcare organization that provides outreach services to Latinos and Native Americans, and the peer-trainers can make adjustments as needed so that the program is culturally sensitive and relevant.

Requirements for Administration

Peer-led memory programs have the potential to reach a considerable number of people in the community. Like other peer-led programs, especially those administered by nonprofit organizations, the limitations or barriers to wide dissemination include staffing, funding, and level of community interest. Administrative activities include advertising the MTP course, screening participants, recruiting, training, and supporting the peer-trainers. The most labor intensive aspects of the MTP program involve managing incoming phone calls after advertisements are placed for either courses or organizing training sessions for new peer-trainers. Identifying new venues to host the course is an ongoing task. Typically, having two to three venues lined up in advance is needed to maintain a steady stream of course offerings.

One challenge common to many volunteer-based programs is the recruitment and maintenance of the volunteers. For the MTP program, we have had many dedicated peer-trainers volunteer for several years. Trainers are recruited through advertisements, word of mouth, and the courses themselves. It is helpful to have peer-trainers commit to presenting three courses per year to reduce volunteer turnover. The time between recruitment of new peer-trainers and their first training venue should be minimized to maintain motivation. In addition, holding periodic trainer appreciation days or continued education is valuable for keeping volunteer peer-trainers involved. In Los Angeles, we maintain an active roster of 35 volunteer peer-trainers. Other organizations have used a combination of volunteer peer-trainers or permanent organization staff. In other self-management peer-led courses (Lorig et al., 1999), peer-trainers sometimes receive stipends.

Course frequency depends upon community interest, venue staffing, and available resources. In Los Angeles, with two part-time staff and an all-volunteer peer-trainer roster, over a 3-year period (2007 through 2009) the program was presented at 61 venues (approximately 20 per year) and reached 1,235 participants (an average of 412 persons each year).

The funding of the MTP program varies. Foundation funding from philanthropic organizations focusing on older adult health, wellness, and other issues is one avenue. Individual donors or self-supported mechanisms such as annual fund raisers are also mechanisms for funding. Venues may be charged a fee to cover expenses for staff time and materials.

In rural locations, a central venue, such as a large senior center, may offer the MTP program for a wide geographical catchment area (e.g., multiple counties), recruit peer-trainers from those areas and then offer the program in the areas where the peer-trainers live to cover a wide area. Some venues have opted to partner with other organizations that act as satellite sites so the MTP program can be held at several locations within a geographical region. In large metropolitan areas, having peer-trainers travel to communities is advantageous for circumventing barriers to access, such as mobility, traffic, insufficient transportation, or travel costs.

Memory Improvement Results from the Program

At three points during the 5-week course (the first, third, and fifth sessions), participants in the MTP program take a memory quiz or memory check, which assesses their ability to learn and remember ten words. The purpose of these memory checks is for participants to observe their progress and gain confidence. To determine if participants are seeing progress, the Longevity Center collected anonymous memory check results on a voluntary basis from participants. We randomly selected a subsample of memory checks from 145 participants and conducted paired t-tests to assess whether performance improved from baseline to the two follow-up assessments. Participants recalled a significantly greater number of words at both follow-up memory checks (session 3, mean [SD] = 8.1 [2.3]; session 5 = 8.3 [2.0]) compared to baseline (5.8 [2.3]), and the effect size from baseline to follow-up was large (ES = 1.17). The ES from session 1 to session 3 (1.10) was larger than the ES from Session 3 to the final session (0.10). The second and third memory checks allowed more time than the baseline memory check (2 vs. 1 min) so that participants had more time to apply the new techniques they learned. Because the length of time is longer for retests, we cannot determine if these results indicate objective improvement, easier test conditions at follow-ups, or both.

The UCLA Longevity Center also tracks participant satisfaction with the MTP program based upon feedback from the peer-trainers and participants. Participants are asked to complete an anonymous evaluation at the end of each 5-week course. Those responses are tallied and reviewed periodically to continuously assess the effectiveness of the program and make necessary changes, adjustments, or revisions to the curriculum or program administration. Participants are asked to complete an anonymous evaluation at the end of the 5 weeks. In the Los Angeles area, from 2007 to 2009, about 61% of the participants completed evaluations. Of those, 95% reported that the information learned in the course helped them improve their memory, while 4% were neutral regarding any program benefit, and 1% disagreed that the program was helpful. Overall, 95% of respondents felt the program was a good investment of their time.

Future Plans

Program Revisions

The Longevity Center staff updates and revises the program on a regular basis. Revisions may include the addition of new material or mnemonic techniques, new topics for education, and adjustments to examples and exercises. In addition to participant feedback from the survey, the volunteer trainers provide ongoing feedback based on their experiences teaching the course, and formal trainer meetings are held to solicit their opinions and then integrate their feedback into subsequent revisions. We recently developed a shorter peer-led MTP program that includes periodic refresher sessions (i.e. "booster sessions"). The course contains new material in addition to many of the tried and true methods presented in the original MTP program. Both programs are now available through the Longevity Center.

Translation and Development of Culturally Specific Programs

Because many non-native English speakers do not have access to memory training, additional efforts could focus on versions of MTP program translated into other languages and developed for other cultures. Currently, translation of the program into Mandarin is underway, as the program has been licensed in Taiwan. Other goals include translation into Spanish language for outreach to the Latino community.

Research

Our preliminary results suggest that the MTP program may improve objective memory test performance; hence, one goal would be to test the effects of the MTP program empirically. Although the memory training strategies in the program are empirically based, we know of no studies that have assessed the effectiveness of peer-led memory training programs. Additional research is needed that demonstrates the effectiveness of memory training in encouraging participants to use memory techniques outside of the classroom so that the program lessons transfer to everyday activities and improve the frequent memory challenges facing people as they age.

Conclusion

Despite evidence supporting the effectiveness of cognitive enhancement interventions in older adults with age-related changes, few if any programs are available in the community that can be administered with ease and high quality, as well as reach a large number of persons. Even cognitive intervention programs that have been effective are not necessarily conveniently available to the general population. Just as peer-led programs have been developed and widely used to promote health awareness, health self-maintenance, and wellness, peers can promote memory awareness and education in community-residing older adults with mild age-related memory concerns. Peer-led memory enhancement and education programs, such as the one developed by the UCLA Longevity Center can make memory education accessible and affordable for a large number of people. Given the many older adults experiencing age-related memory decline and the potential benefits of the intervention, the potential impact of peer-led memory training programs could be considerable.

References

Akbaraly, T. N., Portet, F., Fustinoni, S., Dartigues, J. F., Artero, S., Rouaud, O., et al. (2009). Leisure activities and the risk of dementia in the elderly: results from the Three-City Study. *Neurology, 73*(11), 854–861.

Alcock, G. A., More, N. S., Patil, S., Porel, M., Vaidya, L., & Osrin, D. (2009). Community-based health programmes: role perceptions and experiences of female peer facilitators in Mumbai's urban slums. *Health Education Research, 24*(6), 957–966.

Anschutz, L., Camp, C. J., Markley, R. P., & Kramer, J. J. (1987). Remembering mnemonics: A three-year follow-up on the effects of mnemonics training in elderly adults. *Experimental Aging Research, 13*(3), 141–143.

Baddeley, A. D., & Longman, D. J. (1978). The influence of length an frequency on training session on the rate of learning to type. *Ergonomics, 21*, 627–635.

Ball, K., Berch, D. B., Helmers, K. F., Jobe, J. B., Leveck, M. D., Marsiske, M., et al. (2002). Effects of cognitive training interventions with older adults: a randomized controlled trial. *Journal of American Medical Association, 288*(18), 2271–281.

Belleville, S. (2008). Cognitive training for persons with mild cognitive impairment. *International Psychogeriatrics, 20*(1), 57–66.

Cahn-Weiner, D. A., Malloy, P. F., Rebok, G. W., & Ott, B. R. (2003). Results of a randomized placebo-controlled study of memory training for mildly impaired Alzheimer's disease patients. *Applied Neuropsychology, 10*(4), 215–223.

Cavallini, E., Pagnin, A., & Vecchi, T. (2003). Aging and everyday memory: The beneficial effect of memory training. *Archives of Gerontology and Geriatrics, 37*(3), 241–257.

Chodosh, J., Morton, S. C., Mojica, W., Maglione, M., Suttorp, M. J., Hilton, L., et al. (2005). Meta-analysis: chronic disease self-management programs for older adults. *Annals of Internal Medicine, 143*(6), 427–438.

Craik, F., & Lockhart, R. (1972). Levels of processing: A framework for memory research. *Journal of Verbal Learning and Verbal Behavior, 11*, 671–684.

Craik, F. I. M., & Rabinowitz, J. C. (1984). Age differences in the acquisition and use of verbal information. In J. Long & A. Baddeley (Eds.), *Attention and performance X* (pp. 471–499). Hillsdale: Lawrence Erlbaum.

Craik, F. I., Winocur, G., Palmer, H., Binns, M. A., Edwards, M., Bridges, K., et al. (2007). Cognitive rehabilitation in the elderly: Effects on memory. *Journal of the International Neuropsychological Society, 13*(1), 132–142.

Crook, T., Bartus, R. T., Ferris, S. H., Whitehouse, P., Cohen, G. D., & Gershon, S. (1986). Age-associated memory impairment: Proposed diagnostic criteria and measures of clinical change: Report of a National Institute of Mental Health work group. *Developmental Neuropsychology, 2*(4), 261–276.

Del Ser, T., Hachinski, V., Merskey, H., & Munoz, D. G. (1999). An autopsy-verified study of the effect of education on degenerative dementia. *Brain, 122*(12), 2309–2319.

Desai, A. K., Grossberg, G. T., & Chibnall, J. T. (2010). Healthy brain aging: A road map. *Clinics in Geriatric Medicine, 26*(1), 1–16.

Ercoli, L. M., Crowe-Lear, T., Siddarth, P., Miller, K., Dunkin, J., Moody, T., Kalpan, A., Halabi, C., Halabi, A., Dorsey, D., Byrd, G., Small, G. W. (2005). The effects of memory enhancement training on verbal memory in healthy older adults. American Association of Geriatric Psychiatry Annual Meeting [conference], San Diego, CA.

Ercoli, L. M., Hedberg, J., & Johnson, S. (2006). Community based memory training: A curriculum to sharpen memory skills in healthy adults. National Council on Aging-American Society on Aging Joint [Conference], Anaheim, CA.

Fabacher, D., Josephson, K., Pietruszka, F., Linderborn, K., Morley, J. E., & Rubenstein, L. Z. (1994). An in-home preventive assessment program for independent older adults: A randomized controlled trial. *Journal of the American Geriatrics Society, 42*(6), 630–638.

Fillit, H. M., Butler, R. N., O'Connell, A. W., Albert, M. S., Birren, J. E., Cotman, C. W., et al. (2002). Achieving and maintaining cognitive vitality with aging. *Mayo Clinic Proceedings, 77*(7), 681–696.

Fritsch, T., Smyth, K. A., Debanne, S. M., Petot, G. J., & Friedland, R. P. (2005). Participation in novelty-seeking leisure activities and Alzheimer's disease. *Journal of Geriatric Psychiatry and Neurology, 18*(3), 134–141.

Gammonley, D., & Luken, K. (2001). Peer education and advocacy through recreation and leadership. *Psychiatric Rehabilitation Journal, 25*(2), 170–178.

Hill, R., Backman, L., & Stigsdotter, N. A. (Eds.). (2000). *Cognitive rehabilitation in old age.* New York: Oxford University Press.

Kim, Y. H., & Sarna, L. (2004). An intervention to increase mammography use by Korean American women. *Oncology Nursing Forum, 31*(1), 105–110.

Kocken, P. L., & Voorham, A. J. (1998). Effects of a peer-led senior health education program. *Patient Education and Counseling, 34*(1), 15–23.

Larrabee, G. J., & Crook, T. H., III. (1994). Estimated prevalence of age-associated memory impairment derived from standardized tests of memory function. *International Psychogeriatrics, 6*(1), 95–104.

Lawn, S., Battersby, M. W., Pols, R. G., Lawrence, J., Parry, T., & Urukalo, M. (2007). The mental health expert patient: findings from a pilot study of a generic chronic condition self-management programme for people with mental illness. *The International Journal of Social Psychiatry, 53*(1), 63–74.

Lorig, K. R., Sobel, D. S., Stewart, A. L., Brown, W. B., Bandura, A., Ritter, P., et al. (1999). Evidence suggesting that a Chronic Disease Self-Management Program can improve health status while reducing hospitalization: A randomized trial. *Medical Care, 37*(1), 5–14.

Maticka-Tyndale, E., & Barnett, J. P. (2010). Peer-led interventions to reduce HIV risk of youth: A review. *Evaluation and Program Planning, 33*(2), 98–112.

McCarthy, D. L. (1980). Investigation of a visual imagery mnemonic device for acquiring face-name associations. *Journal of Experimental Psychology. Human Learning and Memory, 6*(2), 145–155.

Nettles, A., & Belton, B. (2010). An overview of training curricula for diabetes peer educations. *Family Practice, 27*(Suppl 1), i33–i39.

O'Hara, R., Brooks, J. O., III, Friedman, L., Schroder, C. M., Morgan, K. S., & Kraemer, H. C. (2007). Long-term effects of mnemonic training in community-dwelling older adults. *Journal of Psychiatric Research, 41*(7), 585–590.

Olofsson, M., & Bäckman, L. (1996). Influences of intentionality at encoding and retrieval on memory in adulthood and old age. *Aging (Milano), 8*, 42–46.

Paillard-Borg, S., Fratiglioni, L., Winblad, B., & Wang, H. X. (2009). Leisure activities in late life in relation to dementia risk: Principal component analysis. *Dementia and Geriatric Cognitive Disorders, 28*(2), 136–144.

Rapp, S., Brenes, G., & Marsh, A. P. (2002). Memory enhancement training for older adults with mild cognitive impairment: A preliminary study. *Aging & Mental Health, 6*, 5–11.

Rogers, E. M. (1983). *Diffusion of innovations* (3rd ed.). New York: Free Press.

Rowe, J. W., & Kahn, R. L. (1998). Successful. *Aging (Milano), 10*(2), 142–144.

Schai, K. W., & Wills, S. L. (1991). *Adult development and aging* (3rd ed.). New York: Haprer Collins.

Scogin, F., & Bienias, J. L. (1988). A three-year follow-up of older adult participants in a memory-skills training program. *Psychology and Aging, 3*(4), 334–337.

Small, G. W. (2003). *The memory Bible.* New York: Hyperion.

Stigsdotter, N. A. (2000). Multifactorial memory training in normal aging: In search of memory improvement beyond the ordinary. In R. D. Hill, L. Backman, & A. Stigsdotter Neely (Eds.), *Cognitive rehabilitation in old age* (pp. 63–80). New York: Oxford University Press.

Stigsdotter, N. A., & Backman, L. (1993). Long-term maintenance of gains from memory training in older adults: Two 3/12 years follow-up studies. *Journal of Gerontology: Psychological Sciences, 48*(5), 233–237.

Stuss, D. T., Robertson, I. H., Craik, F. I., Levine, B., Alexander, M. P., Black, S., et al. (2007). Cognitive rehabilitation in the elderly: A randomized trial to evaluate a new protocol. *Journal of the International Neuropsychological Society, 13*(1), 120–131.

Tulving, E. (1983). *Elements of episodic memory.* Cambridge: Oxford University Press.

Unverzagt, F. W., Kasten, L., Johnson, K. E., Rebok, G. W., Marsiske, M., Koepke, K. M., et al. (2007). Effect of memory impairment on training outcomes in ACTIVE. *Journal of International Neuropsychological Society, 13*(6), 953–960.

Valentijn, S. A. M., van Hooren, S. A. H., Bosma, H., Touw, D. M., Jolles, J., van Boxtel, M. P. J., et al. (2005). The effect of two types of memory training on subjective and objective memory performance in healthy individuals aged 55 years and older: A randomized controlled trial. *Patient Education and Counseling, 57*(1), 106–114.

Verghese, J., Lipton, R. B., Katz, M. J., Hall, C. B., Derby, C. A., Kuslansky, G., et al. (2003). Leisure activities and the risk of dementia in the elderly. *The New England Journal of Medicine, 348*(25), 2508–2516.

Verhaeghen, P., Marcoen, A., & Goossens, L. (1992). Improving memory performance in the aged through mnemonic training: A meta-analytic study. *Psychology and Aging, 7*(2), 242–251.

Wenisch, E., Cantegreil-Kallen, I., De Rotrou, J., Garrigue, P., Moulin, F., Batouche, F., et al. (2007). Cognitive stimulation intervention for elders with mild cognitive impairment compared with normal aged subjects: preliminary results. *Aging Clinical and Experimental Research, 19*(4), 316–322.

Willis, S. L., Tennstedt, S. L., Marsiske, M., Ball, K., Elias, J., Koepke, K. M., et al. (2006). Long-term effects of cognitive training on everyday functional outcomes in older adults. *Journal of American Medical Association, 296*(23), 2805–2814.

Wilson, R., Barnes, L., & Bennett, D. (2003). Assessment of lifetime participation in cognitively stimulating activities. *Journal of Clinical and Experimental Neuropsychology, 25*(5), 634–642.

Wilson, R. S., Mendes De Leon, C. F., Barnes, L. L., Schneider, J. A., Bienias, J. A., Evans, D. A., et al. (2002). Participation in cognitively stimulating activities and risk of incident Alzheimer disease. *Journal of the American Medical Association, 287*(6), 742–748.

Winblad, B., Palmer, K., Kivipelto, M., Jelic, V., Fratiglioni, L., Wahlund, L. O., et al. (2004). Mild cognitive impairment–beyond controversies, towards a consensus: report of the International Working Group on Mild Cognitive Impairment. *Journal of Internal Medicine, 256*(3), 240–246.

Yesavage, J. A. (1982). Degree of dementia and improvement with memory training. *Clinical Gerontologist, 1*, 77–81.

Yesavage, J. A. (1983). Imagery pretraining and memory training in the elderly. *Gerontology, 29*(4), 271–275.

Yesavage, J. A., Rose, T. L., & Bower, G. H. (1983). Interactive imagery and affective judgments improve face-name learning in the elderly. *Journal of Gerontology, 38*(2), 197–203.

Chapter 14
Cognitive Wellness for Diverse Populations

Stephanie R. Johnson

Abstract This chapter discusses beliefs, perceptions, and programmatic methods that should be considered when developing a cognitive wellness program for diverse populations. Perceptions of cognitive health and behaviors that may enhance cognitive well-being are presented first, followed by examples of programs that have included minority older adults in substantial numbers. A final section provides a list of considerations that researchers, organizations, and community programs can utilize for developing cognitive wellness programs for diverse older adult populations.

Introduction

The older population in the United States is expected to diversify significantly over the next 40 years. Researchers project that African Americans will make up 12% of the population and Hispanics 20% of the population by 2050. Currently, there are very few cognitive wellness programs that are targeted toward ethnically diverse elder populations. However, the impending population changes present both a challenge and an opportunity to develop cognitive wellness programs that are culturally appropriate and beneficial to a diverse group of older adults.

Perceptions of Cognitive Health in Racially Diverse Elders

Successful aging may have multiple interpretations that can be objectively measured as a process of continued adaptation (von Faber et al., 2001). However, little is known about diverse communities' perceptions of successful cognitive aging.

S.R. Johnson (✉)
Howard University School of Medicine,
Washington, DC, USA
e-mail: sjohnson@cognitivesolutionsllc.com

To address this issue, the Centers for Disease Control in collaboration with the Prevention Research Centers Healthy Aging Research Network conducted a qualitative study to explore perception of aging successfully among ethnically diverse older adults (Laditka et al., 2009) using focus groups. There were six major thematic areas that emerged as critical variables for successful aging: living to an advanced age, mental attitude, cognition, physical health, social involvement, and spirituality. For purposes of this chapter, only the results for cognition will be discussed. Laditka et al. found that characteristics related to cognitive alertness, having a good memory, and engagement in cognitive activities were important sub-themes for cognition across ethnicities. However, there were some differences cross-culturally for perception of mental alertness. Vietnamese, African Americans, Whites, and Chinese were the ethnic groups that had the most concern for mental alertness. Hispanics and American Indians made very few comments related to this particular issue. The sub-theme of having a good memory was reported as important to successful aging by all ethnic groups. Interestingly, all groups with the exception of African Americans and Vietnamese mentioned that engagement in cognitive activities was important to successful aging.

Another important theme of successful aging from the survey was social involvement/interaction. Although this was deemed important to successful aging by all of the different racial/ethnic groups, the characteristics of social engagement differed across racial groups. Furthermore, the level of importance associated with social engagement and successful aging also differed across ethnicities. Social engagement was mentioned most frequently among American Indians, Whites, and African Americans. Chinese and Vietnamese groups mentioned it with much less frequency. Being involved in church and community events was another important part of social engagement particularly for African Americans, Whites, American Indians, and Chinese participants. Being socially engaged is important for cognition, because research has shown a consistent association between social engagement and maintenance of cognitive skill.

In summary, there are both similarities and differences in how cognitive health is perceived cross-culturally. Memory was consistently identified as an important part of cognitive health for all racial/ethnic groups. By contrast, the perception of mental alertness and its association to cognitive health was differentially affected by race/ethnicity. These data demonstrate the need to consider the diversity of beliefs and perceptions of cognitive health across racial/ethnic groups when developing a program that will target cognition.

Perceptions of Health Behaviors Across Racial/Ethnic Groups

Health behaviors such as physical activity and nutrition appear to play an important role in brain health. However, very few studies have explored the perception of these health behaviors and their role in cognitive health across racially/ethnically diverse elders. An understanding of how these lifestyle factors are perceived by diverse communities can certainly inform the development of future interventions to promote cognitive health and wellness.

One recent survey (Wilcox et al., 2009) explored perceptions and understanding of the link between physical activity and nutrition for maintaining cognitive health across racially diverse older adults. All racial groups agreed that physical activity was paramount to maintaining healthy brain function. However, the level of understanding the correlation between physical exercise and brain health was lower for African American, American Indians, and Hispanics. Whites, Chinese, and Vietnamese participants made explicit references to the link between physical activity and brain health. Whereas, African Americans, Whites, Chinese, and Vietnamese expressed a holistic view of cognitive health as compared to American Indian and Hispanic participants. Moreover, Chinese participants identified specific types of physical exercise to maintain brain health including tai chi, qigong, and yoga.

Wilcox et al. found conflicting views on the role of nutrition/diet for maintaining cognitive health across ethnicities. Whites from urban areas focused on the connection between portion control and maintaining a healthy weight. African Americans mentioned the method of food preparation and its role in decreasing certain diseases that may cause cognitive decline (e.g., diabetes, hypertension). However, only African Americans and Whites discussed the type of food and its association with maintaining cognitive health. It is also important to note that some participants expressed doubt about the link between diet and brain health.

In summary, this study yielded important results that have implications for developing cognitive wellness programs for diverse communities. The authors found that overall, participants had a better understanding of the link between physical activity and brain health versus diet/nutrition and brain health. Differences emerged across racial/ethnic groups' knowledge of the amount of physical activity and the dietary characteristics that are necessary for maintaining brain health. The authors conclude that physical activity and dietary messages may be better received if placed within the context of a specific ethnic group's holistic view and perception of health (Wilcox et al., 2009).

Gender Differences and Health Behaviors

Research suggests that men and women differ in their knowledge and beliefs about the etiology and treatment of various diseases. Wu, Goins, Laditka, Ignatenko, and Geodereis (2009) explored gender differences in the perception and view of cognitive health among a group of older adults living in rural areas. Significant differences were observed between men and women in terms of knowledge seeking behaviors and perception of brain health. Women generally took the lead in providing information about overall health for the family. Women were more concerned about developing Alzheimer's disease and were more likely to seek information on cognitive health. Gender differences also emerged for perceptions and attitudes of social engagement, with women emphasizing social engagement as an integral part of aging. By contrast, social engagement for men was defined by more internally based factors including having a sense of humor, being happy, and having a positive attitude. Men and women also had differing views regarding physical activity. Whereas women endorsed more structured physical activities including dance and group exercise, men discussed employment and manual labor as opportunities for physical activity. Wu et al. hypothesized that some of these findings may be attributed to societal beliefs suggesting that men are more focused on functional activities whereas women typically gravitate toward activities that involve human interaction.

In summary, both men and women are concerned about memory loss. However, women are more specifically concerned about developing Alzheimer's disease and more likely to seek information about cognitive health than men. These gender differences further support the notion that a "one-size-fits-all" approach to developing cognitive wellness programs will not meet the needs of the older adult community.

Cognitive Enrichment and Training with Diverse Elders

Although limited, there are some innovative programs that are beginning to explore the complexities of cognitive enrichment and training for racially and ethnically diverse older adults. One example is the Experience Corp (EC), which is a community-based model of service to improve educational outcomes of children developed by Fried, Freedman, Endres, and Wasik (1997). EC was designed as a social model to increase physical, cognitive, and social activity among seniors through volunteer roles in public elementary schools. The researchers hypothesized that health promotion via engagement in a new, socially useful role could improve certain areas of cognitive function including memory, processing speed, and executive function. These improvements in cognition were also expected to translate into improved activities of daily living. Fried et al. (2004) conducted a pilot randomized trial in Baltimore city. It is important to note that Baltimore has a high African American population thus allowing for a relatively representative sample of African American elders as program participants. One of the findings from the pilot study was that cognitive activity associated with the social health promotion program resulted in improvements for executive function and working memory (Fried et al.). The most significant improvements were greatest for older adults with executive function deficits at baseline. The results of the study lend support for the potential of activity-based interventions to improve certain aspects of cognitive function for a community-based sample. More detailed information about EC is provided in Chap. 27 by Rebok et al.

One of the few empirically based studies that explored the benefits of memory training with minority older adults is the SeniorWise study (McDougall, Becker, Pituch, Acee, Vaughan, & Delville, 2010). SeniorWise is a phase 3 randomized clinical trial that compared the benefits of training in specific memory skills vs. more general health training for improving memory performance. The findings showed that Whites performed better overall, but minority participants showed the greatest improvement in memory function. African American participants and those with less education made the greatest gain on cognition, which continued to the end of the study (26 months).

These two examples demonstrate that cognitive programs can be beneficial for ethnically diverse populations. Under certain circumstances, minority elders may reap greater benefits than their White counterparts. However, more research is needed in order to develop targeted cognitive training programs that will benefit all older adult populations.

Considerations for Developing Cognitive Wellness Programs for Diverse Populations

Communication Methods

Although there are a number of brain health programs currently in existence, most have not considered what might be the best methods for reaching diverse populations. Communication and/or messaging are key to reaching diverse populations that have traditionally been underrepresented in these programs. The development of culturally appropriate communication strategies for older adults and brain health must include a needs assessment, consideration of cultural differences, and cross-cultural preference of how health information is presented.

Friedman et al. (2009) explored older adults' recommendations for effectively communicating brain health information to culturally diverse communities. Most of the participants in this study reported that very little information about brain health was presented by the media. This point was especially emphasized by Vietnamese, Chinese, and African American participants. Participants also emphasized the need to develop cross-cultural messaging and communication that considers the health status of diverse communities. Some communities are plagued by health disparities and environmental variables that have contributed to inadequate knowledge and understanding of health and healthy behaviors. Participants also emphasized the need for brain health resources to reflect the culture through language and cultural traditions. Language-appropriate resources for older adults whose first language is not English are often lacking. Messages about brain health should be made available through the ethnic media (Friedman et al.), and it is important to consider from whom the message comes from. Most ethnically diverse groups agreed that medical professionals were not necessarily the most appropriate group to provide brain health information.

Are Computer-Based Cognitive Fitness Programs the Answer?

In-house "brain fitness centers" are becoming more common in nursing homes, retirement communities, and continuing care retirement communities (Friedman, 2009). Most of these cognitive enhancement centers utilize computer-based programs that complement existing wellness programs (Fernandez, 2008). The Sharp Brains Guide to Brain Fitness (Fernandez & Goldberg, 2009) provides a consumer-oriented checklist to help organizations determine if computerized cognitive fitness programs are an appropriate next step for their clients and facilities. The chapter by Zelinski et al. (Chap. 3) provides additional detailed information about electronically based approaches to cognitive enhancement and support.

Unfortunately, most of the computer-based programs that have been developed so far have paid little if any attention to the role of culture in the development of these cognitive support tools, and at present, it would be difficult to determine whether currently available computerized tools are appropriate for diverse racial/ethnic communities. Researchers and software developers must begin to consider the significant influence of culture on cognitive outcomes. Only then will it be possible to judge the efficacy of these programs for all older adult communities.

For the time being, it would be prudent for older adult communities (e.g., retirement communities, continuing care communities) to consider the demographic of their population and to consider the following questions:

- Will ethnically diverse communities participate in a computerized cognitive fitness program?
- Do the residents feel comfortable using computers?
- Are the programs written for non-English speaking participants?
- Will a computer-based method of cognitive fitness encourage or hinder ethnically diverse populations from participating in the program?
- Does gender play a role in the efficacy of these computer-based cognitive fitness programs?

Toward the Development of Cognitive Wellness Programs for All Aging Adults

Important considerations for developing cognitive wellness programs that reflect the diversity of older adults should include the following:

1. *Health status*: Knowing the current health status of the targeted community will provide a "blue print" for gauging the type of wellness program that will be needed. For example, research suggests that African Americans and Hispanics are at greater risk of developing Alzheimer's disease compared to Whites (Alzheimer's Association, 2010). This highlights the need for a comprehensive cognitive wellness program that targets these two communities that are disproportionately affected by dementia.
2. *Gender*: It is important to consider gender differences in perception of cognitive health. Women gravitate to activities that provide social engagement whereas men tend to focus on functional activities. This is an important consideration when developing cognitive wellness programs that can effectively target the needs of both women and men.
3. *Race/ethnicity*: As this chapter has shown, there are numerous considerations that need to be explored when developing cognitive wellness programs for ethnically

diverse populations. Racial groups have varying levels of knowledge pertaining to brain health. There are also differences across ethnicities in terms of how health behaviors are perceived. And, the messaging/promotion of brain health should incorporate cultural beliefs and behaviors specific to your target population.
4. *Socioeconomic status*: Socioeconomic status plays an important role in both health behaviors and health perceptions. Disadvantaged populations often do not have access to state-of-the-art information pertaining to brain health, which in turn may increase existing health disparities. Cognitive wellness programs should be made accessible for all populations that could benefit.
5. *Geographical representation (urban vs. rural)*: Geographical representation should also be considered, because research has shown that differences in terms of overall health knowledge, accessibility to current health information, and health perceptions exist between older adult populations living in urban vs. rural areas.
6. *Cognitive wellness program methods*: An important theme that emerged from some of the studies exploring attitudes and perception of cognitive health was social engagement, particularly for communities of color and women. This was also demonstrated by the EC model that showed cognitive improvement through an activity-based intervention. Therefore, activity-based cognitive interventions may be more effective for diverse older adults than computer-based programs. This is an area where research is clearly needed.

Conclusions

With the graying of the population in the United States and worldwide, cognitive health is rapidly becoming one of the most important issues that must be addressed. Diversity among older adult populations is of the utmost importance in light of the dramatic increase in ethnically diverse elders over the next 30 years. This presents an opportunity to develop cognitive wellness programs that are appropriate for all older adult populations regardless of race, gender, or socioeconomic status. Going forward, we must begin to reconceptualize how we develop these programs so that maximum cognitive benefits can be achieved by all.

References

Alzheimer's Association. (2010). *Alzheimer's disease facts and figures*. Chicago: Alzheimer's Association.
Fernandez, A. (2008). Brain-health business grows with research and demand. *Aging Today, 29*(2), 10–12.
Fernandez, A. & Goldberg, E. (2009). The Sharpbrain's guide to brain fitness. Retrieved July 2010 from http://www.sharpbrains.com/book.pdf
Fried, L. P., Carlson, M., Freedman, M., Frick, K. D., Glass, T. A., Hill, J., et al. (2004). A social model for health promotion for an aging population: Initial evidence on the Experience Corps® model. *Journal of Urban Health, 81*, 64–78.

Fried, L. P., Freedman, M., Endres, T. E., & Wasik, B. (1997). Building communities that promote successful aging. *The Western Journal of Medicine, 167*, 216–219.

Friedman, D. B., Laditka, J. N., Hunter, R., Ivey, S. L., Wu, B., Laditka, S. B., et al. (2009). Getting the message out about cognitive health: A cross-cultural comparison of older adults; media awareness and communication needs on how to maintain a healthy brain. *The Gerontologist, 49*, S50–S60.

Laditka, S. B., Corwin, S. J., Laditka, J. N., Liu, R., Tseng, W., Wu, B., et al. (2009). Attitudes about aging well among a diverse group of older Americans: Implications for promoting cognitive health. *The Gerontologist, 49*, S30–S39.

McDougall, G. J., Becker, H., Pituch, K., Acee, T. W., Vaughan, P. W., & Delville, C. L. (2010). Differential benefits of memory training for minority older adults in the SeniorWise Study. *The Gerontologist, 50*, 632–645.

von Faber, M., Bootsma-Van Der Wiel, A., van Excel, E., Gussekloo, J., Lagaay, A. M., van Dongen, E., et al. (2001). Successful aging in the oldest old: who can be characterized as successfully aged? *Archives of Internal Medicine, 161*, 2694–2700.

Wilcox, S., Sharkey, J. R., Mathews, A. E., Laditka, J. N., Laditka, S. B., Logsdon, R. G., et al. (2009). Perceptions and beliefs about the role of physical activity and nutrition on brain health in older adults. *The Gerontologist, 49*, S61–S71.

Wu, B., Goins, R. T., Laditka, J. N., Ignatenko, V., & Geodereis, E. (2009). Gender differences in views about cognitive health and healthy lifestyle behaviors among rural older adults. *The Gerontologist, 49*, S72–S78.

Chapter 15
The Role of Physical Activity in Cognitive Fitness: A General Guide for Community Programs

Edward S. Potkanowicz

Abstract This chapter examines physical activity in the context of understanding fitness and preparing for activity as well as practical suggestions for motivating, supporting, and encouraging adherence to exercise regimens. For a more comprehensive review of the exercise–cognition connection, the reader is referred to the Chap. 2 by Boot and Blakely (Enhancing Cognitive Fitness in Adults: A guide for use and development of community-based programs, 2011).

Introduction

Regardless of the bodily system examined, there is an age-related decline in human function over time. Of particular interest to exercise physiologists is the role of physical activity in the mitigation of these declines.

Physical fitness is defined as follows by the ACSM (American College of Sports Medicine, 2010, p. 2):

> …a set of attributes or characteristics that people have or achieve that relates to the ability to perform physical activity. These characteristics are usually separated into either health-related or skill-related components.

While skill-related fitness (i.e., agility, balance, coordination, speed, power, and reaction time) is important, it does not contribute to the current discussion of the preservation of cognition. Health-related fitness, however, does contribute to the discussion. Health-related physical fitness as defined by the ACSM (2006, p. 3):

> …is associated with the ability to perform daily activities with vigor, and the possession of traits and capacities that are associated with a low risk of premature development of

---

E.S. Potkanowicz (✉)
Assistant Professor of Exercise Physiology, Department of Human Performance and Sport Sciences, Ohio Northern University, Ada, Ohio, USA
e-mail: potkanowicz@me.com

hypokinetic diseases (e.g., those associated with physical inactivity, like obesity, diabetes, and hypertension).

Health-related fitness is actually a collection of traits (i.e., cardiovascular endurance, muscular fitness, flexibility, and body composition). Addressed individually as part of a well-designed and comprehensive fitness program, these traits have the potential to significantly impact the older adult's overall quality of life and capacity for independent living. For example, having sufficient muscular fitness makes climbing stairs or lifting grandchildren easier. Flexibility provides for greater range of motion, which makes bending over or looking over your shoulder when driving less difficult. Likewise, maintaining a healthy weight means a lower risk for developing diabetes or cardiovascular disease. Of particular interest to the discussion of maintaining and/or preserving cognition is the improvement of cardiovascular endurance (also referred to as aerobic capacity), which is the focus of this chapter.

Developing Cardiovascular Endurance

Cardiovascular endurance, or aerobic capacity, is improved through participation in aerobic activities. Aerobic activity has generally been defined as an activity that uses large muscle groups, can be maintained continuously, and is rhythmic in nature. Additionally, it is exercise that overloads the heart and lungs and causes them to work harder than they would when resting. There is a seemingly endless list of aerobic activities to choose from (e.g., walking, jogging, cycling, gardening, or swimming). Regardless of the activity chosen, there are guidelines that should be followed so that the experience is a productive and safe one.

In order to promote and maintain cardiovascular endurance, current recommendations from the ACSM and the American Heart Association (AHA) (Nelson et al., 2007) indicate that adults should participate in moderate-intensity aerobic activity for a minimum of 30 min per day for 5 days each week. Or, if capable, the activity can be of vigorous-intensity maintained for 20 min on 3 days each week. The recommendations are listed in their entirety in Table 15.1.

The recommendations also allow for a combination of both moderate- and vigorous-intensity in order to meet these aerobic activity recommendations. Additionally, if the level of cardiovascular endurance is particularly low, one can begin at a level below the recommendations and work up to the minimum recommendations.

Table 15.1 Recommendations for Aerobic Activity

Frequency (days/week)	Intensity	Duration (min)
5	Moderate (defined as 5–6 on a subjective 10 point scale)[a]	30
3	Vigorous (defined as 7–8 on a subjective 10 point scale)[a]	20

[a] Exercise can be started at a frequency, intensity, and duration below the recommended if initial fitness levels are low

These activities are in addition to normal light-intensity daily activities (such as self care and cooking) or moderate-intensity activities associated with everyday life (e.g., walking around the office or walking from the parking lot) that last less than 10 min. Lastly, these recommendations represent minimum levels of involvement with respect to aerobic activity. That said, the older adult should expect to experience the minimum in the way of improvement in aerobic capacity.

Physical Activity

Often there is confusion between what physical activity is and what exercise is. Are they the same? Are they different? Does it matter?

ACSM defines physical activity as:

> ...bodily movement that is produced by the contraction of skeletal muscle and that substantially increases energy expenditure.

The National Institute on Aging (NIA), in their free publication *"Exercise & Physical Activity: Your Everyday Guide from The National Institute on Aging"* (2009), defines physical activity as:

> ...activities that get your body moving such as gardening, walking the dog, raking leaves, and taking the stairs instead of the elevator.

Exercise, on the other hand, is defined by the ACSM and the NIA as being "...planned, structured, and, repetitive..."

While the two terms differ in their specific definitions, the take-home message for the community program coordinator, the exercise leader, or the individual is that being active is beneficial as it relates to cognition (see Boot and Blakely's review Chap. 2). If an older adult is not currently active, he/she should work to become active, and with most active individuals there is room to improve their level of fitness.

Recommendations for Activity

Activity can take many forms. What one chooses to do should be based on a number of considerations such as safety, enjoyment, opportunities for social involvement, and readiness to begin an activity program. With proper preparation and planning, adding regular activity to one's life can be fairly simple.

Safety First

Before beginning any exercise program, older adults should consult with a physician to ensure that they are healthy enough to safely begin an activity program. While most people are sufficiently healthy to begin a low to moderate-intensity program on their own, a physician may have recommendations based on knowledge of the individual's medical history that will make the chosen activity much safer. Although not a substitute for making time with a medical professional, the older adult can begin the screening process on their own. A more recently developed screening tool called the EASY tool, which is an acronym for *Exercise Assessment and Screening for You* (available at www.easyforyou.info), is described as follows:

> …a tool developed to help older individuals, their healthcare providers, and exercise professionals identify different types of exercise and physical activity regimens that can be tailored to meet the existing health conditions, illnesses, or disabilities of older adults
>
> (Resnick et al., 2008).

What makes the EASY tool handy is that it can be completed independently by the older adult or with the assistance of a healthcare or exercise professional. The assessment presents the older adult with six basic health-related questions. These questions address several issues such as chest pain during activity, the presence of high blood pressure, and light-headedness. If the older adult answers "no" to all of the questions, he or she is given recommendations on how to safely begin exercising. If health concerns are identified, the older adult is guided to the safest form of exercise with consideration for his/her condition or is directed to seek a medical consult. However, the authors assert that preexercise screening should not keep people from being active. Rather, given the benefits of physical activity, screening should set people on their way to either starting to become active or significantly increasing their activity level.

What to Do

A number of activities have been identified as being beneficial for developing cardiovascular endurance. The basic criteria are that the activities safely increase heart and breathing rate above resting levels. Examples of this might include going for a casual or brisk walk, jogging, or even in-line skating (Miller, 2003), if balance skills are sufficient! Adult-size three and four wheel cycles and recumbent cycles are growing in popularity. A fun alternative recently developed is the Wii video game by Nintendo®. This gaming system has been used successfully in retirement communities and in residential homes. These games, which include activities such as bowling or tennis, can appreciably increase the heart rate of the player.

Housekeeping activities that can raise heart rate include vacuuming, dusting, shaking out rugs, and scrubbing floors. Outdoor work such as washing the car, sweeping the porch and patio are also considered physical activity. Playful interactions with grandchildren (e.g., hopscotch or hula hoop) are a good way to get the heart rate up as are long walks with a friend. When the weather is inclement, mall walking and walking up and down the basement stairs are acceptable forms of activity. For the more accomplished exerciser, one can include challenging activities such as push-ups (traditional and modified), hiking, jumping jacks, or other calisthenic-like activities.

Regardless of the activity, the format for the exercise session will be the same; i.e., it should include a warm-up period, the activity, and a cool-down.

The warm-up prepares the participant for the activity by safely increasing the heart rate and respiration to levels near to those of the actual activity. This 5–10 min process prepares the body for activity and allows for a safe progression into the actual activity. The warm-up also helps to prevent muscle and joint soreness that might occur during the early adaptive phase of the program. Additionally, the warm-up reduces the likelihood of injury, an important consideration for any participant.

The activity should be one that, as previously mentioned, safely increases heart and breathing rate above resting levels for a given period of time. While the recommendations for cardiovascular fitness suggest a period of 20–30 min at an intensity level of 5–6 or 7–8 on a 10-point subjective rating scale, it is important to note that there are acceptable variations.

An easy method for calculating exercise intensity is the use of what is often referred to as the "Talk Test" (Hartman-Stein & Potkanowicz, 2003). During physical activity or exercise the older adult should be able to carry on a conversation comfortably. The intensity is too high if speaking is difficult (i.e., gasping or gulping for breath). If this is the case, then the intensity should be reduced. However, if the conversation is too easy, the intensity should be increased.

The time spent in an activity can be accumulated; i.e., if initial cardiovascular fitness levels are low, the 20 or 30-min session can be divided into four 5-min sessions, two 10-min sessions, or three 10-min sessions. Setting intensity levels below these recommendations at the onset for the less fit individual is also acceptable. What is important to note is that the goal should be to build on the initial successes associated with the lower intensity and duration levels so as to progress and improve over time.

Activity can be increased simply by changing everyday habits such as parking farther away from the entrance to a store, hanging clothes outside on the line rather than placing them in the dryer, taking the stairs rather than the elevator, or walking to lunch if time and distance permit.

For many, walking, and similar activities, has always been a go-to exercise. However, the definition of what activity is has changed progressively over time. For example, on the National Institute of Health's website for healthy aging entitled "NIH Senior Health" (www.nihseniorealth.gov), the suggested endurance activities listed include not only traditional aerobic activities but also functional activities such raking, sweeping, and gardening. While not commonly included in the traditional list of activities, the lifting, shoveling, bending, and pulling of weeds (without excessive bending and twisting to prevent back injury) during seasonal gardening certainly cause one to breathe faster and deeper and cause the heart rate to increase noticeably.

Often people do not consider hobby-like activities as being exercise because they represent something that they have always done or enjoyed doing. The activity of choice should be enjoyable and fun, stimulate and engage the individual physically and mentally, and be something the participant can do on a regular basis.

There are numerous resources available to help one decide what to do in the way of activity, both in the traditional and nontraditional sense. The National Institute on Aging (www.nia.nih.gov), the National Institutes of Health (www.nih.gov), and the Centers for Disease Control and Prevention (www.cdc.gov/aging) offer free information online and in print. The American College of Sports Medicine (www.ACSM.org), the National Strength and Conditioning Association [NSCA] (www.nsca-lift.org), and American Association of Retired Persons (www.AARP.org) offer free literature and have issued suggestions when developing an activity program.

Researchers at the University of Washington have developed an innovative program, Reducing Disability in Alzheimer's Disease (RDAD) for individuals with dementia (Logsdon, McCurry, & Teri, 2005; Logsdon & Teri, 2010). The exercise component of the program consists of 12-h-long training sessions that include endurance activities (primarily walking), strength training, and balance and flexibility exercises. RDAD is conducted in the home with a trainer who demonstrates the exercise, followed by the individual with dementia practicing it while the caregiver observes and assists. The participant begins by walking at a normal pace and is encouraged to gradually walk at a speed that causes breathing more heavily than usual, but not to the point of shortness of breath. The program is designed so that the caregivers can establish a structured routine that can be continued without a trainer's supervision. The goal of the program is to achieve 20–30 min or more of moderate intensity on most days of the week.

When an activity/exercise is finished, it is important to help the body return to a state near to resting, a cool-down period. During the cool-down, the goal is to reduce the intensity of the activity during the last 5–10 min. Doing so allows the breathing and pulse rate to slowly return to normal. Given the changing face of activity, the cool-down may also take on a different form. For example, the cool-down following a walking session may include slowing the pace or staying on a level surface. After gardening, however, the cool-down might include a stroll around the garden patch to examine your handiwork. While the cool-down after stationary cycling might include a slower pedal rate with less resistance against the flywheel, the cool-down after doing and hanging the laundry might be carrying the now empty basket slowly back to the house. While seemingly different on the surface, the intention and goal are the same, i.e., to safely return the body to a state close to resting.

Strategies for Long-Term Success

While physical activity has numerous benefits for the older adult, what many find to be the most challenging is to remain active over time. Many of us lack the motivation and have trouble adhering to an exercise plan. The following are strategies for staying motivated and keeping physical activity a part of your daily life.

Personal Characteristics

For the healthcare worker responsible for motivating older adults to become more active, consideration should be given to the personal characteristics of the individual such as considering the generation, social/ethnic background, or socio-economic status of the participant. For example, Taylor and Johnson (2008) suggest that many of today's seniors were raised when men and women had very different social and family roles. Men went to work outside the home and women were responsible for the running the home. Because of these gender roles, society did not accept women as regular exercisers until the 1970s or early 1980s. When trying to motivate today's older adults, it is essential to keep in mind that an older adult may not have ever learned how to exercise or had access to a gym in the past.

As mentioned earlier, a resource for the healthcare worker and the older adult is the free NIA publication entitled *"Exercise and Physical Activity: Your Everyday Guide from the National Institute on Aging."* In order to increase motivation, the authors suggest the following.

Make It an Opportunity to Socialize

Physical activity can provide for a great social network. Having fun and being among people whose company you enjoy are often very strong motivators. Combining the social with the physical is a great way to introduce people to physical activity and to increase the likelihood of keeping people coming back.

Make It Interesting and Allow Choices

Activities can vary widely. The key is that the individual finds it interesting and wants to participate. Forcing a particular form of physical activity on an individual only leads to failure. While a structured routine is important (i.e., it should have goals and regular assessments), having the freedom to choose what one wants is important as well see Chap. 6 for review.

Make It Part of Your Routine

Not only should the physical activity have structure and direction, but the activity should also be a regular occurrence in the person's daily routine. Just as brushing teeth occurs each day, physical activity should have a place in the daily schedule.

Make It Easy

Find an enjoyable way to include physical activity into the daily routine. As was mentioned earlier, the definition of physical activity is a moving target. While some people may be perfectly happy on a treadmill in a gym, others may prefer to walk outdoors.

There is a growing body of evidence for the benefits of "green exercise," i.e., that a synergistic benefit occurs in adopting physical activities at the same time being exposed to nature for its stress reducing and relaxation benefits (Pretty, Peacock, Sellens, & Griffin, 2005; Pretty et al., 2007; Mackay & Neill, 2010). Future studies are needed to determine if older adults will increase their adherence to exercise protocols if a nature component is part of the activity, such as exercising by windows with a view of pleasant urban or rural scenery.

Taylor and Johnson (2008) suggest that to increase adherence program coordinators and exercise leaders should consider program enhancers and utilize behavior management techniques.

Program Enhancers

Program enhancers are those things that add variety to the daily routine. For example, adding exercise balls or different types of music, or offering a choice of activities on a given day work to enhance the physical activity experience. Other incentives for regular participation include prizes or certificates of attendance for every 50 visits. The more interesting and novel the program, the more likely the participants will return.

Behavior Management Techniques

By creating a supportive environment, leading by example, and espousing the good guidelines of regular physical activity, the caregiver or staff member in charge of the group can yield significant influence for change.

With the goal being an increase in physical activity, the exercise or group leader can again play a significant role if he or she understands that path to regular physical activity. Changing a behavior usually involves three stages: (1) the decision to change; (2) the early stages of change; and (3) adoption/maintenance of the new behavior. As the participant moves through each of the stages, different strategies are needed to reinforce the new behavior. The exercise leader can incorporate things like dispelling myths to encourage change, suggesting that the participants set their exercise clothes out the night before, solicit support from family and friends, and keep records to document progress.

The RDAD program suggests that a simple checklist be used that can be posted on the refrigerator or other conspicuous location to serve as a reminder. It also provides reinforcement each time the participant checks off completing the exercise (Logsdon & Teri, 2010). As in many behavior change programs, it can be helpful to construct a graph showing the number of days or minutes of exercise. Some participants benefit from the use of a pedometer to count the number of steps, another measure that can be graphed and serve as a reinforcer to document progress.

Summary

The consensus in the literature is that older adults who possess higher levels of cardiovascular fitness demonstrate better cognitive function. While no one mode of exercise has been deemed preferential or more effective, participating in an activity program that has as its goal the improvement of cardiovascular fitness has been shown to be beneficial to the cognitive abilities of the older adult. While there are still many questions that need to be answered, the recommendation for the community program coordinator, the exercise leader, or the individual is that making regular activity a part of the every day life of the older adult is a safe and effective way to positively impact cognitive function. Additionally, activity for the sake of cognition may lead to activity for the sake of health and healthy aging overall.

References

American College of Sports Medicine. (2006). *ACSM's guidelines for exercise testing and prescription* (7th ed.). Baltimore: Lippincott Williams and Wilkins.
American College of Sports Medicine. (2010). *ACSM's guidelines for exercise testing and prescription* (8th ed.). Baltimore: Lippincott Williams and Wilkins.
Hartman-Stein, P., & Potkanowicz, E. (2003). Behavioral determinants of healthy aging: Good news for the baby boomer generation. *Online Journal of Issues in Nursing, 8*(2). Retrieved from www.nursingworld.org/MainMenuCategories/ANAMarketplace/ANAPeriodicals/OJIN/TableofContents/Volume
Logsdon, R. G., McCurry, S. M., & Teri, L. (2005). A home-health care approach to exercise for persons with Alzheimer's disease. *Care Management Journals, 6*, 90–97.
Logsdon, R. G., & Teri, L. (2010). An evidence-based exercise and behavior management program for dementia care. *Generations*, Spring, 80–83.
Mackay, G. J., & Neill, J. T. (2010). The effect of "green exercise" on state anxiety and the role of exercise duration, intensity, and greenness: A quasi-experimental study. *Psychology of Sport and Exercise, 11*, 238–245.
Miller, L. (2003). *Get rolling: The beginner's guide to in-line skating*. Danville: Get Rolling Books.
National Institute on Aging. (2009). *Exercise and physical activity: Your everyday guide from the National Institute on Aging* (NIH Publication No. 09–4258). Washington: U.S. Government Printing Office.

Nelson, M., Rejeski, W., Blair, S., Duncan, P., Judge, J., King, A., et al. (2007). Physical activity and public health in older adults: Recommendation from the American College of Sports Medicine and the American Heart Association. *Medicine and Science in Sport and Exercise, 39*, 1435–1445.

Pretty, J., Peacock, J., Hine, R., Sellens, M., South, N., & Griffin, M. (2007). Green Exercise in the UK Countryside: Effects on health and psychological well-being, and implications for policy and planning. *Journal of Environmental Planning and Management, 50*, 211–231.

Pretty, J., Peacock, J., Sellens, M., & Griffin, M. (2005). The mental and physical health outcomes of green exercise. *International Journal of Environmental Health Research, 15*, 319–337.

Resnick, B., Ory, M. G., Hora, K., Rogers, M. E., Page, P., Bolin, J. N., et al. (2008). A Proposal for a new screening paradigm and tool called Exercise Assessment and Screening for You (EASY). *Journal of Aging and Physical Activity, 16*, 215–233.

Taylor, A. W., & Johnson, M. J. (2008). *Physiology of exercise and healthy aging*. Champaign: Human Kinetics.

Boot, W., & Blakely, D. (2011). Mental and physical exercise as a means to reverse cognitive aging and enhance well-being. In P. E. Hartman-Stein & A. La Rue (Eds.), *Enhancing Cognitive Fitness in Adults: A guide for use and development of community-based programs*. New York: Springer.

Chapter 16
Nutrition and Nutritional Supplements to Promote Brain Health

Abhilash K. Desai, Joy Rush, Lakshmi Naveen, and Papan Thaipisuttikul

Abstract New scientific evidence strongly suggests that a variety of nutritional strategies can promote brain health and slow the course of Alzheimer's disease and related dementias (ADRD). Improving nutrition is, thus, a critical component of any comprehensive strategy to slow the course of ADRD. This chapter presents recommendations designed to meet this objective. Specific goals are to consume a balanced diet with particular focus on increasing consumption of brain power foods. Examples of brain power foods include oily fish (to be consumed at least twice a week), berries (especially blueberries), green leafy vegetables, legumes, and turmeric. In addition, some nutritional supplements (especially vitamin D and vitamin B12) are also necessary to promote brain health. Multinutritional intervention, targeting multiple aspects of processes causing ADRD, instituted as early as possible is likely to have the greatest beneficial effect. Staying physically and mentally active and maintaining a healthy weight can greatly enhance the beneficial effects of nutritional interventions on brain health.

Introduction

Cognitive impairment associated with Alzheimer's disease and related dementias (such as Vascular dementia, Dementia with Lewy Bodies, Parkinson's Disease Dementia, Fronto-Temporal Dementia) (ADRD) causes impairment in daily functioning and significant emotional distress. New scientific evidence has indicated that appropriate changes in a person's diet *can* enhance their cognitive abilities, protect brain from damage, and may counteract the effects of dementia (Morley, 2010).

A.K. Desai (✉)
Medical Director, Geriatric Psychiatry Director, Memory Clinic, Sheppard Pratt Health Systems, Associate Professor, Department of Neurology and Psychiatry, Division of Geriatric Psychiatry, Saint Louis University School of Medicine, 605 N. Charles St., Baltimore, MD 21285, USA
e-mail: adesai@sheppardpratt.org

Nutrition researchers and scientists have identified foods and eating patterns that both increase and decrease the risk of ADRD (Gu, Nieves, Stern, Luchsinger, & Scarmeas, 2010). The effect of brain healthy food can be enhanced by combining it with other healthy lifestyle strategies such as regular exercise and engagement in intellectual and social activities (Kidd, 2008). Clinical trials to date investigating drugs for Alzheimer's disease (AD) have found that 25% of patients with AD do not worsen over 18-month period (Schneider & Sano, 2009). This allows time for nutritional and other lifestyle interventions to be instituted and have their impact.

Mechanisms of Diseases Causing Dementia and Nutrition

Processes that underlie ADRD pathogenesis include oxidative stress, chronic inflammation, accumulation of toxic mis-folded proteins, impaired utilization of glucose by brain cells, mitochondrial dysfunction, toxicity due to excess neurotransmitters (e.g., glutamate), and inadequate blood and oxygen supply to the brain cells (neurons) and brain connections (synapses) (Querfurth & LaFerla, 2010). These processes lead to loss of brain cells and brain connections, eventually leading to memory and other problems characteristic of ADRD. Growing research suggests that several nutritional components (e.g., anthocyanins, sulforaphane, curcumin) can effectively counteract these processes, e.g., by reducing oxidation and inflammation, decreasing accumulation of toxic proteins, promoting membrane formation and formation of new synapses and new brain cells, prolonging life of existing brain cells, improving function of inner lining (endothelial lining) of blood vessels, and thus improving blood and oxygen supply to the brain cells (Kamphuis & Scheltens, 2010). The suggested synergy between nutritional components to improve neuronal plasticity (i.e., capacity of the brain to change with experience and environment) and brain function is supported by epidemiological studies as well as experimental studies in animal models, although randomized controlled trials (RCTs) are lacking (van der Beek & Kamphuis, 2008).

The brain is particularly susceptible to oxidative damage. Brain activity consumes a lot of energy, and the reactions that release this energy also generate oxidizing chemicals. In addition, the brain contains a great amount of oxidizable tissue, particularly in the fatty membranes surrounding nerve cells. Tissue-damaging free radicals (reactive oxygen species and reactive nitrogen species formed during oxidation) become more prevalent as we age and their harmful effects are promoted by accumulation of toxic proteins and decrease blood circulation seen in ADRD (Desai, Grossberg, & Chibnall, 2010). This has led to the attempt to slow the progress of ADRD by using antioxidants (class of chemicals that protect brain cells and other tissues in the body against free radicals). Although research to date using antioxidants in the form of pills (e.g., vitamin E) to treat ADRD has been disappointing, studies to promote brain health through increasing intake of food high in antioxidants (e.g., Mediterranean diet) continue to be encouraging. Fruits and vegetables are the primary source of antioxidants. Over-eating increases oxidative stress on the brain and thus risks undoing the work of antioxidants and exercise. High blood sugar can also cause oxidative stress on the blood vessels and the brain.

Dietary Patterns and Brain Health

Mediterranean diet: The Mediterranean diet is characterized by high intake of vegetables, legumes, fruits, and cereals; high intake of unsaturated fatty acids (mostly in the form of olive oil), but low intake of saturated fatty acids; a moderately high intake of fish; a low-to-moderate intake of dairy products (mostly cheese or yogurt); a low intake of meat and poultry; and a regular but moderate amount of ethanol, primarily in the form of wine, which is generally consumed during meals. The Mediterranean diet has been found to improve cholesterol levels, blood sugar levels, and overall health of blood vessels. It has been associated with longer life, decreased heart disease and strokes, and reduced risk of obesity and diabetes. Recent studies have found that higher adherence to Mediterranean diet was associated with lower risk for both AD and Mild Cognitive Impairment (Scarmeas et al., 2009). Other studies have found that higher adherence to the Mediterranean diet was associated with lower mortality in AD in a possible dose–response effect. The Mediterranean diet may slow the progression to dementia. The potential mechanisms for Mediterranean diet to promote brain health includes antioxidant effect, anti-inflammatory effect, reducing destructive effects of toxic proteins (e.g., beta amyloid and hyperphosphorylated tau in AD), and improved blood supply to brain cells.

DASH diet (dietary approaches to stop hypertension): The DASH diet is a diet rich in fruits and vegetables, and low-fat dairy products, and low in saturated and total fat. The DASH diet comprises 4–5 servings of fruit, 4–5 servings of vegetables, 2–3 servings of low-fat dairy per day, and <25% fat. Besides lowering blood pressure, the DASH diet may also directly promote brain health through its high antioxidant effects.

Specific Food Groups to Promote Brain Health

Fruits, vegetables, and legumes: Fruits, vegetables, and legumes contain a variety of phytonutrients that have strong antioxidant and anti-inflammatory properties. Phytonutrients (also called phytochemicals) are organic compounds of plants that are thought to promote health. Unlike the traditional nutrients (proteins, fat, vitamins, minerals), phytonutrients are not "essential" for life. Some common classes of phytonutrients that have been found to promote brain health include carotenoids, flavonoids (polyphenols), lignans, saponins, and terpenes. All types of fruits, vegetables, and legumes promote brain health. Preliminary research has suggested that certain fruits, vegetables, and legumes may have more nutritional punch in regard to brain health compared to others. Several studies have indicated that regular consumption of 5–10 servings per day of fruits, vegetables, and legumes enhances brain function and may slow cognitive decline. Polyphenols isolated from blueberries have been shown to demonstrate positive effects on cognitive functioning in persons with dementia. Among all fruits, berries have some of the highest amount of antioxidants. Many vegetables (e.g., broccoli) contain chemicals (e.g., sulforaphane) that encourage production of enzymes which protect the blood vessels, and thus promote blood flow to the brain. Among vegetables, tomatoes and green leafy vegetables have some of the highest amount of nutrients (e.g., lycopene, folate) that are needed for brain to function well.

Omega-3 fatty acids (O3FA): O3FA are essential fatty acids (i.e., they cannot be synthesized by the body and need to be obtained from food). There are three O3FA, Docosahexanoic acid (DHA), Eicosapentanoic acid (EPA), and linoleic acid. DHA constitutes 40% of all fatty acids in the brain. DHA is found predominantly in marine fish and algae. DHA has antioxidant and anti-inflammatory properties and enhances synaptic function (function of brain cell connections). DHA provides synaptic membranes with "fluidity" – improved capacity to transmit signals from one cell to another. Therefore, decreased DHA in neuronal membranes may weaken the brain architecture and leave it vulnerable to diseases. Low levels of DHA have been found in persons with dementia. O3FA can improve memory in genetically modified Alzheimer's mouse model. Best sources of O3FA include a variety of oily fish. It is important that fish is consumed either baked or broiled. When fish is fried, the nutritional value is lost (due to loss of omega 3 during the process of frying) and harmful chemicals (e.g., partially hydrogenated fatty acids) are created by frying process that may harm the brain by promoting inflammation. Other sources of O3FA include walnuts, Kiwi, flax seed, and omega-3 enriched food items (e.g., eggs, milk, cereals). It is important to eat a variety of fatty fish. Due to concern about mercury contamination of some fish, we recommend avoiding fish with high mercury content such as King Mackerel, swordfish, golden bass, shark, and tilefish.

Whole grains: Whole grains are another excellent source of phytonutrients. Whole grains pack more nutritional punch and fiber than refined grains (e.g., white bread, white rice). Whole grains are rich in B vitamins, fiber, and antioxidants and thus have significant beneficial effects on brain function. Whole grains include wheat, barley, oats, rye, kasha, bulgar, millet, quinoa, and maize. Commonly consumed food rich in whole grains include whole grain pasta, brown rice, whole wheat bread, and quinoa. We can make breads, muffins, and other home-made goods healthier by mixing whole-wheat flour with white flour. Higher intake of whole grains can help lower amounts of blood sugar, total body fat, and abdominal fat, which may be especially important for individuals with diabetes, obesity, and metabolic syndrome. Not all foods in the grocery store that claim to be "whole grain" are whole grain. Many include refined or enriched white flour. Foods with labels that say "100% whole wheat" (or oats or rye) are recommended.

Monounsaturated fatty acids (MUFA): MUFA, as part of traditional Mediterranean diet, have been found to promote brain health and slow cognitive decline. Animal studies support the concept that extra-virgin olive oil plays a central role in slowing the dementing process. Sources of MUFA include olive oil (preferably first cold-pressed extra-virgin olive oil), canola oil (cheaper than olive oil and equally beneficial) and avocadoes. Regularly adding a few olives in one's salads or other food items is an easy way to improve intake of MUFA. MUFA are high in calories and thus excess consumption should be avoided.

Spices: Spices (e.g., turmeric, cinnamon, cloves, red pepper, black pepper, ginger, garlic) have all been found to contain phytonutrients with potential disease-modifying capabilities. Turmeric, or Indian saffron, is currently the most promising among all spices regarding potential benefits in AD. Several studies have pointed to curcumin, the active ingredient in turmeric, and its anti-inflammatory and antiamyloid properties (Aggarwal & Sung, 2009). Turmeric is an orange-yellow powder commonly used as a spice in curries. Turmeric is present in many Asian curries. High Asian curry consumption has been found to be associated with improved memory and other cognitive functions. Most Asian curries prepared in US restaurants have high salt and saturated fat content and therefore are not good options to promote brain health. A pinch of turmeric may be mixed with home-made healthy curries and sauces. Turmeric is also found in some pickles and in yellow mustard that can be used in sandwiches.

Nuts: Nuts are also an excellent source of many phytonutrients. Tree nuts (e.g., walnuts, almonds, pecans, hazel nuts) have chemicals (e.g., O3FA in walnuts, vitamin E in almonds, MUFA in most of the nuts) that have been known to promote brain health. It is prudent to limit consumption of nuts to small amounts as they contain high amount of fat and thus, high amount of calories.

Green tea: Green tea has high content of polyphenolic flavanoids known as "catechins." Catechin has been demonstated to have potent antioxidant and anti-inflammatory properties. Sugar and saturated fat in many commonly consumed tea drinks (e.g., "chai tea" found in coffee houses) may not only cancel out the beneficial effects but may even be harmful to the brain. Caffeine content of tea can also cause insomnia, anxiety, tremors, and irregular heart beat.

Coffee: Some studies have found that regular consumption of coffee is associated with decreased future risk of ADRD. Sugar and saturated fat in many commonly consumed coffee drinks (e.g., "lattes" found in coffee houses) may not only cancel out the beneficial effects but may even be harmful to the brain. Caffeine content of coffee can also cause insomnia, anxiety, tremors, and irregular heart beat.

Dark chocolate: Dark chocolate (true dark chocolates are bitter) has been found to have beneficial effects on heart health and brain health. Stearic acid in pure chocolate is a saturated fat that acts more like unsaturated fat in that it lowers LDL levels and reduces atherosclerosis. An exact amount is not clear; hence their use is recommended only in very modest amounts. For example, an ounce of dark chocolate (at least 70% cocoa) per day may be appropriate. Note that many "dark chocolates" may not have flavonols (one group of phytonutrients) (removed by their manufacturers because of their bitter taste) but have abundant saturated fat, refined sugar, and calories – all three proven to be harmful to the blood vessels, the heart, and the brain. Even with flavonols present, chocolate lovers should be mindful of the other contents. Those who eat a moderate amount of favanol-rich dark chocolate may need to balance the calories by reducing their intake of other foods.

Sweeteners: Splenda is recommended over other sweeteners such as aspartame or stevia. This is because splenda has been researched the most among all sweeteners and to date, it has not been linked to any adverse direct effects on the brain or body. We recommend using only modest amounts of sweeteners because eating sweet food regularly can train the brain to crave for sweet food which in turn can lead to consumption of calorie dense sweet foods.

Alcohol: Modest alcohol intake has been associated not only with improved heart health but also with reduced risk of future dementia and slower cognitive decline in patients with MCI. However, by the time a person develops dementia, the brain is significantly damaged and thus becomes very sensitive to toxic effects of even modest amounts of alcohol. Brain damage is a common and potentially severe consequence of long-term, heavy alcohol consumption. Even social drinkers who consume more than 21 drinks per week are at high risk for cognitive impairment in the long run. Excessive alcohol use can cause structural and functional abnormalities of the brain. These changes are more severe and other brain regions are also damaged in patients drinking excessive alcohol who have additional vitamin B1 (thiamine) deficiency (Wernicke–Korsakoff syndrome). The more alcohol consumed, the smaller the total brain volume. Thus, the negative effect of excessive, at-risk alcohol consumption and binge drinking habits is of much greater concern than possible beneficial effects of light drinking. At-risk and binge drinking are frequently reported by middle-aged and elderly adults nationwide (Blazer & Wu, 2009). Therefore, advice about alcohol consumption should be tempered by the known risks of excessive use in terms of neurologic and other organ damage as well as increased risk of injury from intoxication. Also, alcohol interacts with many medications routinely taken by middle aged and older adults with potentially serious adverse health consequences. Persons with dementia should be recommended to avoid intake of alcohol. For those adults with dementia who drink regularly and wish to continue, we recommend that men avoid drinking more than 7 U/week (maximum of 1/day). Women should avoid drinking more than 4 U/week (maximum of 0.5/day). All adults with dementia should avoid drinking 3 or more units of alcohol at 1 time. One unit of alcohol is equal to 12 oz of beer, 4–5 oz of wine and 1 oz of distilled spirit.

Medical Foods and "Memory Shakes"

Medical food is defined as a medical product intended for the dietary management of a disease or a specific condition. Medical foods are available by prescription only and should be taken only under the supervision of a physician or a physician extender (nurse practitioner or physician assistant). Axona is the only medical food currently available for clinical management of mild-to-moderate stage AD. Hypometabolism may be involved in the pathogenesis of AD. Hypometabolism involves brain's impaired ability to breakdown and/or utilize glucose as source of energy. Axona is thought to promote brain health by providing an alternative source of glucose that the brain can use for energy. A small study found that there was slower decline in memory and other cognitive functions compared to placebo in subjects with mild-to-moderate Alzheimer's disease who were APOE e4 negative (Henderson et al., 2009).

Adverse effects reported include diarrhea, flatulence, and abdominal distress. We recommend starting with half a packet shaken with milk, fruit juice, or water daily in the morning for a week before trying one packet daily. In individuals with protein calorie malnutrition, Axona can be mixed with health shakes such as Ensure, Boost, or Carnation Instant Breakfast. Patients with uncontrolled diabetes, alcohol abuse, and liver disease are recommended to avoid Axona.

The three compounds – O3FA, uridine, and choline – are all needed by brain cells to make phospholipids, the primary component of cell membranes. Increasing intake of these compounds has been found to dramatically increase the amount of membranes that form brain cell connections. Loss of brain cell connections is believed to cause memory loss and other cognitive impairments seen in ADRD. Souvenaid is a "memory shake" rich in these three compounds. It is currently being studied for potential benefits to persons with AD. There are animal studies supporting its potential effects on memory (Morley, 2010). Preliminary analysis of the study suggested that in patients with early AD, there was an improvement in verbal memory (Scheltens et al., 2010). Benevia is a drink containing lutein and DHA. It is available over the counter and advertised as a "memory boosting" drink. It contains high amounts of sugar, so caution is needed in patients with diabetes. It also contains a good amount of protein and thus may be particularly beneficial to individuals with protein calorie malnutrition.

Nutritional Supplements

Nutritional supplements are often needed to supplement diet in order to promote brain health. They are recommended because even older adults who eat a brain healthy and well-balanced diet may not absorb necessary nutrients because of age and disease-related problems with absorption. There are several widely marketed nonprescription nutritional supplements claimed to be memory enhancers and treatments for cognitive decline associated with ADRD (McDaniel, Maier, & Einstein, 2003). Supplements may promote brain function through a variety of mechanisms including antioxidant, anti-inflammatory, and metabolic regulation. Besides cognition, some supplements (e.g., Vitamin D, O3FA, B12, Folate, Acetyl L Carnitine) may have antidepressant effects (Yashodhara et al., 2009). Table 16.1 lists commonly used supplements, their doses, and common adverse effects. There are also supplement products available that combine a variety of supplements. Studies in animals indicate that some combinations of supplements may decrease oxidative stress and prevent cognitive decline (Suchy, Chan, & Shea, 2009). Caution in using such combination products should be urged due to risks that have not been identified due to a lack of rigorous studies on such products. There is also a potential for many such supplements to interact with prescription medications commonly used by persons with ADRD (e.g., combination of huperzine and antidementia drugs [e.g., donepezil, galantamine, rivastigmine] can lead to vomiting and diarrhea) (Desai & Grossberg, 2003). There are no RCTs to support the use of any herbal remedies and

Table 16.1 Nutritional supplements commonly used to promote brain health

Nutritional supplement	Recommended daily dosage	Adverse effects and toxicity symptoms
Vitamin D	Ranges from 1,000 IU once daily to 50,000 IU once a week depending on how low vitamin D blood levels are	Toxicity symptoms: Excessive thirst, dehydration, anorexia, nausea, vomiting, headache, constipation, weakness, increase levels of calcium in the blood, kidney stones
Vitamin B12	500–1,000 μg	No known toxicity or serious side effects
Folic acid	Ranges from 400 to 1,000 μg/depending on blood levels	Large doses can mask symptoms of vitamin B_{12} deficiency
Nicotinamide	300–500 mg	Toxicity symptoms: increased heart rate, anxiety, bloating, flatulence, nausea, tingling and numbness in extremities, blurred vision
Vitamin B1	100 mg	No known toxic effects from oral intake
Vitamin B3 Niacin	Unclear	Toxicity symptoms: headache, nausea, skin flushing and tingling, sweating
Omega-3	500–1,000 mg of DHA[a] in two divided doses	Adverse effects: eructation, dyspepsia, taste perversion, bleeding time prolonged
Ginkgo Biloba	40–80 mg 3 times/day Standardized to contain 24–27% ginkgo flavone glycosides and 6–7% triterpenes per dose	Adverse effects: nausea, and dyspepsia, prolongs bleeding time and thus avoided in patients at risk of bleeding (e.g., patients taking anticoagulants, or with clotting disorders)
Huperzine A	50 μg 1–3 times/day	Nausea, vomiting, and abdominal distress and interacts with commonly used antidementia drugs
Alpha lipoic acid	20 mg–900 mg/	Low blood sugar, skin rash
Acetyl L Carnitine	500–2,000 mg/ in divided doses; up to 3 g daily have been used	Mild abdominal discomfort, restlessness, vertigo, and headache
Vinpocetine	10–40 mg twice daily	Nausea, vomiting, and abdominal distress

[a] DHA docosahexanoic acid

supplements for the treatment of ADRD. Hence, no supplements are recommended for routine treatment of ADRD. HCPs may consider judicious use of supplements in selected patients with ADRD, especially if there is great interest from the patient and/or the family to try supplements to promote brain health. In patients with ADRD who have documented deficiencies of certain nutrients (e.g., vitamin B12, D), replacement therapy may improve cognitive function and/or slow cognitive decline. Guidance and ongoing follow up from healthcare provider who is knowledgeable about risks and potential benefits of supplements are recommended before initiation of supplement therapy.

1. *Vitamin D (Calciferol)*: Vitamin D helps to maintain normal blood levels of calcium and phosphorus which strengthens bones. Vitamin D is fat soluble vitamin and thus is stored in fat cells. Well-recognized effects of vitamin D deficiency include hip fractures, falls, functional deterioration, muscle pain, and increased mortality. Thus, maintaining adequate levels of vitamin D may improve overall musculoskeletal health and thus, indirectly promote brain function. Recent studies have found that deficiency of 25(OH) vitamin D is associated with cognitive impairment (Morley, 2010). Vitamin D may have a protective role in neurodegenerative diseases. Meeting the recommended daily requirements of vitamin D (1,000–2,000 IU) is a challenge. Foods rich in vitamin D include egg yolks, oily fish (e.g., salmon, sardines), fortified cereal, and dairy products. Sun exposure for about 15 min daily works, too. Salmon has one of the highest natural food sources of vitamin D, with 360 IU per 3.5 oz. Vitamin D deficiency occurs as a result of restricted sunlight exposure, reduced capacity of the skin to produce vitamin D, and reduced dietary intake. The prevalence of vitamin D deficiency is common in elderly, affecting up to 50% of older adults and a much higher percentage of nursing home residents. Hypercalcemia can cause cognitive impairment and vitamin D supplementation may exacerbate hypercalcemia. For this reason, it is essential to measure 25(OH) vitamin D and calcium levels. Most Americans seem to have enough calcium, but vitamin D is a bigger concern. Adequate level should be maintained over 32 ng/mL.
2. *Vitamin B12 (Cyanocobalamin)*: Vitamin B12 assists in making new brain cells and new brain connections. It also prolongs life of existing brain cells, helps production of red blood cells (cells that carry oxygen in the body), and decreases homocysteine levels. Vitamin B12 deficiency is common in older adults and even more prevalent in individuals with ADRD. It is classically on the list of reversible dementia. Other psychiatric symptoms of vitamin B12 deficiency are depression, psychosis, and delirium. Longer periods of deficiency lead to irreversible damage. Vitamin B12 supplements come in injectable, oral, and nasally inhaled form. Whatever the replacement method, vitamin B12 should be monitored to ensure adequate supplement.
3. *Folic acid (folate, folacin, vitamin B 9)*: Folic acid deficiency is uncommon in Americans because of fortification of food (e.g., bread) with folate. Folic acid deficiency can cause cognitive impairment and depression. In addition, deficiency of folic acid results in high concentration of homocysteine through different pathways. An increase in homocysteine level contributes to the AD pathology by vascular mechanisms or as a neurotoxin. A high intake of folate seems to help decrease the homocysteine level. Recent studies in patients with ADRD have found a relationship between low serum folate level and cognitive impairment. A study also found that higher folate intake is related to lower risk of AD. The small number of studies done to date provides no consistent evidence either way that folic acid supplementation, with or without vitamin B12, has a beneficial effect on cognitive function of unselected healthy or cognitively impaired older people (Malouf & Grimley Evans, 2008). In a preliminary study, folic acid was associated with improvement in the response of people with AD to cholinesterase inhibitors.

In another study, long-term use appeared to improve the cognitive function of healthy older people with high homocysteine levels. Folic acid supplementation may exacerbate vitamin B12 deficiency in patients with preexisting, uncorrected vitamin B12 deficiency. Thus, all patients receiving folate supplementation should have vitamin B12 levels checked and if low corrected prior to folate supplementation.

4. *Vitamin B1 (Thiamine)*: Vitamin B1 deficiency is uncommon in patients with ADRD unless they have diabetes or alcohol abuse problems. Thiamine deficiency causes "beri-beri" syndrome, which can involve neurologic and cardiovascular symptoms. Neurologic symptoms include peripheral neuropathy, Wernicke's encephalopathy (confusion, double vision, and impaired balance), and Korsakoff syndrome. Thiamine deficiency often occurs in patient with alcohol addiction. Korsakoff syndrome is characterized by severe memory loss, both anterograde and retrograde, confabulation which is invented memories that are taken as true because of the gap in memories, and apathy which is loss of interest and appear indifferent to change. It may be mistaken for ADRD. Vitamin B1 deficiency induces oxidative stress, increases inflammation, and may exacerbated toxic amyloid beta levels. Treatment of thiamine deficiency involves oral supplementation.

5. *Vitamin B3 (Niacin/Nicotinamide)*: Niacin deficiency is uncommon in individuals with ADRD. Deficiency of niacin can cause "pellagra," a disease with rough scaly skin, diarrhea, muscle weakness, mental confusion, and dementia. Early treatment with niacin can reverse some or all of these problems. Niacin is an effective treatment for high cholesterol and low high-density lipoprotein (HDL) as well. Preliminary data suggest that those with the high intake of niacin were less likely to have developed AD or decline in memory during the 5-year period. In an animal study, niacin was found to restore cognitive deficit in AD associated with tau protein pathology.

6. *Vitamin B6 (pyridoxine, pyridoxal, pyridoxamine)*: Vitamin B6 helps make red blood cells and is important for normal brain function. It helps lower homocysteine levels. It also promotes immune system function. Most Americans do not have B6 deficiency.

7. *Omega-3 fatty acids supplements (O3FA)*: Patients with ADRD who do not eat fish regularly may benefit from O3FA supplements. DHA supplement positively affected weight and appetite in patients with mild-to-moderate AD. Research to date has not clarified its optimal dose. We recommend 500–1,000 mg of DHA per day in divided doses. O3FA can cause abdominal discomfort and slight increase in risk of bleeding. Hence, they should be used with caution in patients on blood thinners (e.g., warfarin). Its use should be discontinued 7–14 days prior to surgery.

8. *Vitamin E (Tocopherol)*: In general, the outcomes of these studies have been disappointing. There is no evidence to date of efficacy of Vitamin E in the prevention or treatment of people with AD or MCI (Isaac, Quinn, & Tabet, 2008). Vitamin E at doses above 400 IU is associated with an increase in all-cause mortality. Vitamin E use was associated with improved survival of people with AD and thus did not support concerns over increased mortality with high-dose vitamin E supplementation in this population (Pavlik, Doody, Rountree, &

Darby, 2009). Vitamin E is associated with increased risk of falls and bleeding. It should be used with caution in patients on blood thinners such as warfarin.
9. *Ginkgo biloba (GB)*: GB is perhaps the most widely used herbal treatment consumed specifically to prevent age-related cognitive decline and slow progression of ADRD. Putative mechanisms of action on brain functioning include vascular effects such as increased blood flow to the brain, decreased blood viscosity (i.e., thinning of the blood so that it is less likely to clot), reduction of oxygen free radicals, and neurotransmitter effects. Evidence to date indicates that ginkgo does not slow decline in memory/cognition in patients with AD, MCI, or older adults with normal cognition (Dekosky et al., 2008; Snitz et al., 2009). There are constraints to the generalizability of research to date due to under-representation in the cohort of individuals with divergent ethnic-cultural backgrounds and relatively few participants with lower educational levels. There are some data to suggest that ginkgo can increase bleeding risk, so people who take antiplatelet drugs (e.g., acetyl salicylic acid, clopidogrel), anticoagulant drugs (warfarin), have bleeding disorders. Patients should discontinue the use of ginkgo at least 36 h and preferably 7 days prior to surgery or dental procedure to reduce potential risk of excessive bleeding. Interaction potential exists between GB and commonly used drugs, such as aspirin and warfarin.
10. *Alpha-Lipoic Acid (ALA)*: ALA is a more powerful antioxidant (free radical scavenger) than Vitamin E. Preliminary data suggest beneficial effects in memory and other cognitive performance in mouse models of AD and human studies (Morley, 2010).
11. *Huperzine A (HupA)*: HupA is an herbal remedy used for centuries in China for its medicinal properties. It has cholinesterase inhibition properties similar to prescription antidementia drugs (specifically cholinesterase inhibitors [ChEIs]) such as donepezil (Aricept), galantamine (Razadyne), and rivastigmine (Exelon) that are currently approved by US FDA for the treatment of AD. Thus, HupA promotes cholinergic neurotransmission that is thought to be impaired in AD. Cholinergic neurotransmission is necessary for optimal functioning of memory and other cognitive processes.
12. *Acetyl L Carnitine*: Acetyl L Carnitine is an amino acid nutrient that has important roles in improving mitochondrial function and thus has potential for cognitive benefits in persons with ADRD.
13. *Vinpocetine*: Vinpocetine increases blood circulation in the brain, and in animal studies has been shown to reduce the loss of brain cells due to decreased blood supply (McDaniel et al., 2003).

A Systematic Approach to Promote Brain Health with Nutritional Strategies

Comprehensive nutritional strategies to promote brain health involve several steps. Please see Table 16.2. These steps need to be individualized and should be in keeping with the goals of overall care. Also, the beneficial effects are greatest if nutritional

Table 16.2 Ten steps to promote brain health

Step 1:	comprehensive assessment of nutritional status
Step 2:	eating a balanced diet
Step 3:	eating food that is appetizing and cooked in healthy ways
Step 4:	increasing intake of brain power foods
Step 5:	reducing intake of food that is bad for the heart
Step 6:	eating frequent small meals with optimal calories to achieve and maintain healthy weight
Step 7:	eating a variety of foods
Step 8:	monitoring food-medication and food-medical condition interaction
Step 9:	proactively addressing unique challenges that dementia poses
Step 10:	focusing on small steps

strategies are initiated in the earliest stages of dementia and combined with active physical, intellectual, and social life. For many individuals with ADRD in advanced stages, liberalization of diet (i.e., providing food that they enjoy irrespective of the nutritional value of the food) may have a better effect on improving their quality of life than food that is brain healthy but not enjoyed by the individual.

Step 1: Comprehensive Assessment of Nutritional Status

Persons with dementia should undergo a comprehensive evaluation of their nutritional status during initial assessment and periodically thereafter (Pepersak, 2009). The goal of such assessment is to identify and treat nutritional deficiencies and disorders early. Such assessment also allows better understanding of the person's food preferences, food habits, and comorbid medical conditions that may influence any future dietary recommendations. Specific nutritional deficiencies (e.g., protein energy malnutrition, dehydration, O3FA deficiencies, vitamin deficiencies [especially Vitamin D, B12, folate, B1, B6, nicotinamide]) may exacerbate pathological processes in the brain that are causing ADRD. In addition, nutritional deficiencies can directly cause memory loss, dementia, and even delirium (sudden onset of confusion). Nutritional deficiencies are common in people with ADRD. Specific nutritional disorders (such as celiac disease) are often overlooked in persons with ADRD. Celiac disease (also called Celiac Sprue/Gluten Sensitive Enteropathy) is associated with many nutritional deficiencies and impaired brain function (e.g., memory problems). It commonly manifests as bloating (especially after eating wheat products), abdominal discomfort, and diarrhea and is often misdiagnosed as irritable bowel syndrome. Treatment of Celiac disease involves avoiding food containing gluten (e.g., wheat products). Hypoglycemia (low blood glucose) and hyperglycemia (high blood glucose) can also cause memory impairment (Morley, 2010). Nutritional problems in individuals with ADRD may reflect years of subclinical malnutrition, possibly paired with nutritional abuse (Baker, 2007). By identifying and correcting nutritional disorders, we have seen dramatic improvement in memory and other cognitive functions of many of our patients with ADRD.

Step 2: Eating a Balanced Diet

To promote brain health, it is important to eat a balanced diet, maintain healthy weight (Body Mass Index between 20 and 25), and consume appropriate amount of calories that are required for weight maintenance. The new Food Pyramid (MyPyramid) for older adults is a useful guide for planning a healthy and well-balanced diet. It emphasizes the importance of consuming nutrient-dense foods (i.e., foods with a higher nutrient value per calorie) by outlining specific recommendations for the basic food groups. Brightly colored vegetables, deep-colored fruits, whole grains and fiber, lean proteins, and healthy types of fats are recommended (http://nutrition.tufts.edu/docs/pdf/releases/071220_ModifiedMyPyramid.pdf). Using packaged (frozen and canned) fruits and vegetables – specifically those without added salt or sugar – can be just as healthy as their fresh counterparts, while also being less expensive and more convenient.

My pyramid also recommends sufficient fluid intake. Adequate daily intake of water is necessary for the brain to function well. Inadequate consumption can lead to dehydration, which in turn can impair the ability to pay attention and remember.

Eating frequent, small meals instead of one or two large meals is recommended. Going more than 3 h without eating should be avoided when possible in order to provide the brain with a steady supply of energy.

The most appropriate ratio of omega-6 fatty acids (O6FA) to O3FA is approximately 4:1 (Rakel & Rindfleisch, 2005). Thus, in order to have a balanced diet, increasing the intake of O3FA and reducing the intake of O6FA are recommended, since the typical American diet is low in O3FA and high in O6FA. Protein content of the diet should be around 12% of the total calories consumed (Baker, 2007). Consuming 21–30 g of dietary fiber per day is recommended. Table 16.3 lists recommended amounts of daily food items for a 1,500-cal intake. Older people simply need fewer calories than younger people, and many individuals with ADRD become physically inactive, in which case energy needs decline further. Adequate consumption

Table 16.3 Brain power foods and daily recommended intake (based on 1,500 cal/day)

Food category	Brain power foods	Recommended intake
Fruits	Berries (especially blueberries), avocadoes	4–6 servings/day
Vegetables	Green leafy vegetables (e.g., broccoli, spinach), tomatoes	4–6 servings/day
Legumes	Beans, lentils, peas	1–2 servings/day
Fatty fish (omega-3 rich food)	Pacific herring (sardine), sablefish (black cod), European anchovies, Spanish Mackerel, wild sockeye salmon, and farmed rainbow trout	2–4 servings/week
Whole grains	Quinoa, barley, oats, maize, brown rice, buckwheat	3–6 servings/day
Spices	Turmeric	A pinch/day
Tree nuts	Walnuts, almonds, pecans, hazelnuts	3–5 pieces
Fluids	Green tea	4–8 oz
	Water	24–40 oz

of calories is critical because brain is an energy hog. Brain consumes 20% of energy despite constituting just 2% of body weight.

Step 3: Eating Food That Is Appetizing and Cooked in Healthy Ways

Many older adults share the common complaint of food no longer tasting as good as it once did. Age and disease-related loss of certain taste functions needs to be addressed to make food more appealing. An example of this can be seen with sweet, which is preserved while there is increased sensitivity to bitter with aging. However, these changes are highly individualistic. Thus, it is important to talk to older adults to find out what specifically they can and cannot sense in a food or dish. This can help design meals that are best suited to their individual perceptions and expectations.

It is important to decrease the salt, sugar, and fat in our menus while not compromising the flavor. Herbs and spices can not only enhance flavor but also have brain health promoting potential. Therefore, herbs and spices can partially or wholly replace less desirable ingredients such as salt, sugar, and added saturated fat in dishes including, marinades and dressings, stir-fry dishes, casseroles, soups, and curries (Tapsell et al., 2006). Vegetables and vegetarian dishes may be more appetizing when prepared with herbs and spices. Researchers have tested extracts of cinnamon, cloves, fennel, ginger, lavender, parsley, rose, rosemary, sage, and thyme and found that simmering, soup-making, and stewing significantly increase the disease-preventing antioxidant capacity of these herbs and spices, while grilling and stir-frying decrease. Allowing fresh garlic to stand for 15 min after crushing it can boost its content of allicin, a phytonutrient that can reduce blood clots and prevent oxidative damage to the brain blood vessels. Some older adults complain of heartburn when they eat onions. Yet swapping sweet for more pungent yellow onions can overcome this without sacrificing the healthful dose of sulfur-containing phytonutrients in this vegetable. Making comfort foods healthier is another good strategy (e.g., putting fresh rosemary and lemon on rotisserie chicken, substituting half of the ground beef for turkey in meatloaf). Replacing sweet potatoes for white or russet or red potatoes, steel-cut oats for instant oatmeal are simple strategies to try out. Cooking pasta *al dente* rather than overcooking it until it is swollen and soft is also a healthier alternative.

Many older adults are open to trying new foods and flavors. Offering them new healthy food options may not only be good for the brain but also be fun!

Step 4: Increasing Intake of Brain Power Foods

Within the category of healthy food items, there are certain foods that are thought to have a higher effect in promoting brain health compared to others. Ensuring consumption of such brain power foods is recommended to further improve the beneficial effects of balanced diet on brain health. Table 16.3 lists brain power foods. Soy has not been shown to have any specific brain health promoting effect but is recommended because it remains a healthy alternative to red meat (as an excellent source of protein).

Step 5: Reducing Intake of Food That Is Bad for the Heart

Improving diet is a critical component of the American Heart Association's strategy to improve heart health (Lichtenstein et al., 2006). Research in the last decade has shown that what is good for the heart is good for the brain and what is bad for the heart is bad for the brain. We recommend reducing intake of saturated fat (less than 7% of daily caloric needs), trans fat (less than 1% of daily caloric needs), cholesterol (less than 300 mg/day) by choosing lean meats and vegetable alternatives, fat-free (skim) or low-fat (1% fat) dairy products and minimizing intake of trans fats; minimizing intake of beverages and foods with added sugars; choosing and preparing foods with little or no salt. Such nutritional strategies can not only promote heart health but also brain health (Lichtenstein et al., 2006; Morley, 2010).

Foods rich in saturated fat and trans fat (e.g., butter, margarine) increase inflammation and lead to elevated levels of cholesterol (Rakel & Rindfleisch, 2005). Elevated cholesterol can cause cognitive impairment through inflammation of the blood vessels and atherosclerosis. The saturated fat found in beef, butter, whole milk, cheese, and other dairy products increases low-density lipoproteins and promotes atherosclerosis (inflammation in wall of blood vessels leading to its narrowing). Trans fats (partially hydrogenated oils) in small amounts occur naturally in red meat. Other common sources of trans fats include packaged baked products such as cookies, cakes, breads, and crackers, as well as fast foods, and some dairy products. Trans fats are even more unhealthy than saturated fats. They directly promote inflammation, besides increasing LDL and worsening atherosclerosis. There is no safe level of trans fat and there are no known health benefits. People also more likely to eat foods high in saturated and trans fats when they have consumed more than healthy amount of alcohol. We also recommend minimizing consumption of fried foods and food with long shelf life. Eating charred, grilled, or burnt foods also increase inflammation. Reducing dietary intake of O6FA(which in US is normally much higher than what is needed for maintaining health) may reduce memory problems because excess amount of O6FA promotes dysfunction in hippocampus (seat for memory formation). O6FA is found in red meat and most vegetable oils.

The American Heart Association recommends reduction in the intake of added sugars to reduce the risk of a variety of metabolic disorders (e.g., metabolic syndrome, diabetes, obesity). Besides promoting oxidation and inflammation, high intake of refined sugars can lead to hypertriglyceridemia. Hypertriglyceridemia can lead to delirium and cognitive impairment in animals and humans (Morley, 2010). A prudent upper limit of intake for most American women is no more than 100 cal/day and for most American men is no more than 150 cal/day from added sugar.

A 330 mL container of a soft drink has on average (unless designed to be sugar-free) the equivalent of ten tea-spoonsful of sugar in it. Simple health promotion campaigns to improve the public's awareness of how much sugar there is in soft drinks is recommended in order to encourage changing to alternatives. Fructose-sweetened foods and drinks (e.g., many yogurts, soft drinks) have a negative effect on body's sensitivity to insulin and its ability to handle fats, increasing the risk of strokes. Many cereals are high in sugar and thus should be selected carefully. Americans are consuming 50 additional calories of sweetened beverages daily compared to 2 decades ago, for an average of about 300 cal daily coming from such drinks. Although less than younger population, baby boomer generation and older adults continue to consume substantial amount of sweetened beverages (12–18% of daily caloric intake) (Storey, Forshee, & Anderson, 2006). Glycemic load and glycemic index are measures for how quickly a serving of food is converted to blood sugar during digestion and how high the spike of blood sugar is. Foods with high glycemic load are digested more quickly, thus rapidly flooding the blood stream with sugar. Sudden high spikes of blood sugar trigger release of insulin to clear the sugar from one's blood. This quick surge of insulin can clear blood sugar dramatically, leaving the blood sugar too low. When our blood sugar is low, we feel hungry and if blood sugar is low soon after a meal, we are apt to overeat. Consumption of refined grains such as white rice, white flour, white bread and pasta (nonwhole wheat varieties), and other foods with high glycemic load (e.g., bagels, cakes, ice-cream, French fries, white potatoes, crackers, soft drinks, refined grains) should be reduced because they also promote inflammation and free radical production.

Low carbohydrate diets may also impair mental acuity and hence not recommended. Glucose is the primary source of energy for brain cells. Intake of food containing coloring agents should be minimized as some coloring agents have been linked to attentional problems. Many soft drinks (e.g, diet coke, diet pepsi) contain advanced glycation end produces (AGEs) that promote inflammation and thus are potentially harmful. Many soft drinks also contain high fructose corn syrup, and high intake of fructose may also lead to excessive inflammation and oxidative stress on the brain. In general, older men (especially those with higher alcohol consumption) are more likely to consume food that is unhealthy (e.g., high in saturated fat and refined sugars) compared to older women (Robinson et al., 2009). In terms of everyday consumption, we recommend reducing intake of food that is bad for the heart. On special occasions such as Thanksgiving or birthdays, there is no need to pass up apple pie or cake. For everyday eating, choosing desserts with less fat and refined sugars is recommended (see Table 16.4).

Step 6: Eat Frequent Small Meals with Optimal Calories to Achieve and Maintain Healthy Weight

It is important to not go more than 3 h without eating, so one's brain has a steady energy supply. Also, to maintain brain health, it is equally important for persons

Table 16.4 Healthy snacks/meals

Examples of healthy snacks
  Hummus with vegetables or whole grain crackers
  Small amount of nuts
  Cottage cheese (fat-free)
  Fruits
  Fat free or low fat (1%) milk (sweetened with Splenda if necessary)
  Oat meal with fruits
  Yogurt
  Trail mix with walnuts and dried fruits
  Some health bars
  Fruit and vegetable juices may be substituted for fruits and vegetables if necessary

Examples of healthy meals
Breakfast
  Skim milk
  Scrambled eggs
  Multibran cereal with raisins
  Pancakes made from multigrain pancake mix
  Fruits (or if necessary, fruit juices)
  Tomato juice (low salt)

Salads
  Avocado, spinach, and lettuce salad, with a scattering of walnuts and toasted crumbled anchovies, and dressed with canola oil and balsamic vinegar
  Broccoli salad with olive oil – balsamic dressing
  Tossed salad with Romaine lettuce, tomatoes, nuts, olives, and low fat dressing

Main course
  Salmon in a curry made with turmeric, broccoli, brown rice served with lentil daal
  Chicken/Turkey sandwich with whole-wheat bread
  Three-grain pilaf with canola oil and mixed vegetables

Dessert
  Dark chocolate with cut up fruits, berries, and almonds

with dementia to maintain healthy weight and to consume appropriate amount of calories that are needed to maintain healthy weight. Weight maintenance is important, even when dealing with those who are overweight or obese. Weight loss within this population is somewhat controversial and not always desirable. Excess amount of calories in older adults who are obese (BMI above 30) should be avoided because it increases oxidative stress and promotes inflammation by increasing body fat stores. Many patients with Fronto-temporal dementia and some patients with AD develop hyperphagia with disabling obesity-related health complications (e.g., impaired mobility). If weight loss is recommended, it can be accomplished through minor changes to the diet and the addition of a light exercise regimen. Modest weight loss strategies (e.g., portion control, replacing calorie dense food with fruits and vegetables) in this group may not only improve mobility but also promote heart and brain health.

Step 7: Eating a Variety of Foods

We recommend eating a variety of brain healthy foods (i.e., variety of fruits, vegetables, whole grains, and fish) to facilitate consumption of a variety of brain healthy nutrients (polyphenols, curcumin). Consuming high amount of only certain foods (even if the food has beneficial effects on brain) can be potentially harmful. For example, nuts in excess amount can dramatically increase total amount of calories consumed and subsequent oxidative stress may override any beneficial effects. In addition, due to potential for mercury toxicity in many fish, a variety of fish should be consumed rather than just one kind on a regular basis. Often, the combination of healthy foods (e.g., unique combination of food items constituting the Mediterranean diet) may have a much bigger impact on brain health than individual food items (Jacobs, Gross, & Tapsell 2009).

Step 8: Monitoring Food-Medication and Food-Medical Condition Interaction

Many food items can interact with prescription and over-the-counter medications leading to harmful consequences. For example, common fruit juices (e.g., orange, apple, grape) have significant brain health promoting effects. However, these juices also have the potential (especially if consumed with medications) to limit the body's absorption of certain commonly prescribed drugs for the treatment of blood pressure, infection, and allergies (e.g., tenormin, levofloxacin, fexofenadine), compromising their effectiveness. Patients with Celiac disease need to avoid food containing gluten (e.g., wheat products). Patients on blood thinners such as warfarin need to minimize intake of food high in vitamin K such as spinach and broccoli. Appropriate precautions should be taken (e.g., input of one's physician, pharmacist) to minimize this risk.

Step 9: Proactively Addressing Unique Challenges Posed by Dementia

In order to create an environment that promotes consumption and enjoyment of meals and snacks by persons with dementia, thoughtful planning and some simple strategies are recommended. Socialization is very important to the elderly and may positively affect the amount of food eaten. However, distractions should be limited to maintain focus on the meal. Televisions ideally should be turned off. Soft music may help to relax those dining. Sometimes, it may be helpful to have everyone seated and ready for the meal a few minutes prior to it being served. This may also help to alleviate any stress or distractions caused during the transition from an activity to mealtime.

As to the actual food that is served, it is usually best to keep the food simple and easily recognizable. Individuals with moderate-to-severe dementia may be more likely to eat something familiar that needs no explanation. Also, the food should be easy to eat. Foods that require tedious manipulation of utensils may not be a reasonable option unless assistance is readily available. Providing utensils that are not only food appropriate, but personally appropriate, is very important. Some may require cups with handles or lids while others may be fine with traditional glasses. Finger foods may also be a good choice, especially if there is limited assistance available to help with feeding. Finger foods also help to maintain some autonomy because no one is really needed to help eat these kinds of foods. Because those with moderate-to-severe dementia tend to be most lucid during the morning with waning alertness throughout the day, breakfast may truly be the most important meal of the day! A full, hearty breakfast should be encouraged daily, even to those who traditionally did not eat in the mornings. Many individuals with dementia suffer from protein energy malnutrition and may need energy-dense foods. This is also helpful to those with early satiety. Foods that can be altered to increase the nutritional content without increasing the actual volume of the food can help better meet their needs.

Step 10: Focusing on Small Steps

Change is hard, especially when it involves changing what we eat. However, even small changes in ones diet (say 20% change) can have a significant effect on brain health (say 80% benefit). Thus, it is best to focus on making small steps (e.g., increasing the amount of fruits and vegetables by one serving per day; adding blueberries to cereal). Adding small amounts of nuts, raisins, and various spices, like cinnamon to one's cereal can dramatically boost their phytonutrient content. Handful of tree nuts or trail mix is a better snack than a cookie made with butter or trans fats. Regular input from a registered dietician at an individual and group level is strongly recommended in order to make changes in daily diet practical and effective. Table 16.5 lists resources (books and websites) we recommend to promote brain health.

Table 16.5 Resources to promote brain healthy nutrition

Healthy eating. A guide to the new nutrition. A special health report from Harvard Medical School. 2006 Harvard Health Publications, Boston, Massachusetts. www.health.harvard.edu

Casey A, Benson H. Mind Your Heart: a mind/body approach to stress management, exercise, and nutrition for heart health. New York: Free Press; 2004

Websites

Pritikin Longevity Center: www.pritikin.com

DASH diet: www.dashdiet.org

Conclusion

Healthy food is essential for all the functions of the body and this is especially true of the brain. Appropriate changes in a person's diet can enhance their cognitive abilities, protect the brain from damage and counteract the effects of aging. Maximizing foods that are brain healthy (e.g., nutrient and fiber-rich fruits, vegetables, whole grains, fatty fish, and legumes) and minimizing foods that put the brain at risk (e.g., fatty meat, high-fat dairy, refined, processed foods) may help to slow cognitive decline in persons with ADRD. It is never too late to make positive changes. Older adults with dementia can make changes today that will improve their brain health tomorrow, which may help them lead a better quality of life.

References

Aggarwal, B. B., & Sung, B. (2009). Pharmacological basis for the role of curcumin I chronic diseases: An age-old spice with modern targets. *Trends in Pharmacological Science, 30*, 85–94.

Baker, H. (2007). Nutrition in the elderly: An overview. *Geriatrics, 62*, 28–31.

Blazer, D. G., & Wu, L. T. (2009). The epidemiology of at-risk and binge drinking among middle-aged and elderly community adults: National Survey on Drug Use and Health. *American Journal of Psychiatry, 166*, 1162–1169.

Dekosky, S. T., Williamson, J. D., Fitzpatrick, A. L., Kronmal, R. A., Ives, D. G., Lopez, O. L., et al. (2008). Ginkgo Evaluation of Memory (GEM) Study Investigators. Ginkgo biloba for prevention of dementia: A randomized controlled trial. *Journal of the American Medical Association, 300*, 2253–2262.

Desai, A. K., & Grossberg, G. T. (2003). Herbals and botanicals in geriatric psychiatry. *American Journal of Geriatric Psychiatry, 11*, 498–506.

Desai, A. K., Grossberg, G. T., & Chibnall, J. T. (2010). Healthy brain aging: A road map. *Clinics of Geriatric Medicine, 26*, 1–26.

Gu, Y., Nieves, J. W., Stern, Y., Luchsinger, J. A. & Scarmeas, N. (2010). Food combination and Alzheimer disease risks: A protective diet. *Archives of Neurology, 67*, 699–706. April 12, [Epub ahead of print].

Henderson, S. T., Vogel, J. L., Barr, L. J., Garvin, F., Jones, J. J., & Constantini, L. C. (2009). Study of the ketogenic agent AC-1202 in mild to moderate Alzheimer's disease: A randomized, double-blind, placebo-controlled, multicenter trial. *Nutrition & Metabolism, 6*, 31.

Isaac, M. G., Quinn, R., & Tabet, N. (2008). Vitamin E for Alzheimer's disease and mild cognitive impairment. *Cochrane Database Systematic Rev, 3*, CD002854.

Jacobs, D. R., Jr., Gross, M. D., & Tapsell, L. C. (2009). Food synergy: An operational concept for understanding nutrition. *American Journal of Clinical Nutrition, 89*, 1543S–1548S.

Kamphuis, P. J., & Scheltens, P. (2010). Can nutrients prevent or delay onset of Alzheimer's disease? *Journal Alzheimer Disease, 20*, 765–777. Feb 24 [Epub ahead of print].

Kidd, P. M. (2008). Alzheimer's disease, amnestic mild cognitive impairment, and age-associated memory impairment: Current understanding and progress toward integrative prevention. *Alternative Medicine Review, 13*, 85–115.

Lichtenstein, A. H., Appel, L. J., Brands, M., Carnethon, M., Daniels, S., Franch, H. A., et al. (2006). Diet and lifestyle recommendations Revision 2006. A scientific statement from the American Heart Association Nutrition Committee. *Circulation, 114*, 82–96.

Malouf, R., & Grimley Evans, J. (2008). Folic acid with or without vitamin B12 for the prevention and treatment of healthy elderly and demented people. *Cochrane Database Systematic Review, 4*, CD004514.

McDaniel, M. A., Maier, S. F., & Einstein, G. O. (2003). Brain-specific nutrients: A memory cure? *Nutrition, 19*, 957–975.

Morley, J. E. (2010). Nutrition and the Brain. *Clinics of Geriatric Medicine, 26*, 89–98.

Pavlik, V. N., Doody, R. S., Rountree, S. D., & Darby, E. J. (2009). Vitamin E use is associated with improved survival in an Alzheimer's disease cohort. *Dementia & Geriatric Cognitive Disorders, 28*, 536–540.

Pepersak, T. (2009). Nutritional problems in the elderly. *Acta Clinica Belgica, 64*, 85–91.

Querfurth, H. W., & LaFerla, F. M. (2010). Alzheimer's Disease. *New England Journal of Medicine, 362*, 329–344.

Rakel, D. P., & Rindfleisch, A. (2005). Inflammation: Nutritional, botanical, and mind-body influences. *Southern Medical Journal, 98*, 303–309.

Robinson, S., Syddall, H., Jameson, K., Batelaan, S., Martin, H., Dennison, E. M., et al. (2009). Current patterns of diet in community-dwelling older men and women: Results from Hertfordshire Cohort Study. *Age and Ageing, 38*, 594–599.

Scarmeas, N., Luchsinger, J. A., Schupt, N., Brickman, A. M., Cosentino, S., Tang, M. X., et al. (2009). Physical activity, diet, and risk of Alzheimer disease. *Journal of the American Medical Association, 302*, 627–637.

Scheltens, P., Kamphuis, P. J., Verhey, F. R., Olde Rikkert, M. G., Wurtman, R. J., Wilkinson, D., et al. (2010). Efficacy of a medical food in mild Alzheimer's disease: A randomized, controlled trial. *Alzheimers & Dementia, 6*, 1–10.

Schneider, L. S., & Sano, M. (2009). Current Alzheimer's disease clinical trials: Methods and placebo outcomes. *Alzheimer's & Dementia, 5*, 388–397.

Snitz, B. E., O'Meara, E. S., Carlson, M. C., Arnold, A. M., Ives, D. G., Rapp, S. R., et al. (2009). Ginkgo biloba for preventing cognitive decline in older adults. A randomized trial. *Journal of the American Medical Association, 302*, 2663–2670.

Storey, M. L., Forshee, R. A., & Anderson, P. A. (2006). Beverage consumption in the US population. *Journal of the American Dietetic Association, 106*, 1992–2000.

Suchy, J., Chan, A., & Shea, T. B. (2009). Dietary supplementation with a combination of alpha-lipoic acid, acetyl-L-carnitine, glycerophosphocoline, docosahexaenoic acid, and phosphotidylserine reduces oxidative damage to murine brain and improves cognitive performance. *Nutrition Research, 29*, 70–74.

Tapsell, L. C., Hemphill, I., Cobiac, L., Patch, C. S., Sullivan, D. R., Fenech, M., et al. (2006). Health benefits of herbs and spices: The past, the present, the future. *Medical Journal of Australia, 185*, S4–S24.

Van der Beek, E. M., & Kamphuis, P. J. (2008). The potential role of nutritional components in the management of Alzheimer's disease. *European Journal of Pharmacology, 585*, 197–207.

Yashodhara, B. M., Umakanth, S., Pappachan, J. M., Bhat, S. K., Kamath, R., & Choo, B. H. (2009). Omega-3 fatty acids: A comprehensive review of their role in health and disease. *Postgraduate Medical Journal, 85*, 84–90.

Part III
Enhancing Cognition Through the Arts

Chapter 17
Enhancing Healthy Cognitive Aging Through Theater Arts

Tony Noice and Helga Noice

Abstract This article reports on 15 years of studies that document the benefits of a short course in acting for theater and film. These studies provide evidence that older adults can experience enhanced memory, problem-solving ability, comprehension, creativity, and sense of personal growth compared to no-treatment controls or those who undergo alternate courses of instruction (visual arts or music).

Enhancing Healthy Cognitive Aging Through Theater Arts

The notion that artistic creativity contributes to healthy aging appears to be gaining credence among those in the gerontological research community. Much of this new interest stems from the work of Dr. Gene Cohen whose seminal research on a wide variety of arts and aging projects brought much needed attention to this underinvestigated area (e.g., Cohen, 2005). Our own efforts have been devoted to one specific art: acting. For almost 15 years, we have been performing a theatrical intervention for older adults designed to improve healthy cognitive aging and lower risk factors for dementia. This eight-session course (two 80-min classes per week for 4 weeks) emphasizes the core principle of the actor's art, namely that good actors never pretend; by analyzing the script, they determine what the character is actually doing and then proceed to do it. That is, if the script calls for Character A to tease Character B, then Actor A teases Actor B. The actor does *not* try to look and sound like someone engaging in teasing behavior, he or she simply teases the other actor *for real*. Each of the eight sessions is more complex, starting with single lines of dialogue

---

T. Noice (✉)
Department of Theatre, Elmhurst College,
190 Prospect Avenue, Elmhurst, IL 60126, USA
e-mail: noicea@net.elmhurst.edu

and progressing to the performance of short scenes, complete with makeshift costumes and props. The intervention has consistently produced robust, statistically significant gains on standard measures of memory, comprehension, creativity, problem-solving, and other cognitive/affective abilities (e.g., Noice & Noice, 2009). We believe the reason for this effectiveness is that the intervention *simultaneously* taps into the main factors that have been shown to promote healthy cognitive aging: novelty, social support, effortful processing, and cognitive-emotive-physiological stimulation. To understand how and why an acting intervention produces such demonstrably strong gains, it is necessary to start at the beginning.

Early Investigations

Throughout our theater research, it was found that actors were generally unaware of the psychological learning principles that lay behind their highly efficient role-preparation strategy. Thus the first phase of the investigation was to identify these principles. A preliminary step was the collection of actors' self-reports on how they commit roles to memory (Noice, 1992). Seven actors, representing a wide range of ages, styles, years of experience, and types of training, were asked to describe their role learning processes. No guidelines were provided so as to avoid demand characteristics. All seven volunteered the information that they did not memorize by rote but rather acquired their dialogue by repeatedly questioning the text to discern the goals and motivations of the character. One of the actors summed up the process this way: "We do things in reverse in the theater. We get the script which is … at the end of the thought process: we have the lines there. Normally in life, you have an impulse and then a thought which you put into words. Well, I have the words. I get the words first in this finished script. And so I have to go back and find out what the thought was, to have you say those words" (Noice, 1992, pp. 420–421). All statements from the self-reports were analyzed for commonalities. Although expressed in highly individualistic ways, there was universal agreement on the overall process of doing repeated readings of the play in order to unearth the ideas behind the literal text, including implied, unstated or, even hidden, agendas of the characters. The only areas of disagreement concerned procedural matters, such as using tape recorders for cuing private rehearsal. To investigate the issues raised in these self-reports, follow-up empirical studies were then conducted.

Basic paradigm. The general paradigm involved giving actors five to seven-page scenes for two characters and having the actors process those scenes under various learning instructions for various lengths of study time. Results were analyzed along many dimensions, including number of elaborations generated, amount of immediate and delayed recall, use of perspective, adherence to temporal ordering, chunking, etc.

Empirical evidence. One experiment (Noice, 1991) used 56 participants (professional actors and psychology students) who studied the same role under the same learning conditions. Immediately following the study period, participants generated retrospective protocols trying to capture all the thoughts they had had. Although all the participants reported producing some elaborations (as would be expected during comprehension of a text), actors produced nearly 3 times as many as novices. In addition, when elaborations were characterized as either explanatory (investigations of the character's behavior) or nonexplanatory (extraneous comments or restatement of scene content without amplification), the ratio of actors' explanatory to nonexplanatory comments amounted to over 13:1, compared to the novices' ratio of approximately 2:1. Furthermore, in generating brief summaries of the scene, actors were significantly more likely than novices to concentrate on the interactions between the characters, to view the scene from a single viewpoint, and to organize the summaries hierarchically rather than sequentially. The depth of processing revealed by these findings was consistent with the self-reports of actors that memory for text is a by-product of exploration of character and not a result of word-for-word memorization. To assess the amount of material retained by actors using their natural (analytical) strategy, a comparison was made with a group of actors who were instructed to use rote memorization (Noice, 1993). Even though rote memorization is often considered the strategy of choice for material that must be retained word for word, the surprising finding was that actors who used their study time exclusively to analyze the motives of the characters retained far more text verbatim than actors who set out to memorize it, $p<0.001$.

The retrospective protocols had shed some light on the overall processes of actors, but such protocols, while ecologically valid, are bound to be incomplete due to some inevitable forgetting between performance and protocol generation. Therefore, we obtained think-aloud (concurrent) protocols from seven additional professional actors to capture on tape each thought as it occurred while the actors prepared a theatrical scene (Noice & Noice, 1994, 1996). These studies revealed that the actors consistently made a fine-grained analysis of the text, attending to both the form (punctuation, grammar, linguistic elements) and the content (character's plans, intentions, motivations) in order to determine the mental and emotional states of the characters and the ways in which these qualities would be made clear to an audience. This intensive background investigation helps fix the exact words in memory without line-by-line memorization. The think-aloud protocols also presented concrete evidence of what had been suggested by our earlier research: that one step in the actors' analysis consists of dividing a script into a series of segments, generally referred to as "beats." In one study (Noice & Noice, 1993), 24 participants (12 professional actors and 12 psychology students) segmented a script, titling each segment. Specifically, actors were told to divide the script as if they were preparing to read the scene at an audition and to label each section using whatever terms they would ordinarily employ. Since the students would not have any experience with this process, they were told to imagine they were going to try out for a role in a college play and to divide the script into whatever they would consider logical segments in order to properly interpret the scene when they read it aloud at the tryout. Results showed that: (a) actors' beats tended to be unique because they were almost always concerned with the characters' intentions as surmised by each individual actor whereas novices' beats were similar to one another, reflecting obvious changes in the story line; (b) actors created far more divisions, resulting in smaller beats; (c) in a surprise recall task after the division into beats, actors recalled significantly more lines virtually word-for-word than students, $p<0.01$. This provided additional evidence that making an extremely fine-grained analysis of the text is a defining characteristic of professional actors and leads to enhanced recall in terms of accuracy and amount, even in the absence of deliberate memorization.

The two stages. Throughout the retrospective and think-aloud protocols, actors referred to a two-stage process of role acquisition. The first is analytical and takes place during initial script study. Most of the early experiments were designed to uncover the details of that process. The second stage takes place during rehearsal and performance. Thus, if the preliminary analysis showed that the character was demanding obedience from another character, the actor would then use the words of the playwright to actively experience the process of demanding obedience. This involvement would necessarily be cognitive (the thoughts that the dramatic situation activates), emotive (feelings of superiority and domination), and physiological (a tightened jaw, aggressive body stance). The particulars would differ from actor to actor and from situation to situation, but the unvarying essence would be that the actor is experiencing the mental-emotional-physical concomitants of the communication and *not* just trying to look and sound like someone demanding obedience. The latter is called "indicating" and is considered a hallmark of bad acting. The concept of genuinely experiencing the on-stage transaction at every performance turned out to have wide application in designing a theater intervention to promote healthy aging. The researchers refer to this concept as the *active experiencing principle* (AE).

The contribution of movement. At various times in this series of experiments, actors have referred to the interdependence of memory for movement and memory for text. The effects of movement on verbal recall have long been of interest to cognitive investigators (for reviews see Cohen, 1989; Engelkamp & Zimmer, 1994; Nilsson, 2000). However, the notion of literal enactment was central to almost all such inquiries. In other words, phrases describing subject-performed tasks (SPTs) such as "move the ashtray" and "throw the ball" were better remembered when actually performed (with real or imaginary objects) than when studied under standard verbal learning instructions. In our previous research, actors have consistently reported that movements facilitate their retention of dialogue (e.g., Noice, 1992) despite the fact that the movements in a play virtually never duplicate the verbal material. The authors refer to this as the nonliteral enactment effect, and it occurs when the verbal material is related to the movement only at a higher-order level. For example, in a play, a husband might suspect that his wife had had lunch with her lover, so he asks her where she ate that day while he casually walks over to the bar and makes himself a drink. There is no literal connection between the stroll to the bar and the question about lunch but there is a goal-directed one: They are both attempts to appear casual while trying to entrap the wife. Despite this difference, an SPT-type effect occurs, showing more extensive and more accurate recall for verbal material accompanied by movement. In one demonstration of this effect (Noice & Noice, 1999), two actors who had finished performing a particular play 3 months earlier were tested on the accuracy of their recall. Using a repeated measures design, it was found that the gain in amount recalled from trial 1 to trial 2 was greater when the second trial was a moving trial as opposed to a sitting trial. (Two alternate explanations of this phenomenon, context effects and hypermnesia, were ruled out by the experimental design.) Two follow-up experiments (Noice, Noice, & Kennedy, 2000) were carried out with six actors, 5 months after the final performance of a play. In Experiment 1, participants recalled two of their scenes either sitting or moving about an empty room that bore no resemblance to the original learning environment. Once again, there was a significant advantage for lines recalled accompanied by movement. In Experiment 2 of the same study, it was shown that lines that had originally been performed while the actors had moved about the stage were better recalled months later than lines that had been performed while the actors had remained sitting or standing in one place on the stage. This finding held true regardless of recall condition (sitting or moving), negating the possibility that input-output similarity was responsible.

Durability of the memory trace. Both the above studies involved long-term recall (3 and 5 months after the final performances). One experiment directly addressed length of retention (Noice & Noice, 2002). Professional actors were tested on previously played roles over retention intervals up to 28 years. Based on fill-in-the blank and recognition tasks, it was found that retention for all the actors was virtually perfect for the first 3 years after they had ceased performing the roles, although presumably they had no reason to retain them. (All the fill-in-the-blank items had been pretested to ensure that the target words could not be guessed from context). After 3 years, accuracy declined (more for some actors than others) but there was still some evidence of remarkable retention (e.g., 87% after 7 years, and 50% after 28 years).

Training of Novices in Actors' Learning Strategies

Given that a number of cognitive learning principles are activated by the actors' analytical strategies, the question was whether these principles were sufficient, in themselves, to explain actors' expert memory performance. If so, nonactors (including older adults) should be able to learn and apply these principles to improve their own memory performance. (For a general model of acting cognition, see Noice & Noice, 1997b).

Studies using college students. Therefore, using college students (with no experience or training in acting) as participants, the investigators began systematically manipulating various learning factors (e.g., elaboration, perspective-taking, self-generation). However, these manipulations (individually or together) failed to produce recall equal to or better than that produced by deliberate memorization (Noice & Noice, 1997a). Previous investigation of these same factors had shown enhanced memory, but not compared with memorization controls, only with read-for comprehension controls (e.g., Anderson & Pichert, 1978; Dooling & Lachman, 1971; Owens, Bower, & Black, 1979; Sulin & Dooling, 1974). Having found that these analytical factors were not sufficient to explain the superior recall repeatedly seen with actors, the investigators examined the second phase of the actors' learning strategy: active experiencing (AE). To test the efficacy of this procedure with nonactors, students were required to actively use the dialogue the way one does in life. They were specifically instructed *not* to try to memorize the material but simply to use the words "for real." Students in the control (memorization) condition were simply told to memorize the same material using whatever strategy they had found useful in the past when material had to be retained with a high degree of accuracy. Participants using an active experiencing strategy remembered significantly more of the text than those using a memorization strategy ($M = 0.641$ vs. $M = 0.445$, $p < 0.001$). These results showed that students, when told *not* to memorize but to use the words actively and tactically (i.e., as the means to obtain a goal), learned significantly more material (word-for-word or within narrowly defined limits) than those who set out to deliberately memorize it. Thus the process of trying to "live" the material rather than just learn it appeared to make a major difference in the results. Subsequent research extended this finding to include expository and narrative material as well as theatrical dialogue (Noice & Noice, 2004).

Movement effects with nonactors. Noice and Noice (2001) tried to isolate the effects of movement using three groups of students. The first group employed the full active experiencing strategy, conveying the meaning of the material by using all channels of communication, including movement. That is, if the text called for a confrontation, one student would walk up to the other, literally getting in his or her face. A second group of students used what was called a partial AE strategy in which pairs of participants sat on chairs facing each other. They tried to become mentally and emotionally involved in the dramatic situation and communicate the meaning of the text using tone of voice, facial expression, etc., but had to remain seated and could not express their intentions through movement. The third group deliberately memorized the same material, but no specific method of memorization was imposed. Three levels of accuracy were assessed: Verbatim, Acceptable Verbatim (which allowed for very minor deviations), and Total Recall (which included paraphrases). Participants in the full AE condition outperformed both other groups at all three levels of accuracy. For example, analysis of the Total Recall data revealed that recall was significantly higher for those students who had processed the scene while moving ($M = 0.76$) relative to students in the other two conditions ($M = 0.46$ and $M = 0.37$ respectively), $p < 0.01$.

Testing the strategy with older adults. Having shown that the actor's learning strategy can help college students enhance memory performance, the investigators examined whether the same benefits might extend to older adults. Furthermore, since the actor's strategy involves highly demanding mental activity that impacts a variety of cognitive skills, the investigators hypothesized that an intervention consisting of a number of weeks of acting training might enhance the overall cognitive functioning of older adults, as opposed to the improved retention of a particular experimental text.

Therefore, the investigators performed an experiment that served as a pilot study for the future interventions (Noice, Noice, Perrig-Chiello, & Perrig, 1999). The participants (ages 65–82) were recruited from the Basler IDA Project in Switzerland, an ongoing interdisciplinary, longitudinal study on aging (Perrig-Chiello, Perrig, Staehelin, Krebs-Roubicek, & Ehrsam, 1996). They were pretested with immediate and delayed recall and recognition tasks, and then were given a 4-week course in acting. The training did not stress memorization but concentrated on teaching the participants basic acting principles, which were then applied to the rehearsal and performance of complete theatrical scenes. The emphasis throughout was on understanding the deep meaning of the dialogue and the motivations of the characters and then using that understanding to experience truthful interactions with one's fellow actors. That is, the pilot study set out to investigate whether older adults' active experiencing of the mental, emotional, and physical actions of dramatic characters would result in demonstrable cognitive improvement. The investigators found an overall significant increase between pre and posttesting despite the fact that nothing in the actors' strategy (which involves identifying with the character's motivations when using a coherent script) should be of any strategic benefit to the recall or recognition of lists of unrelated words. Clearly, no claim was being made that 4 weeks of training would turn these participants into professional-level actors. However, the very attempt to apply expert methodology, even over this short a period, appeared to enhance cognitive functioning. Thus, although this project grew out of expertise research with actors, the aim was not to make novices into experts, but to selectively train participants in those aspects of acting whose application has been shown to increase cognitive efficiency. Although the results of the pilot investigation were positive and encouraging, many questions were left unanswered. The pretest had been performed prior to the investigators' arrival in Switzerland, and consisted of only two measures (recall and recognition). Also, no affective measures were included in the design, and no specific controls were used for this experiment because it was but one in a longitudinal series of studies.

The 2004 NIA Study

Based on the results of the pilot study, the investigative team designed a larger, controlled intervention in the United States (Noice, Noice, & Staines, 2004). Three groups (average age: 72.3 years) were recruited: an experimental group (theater), a no-treatment control group, and a group to control for noncontent-specific effects (art appreciation). They were pretested on three cognitive measures (recall, working memory, problem-solving), and two affective measures: self-esteem, Rosenberg (1965), and a three-component quality of life scale, developed by Ryff and Keyes (1995) consisting of self-acceptance, positive relations, and personal growth. The experimental and the alternative intervention groups received 4 weeks of training (two sessions per week). All three groups took the posttests the day after the final session. Results for the cognitive measures showed that, compared to the no-treatment controls, the theater group improved significantly on recall ($p=0.007$), problem-solving ($p=0.015$), and barely missed significance on working memory ($p=0.056$). The theater group also improved significantly on the quality of life scale ($p=0.002$). In general, the visual art group made fewer gains in fewer areas. Because the no-treatment controls were given a courtesy course following the testing, they could no longer be used for comparison purposes. However, when the theater group was retested in 4 months without any reinstatement of the training, no significant declines were found in any of the measures.

Feasibility Study for Intervention in Continuing Care Facilities

To ensure the practicality of a second intervention, we conducted a short feasibility study (Noice & Noice, 2006) funded by a private charitable organization. It took place in a senior continuing care facility, and was designed to ascertain whether old-olds (average age: 83 years) would be physically and mentally able to partake of the training. Eighteen of the 20 participants who started the course completed it. (The two who withdrew did so because of preexisting health problems.) Furthermore, we strongly encouraged the continuance of the activity by organizing a small theater company with participants who completed the course. They have subsequently put on six plays for their fellow residents, demonstrating the self-reinforcing motivational aspect of the intervention. However, this small pilot study, while answering the feasibility question, left open many important issues that were investigated by the next study.

The Second NIA Intervention

In this study (Noice & Noice, 2009), the participants were no longer living in their own homes and had chosen to reside in subsidized, primarily low-income senior facilities. They were almost a full decade older and far less well educated than previous participants. Many required walkers, wheelchairs, and motorized chairs to move about. In each facility, the participants were randomly assigned to a theater course, a music course (both taught by professionals), or to a no-treatment (i.e. Waiting-list) control group with the one constraint being that women and minorities were not to be underrepresented in any group. The rationale for using music, specifically singing, as the noncontent-specific control, was that the activation inherent in any kind of performance in front of ones' peers might drive the effect rather than the specifics of acting. It was explicitly stated in the consent form that random assignment to a particular topic was an important feature of the study, and that acceptance of the offer constituted acceptance of such random assignment. All participants took the pretest before the intervention started. For the next 4 weeks, the theater and music participants received twice-weekly lessons; then all three groups took the posttest.

Measures

The eight cognitive measures were Word List Memory, Word List Delayed Recall, Category Fluency, Digit Span Forward, Digit Span Backward, Story Recall Task, Delayed Story Recall Task, Means-end Problem solving.

Results

The theater group significantly outperformed no-treatment controls on almost all cognitive measures, as assessed by a multivariate analysis of covariance with group membership as the independent variable (theater, music, no-treatment), age as the covariate, and the eight cognitive variables as the dependent variables (all $ps<0.01$). The only nonsignificant effects were the forward and backward digit span tests. Immediate recall of the East Boston Memory test barely missed significance ($p=0.06$). A similar pattern of results was obtained when the comparison was made with the music group; the theater group outperformed them on almost all variables. An important aspect of all the above studies was that the tests were not targeted to the training but simply assessed abilities necessary or helpful for maintaining self-sufficiency in an aging population. This procedure is relatively rare. In many cognitive interventions, the instruction is specifically targeted, such as training in the method of loci and testing the result with a list-learning task. However, nothing in the theater intervention involves practice on tasks similar to those on the test, nor are the participants taught any test taking strategies. Therefore, the improvements would appear to have been the result of the intense activation experienced by imaginatively becoming immersed in fictional situations and performing them in front of the rest of the class. Of course, some abilities may have been enhanced by abstracting learning principles during instruction. For example, after 4 weeks of monitoring input from the other participants during practice scenes, these older adults may have become accustomed to paying such close attention to even minor clues in the environment that they attended more to the similarities or differences in other cognitive tasks, including processing word-lists or comprehending prose passages. The results of this study (Noice & Noice, 2009), along with those of our previous interventions, demonstrate the efficacy of this approach for promoting healthy cognitive aging.

The Third NIA Intervention

Up until the end of the second study, the intervention had been taught exclusively by the same professional actor-director-Professor of Theater who devised the program. Three important questions were left open. First, was the success of the intervention based on highly individual characteristics of the original instructor or could any qualified acting teacher produce the same results? Second, could activity directors of senior centers/retirement homes without prior theatrical training or experience successfully administer the program? The latter was considered possible because activity directors are highly experienced in running various events in which audience-participation is a key element; therefore, they might be able to learn and administer the various activities involved in the acting intervention. The third question was whether the benefits of the intervention would extend to activities of daily living as measured by the OTDL (Diehl et al., 2005). This measure involves performance of actual tasks such as reading prescription labels and understanding the dosage, balancing a checkbook, or making out medical history forms. This third NIA study is still in progress so only partial results are available. The first question has been answered. An additional acting teacher was recruited. She was able not only to learn the intervention but also to produce almost identical results. Furthermore, her training presented no problems. An email was sent a few days in advance of each session describing the activities for that day, then a follow-up telephone call ironed out any ambiguities. We were on hand to observe all eight sessions, but did not take part in running any of them. In addition to the positive results on the cognitive measures, the newly recruited acting instructor produced significant results on the ODTL tests. The results for the activity directors remain to be seen. However, preliminary inspection suggests that some very positive benefits may be produced by them but not the across-the-board gains observed with professional instructors. We are currently exploring new methods of verifying the impact of acting on healthy cognitive aging including pre and postintervention brain scans of the participants. We are convinced that our "Acting on the Brain" program can significantly contribute to the cognitive health of our aging population.

Author Notes This work was supported by Grants # 1 R 15 AG018266-01, 1 R15 AG026306-01, and 1 R15 AG032120-01 from the National Institute on Aging.

References

Anderson, R. C., & Pichert, J. (1978). Recall of previously unrecallable Information following a shift in perspective. *Journal of Verbal Learning and Verbal Behavior, 17*, 1–12.

Cohen, G. D. (2005). *The mature mind: The positive power of the aging brain.* New York: Basic Books.

Cohen, R. L. (1989). Memory for action events: The power of enactment. *Educational Psychology Review, 1*, 57–80.

Diehl, M., Marsiske, M., Horgas, A. L., Rosenberg, A., Saczynski, J. S., & Willis, S. L. (2005). The revised observed tasks of daily living: A performance-based assessment of everyday problem solving in older adults. *The Journal of Applied Gerontology, 24*(3), 211–230.

Dooling, D. J., & Lachman, R. (1971). Effects of comprehension on retention of prose. *Journal of Experimental Psychology, 88*, 216–222.

Engelkamp, J., & Zimmer, H. D. (1994). *The human memory: A multimodal approach.* Seattle: Hogrefe & Huber.

Nilsson, L. G. (2000). Remembering actions and words. In E. Tulving & F. I. M. Craik (Eds.), *The Oxford handbook of memory* (pp. 137–148). New York: Oxford University Press.

Noice, H. (1991). The role of explanations and plan recognition in the learning of theatrical scripts. *Cognitive Science, 15*, 425–460.
Noice, H. (1992). Elaborative memory strategies of professional actors. *Applied Cognitive Psychology, 6*, 417–427.
Noice, H. (1993). Effects of rote vs. gist strategy on the verbatim retention of theatrical script. *Applied Cognitive Psychology, 7*, 75–84.
Noice, H., & Noice, T. (1993). The effects of segmentation on the recall of theatrical material. *Poetics, 22*, 51–67.
Noice, H., & Noice, T. (1994). An example of role preparation by a professional actor: A think-aloud protocol. *Discourse Processes, 18*, 34–369.
Noice, H., & Noice, T. (1996). Two approaches to learning a theatrical script. *Memory, 4*(1), 1–17.
Noice, T., & Noice, H. (1997a). Effort and active experiencing as factors in verbatim recall. *Discourse Processes, 23*, 51–69.
Noice, T., & Noice, H. (1997b). *The nature of expertise in professional acting: A cognitive view.* Hillsdale: Lawrence Erlbaum.
Noice, H., & Noice, T. (1999). Long-term retention of theatrical roles. *Memory, 7*(3), 357–382.
Noice, H., & Noice, T. (2001). Learning dialogue with and without movement. *Memory and Cognition, 29*(6), 820–828.
Noice, T., & Noice, H. (2002). Very long-term recall and recognition of well-learned material. *Applied Cognitive Psychology, 16*, 259–272.
Noice, T., & Noice, H. (2004). A cognitive learning principle derived from the role acquisition strategies of professional actors. *The International Journal of Cognitive Technology, 9*(1), 34–39.
Noice, T., & Noice, H. (2006). A theatrical intervention to improve cognition in intact residents of long term care facilities. *Clinical Gerontologist Journal, 29*(3), 59–75.
Noice, H., & Noice, T. (2009). An arts intervention for older adults living in subsidized retirement homes. *Aging, Neuropsychology and Cognition, 1*, 1–24.
Noice, H., Noice, T., & Kennedy, C. (2000). The contribution of movement on the recall of complex material. *Memory, 8*(6), 353–363.
Noice, H., Noice, T., Perrig-Chiello, P., & Perrig, W. (1999). Improving memory in older adults by instructing them in professional actors' learning strategies. *Applied Cognitive Psychology, 13*, 315–328.
Noice, H., Noice, T., & Staines, G. (2004). A short-term intervention to enhance cognitive and affective functioning in older adults. *Journal of Aging and Health, 16*(4), 562–585.
Owens, J., Bower, G. H., & Black, J. B. (1979). The "soap-opera" effect in story recall. *Memory and Cognition, 7*, 185–191.
Perrig-Chiello, P., Perrig, W. J., Staehelin, H. B., Krebs-Roubicek, E., & Ehrsam, R. (1996). Well-being, health and autonomy in elderly: Basel interdisciplinary study on aging (IDA). *Zeitschrift fuer Gerontologie und Geriatrie, 29*, 95–109.
Rosenberg, M. (1965). *Society and the adolescent self-image.* Princeton: Princeton University Press.
Ryff, C. D., & Keyes, C. L. M. (1995). The structure of psychological well-being revisited. *Journal of Personality and Social Psychology, 69*(4), 719–727.
Sulin, R. A., & Dooling, D. J. (1974). Intrusion of a thematic idea in retention of prose. *Journal of Experimental Psychology, 103*(2), 255–262.

Chapter 18
Coming Alive: Kairos Dance Theatre's Dancing Heart™ – Vital Elders Moving in Community

Maria DuBois Genné and Cristopher Anderson

Abstract In the emerging arts, healthcare and creative aging movement, Kairos Dance Theatre, founded in 1999 in Minneapolis, is seeking to help pioneer understanding and practices, transform how we think of aging, health care, community and the role of the artist in society, and inspire and guide new programming. Kairos, with a mission to *share the joy of dance and unleash its power to nurture and heal,* is an intergenerational dance company with members from age 4 to 100. Our work draws upon participatory performance art making and brain/body scientific research to catalyze understanding, participation, and health. This chapter describes our program, *The Dancing Heart™ – Vital Elders Moving in Community* and the companion *Memory Care Program,* created in Minnesota in 2005, which are pioneering, national award-winning, evidence-based programs that are transforming the lives of elders, their families, and caregivers in long-term care, memory care, and other health and community settings. These programs are improving quality of life, reducing healthcare costs, building community, and increasing joy and satisfaction.

Introduction

Kairos is a nonprofit organization, consisting of a dancing troupe, ages 4–100, which includes both professional and avocational dancers, office staff, four teaching artists, two apprentices, one intern, and six regular volunteers. We are grateful to have multiyear relationships with forward-thinking corporate, foundation, arts and government funders, and a body of practice, curriculum, and workshops developed over years in real-world health settings. We are attempting to educate others while

---

M.D. Genné (✉)
Kairos Dance Theatre, 4316 Upton Avenue South, Minneapolis, MN 55410, USA
e-mail: maria@kairosdance.org

continuing to pursue our artistic and research goals. In December 2009, we added a *Dancing Heart*™ Apprentice Program and administrative infrastructure to train additional professional artists to facilitate diffusion efforts. We are now seeking to replicate our *Dancing Heart*™ – *Vital Elders Moving in Community* program, a dance, music, and storytelling program led by professional performing artists and support staff.

Inside the Program

"We got carried away with the improvisational music, dancing and story-making, and creative sparks started flying," says Kairos Dance Theatre apprentice teaching artist and puppeteer Margo McCreary about a Dancing Heart™ session at the Ebenezer Fairview nursing home in Minneapolis. One thing had led to another, as they usually do. Margo explains, "We were 'dancing' elders across the circle in their wheel chairs when we got the idea to turn it into a bullfight. The energy was high and the elders were game. Our intern, lively Hannah Smith, jumped in the middle with a red cloth, posturing and daring the 'bulls.' Two elders, with their arms upraised as 'horns,' were incited by the red cloth and made their attacks with help from their wheelchair drivers. There were shrieks, shouts and laughter all around as we did our wild dance of the bull!"

The scene with the bull, described above, is a characteristic example of what we do. We start with the belief that people of all ages, abilities, and backgrounds, dancing together to music we care about, and from personal and cultural stories, are beautiful and make compelling art. We believe that when participants are vitally engaged, with integrity, as full collaborators in a creative process, based on the content of their own lives, with safety, dignity, respect, and fun, then personal, family, and organizational change can happen, as relationships and community are created through these shared experiences.

Bring this artistic drama and community-building expertise into collaboration with professionals in healthcare settings and then the potential for scientifically measurable health and quality of life benefits occurs. Residents, caregivers, visiting family members, volunteers, and even organization executives, if they desire, are all involved in joyful, collaborative, immersion art-making experiences that maximize cognitive, physical, and emotional functioning. Our preliminary evaluation data, described below, suggest that this activity – vital engagement with dance/theater/music/story led by a professional artist – may improve strength, flexibility, energy, balance, memory, socialization, and overall functioning. (See our research data below.) Over time, this activity promotes enjoyment, increased ability to take creative risks, and a sense of belonging in a teaching/learning community for and among participants.

Kairos' professional teaching artists conduct 90-min *Dancing Heart*™ workshops weekly at several adult day care centers, assisted living centers, and five nursing homes in Minnesota. These provide in-depth opportunities for individual artistic development, higher-level physical activity, and community connection. Also included is a 45-min weekly evaluation and coaching session with site staff, volunteers, and Kairos teaching artists in addition to 42 hours of training with Kairos' professional teaching artists for site staff who are part of the support team and help cofacilitate the *Dancing Heart*™.

Sessions include physical and vocal warm-ups, body/brain exercises, dance, theater, storytelling, and choreography. Dances, plays, and stories are built around the elders' memories, life stories, current emotions and creative ideas, and broader cultural references. Improvisation brings surprises and delights. Two to three teaching artists, trained site staff, and volunteers lead each session with 20–25 elders.

The Language of Dance

We notice that participants in our program have cognitive, physical, emotional, and social benefits when they are engaged in becoming more fluent in the "language of dance." This "language" is a universal one and, in our experience, seems to be more complexly integrated into the body/brain system than speech. We work with many people who cannot remember their grown child's name but can dance a fast toe-tapping jitterbug in their chairs while singing the entire lyrics to a Glenn Miller or Andrews Sisters' tune.

The language of dance includes the elements of body, time, space, and energy that as human beings we are familiar because we are constantly moving in space in relationship to the world around us. Dance just formalizes the way we move. We can be reaching, twisting, bending, balancing, moving quickly, moving slowly, moving in a curving pathway, or just moving to the rhythm of our heart. Moving, it turns out, is good for us. Vascular health is key to a healthy mind/body "system." Learning new patterns of movement stimulates the body/brain. Dancing to music that we love seems to open a door to abilities and memories that were forgotten but not lost. We find in *The Dancing Heart*™ that dancing is an invitation for people to connect across different life experiences, abilities, and generations. As a dance artist I invite participants into the process of creative dance as well as learning or remembering formal dance steps.

We start small, value everyone and everything. Personal stories and the storyteller matter. Personal reminiscence and stories find their way into group poems, songs, and dances. With imagination and courage, participants might risk moving a finger. Soon, we might do some easy chair dancing. But, who wants to miss out on the adventures to come – social dancing almost as we remember it, and so much more.

We observe that when people start moving their bodies in new unaccustomed ways, feelings and stories can arise from their personal histories that we can acknowledge and value. The feelings expressed range a spectrum that includes disappointment, fear, anger, shame, grief, delight, wonder, desire, love, and joy.

Dance changes the dynamics of relationships between people, heightening social interactions and dissolving formalized relationships, such as those between care professionals and patients, to ones of peers creating and discovering together. There is no right or wrong way to dance, just many different possibilities. Dance evokes the power of eros in its broadest kinship sense, promoting many kinds of connections. Whether we are creating a chair version of the Virginia reel, dancing the two step with one partner holding on securely to the other more frail partner or creating a "dance of the sea" with silken cloths connecting dancers across the dancing circle, we are creating a community that no longer is limited by time and place, and is enriched by our imaginations.

Working with Elders

Goals for the *Dancing Heart*™ program with elders include health status stabilization such as improving strength, gait, balance, flexibility, stamina, energy, and a range of motion. Psychological goals include mitigating depressive symptoms, building self-confidence in physical, social, emotional and artistic ability, and increasing desire to connect with others. The program helps participants with dementia to improve their focus and attention, decrease anxiety, and enjoy interactions with others. We offer a new vision of elders, emphasizing their vitality and ability, and we help them redefine and explore their artistic gifts. In addition, the program promotes organizational culture change as it builds knowledge for participants, staff, volunteers, and family members regarding the benefits of arts-based programming and encourages everyone to expand their expectations of participant growth, abilities, and value.

We serve elders in the greater Minneapolis/Saint Paul metropolitan area, usually ranging in age from 65 to 100, from broad cultural and ethnicity representation. Also, we are near the end of a 2-year pilot project, funded by Medicaid funds through the state of Minnesota, that includes five nursing homes, two of which are in outstate Minnesota communities, Red Wing and Lake City. Many of these elders cope with an array of health issues, including dementia. We serve high-risk frail elders, and many of them use walkers, canes, or wheelchairs. Management leadership at the sites where we do our program regards our program as highly successful. (Please see data below.) We hope to replicate it in other states.

Some organizations that have embraced the *Dancing Heart*™ model are making dramatic changes in philosophy and programming to align with *Dancing Heart*™ practices. In addition to elders participating, individual staff and family members involved report that the program has been positively life changing for them. In the sessions we strive to affirm family and staff in personal and professional ways, expand their knowledge about brain/body and arts-in-healthcare research, and change their expectations about what elders can do. Everyone has the opportunity to practice taking artistic and interpersonal risks, make artistic contributions from their own impulses and practice new *Dancing Heart*™ ways to relate with each other.

At the Fairview Seminary Home in Red Wing, Minnesota, an Ebenezer Foundation site where we have held weekly sessions for a year and a half, staff members report that they often sing and dance with client elders during out-of-session everyday activities, increasing enthusiasm and enjoyment of both elders and staff members.

We have worked at the Amherst H. Wilder Foundation Adult Day Health Services Memory Loss Program in Saint Paul for 5 years, from 2006 to current. This program, started with seed money from the Society for Arts and Healthcare and Johnson and Johnson, serves older adults who are diagnosed with mid to late stage Alzheimer's and other forms of dementia. When we first began, staff members warned us that we should not permit the clients to get out of their chairs. Now, staff's expectations of what participants can do and what they think is possible for them have changed dramatically.

Director of the program, Sue Ryan, says, "as a result of the *Dancing Heart*™ we've revamped everything. It has elevated the level of activity that we want to provide for people. The sky is the limit as we don't know what people are capable of. We need to encourage involvement in the program and provide an environment that allows for creativity. The *Dancing Heart*™ program has opened the door for self-expression, self-esteem and community building. The program has made staff closer. It has taught staff how to interact with clients in a different way and on a different level. There is so much more joy now."

Here is another example of the *Dancing Heart*™:

We're at Ebenezer Fairview Ridges in Burnsville, Minnesota. After talking about our favorite memories of summer at the fair, Ron, a retired school superintendent with Parkinson's disease, says he can teach us to make the sounds of the merry-go-round. We bring the microphone to him, and, sure enough, he eloquently evokes the joyful experience of the merry-go-round, starting with the musical oom-pah-pah bass beat, then bringing in the classic merry-go-round melody, and then breaking off to give us the mid-way barker who is coaxing us to ride.

We're excited. In our circle, we work up different body, arm, and leg movements we can do on the merry-go-round as animals going up and down; horses will leap, lions will snarl. Two of us will be high school kids "going steady," who are riding together. One of us will hold a baby. One will manage the levers of the controls for the ride. Half the group will do the oom-pah-pah part, the other half will sing the melody, all of us will move as if being animals or riding animals, two will sit hand-in-hand, and one will hold a baby. Ron, with the microphone, will be the barker. The levers are turned. We start singing and moving, cranking up this marvelous big machine, people and "animals" moving. It's a grand time. We note that we almost feel the heat of summer, and smell the caramel corn, straw, and horse manure.

As we're doing this, the children start entering from the on-site preschool. They join us for each session, mid-way through our time together. Hearing and seeing what's going on, they are big eyed, point and sneak whispers to each other. As they take their places alongside elders in the circle, we explain what is happening and ask them to join in. We crank up the marvelous machine again, now with the children involved. Most everyone is thrilled. In a few minutes, as the merry-go-round finally sputters to a halt, one 4-year-old boy, with eyes wide and waving his arm, shouts out, "I know this! We did this! I've been here!" True.

Initial Skepticism Transforms to Enthusiasm

We are accustomed to having professionals in both the arts and medicine being skeptical about the health and emotional benefits that occur for frail elders participating in the Dancing Heart™ program. Health professionals and the lay public in community settings have often thought of artistic pursuits as something only useful to amuse and "kill time," casting elders as passive consumers of these activities. Or, elders get patronized for doing "crafts" and "art work." The fine arts community often has disregard for community programming and a similar attitude toward "crafts" and "art work" of elders. Audiences can be confused by our mixture of the professional and avocational, and usually don't expect deeply affecting art to come from this kind of process and setting.

We love to go against expectations, in our gentle way, and invite everyone into the dance for exciting, inspiring, and nourishing experiences. We imagine that it is a process of culture building without boundaries. We often turn skeptics into enthusiasts who eventually see how this serves to affect individual, organizational, and community health. For example, within 2 weeks of starting to work with the Wilder Memory Loss Program, a family member called staff and asked what was happening on Wednesdays because their mother was starting to initiate communication for the first time in a long while.

Catherine Hoppe, wife of a participant in the Wilder program, said, "When my husband was first diagnosed, his neurologist told me that he would probably have 10 years to live. I was just bleak. It's almost 10 years now, and he is still walking, talking, and eating by himself. He is stimulated in the *Dancing Heart*™ program; he's encouraged to do things. If he were at home, he'd be sitting in front of the TV doing nothing, and he'd be in a nursing home, I swear. I think the *Dancing Heart*™ has helped."

Research on the Benefits of Dance

There is a body of research accumulating that shows dance can positively affect the health and quality of life of older adults by engaging people cognitively, physically, socially, and emotionally. An observational study of older adults living in the community (Verghese et al., 2003) found that dancing ranked high on the list of leisure activities associated with a delay in the onset of Alzheimer's disease. The aim of Dr. Gene Cohen's study (Cohen et al., 2006) was to measure the impact of professionally conducted community-based cultural programs on the physical and mental health and social activities of individuals aged 65 and older. They studied three groups of elders in Washington DC, NYC, and San Francisco, average age 80 years, who worked weekly with a professional artist. This study found that participants had fewer falls, a decrease in doctor visits and use of medication, a decrease in loneliness and depression, and increased involvement in community activities.

Cohen asserts that our later years need not be times of deficit and loss but rather a time of positive emotional and brain development when we are uniquely capable of bridging knowledge and experience in ways that we could not do when we were younger. In his book, *The Creative Age: Awakening Human Potential in the Second Half of Life* (HarperCollins, 2000), Cohen tells many stories about respected elders who come into their full artistic and professional accomplishment in their later years.

Preliminary Findings for Dancing Heart™

Our evaluation of the *Dancing Heart*™ is in early stages, but preliminary findings suggest tangible, measurable benefits in slowing down aspects of the progression of dementia and sustaining the physical, emotional, and cognitive health of participating older adults. In our partnership with Wilder in Saint Paul, 43% of participants in the *Dancing Heart*™ *Memory Care* program showed improvement in both the Mini Mental State Exam and the Sit Stand Fall assessment.

The majority of residents tested maintained or improved balance and cognition, and reduced depression levels. In a population of memory-impaired individuals, results that indicate maintenance of mood, and sitting and standing skills are of clinical significance. Caregivers report maintenance of such improvement translates into significant quality of life improvements and cost of care savings. Weekly narratives on individuals described increasing engagement and new learning. We do not have comparative data for people who did not participate in the Dancing Heart, and we do not know if these results are statistically significant.

In addition to the assessments at the Wilder Memory Care Program, we also have data from five local nursing home sites where staff did an initial baseline measure with all participants in a regular *Dancing Heart*™ program at the onset in October of 2008 and every 12 weeks for three cycles, to continue through January, 2011 (see Table 18.1).

Now we are nearing completion of a 2-year program with the Ebenezer Foundation here in Minnesota, bringing our weekly program for frail elders into five nursing home sites. The table below summarizes the percentage of participants who maintained or improved, compared to those who declined, on measures of depression, cognition (MMSE), and balance over a period of up to 48 weeks. The preliminary findings suggested that the program had an early positive impact on balance, and

Table 18.1 Ebenezer nursing homes program data: *The Dancing Heart*™ model

Assessment tool used	Baseline to week 12		Week 12–24		Week 24–36	
	Maintained (%)	Improved (%)	Maintained (%)	Improved (%)	Maintained (%)	Improved (%)
Balance Sit/stand/fall	34	40.4	27.6	31.0	42.9	28.6
Cognition MMSE	21.4	31.4	18.6	44.2	10.0	30.0
Depression GDS or Cornell	40.8	26.8	24.4	41.5	32.0	40.0

cognition and depression (enthusiasm!) improved over time. Ebenezer staff concludes that these results show positive functional changes in participants. We recognize that this data from Wilder and Ebenezer is preliminary and raw; it is currently being analyzed by researchers at St. Catherine University in Saint Paul. Drs. Dutton, Sullivan and Haertl and graduate students from Saint Catherine University in St. Paul, Minnesota are currently researching the data. Their first quantitative and qualitative study, to be published June 2011, evaluates the impact of *The Dancing Heart*™ on the health and quality of life of participants at the five Ebenezer nursing homes. Initial analysis of the qualitative data using framework analysis suggests that the *Dancing Heart*™ had a positive impact on participants' mood, cognition, mobility, personal validation and creativity. There was also a positive influence on the atmosphere of the long-term care facilities, according to staff.

Dancing Heart™ Program
Summary Data – Year One
Ebenezer Foundation
Five Nursing Home Sites

Test	%Residents Same or better	%Residents Worse
Depression scores change (Cornell)	67	33
Cognition scores change (MMSE)	63	37
Balance scores change (Berg)	72	28

Anecdotal Evidence of the Impact of Dancing Heart™

Sue Ryan, Director of the Wilder Foundation Adult Day Health Services Memory Loss Program, says, "What we see is that, after the [*Dancing Heart*™] group, people's verbalization and socialization increases…." "It carries over into the next thing they are doing, and, for some, it carries over into the whole day…." "We've been able to keep people from not declining, and that's huge."

One day in Red Wing, June, a broad-hearted and quick-to-smile volunteer, age 60, brings her high school prom dress that her mother made for her to show to us. It's beautifully made in white satin, with a powder blue velveteen jacket. She carries it around the circle so we can see it up close, then tells us stories about prom night – how the boy was handsome and brought her a corsage, how they drove in his dad's car, held hands and danced. Then, on the sound system, we play Elvis Presley singing, "Can't Help Falling in Love with You." Teaching artist Peter Podulke comes up behind June and gently taps her on her shoulder. Peter, about 60, is a dancer who has worked most of his life as a bricklayer. He is large and solid, with big hands, straight back, bright face, and big heart. We all enjoy watching his no-nonsense grace and self-effacing dignity. We appreciate his wit and bright cheer. Offering his hand, he asks June if she will dance with him. She agrees and they move together in a slow dance while many of us, misty-eyed, are transported back to our own first experiences of romance.

Reginald Prim, an independent arts activist and critic who previously worked for the Walker Arts Center in Minneapolis as its community liaison, and who now serves on our board of directors, wrote about his experience at a Minnesota Fringe Festival show in 2005 of watching one of our performances for the first time that he titled, "Kairos Dance Theater Makes a World":

"There is something quite moving about watching seventeen people of varying cultural and ethnic backgrounds, ages and skill levels, creating enjoyable, entertaining and even profound dances together. It's as if you're watching a little working model of patience, care and respect. And, you find yourself, for an hour or so, rediscovering your faith in community and believing that art can heal, that dance is ritual and world-making, and that a theater can be a sacred space. I must assume there is a lesson here, a sermon if you will, about how to recover grace and beauty in our everyday lives; how to live artfully despite the limits of our skill and abilities; how to transmute the quotidian into the transcendent. Moreover, the dance here feels like a blessing – an active imparting of Grace into the world, a transfusion of wonder directly to the heart."

What Reggie so eloquently describes is what we try to live up to and what we think is possible in the nursing home, in the community center, and in the world. Our choreographed public performances are often "gee-whiz" experiences for audiences, who, like people in much of our culture, are not accustomed to valuing or having rewarding artistic experiences from performers who are usually marginalized.

Our performances offer provocative images of possibilities of community art-making, start new thinking and conversations, attract performers, advocates and activists, and often bring us invitations to new "off-the-beaten-path" venues, such as libraries, parks, and community centers, for performances and workshops. For example, in Red Wing, Minnesota, we performed at the new band shell in the downtown park.

At the Wilder Memory Loss Program in Saint Paul, we mounted a program for "family night." The participants were focused, articulate, and worked together as an experienced ensemble group in a high energy, musical theater assemblage of story, song, and dance, based on our own biographies and borrowing from traditional Broadway musical forms, bringing tears and laughter, and a good time to everyone. Additional staff members joined us in rehearsals and put time and energy into learning lines, practicing music, and making costumes. After the performance, staff noted that families interacted and sat with other families for dinner. For the first time in the 10-year history of family night, staff cleaned up a full hour later than usual because families stayed to talk with and enjoy each other. This participatory arts program has helped to strengthen positive relationships between elder dancers and their families, between other elder dancers, and between elder dancers and staff. Everyone involved has an experience of the previously marginalized elders as being at the center of community life, and being a source of artistic, social, and emotional content.

A few weeks later, these *Dancing Heart*™ *Memory Care Program* participants traveled for the first time to the other Wilder Adult Day site in St. Paul. Their interactive performance was a hit with clients and staff in the second facility. *Dancing Heart*™ performers had the opportunity to feel a sense of mastery and, as an elder gentleman program participant said, "We put a smile on their faces."

Another few weeks later, the same group performed their poetry and dance piece, "Roses are Red..." at the opening ceremony of a regional Alzheimer's conference of 800 people at the convention center in downtown Saint Paul – to a standing ovation. With family members in attendance, participants enjoyed a sense of social and artistic mastery, and satisfaction that came from this vital engagement with their community. Cohen's research confirms that vital engagement and a sense of mastery are key to promoting the health benefits this work provides (Cohen et al., 2006).

During a Dancing Heart™ session one day near Father's Day, we bring sheet music for a nostalgic and bittersweet song about a daughter remembering her father. Babs, a staff member, offers to play it and is seated at the piano starting to negotiate the music. Fellow teaching artist Carla Vogel and I look over her shoulder and sing the lyrics into the microphone. Then, we take a short time to teach the chorus to everyone. After we've all sung the song through and the poetry of the lyrics has started to sink in, we stop and tell stories about what we remember about our own fathers. Carla copies down these short memories into a notebook.

"He came from Ireland..." one of us says. "He was very handy with his hands – he could do anything..." says another. Stella gets a grim look on her face and says she has nothing good to say about her father. We say that's okay. We know that not all the stories are good ones, but there are many fond memories in the room. Martha has a photo she shows us of her and her father taken on the day she graduated from high school. He is standing next to her and has his arm around her. She says, "He was a beautiful man."

Carla looks at the photo and says to Martha, "And you are beautiful – *you* are beautiful, too!" "Oh, thank you," says Martha.

Then, we do the song again, replacing the lyrics with our own that we made up from our story fragments, which we read from our notes. When we come to it, we all sing the chorus of the song. Then, we go back to our verses, then to the chorus, again. It is very sweet. Some of us dab at tears. At least one of us continues to sit stonily. When we stop, quite a few of us continue sitting pleasantly, eyes lost in thought, one of us mopping up another small tear.

Innovative Role in Society for Artists

The *Dancing Heart*™ comes from Maria's thirty plus years of experience working as a professional modern dancer, choreographer, and teacher with other collaborators, and as the founder of three dance companies. Maria has developed and implemented enrichment programs for people of all ages for schools and other cultural organizations, serving as a "connector" between an organization's traditional programming and audience understanding, enjoyment, and development. Now, *Dancing Heart*™ sponsors – funders, healthcare providers, nursing homes, and community centers – are starting to appreciate the "audience development" power of this program. If the *Dancing Heart*™ is how life is lived here, then this might be the place where we would want to live or where we would want our mother or father to live.

We've initiated a training program for professional artists and site staff and seek to develop a best practice model in order to replicate the *Dancing Heart*™ in new settings. We are neither healthcare providers nor therapists. We don't do what people usually think artists do in nursing homes. We are performing artists who view teaching as a performance art, who engage improvisationally with collaborators, who consider the whole community as our artistic oeuvre, and who include everyone in the community as a participant. What we do nurtures, heals, saves money and positively changes cultures. We seek to collaborate with healthcare providers, care communities, and other groups in a certain way. It is clear to us that in order for programs like the *Dancing Heart*™ to succeed, participant organizations need to enter into a new kind of long-term collaborative relationship with a certain kind of professional community-based artist, with dance at the center of what they do. First and foremost, the art form of these artists must be based on community building.

Our model is based on a radical inclusion and valuing of everyone as a contributor, with a broad acceptance of what is valuable as expression. Everyone is involved in the creative process. All participants have valuable insights, images, sounds, stories, and movements. Our attitude and intention of physical and emotional safety, deep respect, and valuing is paramount. We think this work requires emotional literacy, social ability with varying age groups, as well as artistic finesse.

We accept the sovereignty of each individual, and his authority over his own experience and interpretation. We stay curious about possible connections among creativity, psychology, sociology, human development, spirituality, and pedagogy – valuing dance as the central catalyst. We collaborate with and integrate other art forms – again, with dance and choreography at the center. We create from what is and who is here, from both personal biography and cultural referents. We seek to create intergenerational cross-functional teaching and learning communities, including all stakeholders, based on practice. We trust improvisation, where, out of an encounter with creative chaos can come the time-out-of-time or *kairos* moment – where surprises, discoveries, sounds, movements, stories can leap – the next move toward meaning and connection. In this safe, sometimes deep and fully committed play, we take risks, emotions get freed, tears are shed, laughter is deep and loud, depressions and anxieties "move," muscles get toned and developed, we all belong, and we all matter to each other.

An environment of safety and acceptance is crucial to the success of an arts program for older adults. Each person's gifts are valued and contribute to the ongoing creativity of the group. We believe that, as artists, we can complement the ongoing therapeutic programs at each site. Artists are comfortable working with what quite often looks like chaos, inspired by ideas that often appear in spontaneous and surprising ways. The underlying belief of *The Dancing Heart*™ is that each person has a unique gift that is waiting to be tapped and given expression. It is our job as artists to facilitate each person's artistic growth, no matter their age, background, or ability.

I've always been interested in developing and involving communities in dance theater art-making, and creating experiences for people from entry level to the advanced. In this context, I've always appreciated artistic professionalism, but also I've been willing to respect the depth of content that is often present in the untutored.

Discoveries made by the newcomer often add a freshness and uniqueness that are very exciting and enlivening.

What if a whole community valued this activity? What if every member of this community had a chance to explore his or her potential in this arena? Most of us haven't had an opportunity like this since childhood, when we once knew how to play like everything mattered deeply, anything was possible and we felt so alive. I think this was a time, and can be a time, when we make art out of our lives and put art-making back into the center of our lives. And, now that we are adults, there is so much more richness and material, and we have a better sense of what is at stake.

Perspectives of our Participants

"It's kind of hard to explain," says Margaret Berktold, a resident at Lake City Health Center, in Lake City, Minnesota, a facility of the Mayo Health System. "It's just a feeling of being together. [The *Dancing Heart*™ artists] just make you feel at home. And they don't push us. If we just want to sit there like a bump on a log, we can, but if we want to get into the action, we can. I'm getting limbered up and I walk better than I did. I think we're getting more graceful. We get acquainted – we laugh, talk and sing – and that's good for everyone. I think the *Dancing Heart*™ is good for us."

"There was bewilderment at the very beginning. We didn't know what we were getting into," says Allan Frazier, a resident at Ebenezer Ridges in Burnsville, Minnesota. "Now, we know we're going to go in and act silly, and we know the other people don't care. I enjoy not sitting around with a bunch of long faces all the time."

One day in Red Wing, we share the Martin Luther King quote, "We have flown the sky like birds, swum the sea like fish, but we have yet to learn the simple act of walking the earth as brothers and sisters." Then, we ask the elders to share their legacy – what they've learned from their lives – in the form of a blessing they might have for the good of the world.

"Always find good friends to be with," says Noreen. We hand her the end of a long length of colorful yellow cloth that is then unfurled across the room to the hands of the next person to speak.

"Remember to tell someone you love her," says Ruth, as she takes the end of the cloth.

"Peace in the world," says Bill, starting a new red cloth. As the blessings come, they are physically manifested in the space by the bright cloths criss-crossing from hand to hand. When we're done, the room is ablaze. Then, Rashard, a slight young man from the Minnesota Correctional Facility – Red Wing, leaps up enthused and asks if he can put all this into a song. He is one of 4–5 boys under 18 who come every week from the facility with two staff members to participate in our program – dancing, singing, telling and acting out stories, and making friends. The boys, dressed in the institution issued khaki slacks and dark polo shirts, appreciate the honest admiration of the elders. Handshakes at the end of the session are sometimes slow and heartfelt. Rashard's eyes are flashing. We've never seen him take this kind of risk before. We say, "Sure!" and he eagerly grabs the mike and begins singing. Others of us join in, clapping our hands as he launches into an inspired stylized rap gospel song, using our "blessings" as the lyrics. We're all thrilled, and he finishes to cheers, hoots, and applause.

This day, the elders get a sense of mastery by participating and then having Rashard think that what they said was important enough to put into a song. The song is nervy and beautiful – and startling because our blessings are in it. And, Rashard gets to take a creative risk toward belonging, contributing, and feeling valued.

Future Explorations

The *Dancing Heart*™ has both intrinsic and extrinsic benefits. Many participants think its intrinsic value is reason enough to be involved. But, just like the "secret" of sustainability practices adopted by the business world is that they are good business, the "secret" of the *Dancing Heart*™ arts-in-healthcare program also is that it is good business. And, we think it is apt to think of the *Dancing Heart*™ within the frame of sustainability.

Like other programs we admire that are similar in intention, including Elders Share the Arts in New York City, Stagebridge Theatre in Oakland, California, and Songwriting Works™ in Washington State, professional artists are essential for this work.

Emboldened by the success of the *Dancing Heart*™ with frail elders and the enthusiasm of our institutional partners, we are starting to implement our replication/best practice model training sequence. We continue our intergenerational performing in schools, nursing homes, and assisted living facilities.

Future Programming and Community Involvement

- We've started training local performing artists to give them a foundation for working with older adults.
- We've mounted Dance and Storytelling Residencies that partner us with elementary school children and older adults in explorations of dance and story. One project paired us with children who speak English as a second language, another with children from the Faribault School for the Blind in Minnesota.
- With the Wilder Foundation, we've led programming for people with early stage Alzheimer's disease, their families, and caregivers in what they call Memory Clubs. We would like to find out the effect of the program on persons with early dementia (see Fritsch, Smyth, Wallendal, Einberger, & Geldmacher, 2011).

- We would like to explore integrating more teens and young adults into intergenerational work.
- We want to explore what happens when we participate in more conscious community building involvements in different settings (see Rebok et al., 2011).
- We want to know what happens when we work with people earlier in their life arc, when they are pre-retired or just retired.
- We want to explore how senior centers can become cultural centers – centers of involvement, creativity, inspiration, and enjoyment for people of all ages and all walks of life. Beginning in January 2011, we started Dancing Heart™ programs at four adult day and assisted living sites. Here we are focusing on more active elders who are still living at home, with the goal of delaying or obviating the need for them to be placed in long-term care settings. At the same time, we started a fifth new Dancing Heart™ program in cooperation with the Struther's Parkinson's Program in Golden Valley, Minnesota, with the goal of creating a program specifically for elders with Parkinson's Disease.

Limitations of Our Research

Our data reflect an uncontrolled observational study rather than a randomized controlled trial. In our real world environment, it was impractical to turn down potential participants and put them in a wait list control group, so we accepted every individual who showed interest in participating. A criticism could be made that improvements of clients on MMSE over time may have occurred because of practice effects. We believe that subtle and overt practice changes are arising from our work, but at this point, this remains unproven. We observe that our work is changing the cultures in the facilities where we mount our program. Some of the results are anecdotal evidence and other results are based on program evaluation methods. We are currently working with researchers to improve our documentation of changes in our participants and our research design.

As a performing arts organization, we often surprise audience expectations with our company of professional and avocational dancers, of varying ages and differently abled, often involving audiences in emotionally rich, enjoyable, and inspiring dance theater experiences. We seem to encompass and integrate a broad territory that many people want to divide up into separate fiefdoms. The science and protocol-based health community sometimes has difficulty seeing the *Dancing Heart*™ as an artistic process that has measurable health benefits and significant implications for community building. From our perspective, the dance company and our active involvement with it as professional performers are essential parts of what keeps us alive as artists, and what keeps the *Dancing Heart*™ program vital and useful. Similarly, I hope the fine arts community will recognize that our community-building and social art-making processes involving very diverse and differently abled people can create very good art.

Conclusion

The Dancing Heart™ invites older adults and everyone in our communities to help co-create a new vision of dance theater – one that is inclusive of all ages, all bodies, and many different ways of moving. More evaluation research is needed to fully explore its potential for measurable health benefits, cost of care savings, and community vitality. We bring a vision of what community can be – all ages, all abilities, and all backgrounds dancing together. Much can happen when we dance together.

References

Cohen, G. D., Perlstein, S., Chapline, J., Kelly, J., Kimberly, M. F., & Simmens, S. (2006). The impact of professionally conducted cultural programs on the physical health, mental health, and social functioning of older adults. *The Gerontologist, 46*(6), 726–734.

Fritsch, T., Smyth, K. A., Wallendal, M. S., Einberger, K., & Geldmacher, D. S. (2011). Early memory loss clubs: A novel approach for stimulating and sustaining cognitive function. In P. E. Hartm & A. LaRue (Eds.), *Enhancing cognitive fitness in adults*. New York: Springer.

Rebok, G. W., Carlson, M. C., Barron, J. S., Frick, K. D., McGill, S., Parisi, J. M., et al. (2011). Experience Corps®: A civic engagement-based public health intervention in the public schools. In P. E. Hartm & A. LaRue (Eds.), *Enhancing cognitive fitness in adults*. New York: Springer.

Verghese, J., Lipton, R. B., Katz, M. J., Hall, C. B., Derby, C. A., Kuslansky, G., et al. (2003). Leisure activities and the risk of dementia in the elderly. *The New England Journal of Medicine, 348*(25), 2508–2516.

Chapter 19
Art, Museums, and Culture

Sean Caulfield

Abstract Participation in the arts offers people living with Alzheimer's an outlet to self-expression and personal identity. This chapter will describe how Alzheimer's-specific programs at museums, the cinema, and poetry cafes enable individuals with dementia to have meaningful experiences outside the walls of nursing homes, assisted living residences, and adult day centers. Engaging with society, the author contends, can reduce certain symptoms – such as apathy and anxiety – while simultaneously lessening the stigma that often accompanies a diagnosis.

Introduction

For there to be radical change in the quality of life for people living with Alzheimer's disease there first must be radical, creative imagination. Imagination for what *seems* possible is too limited. Limited imagination has led to where many people living with Alzheimer's find themselves today: stigmatized by society with limited and questionable options for "care," facing insurmountable difficulty obtaining a voice in public affairs, and lacking access to individual expression in the arts. To start the process of "radical change" necessary to change the state of "living with Alzheimer's," we must imagine the *impossible.*

The way an Alzheimer's diagnosis is commonly delivered to an individual and his or her family in our society is the first step in an inevitable negative downward spiral. Often a person arrives with a loved one to see their family doctor or a geriatric

---

S. Caulfield (✉)
ARTZ: Artists for Alzheimer's®, Hearthstone Alzheimer's Foundation,
130 New Boston Street, Suite 103, Woburn, MA 01801, USA
e-mail: Caulfield@thehearth.org

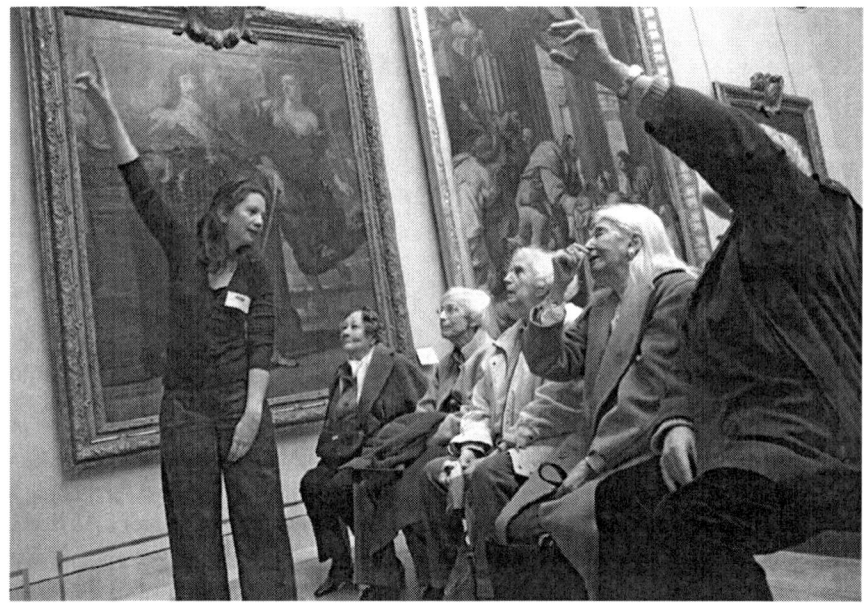
(Photo Caulfield ARTZ chapter- before Introduction)

specialist and receives the news that, "After examining the tests, we can determine that this is most likely a case of Alzheimer's." Delivered with a fatalistic undertone, the diagnosis implies that not much more can be done. The diagnosed individual is given a prescription for the latest Alzheimer's drug and sent on his or her way. With its lack of hope and no options for treatment, a diagnosis delivered this way naturally leads to depression, which makes the symptoms appear worse. Depressed and anxious, this once active individual is soon no longer working, gives up her driver's license, and spends her days isolated and withdrawn from community involvement. Inevitably this leads to a significant decline in cognitive functioning and the individual's inability to care for herself independently. Within a few years, placement in a nursing home or other type of long-term residence becomes the only remaining "care" option.

Imagine a city – let's call it Fable – where the approach to Alzheimer's care is carried out in a way that would currently be considered as impossible. In Fable, the label and diagnosis of Alzheimer's carry no stigma, negative reaction, or fear. A diagnosis of Alzheimer's falls within the category of other treatable conditions such as heart disease and diabetes. Fable's hospitals and medical clinics employ only general practitioners who have undergone extensive training in understanding Alzheimer's. One of the most important lessons is that symptoms can be treated, not only with pills, but with a balance of nonpharmacologic interventions – such as staying active in the workforce, volunteerism, regular exercise, proper nutrition, hobbies, and engagement with programs at Fable's cultural institutions. These include the museum, poetry café, community theater, historical society, amateur sports clubs, horticulture club, and the symphony. Fable's physicians prescribe such cultural "treatments" not because they simply keep patients "active" or give them "something to do," but because these nonpharmacologic interventions have been shown to reduce the symptoms often attributed to Alzheimer's, commonly known as the "Four A's" – apathy, anxiety, aggression, and agitation (Zeisel, 2009).

Case managers work in tandem with physicians to provide access to these resources – discussing with their "client" (not patient) an array of activities that are most appealing and beneficial to their quality of life. Additionally, case managers work with clients and their families to ensure scheduling, arrange transportation and "match" clients with small groups of about seven people with a similar diagnosis and similar interests and abilities. Once formed, these groups develop naturally into informal support groups that regularly meet for coffee at the local café before starting their trip to the Fable Art Museum where they enjoy a private, interactive tour of the newly opened Toulouse Lautrec exhibition. The educators and docents at the museum have been trained and certified to work on Alzheimer's-specific programs as has the staff at all Fable cultural institutions. After the hour and a half guided tour, the group has lunch together in the museum café. After lunch, some members are driven home while others move on to one of two afternoon programs, either an illustrated lecture and discussion at Fable Community College on the "Fashions of the 1940s and 1950s" or a yoga class at Fable High School. Each evening, seven nights a week, there are options to attend an Alzheimer's-related support group held at the home of a person living with dementia, an entertainment program, or an arts and culture event.

Here is an example of a weekly schedule of programs offered in Fable:

Monday	Tuesday	Wednesday	Thursday	Friday
7:30–8:30: Early Birds Walking Club; Fable Mall	7:30–8:30: Early Birds Walking Club; Fable Mall	7:30–8:30: Early Birds Walking Club; Fable Mall	7:30–8:30: Early Birds Walking Club; Fable Mall	7:30–8:30: Early Birds Walking Club; Fable Mall
9–10 a.m.: Coffee and headlines; Lucy's Café	9–10 a.m.: Coffee and headlines; Lucy's Café	9–10 a.m.: Coffee and headlines; Lucy's Café	9–10 a.m.: Coffee and headlines; Lucy's Café	9–10 a.m.: Coffee and headlines; Lucy's Café
10:30: Fable Art Museum, Toulouse Lautrec exhibition	10:30: Fable Historical Society, an interactive tour followed by a discussion on the Great Fable Bank Robbery of 1946	10:30: Painting workshop at the Fable Community Arts Center	10:30: Fable Museum of Photography: factory work during WWII	10:30: Fable Craft Museum: Workshop on Jewelry making
12 p.m. Lunch at museum café	12 p.m. Lunch at Gina's Pizza	12 p.m. Lunch at Arts Center	12 p.m. Lunch at museum	12 p.m. Lunch at museum

(continued)

(continued)

Monday	Tuesday	Wednesday	Thursday	Friday
2 p.m. (A) Lecture/group at Community College; Topic: President Kennedy	2 p.m. (A) Lecture group at Community College; Topic: How Henry Ford changed America	2 p.m. (A) Lecture group at Community College; Topic: the 1950s	2 p.m. (A) Lecture group at Community College; Topic: How Fable survived the Great Depression	2 p.m. (A) Lecture group at Community College; Topic: The Marx Brothers and Comedy in the twentieth century
(B) Yoga class at YMCA	(B) Nature walk at the Fable Preserve	(B) Strength training at the YMCA	(B) Tai-chi class at the YMCA	(B) Breathing and Meditation Workshop: Fable Zen Center
7 p.m. (A) Support group at Tom and Linda Landry's home	7 p.m. (A) Support group at Gina and Phil Talbot's home	7 p.m. (A) Support group at Gary and Suzanne McCarthy's home	7 p.m. (A) Support group at Wilma and Ned Johnson's home	7 p.m. (A) Support group at Sarah and Syd's house – pot luck dinner
(B) Open-mic poetry session at the Fusion House of Blues	(B) Folk-music night at Crazy Larry's Music Shack	(B) Cabaret Fundraiser for Alzheimer's Research at Liza's Lounge	(B) Ballroom dancing class at O'Houlihan's Dance Hall	(B) Movie night at the Fable Cinema: A Walk Down Memory Lane: classic clips from the twentieth century
(C) Bowling Club at the Fable Bowlorama	(C) Square dance at Barney's Giddy-up Bar and Grill	(C) Kitchen renovation ideas; Workshop; Fable Home Depot	(C) Cooking Seminar: Hors d'oeuvres for your next house party; Fable Culinary School	(C) Friday Night Book Discussion Club; Tuesday's with Morrie; Fable Barnes and Noble

Of course, not everyone will be able or want to attend all of the available programs, but just having options available brings hope to those living with Alzheimer's and their partners. This model of treatment through "action" is both highly positive and engaging. It demonstrates to people living with Alzheimer's that although they may have a disease, if they remain active, stay intellectually curious, and use their unique creativity, they have the best chance to maintain a high quality of life. It is imperative that people living with Alzheimer's disease – and the community at large – realize that Alzheimer's is a condition that people *live with* – not *die of*. Many people exhibit symptoms of Alzheimer's for 15 years or more. That is not a death sentence. Seen in the best possible light, a person diagnosed at an early stage can see this as the next chapter in their life – one that will certainly have its share of challenges – yet one that can be lived to the fullest.

Fable is an imaginary town, but the activities described are not imaginary. Such initiatives can be realistically carried out cost-effectively in every town, city, and country in the world; we have seen them in action in New York, Boston, London, Madrid, and Paris. Since 2001, ARTZ: Artists for Alzheimer's®, an organization I cofounded, has helped bring people living with Alzheimer's from nursing home beds to standing in front of the Mona Lisa at the Louvre; from playing bingo in a day center to reciting poetry in a New York City club; and from an inpatient geriatric psychiatric hospital to attending the premiere of a movie at the Tribeca Film Institute. ARTZ is doing what less than a decade ago was considered impossible: treating dementia by integrating people living with Alzheimer's into society – not by herding them into a locked nursing home Special Care Unit. The only way to create quality of life for people living with dementia is to change ourselves and society's view of the condition rather than trying to change those with the diagnosis.

History of ARTZ

ARTZ: Artists for Alzheimer's®, founded in 2001, is a 501(c) (3) initiative of the Hearthstone Alzheimer's Foundation. Its mission:

> To enrich the cultural life of people living with Alzheimer's disease, enable them to express their inner-selves, and lessen the stigma that often accompanies a diagnosis.

Drawing on the support and collaboration of artists and cultural institutions as a collective resource to share, educate, and inspire, ARTZ has developed and itself inspired Alzheimer's-specific cultural access programs at some of the world's most respected cultural institutions. These include the Louvre in Paris, the Peabody-Essex Museum in Salem, MA, the Big Apple Circus (BAC), the Museum of Modern Art in New York City, the Kohler Arts Center in Wisconsin, the Harvard University Natural History Museum in Cambridge, MA, the Coolidge Cinema in Brookline, MA, the National Gallery of Australia (NGA), the Tribeca Film Institute, and others.

Born in Boston, heavily influenced by the theories and research of sociologist and author, John Zeisel, ARTZ has developed Alzheimer's-friendly tools and professional training enabling cultural institutions to provide research-based, Alzheimer's-specific access programs for their membership and the general public. The expanding ARTZ network has organized and promoted hundreds of community events, encompassing thousands of people living with Alzheimer's and related dementias in Boston, New York, London, Melbourne, Paris and Madrid, among other cities. What was thought an impossible ideal in the lives of people living with Alzheimer's is achievable.

What ARTZ Does?

The organization and its chapters
- Partner with museums, symphony orchestras, poetry clubs, the circus, movie theaters, and other community cultural institutions to provide specialized access programs for people living with Alzheimer's disease and their families living at home, in assisted living residences or in nursing homes.
- Implement art-training programs for clients of adult day centers and senior centers and residents of assisted living residences and skilled nursing programs.
- Promote affordable cultural events with accessible transportation that are open to all people living with Alzheimer's disease and their loved ones in a community.
- Organize art exhibitions at galleries and public spaces featuring exclusively the artistic expression of people living with Alzheimer's disease.
- Conduct research on the efficacy of the "art experience" as a nonpharmacologic treatment for symptoms of Alzheimer's disease and related dementias.

Why Art Works as a Treatment for Alzheimer's Symptoms?

Whether painting, writing poetry, or attending the symphony, art participation is a powerful form of treatment for people living with Alzheimer's disease and related dementias. Whether the organization is ARTZ, the Society for Arts and Health, the Longwood Symphony Orchestra, the Alzheimer's Poetry Project, Ladder to the Moon, or self-organized tours in a local museum, art participation can significantly reduce the four "A" psycho-behavioral symptoms often associated with dementia – anxiety, aggression, agitation, and apathy. Access to art and culture contributes to maintaining cognitive functioning, optimizing remaining capacities, and utilizing areas of the brain that are often overlooked or ignored without emotionally engaging artistic stimulation. Oliver Sacks observed just this:

> I have myself seen all sort of skills preserved or largely preserved, even in advanced stages of dementing diseases such as Alzheimer's. Indeed, I think this preservation, if not of artistic skill, at least of aesthetic and artistic feeling, is fundamental....A colleague of mine specializes in this and has some remarkable paintings done by people living with Alzheimer's so advanced that they have become incapable of verbal expressions. Such paintings are not mere mechanical facsimiles of previous work but can show real feeling and freshness of thought (Stevens & Swan, 2004).

While Alzheimer's disease clearly affects short-term memory and the ability to complete complex sequential tasks such as cooking a gourmet meal or driving an automobile, it has far less impact on perception, emotional awareness, and creative sensibilities. A person living with Alzheimer's can comprehend visual art, music, and performance art on a deep, emotional level even though it may not be apparent to a casual observer. In many ways, individuals with Alzheimer's are more "in tune" with the subtleties and multi-layered complexities that art can convey because of their emotional sensitivity and openness. Simply put, art is a conduit that helps restore a sense of self, dignity, and connection with the outside world.

Observations and evaluations of ARTZ programs have shown improvement in participants' access to memories of recent events as well as events long passed, increased verbal expression, ability to focus attention for longer periods, heightened mood, more engaging social interactions, and a greater sense of self. We have also seen memories of art experiences stay with people living with Alzheimer's in an incredible way. The link between art and quality of life among those living with Alzheimer's seems self-evident and deserves to be made more profound. Every program that makes available and accessible existing cultural institutions and public programs is a relatively inexpensive form of treatment.

Benefits of Particpation in the Arts

Some of the many benefits of experiencing the arts have clear cost-benefits. Such experiences reduce the need for prescription drugs, most notably anti-psychotic medications that are commonly prescribed for Alzheimer's patients, and reduce the need for premature hospitalization and nursing home placement. The most meaningful benefit may be that public culture and art participation reduce the negative stigma around Alzheimer's, encouraging more people to seek out a diagnosis and to understand that while Alzheimer's keep as is not presently curable, it is in fact treatable. This enables people with a diagnosis to avoid "hiding" from their neighbors and the greater community – significantly reducing social isolation, depression, and care partner "burnout" at home.

The Benefits of Volunteering

The following description by Diana Leroux is typical of the many stories of personal growth we hear when artists volunteer in Alzheimer's programs. Starting as a volunteer, Diana became an intern with ARTZ and eventually a Program Director in an assisted living program for peole with dementia.

> As a recent graduate with an Art Therapy Degree from Endicott College and a new ARTZ volunteer, I was unaware of the challenges I would face while working with people who have dementia. This became evident the first day when I attempted to lead a group through still-life watercolor painting. I quickly discovered that my approach would have to change dramatically for the program to be successful. My initial goal of creating a finished painting was redirected to simply having the participants hold their brushes in an appropriate way. Also, my way of communicating directions was sometimes taken so literally that when I instructed one participant to put his paintbrush down onto the paper (to make a

mark), he released the brush onto the table completely. I began to spend more and more time with the residents throughout the month, sometimes for two or three hours at a time. With continuous watercolor painting practice, participants began not only to hold their brushes appropriately, but were able to initiate the process without me reminding them of how to begin. Each individual's progress could be seen week to week in the artwork they created. Marks on the paper became lines and lines became forms which resembled the subject matter that we were trying to capture. This experience convinced me that people with dementia do have an ability to learn skills through artistic memory, even when their short term memory is damaged.

Much of the work itself was highly original, expressive and self-revealing. It taught me lessons I never would have learned in my four years of college—namely, that everyone, regardless of how compromised their cognitive abilities may be, has a deep reservoir of personality and spirit; it just needs an outlet to find its own way.

Museums

There is a dire need for qualified, research-based Alzheimer's-competent museum programs to provide truly therapeutic museum experience for the tens of millions of people worldwide living with dementia. For most cultural institutions, people living with Alzheimer's are thought of as a disability group to be catered to, rather than as participants or members. This may stem from a lack of education about the realities of Alzheimer's disease, societal stigma, or the presence of a misinformed media that as a rule inaccurately portrays Alzheimer's as a hopeless, untreatable condition.

The ARTZ Museum Partnership Program develops, inspires, and guides interactive, educational museum programs for people living with Alzheimer's disease and related dementias. In the program ARTZ sets up and guides, it employs a comprehensive training program and a systematic research-based artwork selection process. The first museum program ARTZ developed was at the Museum of Modern Art in New York City now known as "Meet Me at MoMA…and Make Memories." This extremely successful joint initiative that MoMA now conducts independently has garnered worldwide attention and acclaim with MoMA docents leading multiple tours each month. Most importantly this program has positively influenced the way in which the general public views Alzheimer's as a treatable condition. This same initiative has been realized at the National Gallery of Art in Australia, the Louvre in Paris, and museums in Spain, the UK, throughout the US and beyond.

Museum of Modern Art (MoMA in New York City): In 2003, ARTZ approached the Community and Access Programs Department at MoMA and proposed the idea of developing an Alzheimer's-specific access program. After several meetings and discussions, MoMA and ARTZ decided to work together to create "Meet Me at MoMA…and make memories." During the 2 years of program development, ARTZ provided research and facilitated focus groups with Alzheimer's participants, all of which contributed to the training of MoMA docents and staff that ARTZ facilitated. The MoMA staff who went through these ARTZ workshops received an ARTZ certificate of training – distinguishing them as the first museum in the world to receive such a comprehensive Alzheimer's-specialized education. The program was opened to the public in January of 2006 and is now self-sustaining.

NGA: Collaborating with the Health and Arts Research Center, in Australia, and the New South Wales Alzheimer's Association, ARTZ selected artworks and trained volunteer docents and in a pilot program with the NGA, in Canberra. ARTZ staff selected paintings for the tours based on responses of people living with Alzheimer's from home and care homes, and trained museum educators on these paintings. The research model developed to evaluate this program included videotapes of the tours, focused interviews, and linguistic analysis of the videotaped discussions – all geared to identify changes in participants and staff. Evaluation results indicated remarkable levels of engagement (MachPherson et al. 2009).

The Louvre (Paris, France): The Louvre, arguably the world's greatest museum, has partnered with ARTZ to create Europe's first Alzheimer's-specific museum program. The Paris staff, overseen by ARTZ Paris Director Cindy Barotte, PhD, visited the Louvre with residents from local hospitals and senior residences to select and experiment with different art objects to be part of the tour. ARTZ Paris is employing Research Methods that ARTZ has developed in addition to research tools developed in Paris to test the efficacy of the museum visits. Collaborating in the effort are two doctors with expertise in dementia from two Paris Hospitals – Joel Belmin from Hospital Charles Foix and Olivier Drunat from Hospital Bretonneau and researcher Kevin Charras, PhD. The guided visits started in the Louvre's French historical painting gallery with most visits documented on film, allowing the research team to study the different approaches within the program design.

The Massachusetts ARTZ Museum Network

ARTZ formed the Massachusetts Museum Network in 2007 to develop a network of research-based, Alzheimer's-specific access programs at Massachusetts museums and cultural institutions. Funded through a generous grant from the McCance Family Foundation, the network seeks to enhance and improve the quality of life for people living with Alzheimer's, including care partners, family, and friends. ARTZ formed the coalition of five Massachusetts museums, each of which participated in a sponsored 6-month research pilot program culminating in the public opening in 2008 of the Massachusetts ARTZ Museum Network. Participating museums include the Peabody Essex in Salem, Fuller-Craft in Brockton, DeCordova Museum and Sculpture Park in Lincoln, Museum of National Heritage in Lexington, and the Harvard Museum of Natural History in Cambridge. ARTZ schedules guided tours at one museum each week of the year on the same day and the same time so that people living with dementia and their partners can anticipate and plan for a standard outing each week. Each museum participates in 10 yearly visits so that the program runs 52 weeks of the year.

The ARTZ Massachusetts Museum Network offers free weekly tours at one of five museums, enabling people living with Alzheimer's disease to get out and experience their community and great art, and delivers Alzheimer's-specific training for museum staff and volunteer companions. All this provides much needed respite for care partners who are often profoundly affected and need protection from "care giver burnout" and reduces the negative stigma of the Alzheimer's condition by demonstrating to society that tour participants are first and foremost individuals with their own personalities, opinions, and world view and second that they are *living not dying* with dementia. As Avis, an 83-year-old woman from a local skilled nursing facility, was leaving an extravagant fashion exhibition by designer *Iris Apfel: A Rare Bird of Fashion* at the Peabody Essex Museum, she turned to museum educator Ellen Soares and ARTZ Guide Peggy Cahill, sating, "I guess I need to postpone dying, there is so much more I need to see."

Facts and Figures

In 2009, 626 people living with Alzheimer's disease from 39 towns and cities participated in this 5-museum Museum Network. Similar figures are likely to be found where other museum tours for people living with Alzheimer's have established reputations. Participants cross all socio-economic backgrounds and come from settings that include private home, assisted living memory residences, skilled nursing facilities, adult day health programs, early-stage Alzheimer's support groups, private geriatric care management organizations, hospice, and visiting nurse agencies.

Popularity/Need/Demand

Every month since its inauguration has seen an increase in attendance. As word of mouth and awareness of the program has spread within the Alzheimer's community, tours are fully reserved at least 2 months in advance.

The Museum Network clearly fills a service gap in the Alzheimer's care community in Massachusetts, as do similar programs in other cities in the US, Europe, UK, and Australia. A common response from participating groups is, "I wish all cultural institutions offered programs like this" or "It would be great if our residents could take advantage of this every week." Partners also benefit from coming to the museum together to experience things as a couple without worrying about arrangements, environmental challenges at the museum, and lack of staff education. Janet Washington and her husband Willie, who has the diagnosis, have attended museum tours since the program first began. Janet reports:

> ARTZ programs for persons diagnosed with Alzheimer's disease and related dementia were eye opening for me as the care partner for my husband. The knowledgeable docents modeled how to present art information and elicit responses and that it is necessary to allow time for participants to engage with the art in different settings. In two visits at Harvard University's Museum of Natural History I understood for the first time that my husband was connecting in a different way with art since the diagnosis. Seeing with different eyes, Willie explained to me: "My way of coping with the disease is to focus on beauty…What makes life better is latching onto the art." He loves art, architecture and nature.

At the DeCordova Museum & Sculpture Park another participant seamlessly slid into a dance after viewing an exhibit. Willie was captivated by this experience and we talked about it for. We recently took an art class with our daughter, and Willie was surprised at 'how easy it was to paint.'

Establishing an Alzheimer's-Competent Evidence-Based Museum Program

To be effective in reducing symptoms, especially among participants further along in the Alzheimer's journey, is not easy. Museum Partnership training and tour development must be conducted intensively for several days and include the following linked steps. First, there needs to be a visit to the museum collection by someone trained in museum tours of this sort. This visit is used to select an initial set of artworks for the eventual guided tour. It is essential to choose the artworks for the tour carefully so that participants are engaged during the discussions as the guides lead at each artwork.

Our previous experience and research with artworks from other museums (Zeisel, 2009) indicate that artworks that contain a story with strong emotions, elicit moral judgment, and generate personal memories are particularly engaging.

Initial selection will necessarily be only partly on target because no one with dementia has so far been consulted. Focus interviews with a sample of potential participants living in Alzheimer's assisted living programs pare down the choice. Interview topics for this interview form part of the ARTZ training program. The final paring down of artworks is accomplished during pilot tours with actual participants in which not only the artwork but also the tour questions are tested and responses observed. When an artwork or a particular discussion topic does not engage participants, this is clearly evident. These tests always bring surprises in the perceptiveness of participants. Selecting artworks is a dynamic participatory process.

Just as artworks must be selected carefully, the pathways followed by tours must be carefully selected and tested to create a discovery sequence of 5 or so artworks. We learned this particularly at the Louvre where Cindy Barotte had to create several pathways for several groups of paintings in what turns out to be a complex set of corridors, elevators, stairways, and escalators. This is similarly done first by educators alone and then with groups of participants. In order to use this selection process as a training tool, we encourage museum educators to participate in a debriefing critique to share their impressions, to discuss how they are affected emotionally, and to refine details.

When we train museum staff and educators to kick-off the program, we present to them the brain's creative capacities even with Alzheimer's, the relationship between art and Alzheimer's, Alzheimer's-friendly communication techniques, understanding the effects of the museum's environment and layout on participants, and an overview of the selected collection from an Alzheimer's perspective including results of focus interviews and pilot tours. We translate scientific knowledge into simple and operational language. We explain how the person can be present to artistic experiences and we show that they can learn and remember if we know how to reach their procedural and episodic memory. The goal of all this is that the art experience works as a treatment for the condition.

But training can't stop there. It continues during the first few museum tours conducted with invited participants living with Alzheimer's and even tours once the program is in full swing. Postcritiques held at the conclusion of each tour enable everyone to voice their views on the tours and suggest improvements. Our trainers together with museum education staff collaboratively arrange the final museum tour, employing the techniques from the training program.

The final tour process starts when participants step out of a car or bus when they arrive at the museum and ends when they leave the museum. We predict as many barriers as possible and predict and identify toilets, elevators, and other vital elements. A bench or several stools placed in front of the artwork not only improves comfort but also makes the situation more legible and understandable for participants; prepared seating indicate the artwork that will be viewed by the group. Tour leaders focus on discussion topics that stimulate emotional memories and increase feelings of competence.

A final set of preinauguration tours is carried out to test the actual program in action. Much like a ship's shake-down cruise before the ship is officially commissioned for its maiden voyage, each museum inaugurates and carries out this pilot program to work out the bugs in the program with participants whom we recruit from local Alzheimer's Association early stage support groups, Adult Day Health programs, and assisted living and skilled nursing home facilities. Final program modifications are based on these pilot tours. Generally, programs are officially inaugurated with attendant local and national publicity.

We present an *ARTZ Certificate of Museum Training* to the museum after successful completion of the program and invite staff to register for the annual follow-up in order to train new staff, update staff on the latest evaluation methodologies, learn from other members, and generally maintain high quality tours.

Research and Evaluation

If museum programs such as these and others are to become established as both treatment for symptoms and ways for those early in the Alzheimer's journey to slow its progression, research demonstrating outcomes, not just participant satisfaction, will be necessary. If all museums were to employ the same evaluation methodology, an effective and compelling critical mass of data could be generated. Unfortunately ARTZ can only guarantee that its member museums cooperate on evaluations. A commitment to take part in ongoing evaluation of the visits is part of the agreement with museums who take part in this program. A standardized questionnaire is distributed to museum participants in the training, and to family members who take part in the test tours. The elements that make the final tour program an established part of the museum's repertoire are cataloged and news clippings that demonstrate the public outreach effects of this program are tracked. The tours are videotaped and the videos analyzed to establish measures of engagement, attention, and affect of those living with Alzheimer's who attend the museum tours. Care partners and tour observers also fill out the *ARTZ Stigma Questionnaire* which identifies any changes in attitudes that may occur during the tour process.

This process evaluates the art experience not only on those living with Alzheimer's but also equally on the educators and the public. The effects of implementing such a project encourages, among other things, questioning preconceived and stereotyped ideas that people have about the illness – tested with the ARTZ Stigma Questionnaire. Observing the museum tours demonstrates that those living with Alzheimer's can understand the world around them, communicate appropriately, participate openly in such an activity, and can remember it.

Museum Educator and Activity Director Observations

We pay close attention to direct feedback from museum educators and activity directors. The following quotes are from feedback questionnaires they have filled out:

> As they look at art and start responding to what they see, we are able to get a sense of who they are. I recall a man looking at a maritime painting and talking about the seaside town he grew up in and the history of whaling he had learned from living there.
>
> As someone who works in an art museum I believe that art has the power to transform someone's life. It is amazing when you can see how looking at and talking about art provides an avenue to successful engagement and conversation that is completely different from what one might expect from someone with Alzheimer's disease.
>
> A memory that particularly stands out occurred during the first pilot tour. Upon arriving at the sculpture Two Big Black Hearts by Jim Dine, one of the tour participants immediately rose from his wheelchair to feel the sculpture. The surfaces of these two large heart sculptures are filled with relief representations of objects symbolizing the artist's passions, many of which are tools (saws, hammers, wrenches, etc.). This particular tour participant was noticeably drawn to the tools of this sculpture, as he rose and wrapped his hands around the base of the hammer.
>
> People (residents) had more of a normal affect at the museum, they socialized, got excited, and were so happy – it's a place of honor. It honors their past and their intellect.

The "It Takes a Village" Project

"It takes a village to live with Alzheimer's." No one individual can successfully cope with the daunting challenges of raising a child, dealing with addiction, or generally navigating through life without the assistance of neighbors, friends, and the community in which they live. The same is true for coping with the journey of Alzheimer's. The "It Takes a Village" Project creates networked community-based Alzheimer's-competent arts and culture venues that collectively provide once-a-week events in a region or city where people at all stages of Alzheimer's and their care partners can access arts and culture community resources 52-weeks a year.

The "It Takes a Village™" Project links numerous arts and culture offerings in a geographic area, trains each to be Alzheimer's-competent, and provides programs specially designed for people living with Alzheimer's disease and related dementias. "It Takes a Village" schedules events at these venues at the same time and day of the week on a weekly basis (one event at one partner's setting each week, not one event per venue each week), publicizes this network to the Alzheimer's community, and establishes a reservations and transportation system to link those in need with the opportunities presented

Success of "It Takes a Village" Projects to Date

Since 2003, ARTZ has piloted the "It Takes a Village" Project in New York City with venues including museums, the circus, the cinema, and a poetry club, all of which are regularly attended by people living with Alzheimer's, loved ones, care partners, and healthcare staff. Other venues in NYC – a cabaret, an improvisational theater group, a musical group, and a sports club – are being recruited as new "It Takes a Village" Partners.

In Massachusetts, the ARTZ Museum Network is a de facto "It Takes a Village" program. Each of the five established museums all within half an hour of Boston partners with ARTZ to offer a specially designed museum tour for people living with Alzheimer's on Thursday mornings at 10 a.m. each week 52 weeks of the year.

"It Takes a Village" Program Partners

Each "It Takes a Village" Program comprises several arts and culture centers within a given region or city, each of which has a specialization – café discussion, sports, historical or art museum, music, theater, film, and so on. Each center offers a program 5 times a year the same time of day and day of the week ensuring a diversity of choice and frequent opportunities for participation. If fewer Partners join an "It Takes a Village" Project in a particular geographic area, each holds an event more frequently. With more Partners, parallel events are held at the same time, offering greater choice and opportunity.

"It Takes a Village" arts and culture settings	
Museum/gallery	Classroom/university
Cinema	Park/nature preserve
Conversation Café	Sports event
Live theater	Golf club (putting green)
Poetry Café	Circus and the Vaudeville arts
Comedy club	Fitness center
Cabaret	Zoo
Music/concert	Improvisational theater
Dance performance	

A Local Organizational Partner

When the ARTZ "It Takes a Village" Project forms an organizational partnership with an established local Alzheimer's service organization in a region or a city, efforts of participant recruitment, publicity to members of the Alzheimer's Community, and so on can be shared rather than duplicated.

Expected Measurable Outcomes and Evaluation

Based on our experience in New York and Boston, and on the research we and others have carried out, it is clear that programs like "It Takes a Village" can measurably improve quality of life for participants by reducing social isolation, depression, and care giver burnout. In addition, the more public and publicized the program is, the more public stigma surrounding the condition and disability of Alzheimer's and related dementias is reduced. Outcomes for each event can be measured in two ways: improvements in degree of engagement, focus of attention, use of language, and mood; and reduction of negative behaviors – apathy, anxiety, agitation, and aggression. Cooperative and systematic evaluation of programs like the "It Takes a Village" Project needs to be part of each program, as it needs to be part of each museum program.

Ladder to the Moon

> Drama grabs the attention of people living with Alzheimer's, both when they are part of a theater audience and when they are acting in plays. Drama conveys feelings and ideas more forcefully than any formal lecture can.
>
> John Zeisel, "I'm Still Here"

I first encountered the Ladder to the Moon Theatre Company (LTTM) in the fall of 2009 while consulting on an arts and Alzheimer's initiative in Barnet, a borough in North London. The goals of this remarkable program are to:

- Increase residents' self-esteem by empowering them to think creatively and influence what happens within each performance.
- Alleviate isolation by facilitating socialization among other residents, staff, and performers.
- Enable staff to deliver the highest standard of care by accomplishing the following:
  - To see the residents in a totally "new light," aka as normal people who have potential and the ability to contribute creatively and to engage in relationships.
  - Increase staff's self-confidence and a sense of camaraderie.
  - Improve empathy and communication skills with residents.
  - To see themselves as part of a community that is on equal footing with the persons living with dementia, administrators, family members, etc.
  - Giving staff and visitors alike, a positive shared experience that they can relive with the residents.

Along with ARTZ cofounder John Zeisel, I met with Chris Gage, the LTTM Artistic Director, at the October Gallery in London. At Chris' invitation I attended my first LTTM event at a skilled nursing facility located on the outskirts of the city. The facility itself was not impressive – just your basic, run-of-the-mill nursing home model, with linoleum floors, bad lighting, and that certain smell that one often associates with such places. I entered a large common area to find about 30 elderly residents in a wide circle. Also in the room were care staff, nurses, and in the middle of it all, two actors dressed in full Shakespearean splendor. What I saw over the next 60 or so minutes was one of the most joyful, uplifting, and creative programs I have ever witnessed.

Before the production began, I had time to talk with and mingle with the residents who would be attending the LTTM performance. Most of these individuals, (who unsuspectingly turned out to be participants/performers within the production) were in wheelchairs, had difficulty in maintaining coherent conversation, and could loosely be defined as having "advanced dementia." As soon as the LTTM production began in this common room without a stage at the eye level of each resident/participant, there was an instantaneous change in the room. The actors, performing a scene from Shakespeare, began speaking to the residents/participants – addressing them cordially and with a tinge of the dramatic – developing awareness within the room that something "special" was going on. A hushed silence came over the residents/participants, along with a level of concentration and focus on the performance already underway. Within 5 min, the actors had found ways to incorporate their lines and the story itself with the reactions and comments from the participants. I write "participants" now, as the individuals with dementia ceased to be mere residents observing a show. Each person was contributing, whether it was holding a small light-weight flag, or an elderly gentleman kissing the hand of the female performer who held it out to him. There was intense laughter and interplay among the participants, and the actors no matter what was said or shouted out to them were always able to improvise and work each of the participant's contributions into the performance. It was completely failure-free and the concept of time seemed to simply vanish; as is often the case when people living with Alzheimer's (and those without Alzheimer's) are completely "in the moment" and not focusing on the struggle to merely get by, minute by minute.

An outsider watching this group would not have the impression that any of these people were cognitively impaired because there was such a high level of competence, humor, and social interplay for that one magic hour – especially when contrasted with the period before the performance began. During the performance, the room was full of people experiencing life – human beings simply being human. Why? The symptoms related to Alzheimer's and related dementias were not "tested" during that period. If the symptoms do not manifest, the disease does not appear; the disease fades into the background and the person and their self-identity come to the forefront. When these moments happen, it is as though "there is no Alzheimer's in the room." No pill or any type of Alzheimer's drug presently available can match these effects.

The Ladder to the Moon Process

Professional actors trained in relationship-theater by the LTTM Theatre Company perform the plays with residents with dementia, all of whom become participants and each of whom has a part in the performance. Some people have more significant roles and others have supporting roles, such as holding a flag or a tambourine. Performances take place in a common space where the residents/audience can be at eye level with the actors. The play itself is very malleable – all of the props fit into a suitcase and the scenery is minimalist to the extreme – letting the play be performed in a large living room or a small theater. The plays are written and chosen according to their ability to bring about audience participation and self-expression. All the plays Ladder performs involve content rich in emotional expression. Although people living with Alzheimer's disease undergo a cognitive decline, it is worth noting that there is a growing body of research that suggests that certain cognitive capacities, such as perception/emotional intelligence and artistic interpretation, can actually be enhanced (Basting & Killick, 2003). Residents/participants are therefore very much "in tune" with the play and its essence.

The level of participation varies according to each participant's abilities and desire to contribute. Before each performance, the actors dressed in street clothes meet with the staff and are introduced to the residents/participants who will be attending the play later on. This gives the staff and the actors a chance to assess residents for different roles in the play. Once chosen, that particular resident becomes one of the characters already written into the play.

When the actors enter the home, they proceed to a large common room where most of the residents spend their time. They start by putting on music and begin to dress the space with decorations hanging from the ceiling and on the walls. At this point, they begin to introduce themselves to the residents and explain that a play will be starting soon.

When the residents are seated in a circle, the actors return to the room dressed in costume and hop right into the play. They start to perform in character and slowly introduce those in the room to the other characters – residents to whom they assign roles. They don't so much ask if someone would like to be "Prince Charming," but instead address the resident as "Prince Charming" and his reaction tells them whether or not he accepts the role. This method of assigning roles continues throughout the play as new characters are introduced. Both actors and residents playing roles remain in character throughout the entire performance.

As the play progresses, the actors serve as the string that keeps all the conversation in the room connected as well as keeps the play moving forward. They speak with each resident and involve everyone in the room including staff and some family members. Some residents refuse to be involved in the beginning, but the actors reapproach them so that by the end of the play, most everyone is involved.

The actors also pass out props. LTTM actors find that residents/participants truly enjoy wearing a crown, or holding "an infant." The props, although small and inexpensive, add much life to the play helping residents step into their character. For instance, one gentleman playing a king with a crown addressed the queen a number of times, simply because she was also wearing a crown. When the actors change their hats or put on a bracelet during a scene change, they ask the residents to help them.

The actors direct attention to the different residents, and with the exception of a handful of "scripted" conversations they take what the residents say and address their words and actions in the context of the play. This happens too with residents repeating their role after that scene has passed. For instance one woman, asked to "look after this child until she is grown," got up and started dancing with the baby/doll. As the play went on, another resident/participant was assigned to be the "grown child." At this point, the lady with the baby began dancing again and the actors just danced with her proclaiming "there has been another baby!"

The play ends with a finale, in which everyone in the room takes part, each holding a prop – a flag, a light musical instrument, or a hat. When the play ends, the professional actors take a bow and present each character in turn, encouraging everyone to applaud. As the professional actors undress the room, the music comes back on and the residents continue to talk and laugh together.

Chris Gage, Ladder to the Moon's Executive and Artistic Director, stresses the importance of evaluating the programs he develops. In partnership with the London School of Economics, the Public Engagement Foundation, and the University of Bath – overseen by Naidoo Associates – Ladder is evaluating the social and economic impact of the plays on the residential care homes and the individuals who live and work there. The data from their original work, evaluated by Maria Parsons from the Oxford Research Association, has been published through the Central and Cecil Housing Trust, in London (Parsons & Naidoo Associates, 2009).

Cinema

In partnership with the New York City-based Tribeca Film Institute and the Coolidge Corner Theatre Foundation in Boston, ARTZ has produced a cinematic educational program specifically designed for people living with Alzheimer's and related memory loss. *Meet Me at the Movies...and Make Memories*™ was first performed at the Tribeca Cinema in 2007 and features iconic film clips specifically selected to prompt long-term memories and self-awareness in individuals living with Alzheimer's and their family members and partners.

This program gives those living with memory loss an expressive outlet and forum for dialog by viewing preselected film scenes, immediately followed by group discussion. Volunteers from ARTZ work with audience members to engage in reminiscence and to highlight themes, such as family, love, the Great Depression, World War II, and Old Hollywood. Focusing in depth on icons from Hollywood's Golden Age, the program includes performances by legendary stars Jimmy Stewart, Humphrey Bogart, Judy Garland, and Lucille ball among others. During the film programs, people seem to thrive and achieve a greater sense of selfhood, and their partners experience this as well.

With my colleague and ARTZ cofounder John Zeisel, we developed this program by conducting focused group interviews with potential participants to determine which films would most resonate with the audience. Volunteers acting as ushers and welcomers are given special training to learn about the effects of Alzheimer's and to develop specific approaches to keep participants' attention focused.

This replicable cinematic treatment program for people living with Alzheimer's disease appears to reduce anxiety, agitation, aggression, and apathy through reminiscence and image recognition. The program has been performed successfully for over 4 years at senior centers, theaters, universities, Community Centers, Adult Day programs, and assisted living residences. Before and after each of ten 4-min film clips projected during the performance, two "guides" on stage gently coax memories, opinions, and feelings from the audience, leading to increased focus of attention and engagement.

Evaluation of the program has employed two main methods: Focus groups of participants with Alzheimer's at Alzheimer's adult day and assisted living programs in New York City and Massachusetts, and postperformance group interviews with program staff. These methods have demonstrated the effectiveness of each film clip and helped to fine-tune and shape subsequent performances.

Poetry

The Alzheimer's Poetry Project and its founder Gary Glazner pioneered poetry events for people living with Alzheimer's. Since 2007, in collaboration with Gary, ARTZ has held public poetry events at the Bowery Poetry Club in New York City. Participants come from assisted living memory programs, skilled nursing centers, Adult Day centers, and private homes throughout the city. Some take part reciting their own original works or poems that are their favorites – the ones that spark memories and draw upon their emotional "self." Others watch actively as ARTZ/NY Coordinator Lauren Volkmer, Gary's students, and Gary perform. Gary generally facilitates the process, leading participants and attendees in group readings, group poetry writing, conversations, discussion, and interactive performance. There is something special about hosting these programs in "real" settings. When participants arrive at the Bowery Poetry Club on second Avenue just north of Houston Street in Manhattan, their brains recognize that this is a performance space. The sights, the smells, the lighting, and the stage all provide environmental "cues" they understand – allowing the persons living with Alzheimer's to "know" where they are. And when they know where they are and what their role is there (which we emphasize and remind them), they cease to exhibit many of the symptoms related to Alzheimer's. They simply become a person attending and participating in a cultural event leading to an increase in self-confidence, expression, and a willingness to communicate their feelings and opinions.

Lauren Volkmer, who began her affiliation with ARTZ back in 2004 as a volunteer poet and Artist-in-Residence, clearly sees the difference between the Bowery Poetry Club performances and readings inside a residence. The in-house readings are usually small groups – six people or so in a small familiar room. The public events, produced in collaboration with Gary Glazner and the Alzheimer's Poetry Project, can have as many as 40 people in a space they are not used to but with sensory clues as to what this room is. There is colorful art, dim lighting, and exposed brick walls. There are small café tables and chairs grouped around them. There is a stage with a microphone – what happens on that stage? There is soft music coming through the speakers. This is a creative environment, a place where people come to talk and share ideas. There may be some anxiety as the person becomes accustomed to this environment, she says, and adds that staff and family members can ease the anxiety by talking reassuringly about why everyone is there and what will be happening. Some people may be worried that something out of the ordinary will be expected of them. They need to be reassured that they are here to be entertained and involved in a failure-free creative process.

Gary's model of poetry performance is a musical one. He emphasizes rhythm and high-energy interaction with the audience. He uses call-and-response techniques and encourages participation in the form of assembling a "group poem," with suggestions from the audience around a specific prompt (Glazner, 2005). People living with Alzheimer's become extremely engaged during his performances, especially when he takes their hands in his and sways to the rhythm of the poetry. He recognizes and uses their strengths and remaining abilities. At a recent event, Lauren brought in a large print, short version of famous poems. Those who were able stood up and read the lines aloud. The rest of the participants echoed the lines back, call-and-response style. Looking around, Lauren reports she saw smiling, engaged faces: proud of their accomplishments, not focused on their impairments. Mission accomplished!

In this country, schoolchildren used to be required to memorize and recite poetry. Families often shared poetry with each other and it was far more of a national pastime than it seems to be today. For those who were already familiar with a certain poem, like Joyce Kilmer's "Trees," the rhythm and rhyme of the poem seem to share a similar retrieval method as familiar music. Time after time Lauren has read famous poems aloud and has seen people living with Alzheimer's who could not tell you what they had for breakfast, or even what they were doing 20 min ago, spontaneously recite lines along with her. They tend to brighten up when this happens – there is a sense of pride that they can remember these words and a comfort in hearing them spoken aloud.

Other poems that may not have been memorized but still contain vivid imagery and repetition, like "Sea-Fever," tend to elicit more reactions during discussion. "Has anyone been sailing? What did it feel like? Did you want to do it again?" Other poems tell a story, like the baseball poem "Casey at the Bat." Some people resonate with beloved poems that they read to their own children when they were young, such as "The Owl and the Pussycat." Those who were not born and educated in this country or whose first language is not English might not have been exposed to these particular poems previously, so poems in their native language or English-language poems with strong imagery and straightforward language work best. The most important thing to remember is that the choice of poetry, like all interactions with people living with Alzheimer's, must be individualized. It depends on that person's interests, education, and family history. Generally, through trial and error and, if necessary, with input from staff and family members, you will find something that they enjoy and can respond to.

Lauren Volkmer's recommended poetry list	
Wynken, Blynken, and Nod	Field
I Wandered Lonely as a Cloud	Wordsworth
I Hear America Singing	Whitman
Sonnet #18	Shakespeare
Sea-Fever	Masefield
The Arrow and the Song	Longfellow
The Owl and the Pussycat	Lear
The New Colossus	Lazarus
The Road Not Taken	Frost
Stopping by Woods on a Snowy Evening	Frost
I'm Nobody—Who Are You?	Dickinson
How Do I Love Thee?	Browning
The Tiger	Blake
He Wishes for the Cloths of Heaven	Yeats
The House with Nobody in It	Kilmer
Trees	Kilmer
In Flanders Fields	McRae

Circus and the Vaudeville Arts

Since 2006, ARTZ has had the pleasure to partner with the world renowned Big Apple Circus (BAC). The program began with a pilot group of five participants with Alzheimer's in Massachusetts, when the BAC was performing in downtown Boston.

Along with BAC founder Paul Binder and ARTZ cofounder John Zeisel, I attended the performance with the pilot group and witnessed the positive impact the vaudeville acts made on the demeanor of participants. Initially, before the project began, we had trepidation regarding whether a 2-h performance was too long. There is a widely held belief that people with mid to late-stage Alzheimer's have difficulty with concentration and that most art and culture experiences should be limited to 1 h. Our plan for the pilot performance in Boston was that we would leave during intermission after 1 h – in the event that participants showed a lack of attention and focus. What we observed, however, was that attention, focus, and level of engagement were sustained during the entire show. A sense of anticipation, joy, and excitement ran throughout the 2 h even during intermission. Participants recalled memories from their own childhood, as well as times when they took their own children to the circus.

Since that first pilot performance in 2006, the BAC has annually donated tickets to circus events at their permanent NYC location at Lincoln Center. ARTZ coordinates travel, arranges seating based on physical and cognitive issues, and has trained staff at each event to respond to participants' needs. A similar circus event was held at Cirque du Monde in Paris with residents of Hospital Bretonneau, with similar increases in focus of attention and attention span. Each circus event now serves about 40 participants living with Alzheimer's and their care partners and family members from all over New York. One of the reasons ARTZ sought out the BAC as a partner is that the Circus' programming and mission go beyond the boundaries of mere entertainment, crossing into the realm of healing and self-discovery through other programs like their Clown Doctors program in pediatric hospitals.

Summary

In sum, arts and cultural events are now increasingly being made available to people living with dementia. The positive results are clearly observable. A great deal more research is needed to demonstrate that these results are generalizable to others, so that societal change can come about obliterating the stigma surrounding Alzheimer's and dementia that dominates in society today. The cultural and arts programs that the Hearthstone Alzheimer's Foundation and its Artists for Alzheimer's® program have developed are just a start. We have been fortunate to develop programs at museums, cinemas, poetry clubs, theaters, and circuses in cooperation with other adventuresome mission-driven organizations. Many of these, primarily the museum programs, have been adopted by other organizations not only in North America but also throughout Europe, Australia, and beyond. While parts of Fable City actually exist in many real cities, unfortunately Fable City is not fully realized anywhere – yet.

References

Basting, A., & Killick, J. (2003). *The arts and dementia care: A resource guide*. Brooklyn: The National Center for Creative Aging.

Glazner, G. (2005). *Sparking memories: The Alzheimer's poetry project anthology*. Santa Fe: Poem Factory.

MachPherson, S., Bird, M., Anderson, K., Davis, T., & Blaire, A. (2009). An art gallery access programme for people with dementia: "You do it for the moment". *Aging & Mental Health, 13*(5), 744–752.

Parsons, M., & Naidoo Associates. (2009). *Over the moon: Effectiveness of using interactive drama in a dementia care setting*. London: London Centre for Dementia Care, University College London, for Central & Cecil Housing Trust of London.

Stevens, M., & Swan, A. (2004). *De Kooning: An American master*. New York: Alfred A. Knopf.

Zeisel, J. (2009). *I'm still here: A breakthrough approach to understanding someone living with Alzheimer's*. New York: Penguin/Avery Books.

Chapter 20
The Songwriting Works™ Model: Enhancing Brain Health and Fitness Through Collaborative Musical Composition and Performance

Judith-Kate Friedman

Abstract The author began developing the Songwriting Works™ method 20 years ago. More than 3,000 older adults across the cognitive spectrum have participated to date; they have composed and performed more than 300 songs. This chapter outlines basic principles of the Songwriting Works model and the practices through which its outcomes are fostered and measured. Case studies illustrate impacts of the collective songwriting experience within culturally and cognitively diverse communities. Research underlying and supporting Songwriting Works' methodology, including Dr. Theresa Allison's music's study of the model in a skilled nursing context, is cited. Implications and applications are explored.

Introduction: The Music of Being Human

Beauty's Reflection

It is a spring day at an Alzheimer's day center. Twelve elders are gathered for a songwriting session, seated in a circle opposite a large easel. The facilitator is in the middle, colored markers in hand, guitar at the ready, leading discussion. A man begins to reminisce about holidays. Soon the group is alive with memories: family vacations, honeymoons, and adventures. Conversation turns to Hawai'i, a place where many have traveled. "Ah," a woman says, her face lighting up. She has been quiet and apparently disoriented for most of the hour and now speaks for the first time. She describes the beauty of that place; how much

---

J.K. Friedman (✉)
Songwriting Works™ Educational Foundation, 2023 East Sims Way #271,
Port Townsend, WA 98368, USA
e-mail: director@songwritingworks.org

she loves it. The facilitator sings her words back to her. The woman grins, widely: "I don't know who said that" she says, " – but I sure do feel that way!" The group sings together, weaving a chorus, threading each other's stories into song. (Friedman, 2004)[1]

Music is a full-bodied experience and a whole-nervous system activity; it involves nearly every part of the brain (Parsons, 2009). As such, it belongs in any "use it or lose it" cognitive fitness and health program. Music aids in cognition. It sparks memories *and* new ideas, and helps sustain brain function as it builds social *and* neurological relationships. Humans are built to engage musically. The importance of developing musical intelligence in young minds (Gruhn & Rauscher, 2002; Rauscher, 2001; Weinberger, 1998) continues to the very end of life, even for those whose ability to think and communicate is limited by brain illness or injury (Allison, 2010; Sacks, 2007). Older adults who regularly participate in step-by-step learning with music professionals, in a community of peers, experience significant increases in their physical, mental, emotional, and social health (Cohen et al., 2006). Family caregivers and their loved ones with dementia report greater satisfaction and communication when they are making music together (Clair & Ebberts, 1996).

Songwriting Works™: Enhancing Brain Health Through Song

I've never sung before in my life and now I'm singing. –E.N., age 90 (participant, 2001)[2]

Songwriting Works™ is a collective musical experience that springs from the Oral Tradition. It starts with the premise that all human beings are inherently intelligent, musical, and cooperative and that making one's own music is a healthy, normal part of biological as well as cultural expression (Hodges, 2000; Wallin, Merker, & Brown, 2000). In the United States today, listening to music – rather than originating it – has become the norm. Yet over the course of history, in all times and places, singing and "making up tunes" has occupied a central, if not pervasive, function in human life very much as musical intelligence has occupied a distinct role in human cognition (Gardner, 1983). When the experience of collectively composing songs – integrating original thought, feeling, words, melodies, and rhythms – is reintroduced, the results can be transformative. As medical doctor and ethnomusicologist Theresa Allison concluded in her 9-month study of Songwriting Works: "Songwriting in the nursing home is not a mere activity – it is an opportunity for intellectual, artistic, relational and spiritual growth. As such, it fosters a real sense of neighborhood and transcends the artificiality of the institutional life." (Allison, 2008).

---

[1] *From a workshop held at Senior Access' Corte Madera Alzheimer's Day Program, 1995. Senior Access was a Songwriting Works partner site between 1994 and 1999 (Marin Arts Council). A version of this story appeared in different form in Friedman, 2004, Freeing the voice within, op. cit.*

[2] Erna Neubauer speaking to filmmaker Nathan Friedkin in his documentary "A 'Specially Wonderful Affair." (Friedkin Digital, 2002). The film tells the story of the making of the Jewish Home elders' debut CD "Island on a Hill" during the week of September 11, 2001. www.fdigital. net link: documentary.

Access to Musicality

> Those who didn't know they could, collaborate with energy they didn't know they had.
>
> Marcia Perlstein M.S.W. L.M.F.T.[3]

Songwriting Works began as an artist-in-residence project serving ethnically diverse communities of elders[4] through Artworks (now CEYA: Center for Elders and Youth in the Arts) at San Francisco's Institute on Aging in affiliation with Mt. Zion/UCSF hospital with funding from the California Arts Council.[5] Artworks' then-director Robert Rice informed Songwriting Works' methodology in terms of authenticity: if an experience were to be compelling for participants and sustaining for the artists leading it, the process would need to ignite the imagination and passion of both. Rice trained his artists to find their own esthetic voice *in service* to the collective. He taught that songs (and other works of art) created in this way have equal benefit for their makers and for all who hear them.[6]

> You help humanity be themselves by putting a lilt on it.
>
> D.H., age 87[7]

Each year, hundreds of older adults, family/kinship caregivers, and professionals in arts and health care participate in Songwriting Works' collective song composition and performance workshops. To date, more than 3,000 have composed 300 songs. Songwriting Works Educational Foundation now operates as a nonprofit organization based in Port Townsend, WA, and offers workshops, trainings, and concerts internationally. In 2009, with support from the National Endowment for the Arts, Songwriting Works launched a facilitator certification training program for professional songwriters and a pilot program in which caregivers and their loved ones wrote songs together (see Case Study 3). In 2010–2011, in conjunction with the Washington Health Foundation, Songwriting Works is developing music-for-wellness tools to give homebound elders, families, and music lovers of all ages increased access to making original music.[8]

---

[3] Marcia Perlstein, psychotherapist and member of Songwriting Works Olympic Peninsula elders advisory council, stating her observations of Songwriting Works in a 2008 letter of support for funding.

[4] Songwriting Works uses the honoric "elder" to refer to any participant over the age of 60.

[5] The author founded and developed the Songwriting Works method between 1990 and 1997, first as California Arts Council artist-in-residence at Artworks (1989–1992 CEYA: http://ceya.ioaging.org/) and then through a series of Marin Arts Council grant projects (1994–1999).

[6] Robert Rice, a painter, dancer, teacher and visionary advocate for the arts and spirituality in healthcare, served as director of the San Francisco Institute on Aging's Artworks program from 1986 to 1991. The author trained with Rice as part of Artworks' California Arts Council artists-in-residence team of professional musicians, painters, actors, poets, textile artists, dancers and vaudevillians. Twenty years later, most of these artists continue working with elder adults. Rice passed away in 2008 at the age of 71. *This chapter is dedicated to him, with gratitude.*

[7] Artworks client, testimonial 1991.

[8] For more information on Songwriting Works' Facilitator Certification and other trainings for arts and health professionals and family caregivers contact: http://www.songwritingworks.org/programs/training.htm.

I've always been a 'listener' – I found out that I can be a singer, too.

L.W., age 88[9]

Inclusion Is Key

Twenty percent of Songwriting Works' workshops are held in community locations with a majority of well and cognitively alert older and elder adults; 5% of these programs are broadly multigenerational.[10] Eighty percent of workshops take place in healthcare settings (skilled nursing, dementia care, gero-psych, adult day programs) and continuing care residential communities (retirement, independent and assisted living). In these, participants are average age 87; 90% have some level of physical disability; 70–85% have some degree of memory loss or cognitive impairment due to neurodegenerative disease including early through later-stage Alzheimer's and other dementias, poststroke aphasia, apraxia, Parkinson's, Multiple Sclerosis, brain injury, and depression.

> The woodpecker knocks at the door of our dullness and awakens us into life through our ears.
>
> Robert Rice (2008)

Songwriting Works' organizational structure mirrors its programmatic commitment to inclusion, reciprocity, and honoring each voice: An *advisory council of elders* oversees project design ensuring community relevance. *Professional songwriter-performers* are trained and certified to facilitate workshops with *elders and families*. *Arts, health and aging services partners* host and publicize events within their communities. Sessions are digitally documented and analyzed in collaboration with *researchers in medicine, gerontology, public health, arts, and aging*. Workshop series culminate in *community celebrations* where participants share their songs. Those who are able, perform. Those who were not a part of songwriting may join their friends in performance. These events give elders and families new ways to be heard and seen, to leave legacies, and to raise public awareness (and funds).

International Audiences

Once composed, songs reach international audiences through publications, film, broadcast media, and the internet. Inclusion is also part of the publication experience. For example: two dozen Singers & Songwriters of the Jewish Home San Francisco formed a production steering committee for their "Island on a Hill" debut CD. With mentors, they juried songs, suggested musical arrangements, auditioned

---

[9] Jewish Home participant, testimonial 2007.
[10] Most all Songwriting Works events span ages 50–100. The 5% figure reflects youth-specific participation in workshops where ages 5 to 100+ years compose songs. Three and even four generations may participate together.

for parts, gave interviews to press, rehearsed, sang and recorded stories behind the songs, and provided input into mixing the record.[11] They then performed with guest artists in concert and in Nathan Friedkin's documentary "A 'Specially Wonderful Affair," (Friedkin, 2002) and received a standing ovation from an audience of 900 at its San Francisco Jewish Film Festival premiere (Ford, 2002).[12] Songwriting Works' program and publications have won awards[13] and sparked new collaborations including a sacred music composition program – Psalms, Songs & Stories™ (see below) – and the Jewish Home's comedy clinic.[14]

> The lyrics did some cathartic mending of places deep in my heart.
>
> Jonathan Toste[15]

At Any Age, in Any Rhythm: The Songwriting Works™ Experience

> The impact of the songs goes beyond the individual to contribute to a higher standard of care.
>
> Kelly Philpott Brisbois[16]

Musical Mural Painting

In the Songwriting Works model each participant has a voice. As in a mural or quilting project, every song contains unique elements that contributors recognize as their own while the whole serves as a portrait of community. Professional songwriter-facilitators use the same framework, materials and principles for all groups,

---

[11] The "Island on a Hill" (2002, Jewish Home/Composing Together Works) CD project was funded by the Jewish Home of San Francisco's board of trustees, under the leadership of Peter E. Rosenberg and Dr. Emanuel Friedman. The Marcus Music Fund, a named fund of the Jewish Home, provided a significant gift toward this effort. Additional funding was provided by the family and friends of Betty Ginsberg and by the California Arts Council as part of Judith-Kate Friedman's artist-in-residence year.

[12] The film premiered at the San Francisco Jewish Film Festival, Castro theater, August 2002.

[13] Program awards include the MetLife/American Society MindAlert Award (2007), and the Society for the Arts in Healthcare Blair Sadler International Healing Arts Award (2008). Publication awards include Just Plain Folks International Best Song, Jewish Music category (2004) and Best Video (2006).

[14] Comic and Comedy Producer Lisa Geduldig met Esther Weintraub, then 87 through Weintraub's performance in "A Specially Wonderful Affair" (Friedkin, 2002). Their legendary friendship sparked Geduldig's founding of a Comedy Clinic at the Jewish Home and Weintraub's finding new audiences as a stand-up comic. See, Geduldig's film, "Esther and Me" (2010).

[15] Testimonial, Jonathan Toste, benefit concert host, 2005.

[16] Testimonial, Kelly Philpott Brisbois, oral historian and past president of Eldercare Advocates of Marin, 1999.

irrespective of an individual's cognitive, physical or verbal ability, their educational background, language, culture, knowledge of songwriting, prior participation, or even mood. The intention is to write a memorable song that is easy to sing, yet sophisticated and emotionally potent enough to sustain repeated listening and group attention. A good song will satisfy *both* the most alert and discerning *and* the cognitively challenged. The prospect of sharing their completed work further serves to increase participants' empowerment.

Facilitators set a tone of collective musical discovery creating a "failure free zone." Groups sit in a circle around a white board or flip chart. Musical instruments – guitar, mandolin, harp, piano – are at hand. First-time groups warm-up by singing a familiar tune; ongoing groups sing their most recent song or one in progress. Those present who helped write the song are acknowledged, even if they do not recall their participation. Those who hesitate or claim they are "not creative" are invited to listen and *give an opinion*. There are no wrong answers. Fear, judgment, and competition are dispelled. Individuals are encouraged as they find multiple ways to solve a collective puzzle: *to compose a song strong enough to carry a message they deem important, interesting or beautiful.*

Cognitive Playground

In cognitive terms, this experience stimulates neurogenesis, dendritic sprouting and glial cell formation through multiregion brain function, free associations, memory retrieval, and meaningful social interaction (Cohen, 2005a, 2005b). Songs take shape in the course of conversation. Idiom, whimsy, melody, and meaning arise spontaneously through storytelling, improvisation and life review. Participants direct all artistic decisions. They may determine musical genres in advance ("Let's write a Polka!" "My favorite is Country & Western") or one person's spoken cadence (rhythmic phrase) may suggest a tradition such as gospel for "you can serve your God under your own fig tree" or klezmer for a Chanukah song. Facilitators stay true to participants' musical inflections, including those expressed through tapping feet or moving hands. Catchy, funny or poignant lines, and illuminating side comments are gathered verbatim and scribed for all to see. Words are recapped, sung, rhymed, and repeated. Pitch (note and key) changes – even in spoken speech (see Case Study 2, 3) – are recorded and re-sung. Rhythmic entrainment further increases neural connectivity and availability of expression, spirit, and thought.

> What have I learned? Can you put a count on a sunset?
>
> J.D., age 87[17]

The songs tell stories, true and imagined ("Dancing with the Daughter of a Flower Rancher," "Don't Forget Me"). They may collect reminiscences ("Summer," "The Jazz Age") or offer new views on love, peace, work, faith, and family. Time of

---

[17] Testimonial, Artworks participant, 1991.

year or day may inspire tributes to seasons, holidays, new grandchildren, or community events ("A Special Day for Moms," "the Butterfly Song" to celebrate a new garden[18]). Consensus on editing and polishing can be tested by vote but is more often revealed in bursts of laughter and excitement, nonplussed silence, or agitated boredom. Pleasing punch lines, melodic grooves or "hooks" send ripples of mutual agreement through a group. A communal 'yes' or 'aha!' follows a good story. Spontaneous unsolicited repetitions "stick," or parts are shed or adjusted when a majority unconsciously skip phrases or avoids less singable stumbling spots. An experienced elder may simply say "Enough! That's it! We're done!" Cultural preferences are always honored (Bartlett, Kaufman, & Smeltekop, 1993). Song styles have included folk, country, gospel, nueva cancion, rock, jazz, swing, and a choral cantata about WWII Homecoming (Case Study 3). The social context further boosts self-esteem, cognitive engagement, positive affect, and immune system response (Cohen et al., 2006; Glass, Mendes deLeon, Marottoli, & Berkman, 1999; Lachman & Weaver, 1998; Rodin, 1989).

Recipes for Heritage

> Through my experience as a facilitator in training, I have already witnessed the impact Songwriting Works has made on a regional level. I have seen painful edges softened between a father with dementia and his daughter as they cocreate together. I have witnessed women in their 90s revitalized by the participatory process of writing a song about cooking in the kitchen!
>
> Keeth Monta Apgar[19]

Gefilte Fish

On the psychiatric care unit at San Francisco's Jewish Home, a song about the Coney Island and Santa Cruz boardwalks leads a man to reminisce about the Long Beach pike, an amusement park from childhood.

> "Pike? What are you talking about the beach?" asks a man, originally from England. "A pike is a spear the guards carry at the Tower of London!"
>
> "Huh? A spear?" a woman, over the age of 100 laughs. "Pike? Is a fish! White fish! You use in making gefilte fish!"

So begins a series of sessions in which the group gathers and argues over proper recipes for the Jewish delicacy. One of the most buoyant composes the chorus:

---

[18] The Rosenberg Garden at San Francisco's Jewish Home. www.jhsf.org.
[19] Keeth Monta Apgar of the band Harmonica Pocket, apprentice facilitator, in a 2010 letter of support to funders.

> Gefilte fish, gefilte fish – There is no dish quite like it.
> If I could wish for any wish, I'd wish for some – gefilte fish!
>
> (Jewish Home and Composing Together Works, 1998)[20]

The song – a waltz – becomes a "hit" throughout the Home and later on film and CD. As significant, however, is a nurse's comment that the songwriting process has brought two elders, who normally have difficulty being in the same room, into the same conversation. (Friedman, 2004)

Chopped Liver

To open a first time songwriting session at the Inn, an assisted living residence at Madlyn and Leonard Abramson Center for Jewish Life near Philadelphia, the facilitator opens with a familiar Hebrew song about community. She then proposes the idea of songwriting by singing the "Gefilte Fish" song. In a moment of friendly East vs. West Coast rivalry, a woman sitting with her husband asks:

> Gefilte fish? They wrote it just like that? …Well if they can write a song about gefilte fish – WE can write a song about chopped liver!

The room erupts in laughter and clear consensus. By the end of the week they have written their first song, a Swing number called "A Forshpayz, A Machaya!" (An Appetizer, A Pleasure!), providing lessons in cooking and Yiddish:

> Gehakte leber means chopped liver,
> You can picnic on it by the river,
> Serve it with a Spanish radish,
> mit a bisl zaltz und feffer (salt and pepper),
> You'll be floating on… a… zephyr!
> …Put it on a platter, Put it in a knish –
> It really doesn't matter – This dish is delish…[21]
>
> (Composing Together Works and Friedman, 2005)

Most songwriting workshops begin with open-ended questions ("What would you like to write about today?" or the less abstract "What keeps you going?"). On occasion site staff, family, or overriding events may suggest a theme (i.e., "I'm 100 Years Old" in honor of a participant's birthday, "Para Siempre Queremos Paz/For All Time We Want Peace" at the start of the 1991 Gulf War).[22] Agencies may invite Songwriting Works to help address social issues:

---

[20] *Gefilte Fish ©1998, (P) 2002 Composing Together Works/Jewish Home. Words and music by elders of the Jewish Home San Francisco and Judith-Kate Friedman, California Arts Council artist-in-residence. All rights reserved. The song is performed by its composers on "Island on a Hill" CD (www.cdbaby.com) and in "A 'Specially Wonderful Affair." (www.fdigital.net, www.songwritingworks.org). A version of this story appeared in different form in Friedman (2004), Freeing the voice within, cited below.*

[21] *Elders at the Abramson Center's Inn (assisted living) and Residence (skilled nursing) composed 20 songs in 24 days over the course of a year long artist-in-residence project 2005–2006. A Forschpayz, A Machaya! © 2005 Composing Together Works. Words and music by elders of the Abramson Center for Jewish Life and Judith-Kate Friedman guest artist-in-residence. All rights reserved.*

[22] A full catalog of Songwriting Works songs is available on-line: www.songwritingworks.org.

Free at Last

It is early spring in San Francisco. A social worker wonders if songwriting might bridge a cultural gap at an adult day center where 50% are Russian-speaking Jewish immigrants from the former Soviet Union and 50% are elders of African heritage who came to the Bay Area from the Southern U.S. in the 1940s and 1950s. As she puts it "one can draw a line through the center of the room." Songwriting Works schedules four workshops in the weeks leading up to Passover and Easter. Working with a Russian interpreter, the facilitator opens with familiar Old Testament spirituals ("Go Down Moses" "Oh Mary Don't You Weep") then speaks to common themes of the season: freedom, springtime, and liberation. She interviews each person, zig-zagging between cultures: "Where are you from?" "Mississippi, Houston, Odessa...." "Why did you come to San Francisco?" "To work at the shipyards in WWII" "To escape from oppression" "To find new opportunities" "To leave bigotry" "To find a good life for my children" "We had only one light in our house, we were poor." As each hears their common experience, they compose a gospel song in Russian and English:

> The spirit of my people says we gotta be free, gotta be free, gotta be free at last.
>
> (Composing Together Works and Friedman, 1992)[23]

Research: Toward an Evidence-Based Model

> Creating and performing original songs improves quality of life and enables institutionalized elders to remain vibrant and creative despite the progression of physical and cognitive challenges.
>
> Dr. Theresa Allison (2008)

> Songwriting Works has resulted in quite dramatic improvement in depressive symptoms such as isolation, tearfulness and poor appetite. I am also convinced that it has helped stave off depression in individuals who are at very high risk.
>
> Dr. Jay Luxenberg (in Sadler and Ridenour, 2008)

In 2007, Theresa Allison, M.D., M.Music, studied the impact of Songwriting Works participation for elders residing in a skilled continuing care nursing home serving 420 older adults. She followed 40 elders, average age 87, over the course of 9 months in sacred and "secular" songwriting contexts, observing sessions with cognitively alert participants and those with early to later-stage dementia (Allison, 2008). At the time the study began, the author had been conducting Songwriting

---

[23] *The Spirit of My People (Gotta Be Free At Last)* © *1992 Composing Together Works. Words and Music by elders at Ruth Anne Rosenberg Center and Judith-Kate Friedman, California Arts Council artist-in-residence with Artworks/Institute on Aging. All rights reserved.*

Works for 8 years; and Psalms, Songs and Stories™ for 4 years (Marder, 2005).[24] More than 250 elders had participated and the aforementioned CD and film had been released.

Dr. Allison observed that participants with short-term memory deficits due to dementia retained words and music to the original songs that they and/or their community had collectively composed; their songs entered the repertoire of the institution. Even those with advanced cognitive decline were able to generate fresh, creative, memorable lyrics, melodies, images and word choices, and sing lines to the choruses of songs they helped compose without prompting (Allison, 2008, 2010). Repeated participation had demonstrated cumulative and lasting impact on cognition and socialization. Through songwriting, elders were able to break through isolation and forge new relationships. Their singing of original Psalms for the dedication of a new synagogue transformed institutional spaces (the synagogue, the Home) and their relationship to them.

> Songwriting provides [elders] an opportunity for the creation of heritage, the development of community, the ability to become productive and contributing members of the institutional village in which they reside. Through engagement in songwriting, elders tap into rich stores of memory, combine them with new skills and techniques, and produce tangible cultural products for dissemination within and outside the nursing home. In this way, they are able to transcend the boundaries of the institution both by bringing in memories and relationships that exist outside the physical space of the nursing home and by creating meaningful music that permeates the nursing home and also transcends it – being heard outside the physical space through professional recordings and live performances. ....
> Through physical products, concerts, memories, and moments of sacred transformation, the elders continue to grow and expand in ways quite unexpected in an institutional setting. To quote one of the songwriters: "It's life-long learning all the time."
>
> (Allison, 2008)

Singing into the Field: Other Research Supporting the Songwriting Works Model

> Creativity is our species' natural response to the challenges of human experience.
>
> Adriana Diaz (Diaz, Miller 2010)

> We're learning to treat diseases because we're learning to listen. Not only to our patients but to single cells in the brain. If we listen carefully, they tell us a story... How fast they're talking, the pattern of how they talk ...Each of us has many different subplots going on within our brain. Sometimes those subplots are not unfolding in such a way that they result in beneficial symptoms. We call that disease. ....We've learned that if we can disrupt this chatter and normalize it – we can improve disease. – Michael Okun
>
> (in Cavenaugh and Drewry, 2008)

It is an exciting time to be working at the crossroads of musical creativity and brain health. Research in diverse arenas of study and practice are converging as publications

---

[24] In 2003, the author and the Home's chaplain, Rabbi Sheldon Marder, founded and co-direct Psalms, Songs & Stories™ a program that blends the original Songwriting Works workshop model with intensive text study of Psalms. Collective songwriting becomes a means of reflecting upon the text and a doorway into pastoral care. See Rabbi Sheldon Marder, 2005.

of findings proliferate and filter into popular consciousness. Studies confirm the challenge of pinpointing complex levels of brain activity involved in vocal singing and musical improvisation; while functional MRIs, EEG, MEG, and PET scans make closer investigation possible. Knowledge has exploded over the last 20 years, and even 5 years, supplying answers and opening unforeseen, fascinating paths of inquiry. Case Study 1, summarizing the composition of "Out On the Water," is interwoven here with findings from other research that support the Songwriting Works' model.

Case Study 1: "Out on the Water" – Lessons of Place and Time

On a summer afternoon at an Olympic Peninsula care center seven women in their 70s and 80s gather to write a song for the first time. All have mid- to later-stage dementia. The facilitator has conducted hundreds of workshops in dementia care for more than 15 years in urban and suburban settings. No single workshop for a group with a significant degree of cognitive impairment has gone longer than 60 minutes. Here, in a rural seaport town – with few available interactive music programs other than sing-alongs – the host agency has planned a 2-hour session. After introducing herself and greeting each person by name, the facilitator asks about favorite music.

After a long silence the activity director, a man, jumps in: "Cowboy songs!"
"Opera!" a woman replies in turn. "Western." "Elvis!" …"Jazz"

At the start of each workshop, Songwriting Works solicits musical preferences. Bartlett, Kaufman and Smeltekop's research exploring positive immune systems outcomes for music listeners found that "preferred music types, in particular, tend to increase the likelihood of obtaining positive sensory experiences, and possibly for evoking chemical changes" (Bartlett et al., 1993). In other words, on a biological as well as psycho-social level, opportunities to have one's esthetic preferences respected and brought to the fore of interactivity may be key in optimizing beneficial outcomes for individuals and programs.

The group warms up with a familiar cowboy song; most sing. However, two women sit quietly, staring past the facilitator, apparently quite disengaged. They remain this way for the next hour, while the session unfolds:

Facilitator: "What shall we write about today?"
After a long pause a woman smiles heartily: "Being out on the water."

In this town surrounded on three sides by water the theme hits home. Others begin to add thoughts and images, slowly filling the easel with words:

"It's nice to be on a boat on the water"
"A blue motorboat"
"Round about this time"
"Food"
"It's so peaceful"

The facilitator goes back and forth asking open questions, sometimes reframed from new angles:

"What's it like in that boat?" "What do you do when you're there?"

After each question she respectfully leaves time for responses. There are no wrong answers; rather, a welcoming space is made evident through facial expression, body language, pace, eye contact, well-articulated speech, and genuine patience. Contributors' words, images, ideas, and phrases are scribed, repeated and recapped; each is acknowledged by name.

Respect is a pre-requisite when seeking authenticity and providing access to those with diverse needs. Dignity is of the utmost importance, especially for those who have been marginalized or isolated due to age, cultural, or cognitive prejudice. For those with cognitive deficits who can no longer easily communicate, dignity seems to be "grasped" one could say, in "meta-awareness."

> "What's being on the water like?" the facilitator asks again.
> "Soothing" comes a thoughtful reply.
> "I meditate" says another.
> "Crying – sometimes" says a third.
> Addressing this woman directly, the facilitator asks, gently: "Say more?...."
> "You think about old times… think about sad times"
> "Sing!" the woman who had the initial song idea says loudly.
> Another adds in an even tone: "Think of all the good things that have happened to you."

Music therapist and researcher Alicia Ann Clair, Ph.D, RMT-BC has extensively studied the impacts of making music with and for elders with late-stage dementia. One study measured responses to a series of specifically replicated 2-minute music therapy interventions including unaccompanied singing, silence, and reading. Sessions took place over a series of days. Clair noted that given proper respect and support, "persons who are in very late-stage dementia are still capable of responding to stimuli in their environment. …Extremely long response latencies may require stimulation over time. …It is possible that these persons respond slowly over time and any attempts to determine their response patterns must be done in a series of sessions…" (Clair, 1995, 1996a, 1996b). These findings suggest that greater responsiveness is aided by relationship building.[25]

The session is now at 50 minutes staff and facilitator meet eyes acknowledging a subtle shift in the room. The women's sentences are growing longer; there is more interactivity.

> "Enjoying the quiet."
> "I'd have my radio going, lie down and just listen to it."
> "I sooner be on water than on land"
> "I prefer a sailboat."
> "Not hearing so much noise as you do on land."
> "I'd rather be watching from the shore."
> The most outspoken women adds: "I like it when its rough; The boat goes up and down up and down."
> Another says (possibly in response, though this cannot be ascertained): "You should never go on in life having no idea what so ever."

---

[25] Additional links and abstracts on music therapy in dementia care can be found at http://www.mtabc.com/page.php?58 Cited 9/12/10.

Later as lyric and music take shape, the facilitator offers a format of couplets which can accommodate diverse viewpoints:

> Out on the water, cool clear water – In my sailboat, with the radio on.
> Out on the water, cool clear water – Peaceful, soothing, we enjoy the quiet....
>
> (Composing Together Works and Friedman, 2007)[26]

As noted, facilitators are trained to model cooperation and respectful exchange across cultural and other differences, countering gossip and stereotyping and accommodating cognitive variances within the group. Their genuine interest helps dissolve social barriers. Likewise, the physical setting is arranged to maximize eye contact and rapport.

Following a snack break, the facilitator asks for a melody to match the words "cool clear water," steering clear of the first melodies offered which resemble the cowboy classic "Cool Water" by the Sons of the Pioneers. Originality is elicited by sharing the composition: sung pitches are gathered from one for "on the water," and another for "cool clear water." The group's enthusiasm confirms the melody for the song's refrain.

> On the water, water, cool clear water...'

As the session reaches 70, then 80, minutes the two women who have been seemingly unengaged throughout the workshop begin to contribute.

> "Sleep"
> "Happy as a bird"
> "I see seagulls"
> "Take cover!" the raconteur banters in response, "I'll rush for shore"
> Another who has become more and more active throughout says: "Take it any way it comes"
> Another: "It makes me anxious to watch it."

Time constraints – quite rigid in most healthcare delivery systems, classrooms, and workplaces – fall away as "progress" in songwriting is not something to be expedited. While facilitators are aware of time, songs evolve organically from a group's expression; time "flies by" for those deeply engaged. The principles of "timelessness" and openness foster spontaneity. In their pioneering work on the Eden Alternative and Green House projects Dr. William and Jude Thomas' name *spontaneity* as a key to turning institutional living environments into humane habitats (NCPAD Monograph, 2010; Thomas, 1996).[27]

> The session closes with singing the group's song "Out On the Water" and thank yous all around. Afterward, the activity director comments that he thinks it may have taken the two women seventy or more minutes to orient to the process and find their place in it.
>
> (Friedman, 2007)

---

[26] *"Out on the Water"* © *2007 Composing Together Works. Words and music by elders of Kai Tai Life Care Center with artist-in-residence Judith-Kate Friedman. Sponsored by the Arts to Elders program of Northwind Arts Alliance, Port Townsend, WA. All rights reserved.*

[27] For more about the Eden Alternative see www.edenalt.org.

Songwriting Works evaluates impacts by measuring participants' level of interactivity, frequency and quality of responses, repeat engagement in the same and subsequent sessions, solicited and unsolicited testimonials, surveys and interviews with participants, family members, staff, facilitators, and audiences, and when possible, outside evaluation and collaboration with researchers. The 2-hour time frame, noted above, has proved successful and is now Songwriting Works' standard practice.

> I'm impressed. We're learning a lot.
>
> – F.G., age 84[28]

Music and the Brain: Speech, Song, Rhythm and Memory

> Music is one of the most effective mnemonic devices. It enables preliterate societies to retain information – not just facts but the feelings that accompany the facts... Poems, songs, and dances are primary vehicles for the transmission of a heritage.
>
> Donald A. Hodges (2000)

> Music engages huge swathes of the brain - it's not just lighting up a spot in the auditory cortex.
>
> Dr. Aniruddh Patel (2010)

Multiple parts of the brain (areas, clusters, networks) become engaged when words are accompanied by melody, as occurs in singing (Peretz & Zatorre, 2005). Auditory training has been shown to improve neural timing in the human brainstem (Russo, Nicola, Zecker, Hayes, & Kraus, 2005). A yet greater number of brain functions are activated when musical pitch, words, *and purpose of expression* are combined. Often cited by choral directors, educators, and drum circle leaders around the world, pioneering music and brain health neurobiologist Norman M. Weinberger summarizes the reasons innovative music and wellness programs such as Songwriting Works and Remo, Inc.'s HealthRhythms are meeting with replicable success in terms of cognitive fitness (Remo, Inc, 2010; Yamaha.com, 2010)[29]:

> Music making is thought by some researchers to be the most extensive exercise for brain cells and for strengthening synapses. Brain scans of musicians reveal that nearly all of the cerebral cortex is active during performance. It would be difficult to find another activity that engages so many of the brain's systems.
>
> Norman Weinberger (1998)[30]

---

[28]Testimonial, Madlyn and Leonard Abramson Center for Jewish Life participant, 2005.

[29]Musical instrument makers and manufacturers have contributed extensively to research, discussion and the practice of music-making and health. See links to research on stress reduction benefits of playing music. (Remo, Inc and Yamaha Institute, cited below.)

[30]Norman M. Weinberger, professor and fellow of the Center for the Neurobiology of Learning and Memory, UC Irvine, serves as Executive Director of the International Foundation for Music Research and is co-founder and director of MuSICA – The Music & Science Information Computer Archive. Quotes are reproduced with permission of Dr. Norman M. Weinberger and the Regents of the University of California.

While a more thorough overview of research on music and the brain is beyond this chapter's scope, many areas of study are relevant to the Songwriting Works model. These include: investigation of similarities and differences in spoken vs. sung speech, in vocal vs. instrumental music-making and music listening, and in performing music of one's own composition vs. that of another composer; the impact of emotional and spiritual lyric and melodic content on perception, cognition and brain function; distinctions due to, and degree of variance in, cognitive response and outcomes based upon *contexts* occasioning group song composition and performance.

Cognitive Benefits of Musical Improvisation

> The process of improvisation is involved in many aspects of human behavior beyond those of a musical nature, including adaptation to changing environments, problem solving and perhaps most importantly, the use of natural language, all of which are unscripted behaviors that capitalize on the generative capacity of the brain.
>
> Charles J. Limb and Allen R. Braun (2008)

Limb and Braun's 2008 study of improvising professional jazz musicians suggests that instrumental music improvisation – including that with a biographical and/or emotional component such as the reminiscence-based spontaneous melodic expression that occurs in the Songwriting Works process – has been found to increase the level of complexity in brain activity. Improvising was found to simultaneously activate and deactivate different brain regions. This suggests that the *relationship between* activation and deactivation may be a key to understanding how creativity blossoms when conscious control is relaxed.

Leaping into Aging

To illustrate cognitive fitness and the brain's capacity for neural growth and engagement even amidst significant decline, Dr. Gene Cohen used the image of squirrels leaping between trees:

> In a brain with fewer dendrites the leaps between synapses would be like leaps between bare-branched trees. The spaces on bare-branched trees would be wider to navigate, the leaps more difficult to make. In contrast, in a brain [with] many branches and connections – a great number of dendrites – a person's thoughts and responses, like our leaping squirrel, could move with more facility between ideas and associations. The more bridges or branches there are, the more connectivity and communication.
>
> (Cohen, 2005b)

Cohen's groundbreaking "Creativity and Aging" study demonstrated significant health impacts for community dwelling older adults, average age 80, who attended weekly professionally-conducted arts programs (choral ensemble, theater group, painting class) in three U.S. cities (Cohen et al., 2006).[31] At the end of 3 years, participants had experienced significantly fewer falls, fewer doctor's visits, reduced need for medication, improved scores on loneliness and depression scales, and increased social engagement beyond the time of the study, compared to those in a control group who did not participate in similar programs. Cohen had hypothesized that master teaching artists – those adept at breaking down complex learning activities into accessible increments for their students – might create conditions for health by engendering in learners a greater sense of mastery (Lachman & Weaver, 1998; Rodin, 1989) while positively engaged in a social context (Glass et al., 1999).

Methodology: Eight Principles that Support Healthy Creative Engagement

> Everybody felt they were a part of the program for the day. It was very good for us.
> Better than pills!
>
> C.G., age 80[32]

The Songwriting Works model is founded on these eight "best practice" principles:

1. Access
2. Inclusion
3. Originality
4. Authenticity
5. Respect
6. Reciprocity
7. Restoration
8. Celebration[33]

These practices are illustrated with examples in Case Study 2, presented here in a condensed transcript from Einat Kapak's film (Kapak/Ziv Tzedakah, 2006). Additional supporting research is cited.

---

[31] Cohen's 3-year study funded by the National Endowment for the Arts, the National Institute on Mental Health and others, followed participants in professionally conducted arts programs Elders Share the Arts (theater, Brooklyn, NY), Center for Elders and Youth in Arts (painting, San Francisco, CA), and the Levine School of Music (choir, Washington, D.C.)

[32] Testimonial, Caroline Kline Galland Home participant in an interview with filmmaker Einat Kapak (cited below) in her documentary "Between Heaven and Earth, Vol. II, (Ziv Tzedakah Fund, 2006), Songwriting Works segment.

[33] An earlier version of these principles appeared in Songwriting Works Training Manual, © 2008 Judith-Kate Friedman, and in the Songwriting Works American Society on Aging/MindAlert webinar 3/10/2010 and trainings 2007–2010.

Case Study 2: "The Eye of the Storm" – Songwriting as Life Review

At Heritage House at the Market, a Providence Health and Services assisted living residence in downtown Seattle, a first time songwriting session takes place on a sunny afternoon. Most participants have memory loss; some advanced hearing loss. The facilitator [JK] has been asked to come in "cold" for the purpose of filming a demonstration of initial impacts. She has no information about individuals and little about the culture of the facility. She circles the room, greeting each person with a handshake: a moment to connect one to one before the formal program.

Access

> JK: "Have you been making music in your life?"
> Participant A: "When I was young – but then I lost my hearing."
> JK: 'Ah…"
> A, making more intent eye contact: "Well, in the beginning it was silent anyway."
> JK, meeting A's eyes, repeats gently: "In the beginning it was silent anyway."
> A, vigorously shaking her head in affirmation : "Yes…"
> JK: "That's a beautiful perspective."

Accessibility is a baseline for all Songwriting Works events. From a creative viewpoint, cognitive and physical limitations are not seen as deficits; they are simply the realities and challenges of a given situation on a particular day. In an improvisational context everyday fluctuations and surprises precipitated by flickering memory, effects of medication, pain and exhaustion, and the social ins and outs of group dynamics are easily accommodated. While impacts of this level of openness and acceptance have yet to be measured in clinical trials, observational study has shown a palpable connection between sincere interest and engagement on the part of a facilitator and the increased involvement and positive affect on the part of elders, including individuals who have advanced dementia, and family caregivers who initially appeared reticent to participate.

Inclusion

JK walks up to the microphone and sings "This Little Light of Mine" (Dixon Loes, cf. 1920); she solicits words for each verse and so doing, gets a "read" on individuals' initial level of interest and cognitive engage-ability.

> JK: "We're going to get a chance to write a song… What should we write about?"
> Participants B, C, D: "Love" "Springtime" "Atmosphere"
> JK: "Love, springtime, atmosphere…" Looking to others: "What else should we write about?"
> Participant E: "You always hear something about the eye of the storm."
> JK: "Okay – The eye of the storm…(scribes)"

> E: "It's a wonderful place"
> Participant F: "That's the best"
> JK: "F says 'the eye of the storm' that's the best. Is that a topic that we should discuss... and...write something about?"
> Participant G: "It's just the most awful thing you've ever been through. You can't stop anything."
> Participant H: "Life is filled with chaos....No jobs...and people are hungry."
> JK scribes all words verbatim, then feeds them back to group.

Facilitation that "levels the playing field" opens the way for honest interchange. Unexpected inspirations are welcomed. Personal stories are received with sensitivity; shared material is held in confidence and recounted anonymously unless participants (or their guardians) agree to be publicly credited. With repeated participation in a workshop or series, individuals often become more willing to try new things (give input, improvise melody, reveal life history). Likewise the group "tone" becomes more inclusive; peers begin to uphold principles of access and inclusion for one another (Friedman, 2009).

Originality

Twenty-five minutes into the session E has recounted her personal experience as a tornado survivor. G has noted that she is from New Orleans. It is now clear that although Hurricane Katrina hit the Gulf Coast 9 months earlier, the topic has evoked feelings about that disaster and its aftermath. Whether participants are thinking about a specific storm or not, nearly all are now responding to the theme. JK turns to those who've yet to speak.

> JK to Participant J: "J?"
> J: "No."
> JK addressing J and the group: "There's no right or wrong answer, you know that?"
> Participants on the side laugh quietly.
> JK: "It's all about our understandings, our feelings, our imagination. Everything is the right answer."

Reading from the easel JK recaps, affirming each participant as she repeats their contribution.

> Participant K, speaking slowly, with some difficulty due to a speech or cognitive disability: "Afterward.... I remember.... children would go out and play in the street.... and get all wet.

Participants laugh gently with recognition.

> JK recaps, scribing: "The children.. get wet..." Turning to all: " – We're having a deep conversation, aren't we?"

Participants learn to honor, hear, and recognize their own and the "group voice" as facilitators affirm originality aloud. In a society that rarely assumes that a group (of "non-musicians") can make good music *from scratch,* this approach allows fledgling creativity to develop and grow.

Authenticity

Everyone has a unique viewpoint. By capturing verbatim speech and melodies as they arise, and testing for group consensus, songs accurately reflect their makers. Participants recognize themselves in their music and can be recognized in turn.

> JK to F, one of the most engaged in the group: "What do you think the eye of the storm feels like?"
> F, quietly: "Oh... Tossed about in life?"
> JK scribing, speaking slowly, amplifies: "Tossed about in life."

A flurry of responses follow this rhythmic phrase. The whiteboard is soon full of lyric ideas.

> JK: "Anybody got a melody?"
> E who initiated the topic, sings in a plaintive southern folk style: "Tossed about in life."
> JK echoes E's words, melody, cadence and tempo, a cappella: "Tossed about in life."
> E adds a next melodic and lyric line, singing: "Like a ship without a rudder."

Songwriting continues. JK stands in front chording the guitar; she solicits images to fit with the newly composed lines. Repeating the verse in progress, she sings directly to E, then turns toward the page and embodies her speech as if to "follow the bouncing ball" and physically convey to the larger group: A song is on the board, melody is in the room, words and melody are being joined....

> JK (singing): "Tossed about in life, like a ship without a rudder,
> Blown and pushed over from one end to another."
> K with enthusiastic, although labored, speech follows: "Oh, how the wind can blow-oh!"
> JK to K, approximating the melody to pitches of K's spoken voice: "Oh, how the wind can – "
> K repeats the phrase with more pitch emphasizing two beats or syllables: "...Blow-oh."
> JK sings the exact phrase, encouraging group participation:
> " 'Oh – how the wind can blow – oh' – Everybody..."
> Participants, sing: "Oh how the wind can blow–oh."

JK repeats the refrain which has now taken hold. Others join in, including K who is beaming:

> "Oh how the wind can blow–oh."
> As the refrain closes K jumps in, in rhythm: "Wow! – "

Respect

JK appreciates the humor of K's "Wow!" but holds back her personal view to solicit group response. G from New Orleans is concerned that the situation be taken seriously. She and several others get into animated debate regarding the appropriateness of "Wow" for the song. JK, offering options, sings "wow" softly and "WOW!" vigorously as K originally delivered it, then omits it. Participants settle into comfort with three repetitions of "Oh how the wind can blow": once without "wow," then with an understated "wow" followed by a final big one. By time they sing the ending (coda) with a resounding "Wow!" G is laughing heartily.

As noted above, dignity and respect are essential conditions for cognitive, social, and creative musical collaboration. Facilitators adjust pace and patience to foster full participation. Any criticism or narrow set of "shoulds" are suspended in favor of wonder and the most satisfying consensus possible.

Reciprocity

> JK: "That's great! Here we go – "
> All sing: "Oh, how the wind can blow.
> Oh how the wind can blow, wow.
> Oh how the wind can blow –
> WOW!"

Peels of laughter abound; the guitar keeps time. Chuckles, and a sense of relief and completion ripple through the room – confirming the group has reached consensus.

Reciprocity is key to achieving inclusion and consensus in songwriting. What is good for participants must have meaning for the musician-facilitator and vice versa; thus, keeper lines, song sections and final works are determined. Evaluation of process, song and program occur instantaneously as participants augment and edit – and facilitators "course correct" – as they go.

Restoration

> Trust is the basis of all human social endeavors, and a case is made that it is created through the practice of music. How and why, in biological terms, can music and dance bring humans together with a depth of bonding that cannot be achieved with words alone?
>
> Walter Freeman (2000)

With 10 minutes left in this one-time session, JK moves the group toward completion. She gestures to the easel, recapping collected ideas and phrases yet to be used in the lyric. "Faith" and "brings us home" get strong response.

> JK (offering a pairing of words): "The faith that we have brings us home."

The group approves. JK quickly solicits new words (see underlined below) in the manner of a zipper song.[34] The lyric is put in sequence by consensus. Due to shortness of time this coda is spoken rather than sung:

> JK: "The <u>trust</u> that we have brings us home.
> The <u>faith</u> that we have brings us home.
> The <u>love</u> that we have brings us home.
> All, singing: "Oh how the wind can blow.

---

[34] *For a description of a zipper song see* http://www.uua.org/religiouseducation/curricula/tapestry-faith/makingmusic/chapter6/129370.shtml *Cited on 9/14/10.*

> Oh how the wind can blow, wow.
> Oh how the wind can blow – Wow!"
>
> (Composing Together Works, 2006[35])

Restoration occurs at several levels: Participants and communities (re)engage in the physiological and cognitive experience of music-making and vocal (sung, recited) expression. Honor is restored as individuals' precise creative input is incorporated and repeatedly validated. Recognition later extends in public celebration. Feedback from surveys and interviews suggests that the experience affirms elders' and caregivers' sense of usefulness, belonging, value, and overall well-being (see Case Study 3).

Being recognized as a contributor, and as an integral part of one's family and community, leads to increased learning, self-esteem and school retention for youth-at-risk (Heath & Roche, 1999),[36] enhanced communication and cognitive facility among elders with dementia (Allison, 2008, 2010), heightened job satisfaction and happiness among successful CEOs (Dean & Stevenson, 2004),[37] and a deepened sense of well-being and purpose for retirees. (Mark & Waldman, 2002).

Cognitive psychologist Barbara Rogoff describes a "social matrix of purposes and values" that is created as humans define, discover, solve and learn from problems they encounter; they collectively respond, in part, by developing more resources (social structures, strategies, technology, tools). This social contextualization further catalyzes engagement and cognitive development (Rogoff, 1990, 1998). In both song composition and performance, the Songwriting Works' model helps create this type of "social matrix" for growth.

Celebration

> When they see – it makes me cry and I can't talk. I'm going to take this (songbook) home and show it to my children
> so they can take it to my grandchildren.
>
> B.C., age 86[38]

---

[35] *The Eye of the Storm* © 2006 Composing Together Works. *Words and music by elders of Providence Heritage House at the Market with guest artist Judith-Kate Friedman. All rights reserved. The session was held as a demonstration session. Transcript cited is from an edited film clip documenting Songwriting Works for the Ziv Tzedakah Fund's film "Between Heaven and Earth" profiling grant recipients. An excerpt of the film, Einat Kapak dir., is posted on Songwriting Works' You Tube site (search at www.youtube.com).*

[36] In their 10 year study of youth identified as "at-risk" who engaged in after-school arts programs, Shirley Brice Heath of Stanford University and Adelma Roach of the Carnegie Foundation for the Advancement of Education found significant increases in academic participation and performance, self-esteem and empowerment, enhanced confidence in life-planning, likelihood to pursue higher education, and a greater ability to envision a positive future (op. cit).

[37] Harvard Business School researchers Laura Dean and Howard Stevenson interviewed hundreds of top executives to find their recipe for, and definitions of, success. They found four irreducible categories representing conflicting human needs between which successful leaders were able to achieve balance. "Significance" and "Legacy" accounted for 50% of the equation, along with "Achievement" and "Happiness" (op. cit).

[38] Testimonial, participant at the Madlyn and Leonard Abramson Center for Jewish Life, 2005.

Community celebrations, concerts, and publications are key to bringing reciprocity, dignity, and honoring full circle. When song-makers access new audiences and find new ways to leave a legacy, additional "meaning-making" can occur. As community builds, isolation dissolves; possibilities open; new awareness – and liberation – can result (Cohen, 2001).[39]

Applications, Implications, Questions: Restoring Health and Community Through Songwriting

Music as a Key to Cognitive Intelligence

> If you can walk you can dance, if you can talk you can sing.
>
> Zimbabwean Proverb

> It is reasonable to suppose that musical skills played a major role early in the evolution of human intellect, because they made possible formation of human societies as a prerequisite for the transmission of acquired knowledge across generations.
>
> Walter Freeman (2000)

Songwriting Works' mission is to restore health and community through reintegrating musical practice and original sung expression into daily life. Through their songs and performances elders' and others' presence – their voices and value – are reintroduced into the culture aiding in "transmission of acquired knowledge across generations." It is well documented that musical memory is one of the last aspects of memory to deteriorate in elders with debilitating late-stage dementia. Extensive study of the singing of popular songs with such elders has demonstrated that vocal musical engagement is an effective aid in increasing communication, cognition, and well-being (Clair, 1996a, 1996b; Götell, 2003; Götell et al., 2009).[40] Songs entering the "musical memory bank" early in life appear to be the last memories depleted.

Could it be that a similar phenomenon operates for humans *as a species?* Might the earliest input of vocal musical function – which some theorize preceded plain speech in human evolution – have set neurological architecture in place for retention of music in the brain as an overall foundational component? Might vocal music, if considered an elemental 'blueprint' or template in neurological structure, underlay or foundationally interact with additional neural networks or areas in ways that serve as keys to function within, or communication between, any number of neural locations?

---

[39] For discussion of developmental stages in the second half of life, including the "Liberation" and "Encore" phases see Gene Cohen, M.D.'s books, (op. cit).

[40] Claire and Götell have each well-documented the phenomena of re-engagement that can take place when singing is intentionally used to enhance communication with persons diagnosed with Alzheimer's Disease and other dementias and their caregivers. For links to Götell articles and music and caregiving research see: http://www.dementiacaresinging.com.

> It doesn't surprise me that people with dementia compose songs, but it does surprise me that they remember them.
>
> Jewish Home Geriatrician (Allison, 2008)[41]

Songwriting Works has found, and Dr. Allison's research (2008, 2010) has confirmed, that persons with severely limited short-term memory capacity are yet able to retrieve *new music* – words and melodies – which they helped to compose. To this author's knowledge, there has yet to be a longitudinal study that measures *how and under what conditions newly composed and performed material* gets stored in brains with significant neurological decline, and how, once stored, these moments of paired melody, language, and expression may become retrievable.

In 2009, the National Endowment for the Arts funded Songwriting Works to bring its model to the rural Olympic Peninsula in conjunction with Arts Northwest, the Olympic Area Agency on Aging, and more than two dozen agencies and regional leaders. As part of this year long "Creativity and Aging in America" initiative, a pilot program brought thirty elders diagnosed with Alzheimer's disease and their family care partners together to compose original songs. A series of seven weekly 2-hour workshops and a culminating concert celebration were held at Dungeness Courte, a Northwest Care Management memory care residence, in Sequim, WA. Survey questionnaires were designed in consultation with Critical Junctures Institute at Western Washington University/St. Joseph PeaceHealth hospital. Written and interview testimonials were collected from family members and participating elders, host-site staff, and Songwriting Works' apprentice-facilitators after each session and during and immediately following the culminating concert. The host-site administrator also reviewed and summarized relevant medical data collected from elder participants' charts at the start, midpoint, and 2 months following the series (coded to retain anonymity).

The sequence of activities within each workshop followed Songwriting Works' model as in Case Studies 1 and 2, above; all sessions were digitally documented (audio). The following Case Study (#3) details highlights of composing a World War II Homecoming song as part of the 2009 NEA pilot project. Implications and questions arising from initial project findings are noted.

Case Study 3: "The Big Day is When the Ship Comes In" – Songwriting with WWII Veterans and Caregivers

> One knows that there is still a self to be called upon, even if music, and only music, can do the calling.
>
> Oliver Sacks (2007)

> We have seen the Alzheimer patient, who no longer uses spoken language, come up with a line of melody that perfectly fits the phrase just spoken by another. We have borne witness as people who claimed they were 'never creative', who were told that they were 'listeners,

---

[41] As quoted in an interview by Theresa Allison, M.D., M. Music (op. cit).

not singers', morph into poets and tunesmiths. We have heard and transcribed stories as diverse as cooking and coming home war.

Paula Lalish[42]

It is week 5 of 7 at a residential care facility where several dozen elders diagnosed with Alzheimer's disease have been writing songs with their loved ones. Upon finishing the second of two light-hearted original songs, Songwriting Works' team suggests the group revisit a story that has been collected and scribed but has not yet been used. Site staff has informed the team that a day program participant (here called Veteran 1) who contributed his story, has been telling his daughter he "just can't believe (they've) put his words up on the wall" and are taking him seriously.

> On the way over in World War II, with my twin brother in the Marines, I went – all over.
> Shipped out again to the Philippines, Africa, China, Korea, Japan – South Pacific…
> The war got over – We came back home – Both alive![43]

As the group is polled about their interest in setting these words to music, three gentlemen who reside at the center come forward with their stories. They are also former WWII Marines. (Here called Veterans 2, 3 and 4). Veteran 4 has little verbal ability due to advancing dementia. He seldom speaks; when he does his words are sometimes poetic but have no discernable connection to group conversation. However, he can sing.

Alicia Ann Clair's above-cited research (1995, 1996a, 1996b) demonstrated increased engagement for elders with late-stage dementia in which unaccompanied singing took place in *successive* sessions. Beginning in 2007, Songwriting Works and host-site staff had begun noting impacts of relationship building between facilitators, caregivers, and elders with late-stage dementia *within a single 2-hour session* as well as throughout workshop series. Initial analysis of data from the 2009 NEA pilot project suggests that 2 h seems an effective session length for those with dementia-related long response latencies (Friedman, 2009, 2010). There is also a positive cumulative impact of engagement over a series of weekly 2-hour sessions. For example:

In session #1, Veteran 4 stayed at the edge, wheeling himself in and out of the room with expressed agitation throughout most of the 2 hours though he returned and connected with facilitators at the session's end. In session #2, staff and facilitators observed he had more sustained attention. At session #3 he had begun sitting more closely to the facilitators and easel where stories were scribed (he moved around during the session but did not leave the room for any extended time). On week #4 and at all subsequent sessions, Veteran 4's daughter accompanied him and was present when he provided formative melodic input for the composition.

The group enthusiastically agrees to write a song about WWII Homecoming.

---

[42] Paula Lalish, apprentice facilitator, in a letter to funders, 2010.

[43] WWII Homecoming Song © 2009 Composing Together Works. Words and music by elders of Dungeness Courte, family members, and staff with Judith-Kate Friedman, Paula Lalish, Andrew Wheatley, Matt Sircely, and Keeth Monta Apgar of Songwriting Works. A project of Songwriting Works on the Olympic Peninsula in conjunction with Arts Northwest and the Olympic Area Agency on Aging with support from the National Endowment for the Arts. All rights reserved. For more information contact: 360.385.1160 or visit the song gallery at www.songwritingworks.org.

20 The Songwriting Works™ Model: Enhancing Brain Health and Fitness... 349

> Facilitator (recapping Veteran 1's words): "....Africa, China, Korea, Japan – South Pacific...
> The war got over – We came back home – Both alive!"
> Veteran 1: "The big day is when the ship comes in."
> Veteran 4 responding immediately, singing without words: — — — — — — — — —

Veteran 4 delivers sung tones that perfectly match the rhythm of Veteran 1's words; he sings directly to the facilitation team with vigor, volume, and emotional intensity, drawing the full focus of all in the room. The team leader sings this melody back to him and the group, adding the lyric:

> The big day is when the ship comes in.

The session continues as participants match this rhythmic phrase with another.

> Veteran 1: "We fly to Hawaii to meet the ship..."

Once the men have added their stories and sounds, the women of their generation speak up. In the remaining time and in the following week's session they add tales of awaiting brothers, husbands, and nephews who served, mourning losses and celebrating good fortune "on the front porch with some moonshine" when families reunited. Images are summed up and polished by consensus (as in above Case Studies): "Wives have been waiting, children waiting, family waiting –

As the song is reviewed, melody added and sung to these words, a resident who has been walking by, and has never before participated, rolls into the room leaning on her walker. She observes the group for a second; looking non-plussed she throws up her arm and sings four notes: "Ah———" in a dramatic-operatic series of intervals. Again the room is riveted to the sound. Although this woman quickly leaves the room (and never again participates in a session), her melody is added to the lyric line. There is gentle laughter and humor in the incident, and the group agrees that the haunting sound carries the spirit of the song.

> On the way over in WWII with my twin brother in the Marines I went – all over.
> Shipped out again to the Philippines – Africa, China, Korea, Japan
> South Pacific – The war got over – We came back home – Both alive!
> Hallelujah!

> The big day is when the ship comes home
> We fly to Hawai'i to meet the ship
> Wives have been waiting, Children waiting, Families waiting – Aaaah....
> Seventeen months in one stretch – I don't want to go over again
> Aaa – ah
> (Instrumental break)
> The big day is when the ship comes home
> We wait on the dock to meet the ship
> Family together, Celebrating, Home on the front porch, Big orange soda
> And some moonshine – Aaaah....
> Home Again
> Hallelujah!
> Hallelujah!
> Hallelujah!
>
> (Composing Together Works and Friedman, 2009)

> As a direct result of the Songwriting Works program our residents have a better quality of life. Residents that were not verbal prior to this program continue to have a voice in our

community. Caregivers learned new ways of listening and accepting resident input and most importantly, families are able to share laughter and joy again.

Kathy Burrer, administrator, Dungeness Courte[44]

Over the three WWII Homecoming song sessions, Veteran 4 contributes 70% of the melody for the piece – a cantata. Songwriting Works' facilitators acknowledge and welcome his passion and musicality throughout the pilot series; they include him as a leader in the musical composition despite his inability to communicate through words. Mid-series, the lead facilitator inquires with staff about Veteran 4's level of engagement and his seemingly increased interest, or perhaps trust. The activity director notes: "I don't know if he's connecting with that but there's a possibility he is. When he first he had a real strong beautiful tenor voice." And after the next session: "He's very musical…he's always had random songs… You're validating the noises he's making, turning them into songs instead of saying "okay." (Friedman, 2009)

After the final concert, Veteran 4's daughter sitting beside her father remarks: "Dad doesn't usually participate in things like this. I think he really liked the idea that you could take his song, his rhythm, and you used it immediately…. I think he stayed with it because it came from him… he could contribute to it. When he's in choirs they usually tell him to tone it down…. And you keep telling him to turn it up!" Hearing this, the lead facilitator shakes Veteran 4's hand: "You've contributed so much music." He answers: "You're welcome." And smiles. The activity director later comments: "Taking everyone at face value, it looks like he's beginning to trust that he's going to be heard. He's looking me in the eye more…." (Friedman, 2009)

According to survey data, the experience for family and kinship caregivers was overwhelmingly positive. Sixty percent of the elders with dementia were joined by loved ones in cowriting three original songs. Once they attended, 75% of family caregivers participated in every subsequent session, or sent another family member. Many identified the experience as respite. The daughter of Veteran 3 wrote:

> The program opened my eyes to the vast potential of the human brain including (those with) dementia. Being new it helped me get to know the staff. It was a positive experience for an otherwise previously uncomfortable and depressing environment. Now I'm OK with Dad being in the care center.

(Friedman, 2009)

Of initial project findings one of the most striking is families' reports that they gained awareness of their loved one's needs through the Songwriting Works process. The daughter of Veteran 1, the man whose story sparked the Homecoming song, wrote to the team 5 months after the series:

> It was very difficult for me to let go and return my Dad to Ohio. Other than serving during WWII, he has never lived anywhere else. As you know from the song, he and his twin served

---

[44] Kathy Burrer, administrator at Dungeness Courte Memory Care, Sequim, WA evaluating NEA-funded Songwriting Works on the Olympic Peninsula pilot project in which elders with dementia composed songs with their family and kinship caregivers. As quoted in Friedman, Judith-Kate (2009, 2010) *Creativity and Aging in America grantee evaluation and report to the National Endowment for the Arts* (op. cit)

together...the longest time they were apart was while he lived with me in Washington (state). My Dad's twin does not have dementia and missed being with (him) ...When Dad opened up to help write the WWII song it made me realize I couldn't keep those twins apart any longer.[45]

Further research is needed to measure the impact of songwriting for veterans' and to gauge benefits for families engaged in sharing *memories* and discovering what is possible for and with their loved ones – creatively and cognitively – *in the present*.

The Power of Association

Associative processes have a surprising richness. They include far more complex processes than simple conditioning and they exhibit a remarkable ability to account for many "higher cognitive" processes such as categorization and concept formation.

Norman M. Weinberger (2010)

The body of multidisciplinary research to date strongly suggests that artists hold keys to understanding processes that involve particularly complex cognitive function, and the relationship of arts processes to learning, socialization, and health. Artists in all disciplines have, or develop, the facility to make associative "leaps," maneuvering between abstract and concrete, concepts and materials, infinite and defined sets of choices, planned and instantaneous, as they explore, invent, and produce new outcomes – "the very definition of creativity" (Cohen quoting Rollo May, 2001). "New outcomes" may be tangible end-products such as a replicable song, or more ephemeral as in musical improvisation or new insights participants share about one another.

When we open our eyes...when we change our state of consciousness, [these are] momentous events on the neuro-physiological basis....[This] is brought about, usually, by rhythmic stimulation...by singing, by clapping....

–Felicitious Goodman (2009)

Music is highly effective at promoting simultaneity of different parts... promoting cooperative group performance and interpersonal harmonization. In addition, musical meter is perhaps the quintessential device for group coordination, one which functions to promote interpersonal entrainment, cooperative movement, and teamwork.

–Steven Brown (2000)

In addition to studying the complexity of the artist's internal creative process, the relationship between artist, audience and cognition also bears further study. In collective musical experiences, complexity of many voices and viewpoints can be held at the same time as unity of feeling, intention, and perspective. The Songwriting Works process reveals and relies upon phenomena of patterns emerging in seeming randomness in nature (Strogatz, 2003) and of rhythmic gravitation to a pulse (entrainment) (Halprin & Kaplan, 1995). Understanding collective physiological and psychosocial responses to music may begin to explain the increased level of participation

---

[45]Testimonial excerpted from family caregiver letter, Dungeness Courte, 2009 (see Friedman 2009, 2010).

for elders with dementia and the increased insight and engagement that caregivers and their loved ones experience together when they share in song composition.

Pastoral Care: Adding a Spiritual Dimension to the Model

> I just never thought this was possible for me in my lifetime. Participant, age 88 describing her experience of performing original songs for the dedication of her synagogue
> (Allison, 2008)[46]

In 2003, the author and Rabbi Sheldon Marder cofounded Psalms, Songs & Stories™, a program that blends the Songwriting Works experience with intensive text study and reflection upon the Psalms. The program, as noted in Dr. Allison's research, seeks to awaken personal and communal intelligence through spiritual study, self-inquiry, collective collaboration, and musical exploration. Workshops engage groups with mixed cognitive ability; 60% or more have some level of dementia. Their average age is 88. The replicable Psalms, Songs & Stories model deserves mention in a cognitive fitness context, particularly since the construction and intention of Psalms can be profoundly reorienting for participants (Marder, 2005). Reorientation appears to occur irrespective of individuals' prior religious background or familiarity with the text. Though this has yet to be formally studied, observers have noted that participants in this program tend to break into spontaneous singing and melody "finding" through improvisation more frequently than in the original Songwriting Works model. The founders speculate that this may be due in part to an increased sense of spiritual mission or permission.[47]

Musicians in Service Across Generations:
Cost Effective Social Innovation

> Data sources across a wide spectrum conclude that creative arts applications have a positive impact on quality of life and demonstrate that creative arts interventions provide a marked benefit through cost savings potential and improved response to health and wellness programs.
> National Association of State Art Agencies Arts Brief (2010)

> What Songwriting Works proposes – giving performers of the highest caliber, their audiences and community volunteers an opportunity for a type of service-through-music – is new to this region.
> John McElwee, Executive Director of Centrum (2010)[48]

---

[46] As said to Theresa Allison, M.D., M. Music (Allison, 2008, op. cit).
[47] Conversation between Psalms, Songs & Stories™ co-founders Rabbi Sheldon Marder and Judith-Kate Friedman (2009). For more information about the project: http://songwritingworks.org/programs/diversity.htm.
[48] John McElwee, Executive Director of Centrum, Western Washington's premiere Arts & Education Center at Fort Worden State Park, in a 2010 letter of support to funders.

If proven programs such as the one detailed here are to be sustained, shifts in perception of their value must lead to integration into health delivery systems (current and new) with adequate funding. Research shows direct health-cost savings resulting from music/arts participation (for individuals, providers, employers, insurers, et al.) may range in the millions, and potentially billions, of dollars (Bittman et al., 2003; Cohen, 2006).

Health facilities are beginning to incorporate professionally facilitated music and arts engagement programs in their annual budgets. Arts, health, and education partners are collaborating locally, regionally, and nationally toward increasing public access to proven music-for-health programs. Teaching artists are finding increasing numbers of allies, and new avenues of training and prospective employment through the advocacy movements of arts-in-health care, creative aging, civic engagement, lifelong learning, culture change within long-term care, positive aging, and family caregiver support. As the population ages, greater numbers of trained artists and effective brain fitness enhancing arts programs will be needed to serve those with physical and cognitive deficits and those seeking to sustain cognitive and overall health.

Conclusion

> It's clear that [Frederico Garcia] Lorca is often leaping from one brain to another.... Lorca pulls an image out of the memory bank of the mammal brain: "The creatures of the moon sniff and prowl about their cabins," and then immediately follows with an image from the memory bank of the reptile brain, "The living iguanas will come to bite the men who do not dream", and then an image from the memory bank of the new brain comes in: "The man who rushes out with his spirit broken..." He doesn't do it deliberately – that's simply how the brain works when it is confident and excited.
>
> Robert Bly (1990)

Songwriting Works excites parts of the brain and makes connections where verbal, musical, rhythmic, gestural, and imaginal processes take place. It does this while offering participants and practitioners alike new avenues of mastery and confidence on the health-enhancing path of creativity. Multivalent stimulation offered in the act of collective songwriting increases neural activity and growth. Research on the specific impacts of the Songwriting Works experience and brain function, especially for those elders with dementia and other neurodegenerative illness, has yet to take place. Nevertheless, what *is* known, without doubt, is that intentional cultivation of group musical resonance consistently builds community, promotes self-esteem, and creates conditions for improved cognition as well as physical, mental, and spiritual well-being.

With age, and even with deterioration and illness, the human body, mind and spirit remain attuned to our inherent human proclivities: to learn, to participate, to express, and to give. When these processes are activated, health and wellness significantly improve for the individual and the collective (Cohen et al., 2006). Communal musical interactions which contain depth of meaning for elders have profound positive impacts on their physical and social well-being and can transform the culture in which they live (Allison, 2008, 2010).

> When I grew up we didn't have TV. We didn't sit around. People played music and they sang. Just because you may not get to Carnegie Hall doesn't mean you can't have the experience of playing music.... The music is the medicine.
>
> –Andy Mackie, Andy Mackie Music Foundation[49]

As music composers and group facilitators it is our job to maximize engagement, to welcome elders onto a playground of possibility – drawing out story, word, gesture, idiom, emotion, image, sound, and musical shapes. In this way different parts of the brain, including storage zones of reminiscence, springboards of imagination and the mysterious "breeding ground" of curiosity can be engaged. Through this work we heal the culture; we restore dignity to people of all ages and abilities, and awaken and welcome the dormant and marginalized musical intelligence in individuals and communities.

Humankind is neuro-biologically "wired" for making music (Wallin et al., 2000). Music is, as all art-making, a natural expression of the human process of making sense of, and relating with and to, our surroundings (Dissanayake, 2000; Hodges, 2000). We appreciate music, dance to its rhythms, identify with symbols, shapes and sound colors, create and attune to language, tonality, and pitch. It moves us and we join in. Hence, any cognitive fitness and health program should include active musical engagement.

If we have lost a sense of empowerment or feel we're "out of practice" the good news is: we already know how to do it. Throughout the life cycle, at any point on the continuum of aging and of physical, emotional, spiritual and cognitive health, musical experiences and support for our remembering are readily available. All that is needed is opportunity, patience, and a context of practice to be restored.

> We all hunger for stories, both the telling and the hearing. They are how we come to make sense of the world. When stories are told and songs sung, the generational differences disappear. Now, late in the game, these elders' gifts to us are their stories. Our gift to them is to listen, with respect and care, and to midwife those stories into birth as songs.
>
> Paula Lalish[50]

The author thanks Nancy Horowitz Moilanen, Dr. Theresa Allison, and Daniel Deardorff for conversations about music and medicine, and Paul Kleyman and Daniel Deardorff for their help in editing this chapter. Dedicated to the work and memory of Robert Rice.

---

[49] Andy Mackie, music educator, instrument maker, philanthropist and holder of the Guinness World Book of Records title for the world's largest harmonica band, is a founding member of Songwriting Works' Olympic Peninsula elders advisory council. He is quoted here from an interview with Songwriting Works' Aimée Ringle, 1/8/2010.

[50] Paula Lalish, apprentice facilitator, quoted in Songwriting Works' Quarterly News 1:1, www.songwritingworks.org.

References

Allison, Theresa. (2008). Songwriting and transcending institutional boundaries in the nursing home. In Ben Koen (Ed.), *Oxford handbook of medical ethnomusicology* (pp. 240–243). Oxford: Oxford University Press.

Allison, T. (2010). The nursing home as village: Lessons from ethnomusicology. *Journal of Aging Humanities and the Arts, 4*(4), 276–291.

Allison, T. (forthcoming). *Transcending the limitations of institutionalization through music: Ethnomusicology in a nursing home.* Doctoral dissertation in Musicology, Advisor Professor Bruno Nettl. University of Illinois at Urbana-Champaign.

Barry, B., Berk, L. S., Felten, D. L., Westengard, J., Simonton, O. D., Pappas, J., et al. (2001). Composite effects of group drumming music therapy on modulation of neuroendocrine-immune parameters in normal subjects. *Alternative Therapies in Health and Medicine, 7,* 38–47.

Bartlett, D., Kaufman, D., & Smeltekop, R. (1993). The effects of music listening and perceived sensory experiences on the immune system as measured by interleukin-1 and cortisol. *Journal of Music Therapy, 30,* 194–209.

Bittman, B., Bruhn, K. T., Stevens, C., Westengard, J., & Umbach, P. O. (2003). Recreational music-making: A cost-effective group interdisciplinary strategy for reducing burnout and improving mood states in long-term care workers, *Advances in Mind-Body Medicine, 19,* 3–4.

Bly, R. (1990), *Leaping poetry: An idea with poems and translations*, (p. 72). Boston: A Seventies Press Book/Beacon.

Brown, S. (2000). The 'musilanguage' model of music evolution. In N. L. Wallin, B. Merker, & S. Brown (Eds.), *The origins of music* (p. 297). Cambridge: The MIT Press.

Cavenaugh, J. & Drewry, D. (2008). *Healing words: Poetry and medicine.* DVD, Healing Words Productions/PBS.

Clair, A. A. (1995). *Quoted in proceedings of the National Association for Music Therapy annual conference*, Houston, Texas, November, 1995.

Clair, A. A. (1996a). The effect of singing on alert responses in persons with late stage dementia. *Journal of Music Therapy, 33,* 4.

Clair, A. A. (1996b). *Therapeutic uses of music with older adults.* Baltimore: Health Professions Press.

Clair, A. A., & Ebberts, A. (1996). The effects of music therapy on interactions between family caregivers and their care receivers with late stage dementia. *Journal of Music Therapy, 34,* 148–164.

Cohen, G. (2001). *The creative age: Awakening potential in the second half of life.* New York: Harper.

Cohen, G. C. (2005a). *Staying sharp: Proceedings from the 2005 American Society on Aging brain health seminar*, disc 2, track 3.

Cohen, G. (2005b). *The mature mind: The positive power of the aging brain.* New York: Basic Books.

Cohen, G., Perlstein, S., Chapline, J., Kelly, J., Firth, K. M., & Simmens, S. (2006). The impact of professionally conducted cultural programs on the physical health, mental health, and social functioning of older adults. *The Gerontologist, 46*(6), 726–734.

Dean, L., & Stevenson, H. (2004). *Just enough: Tools for creating success in your life.* Hoboken: Wiley.

Diaz, A. (2010). As quoted on http://memory.ucsf.edu/Art/director.htm, the *website of the University of California's Memory and Aging Center*, Bruce Miller, M.D., Clinical director. Cited online 9/5/2010.

Dissanayake, E. (2000). Antecedents of the temporal arts in early mother-infant interaction. In N. L. Wallin, B. Merker, & S. Brown (Eds.), *The origins of music* (pp. 399–402). Cambridge: MIT Press.

Dixon Loes, H. (1920). *This Little Light of Mine*, as cited online in wikipedia. Retrieved September 4, 2010 from http://en.wikipedia.org/wiki/This_Little_Light_of_Mine

Ford, Dave (2002). Singer stirs seniors' creativity, they write their own songs of hope, *San Francisco Chronicle*, Friday August 2, 2002.
Freeman, W. (2000). A neurobiological role of music in social bonding. In N. L. Wallin, M. Bjiorn, & S. Brown (Eds.), *The origins of music* (pp. 412–422). Cambridge: MIT Press.
Friedkin, N. (2002). *A 'specially wonderful affair*. Friedkin Digital. www.fdigital.net. (The film tells the story of the making of the Jewish Home elders' debut CD "Island on a Hill" during the week of September 11, 2001).
Friedman, J. K. (2004). Freeing the voice within: the healing art of songwriting with elders diagnosed with alzheimer's disease and other cognitive disorders. *Signpost: Journal of Dementia and Mental Health Care of Older People, Spring*, 12–15. UK: Cardiff and Vale University, National Health Service of Wales (An abridged version appeared as Freeing the voice within: The healing art of songwriting" in *Aging Today*, American Society on Aging, November-December 2004: 14–15).
Friedman, J. K. (2007). Field notes and transcriptions, Arts to Elders sessions at Kah Tai Life Care Center, Port Townsend, WA.
Friedman, J.-K. (2008). *Songwriting Works™ introductory training manual*. Port Townsend: Songwriting Works Educational Foundation.
Friedman, J. K. (2009). Field notes, interviews and transcriptions, NEA pilot project sessions at Dungeness Courte Memory Care, Sequim, WA.
Friedman, J. K. (2009, 2010). *Creativity and Aging in America grantee evaluation and report to the National Endowment for the Arts*. Songwriting Works Educational Foundation, Port Townsend.
Gardner, H. (1983). *Frames of mind: The theory of multiple intelligences*. New York: Basic Books.
Geduldig, L. (2010). Esther and me. Project comedy. www.estherandme.com Documentary. Trailer: http://www.imdb.com/title/tt1630552/. Cited 11/23/2010.
Glass, T., Mendes deLeon, C., Marottoli, R., & Berkman, L. (1999). Population-based study of social and productive activities predictors of survival among elderly Americans. *British Medical Journal, 319*, 478–483.
Goodman, F. (2009). On-line, Retrieved 10/9/09 from http://www.youtube.com/watch?v=jkCPo93BcUo
Götell, E. (2003). *Singing, background music and music-events in the communication between persons with dementia and their caregivers*. Thesis defended in Stockholm, 2003 (Neurotec Department, Center of Excellence in Elderly Care Research, Krolinska Institutet, Huddinge, Sweden/Department of Health, Science and Mathematics, Blekinge Institute of Technology, Karlskrona, Sweden).
Götell, E., Brown, S., & Ekman, S.-L. (2009). The influence of caregiver singing and background music on vocally expressed emotions and moods in dementia care: A qualitative analysis. *International Journal of Nursing Studies, 46*, 422–430.
Gruhn, W., & Rauscher, F. H. (2002). The neurobiology of music cognition and learning. In R. Colwell & C. Richardson (Eds.), *Second handbook on music teaching and learning*. New York: Oxford University Press.
Halprin, A., & Kaplan, R. (1995). *Moving toward life: Five decades of transformational dance*. Hanover: Wesleyan University Press.
Heath, Shirley Brice with Roach, Adelma (1999). Imaginative actuality: Learning in the arts during the non-school hours. In *Champions of change: The impact of the arts on learning*. Washington D.C.: The Arts Education Partnership, the President's Committee on the Arts and Humanities, the GE Fund, and the John D. and Catherine T. MacArthur Foundation. Download online: http://aep-arts.org/files/publications/ChampsReport.pdf
Hodges, D. A. (2000). Support for an evolutionary theory of human musicality. *Proceedings of the Sixth International Conference on Music Perception and Cognition* (pp. 1–6). Keele: Keele University. Retrieved from http://www.uncg.edu/mus/faculty/musEd.html. Cited on 9/5/2010.
Kapak, E. (2006). Between Heaven and Earth, Vol. 2. Ziv Tzedakah Fund. Documentary profiles twelve projects funded by Danny Siegel's Ziv Tzedakah fund. The Songwriting Works segment

was filmed in Seattle at the Caroline Kline Galland home and Providence's Heritage House at the Market. Retrieved from http://www.songwritingworks.org/portfolio.htm. Cited on 9/30/2010.

Lachman, M. E., & Weaver, S. L. (1998). The sense of control as a moderator of social class differences in health and well-being. *Journal of Personality and Social Psychology, 74*(3), 763–773.

Limb, C. J. & Braun, A. R. (2008). Neural substrates of spontaneous musical performance: an fMRI study of jazz improvisation, doi: 10.1371/journal.pone.0001679 published online February 27, 2008 http://www.ncbi.nlm.nih.gov/pmc/articles/PMC2244806/.Online (download) cited 9/1/2010.

Luxenberg, J. as quoted in Sadler and Ridenour (2008) *Transforming the healthcare experience through the arts* (p. 138). San Diego: Aesthetics.

Marder, R. S. (2005). God is in the text. In D. Friedman (Ed.), *Jewish pastoral care* (2nd ed.). Woodstock: Jewish Lights Publications.

Mark, M., & Waldman, M. (2002). *Recasting retirement: New perspectives on aging and civic engagement*. San Francisco: Civic Ventures/Temple University Center for Intergenerational Learning.

Miller, Bruce (2010) Website of the University of California's Memory and Aging Center. Retrieved from http://memory.ucsf.edu/Art/director.htm. Cited online 9/5/2010.

National Association of State Art Agencies (2010). *Arts in healthcare: Strengthening our nation's healthcare through the arts*. Downloadable pdf online at: http://www.nasaa-arts.org/Advocacy/Federal-Updates/ArtsIssueBriefHealthcare2010.pdf. Cited 9/30/2010.

National Center on Physical Activity and Disability (NCPAD). (2010). *An Eden alternative: A life worth living* (monograph) profiling the work of Dr. William and Jude Thomas. Retrieved from http://www.indiana.edu/~nca/ncpad/eden.shtml (on line, 9/14/10).

Okun, M. O. (2008). speaking in *Healing words: Poetry and medicine*, dir. James Cavenaugh and David Drewry, DVD, Healing Words Productions/PBS.

Parsons, L. (2009). Speaking at *Notes and neurons: In search of the common chorus*, World Science Festival, Gerald Lynch Theater, John Jay College, June 12, 2009. Part 2. Viewable online: http://www.worldsciencefestival.com/video/notes-neurons-full (cited on line, 9/12/2010).

Patel, A. (2007). *Music, language and the brain*. USA: Oxford University Press.

Patel, A. as quoted by Victoria Gill (2010). Singing 'rewires' damaged brain, BBC Feb 21, 2010. Cited on line 8/20/10.

Peretz, I., & Zatorre, R. J. (2005). Brain organization for music processing. *Annual Review of Psychology, 2005*(56), 89–114.

Rauscher, F. (2001). Current research in music, intelligence, and the brain. In M. McCarthy (Ed.), *Enlightened advocacy: Implications of research for arts education policy and practice* (pp. 5–16). College Park: University of Maryland Press.

Remo, Inc. (2010). HealthRHYTHMS® program: http://www.remo.com/portal/pages/hr/research/index.html. Cited online 9/5/2010.

Rice, R. (2008). *Autobiography*. Retrieved from http://robertriceart.com, (cited August 30, 2010).

Rodin, J. (1989). Sense of control: Potentials for intervention. *The Annals of the American Academy of Political and Social Science, 503*(1), 29–42.

Rogoff, B. (1990). *Apprenticeship in thinking: cognitive development in social context* (p. 6). Random House: New York.

Rogoff, B. (1998). Cognition as a collaborative process. In W. Damon (series Ed.) & D. Kuhn & R.S. Siegler (vol. Eds.), *Handbook of child psychology* (vol. 2: Cognition, Perception, and Language, pp. 679–744), New York: Wiley.

Russo, N. M., Nicola, T. G., Zecker, S. G., Hayes, E. A., Kraus, N. (2005). Auditory training improves neural timing in the human brainstem, *Behavioural Brain Research 156*, 95–103. Online download 9/5/2010.

Sacks, O. (2007). *Musicophilia: Tales of music and the brain* (p. 346). Knopf: New York.

Sadler, B., & Ridenour, A. (2008). *Transforming the healthcare experience through the arts*. San Diego: Aesthetics.

Songwriting Works Educational Foundation. (2010). Songwriting Works Quarterly News, 1:1. Retrieved from http://www.songwritingworks.org.

Strogatz, S. H. (2003). *SYNC: The emerging science of spontaneous order*. New York: Hyperion.

Thomas, W. H. (1996). *Life worth living: How someone you love can still enjoy life in a nursing home*. Acton: Vanderwyck and Burnham.
Thomas, W. H. (2004). *What are old people for?: How elders will save the world*. Acton: Vanderwyck and Burnham.
Wallin, N. L., Merker, B., & Brown, S. (2000). *The origins of music*. Cambridge: MIT Press.
Weinberger, N. (1998). The music in our minds. *Educational Leadership, 56*(3), 36–40.
Weinberger, N. (2010). The cognitive auditory cortex. In *The Oxford handbook of auditory science: The auditory brain*, (p. 443). New York: Oxford University Press.
Yamaha Music and Wellness Institute. Retrieved from http://www.yamahainstitute.org/. Cited online 9/5/2010.

Part IV
Cognitive Wellness Interventions for Adults with Memory Impairment

Chapter 21
Supporting Cognition and Well-Being in Older Adults with Mild Cognitive Impairment: A Pilot Intervention

Asenath La Rue

Abstract About one in five older adults in the community have cognitive impairments greater than expected for age, but less severe than dementia. Activity-based interventions tailored to this important "in-between" group may help to extend continued independence in everyday functioning while sustaining mood and well-being. This chapter reviews research on cognitive wellness interventions for persons with mild cognitive impairment (MCI) and describes a 1-year pilot intervention based on individualized plans for increasing cognitive and physical activity. The need for controlled trials of MCI interventions with follow-up and measurement of impacts beyond cognition (e.g., well-being and everyday function) is discussed.

Mild cognitive impairment (MCI) is an early stage of cognitive difficulty that often precedes dementia. Between 3 and 19% of adults 65 years and older have cognitive problems consistent with MCI (Gauthier et al., 2006). Prevalence rises with age, to an estimated 20% at age 75, 30% at age 80, and 42% at age 85 (Yesavage et al., 2002). Individuals with MCI function well in most everyday activities and are usually aware of, and often worried about, their cognitive changes. As such, they may be a high priority group for developing programs to sustain well-being and support cognition and everyday function.

This chapter describes a pilot intervention called Take Charge that encouraged activity and lifestyle changes to support well-being and cognitive function for individuals with MCI. The initial section discusses how MCI is identified, reviews relevant research, and describes new programs designed for persons with MCI. The second section summarizes the rationale, procedures, and findings of Take Charge.

A. La Rue (✉)
Wisconsin Alzheimer's Institute, University of Wisconsin, 7818 Big Sky Drive, Suite 215, Madison, WI 53719, USA
e-mail: larue@wisc.edu

The final section discusses lessons learned from Take Charge and looks ahead at what is needed for a better understanding of the role of training and lifestyle support for persons with MCI.

Diagnostic Criteria and Clinical Research

Identifying MCI

Individuals with MCI have cognitive problems that exceed what is expected for their age and background but are not severe enough to warrant a dementia diagnosis. Key features in diagnosing MCI are as follows (Gauthier et al., 2006; Winblad et al., 2004):

- Individuals with MCI are not demented, but their cognitive abilities are lower than expected for age and background…it's a mental "in-between" stage
- There is objective evidence of cognitive decline over time, or
- If the person is being seen for the first time, performance on cognitive testing is lower than expected for age, and the person, or a close informant, believes that his or her cognition has declined
- Basic activities of daily life are preserved, and complex instrumental activities are either intact or minimally impaired.

Some individuals with MCI have had a lowering of memory only (amnestic MCI), while others have selective declines in a different cognitive area such as language or visuospatial ability, or mild declines in several areas (multiple domain MCI) (Petersen & Morris, 2005). Amnestic MCI has received the most attention among researchers, because it is most likely to progress to Alzheimer's disease (AD).

New criteria for diagnosing MCI have recently been proposed (see http://www.alz.org/research/diagnostic_criteria/mci_reccomendations.pdf). The proposed criteria retain the basic features noted above; they also define different levels of severity and address the role of biological markers in identifying MCI.

MCI is a risk factor for developing AD or other dementias. It is often considered a preclinical stage of dementia, but not everyone with MCI goes on to develop dementia. In community surveys where MCI is identified on the basis of brief cognitive tests or questionnaires, the diagnosis is often unstable, with a substantial proportion of cases reverting to normal cognitive performance on follow-up (Bruscoli & Lovestone, 2004; Perri et al., 2009). The diagnosis is more likely to have predictive significance when it is identified through a work-up at a memory diagnostic clinic or by other dementia specialist assessment. On average, persons diagnosed with MCI at memory clinics develop dementia at a rate of 16–18% per year, with some studies showing progression rates as high as 40% per year (Gauthier et al., 2006). Memory clinic clients may have greater impairment – enough to motivate them to seek medical attention – based either on their own concerns or those of family members.

There is no way yet to know which individuals with MCI will develop dementia and which will not. However, those with more severe cognitive deficits, an apolipoprotein epsilon 4 genotype (APOE e4) or smaller hippocampi on neuroimaging are at increased risk for developing AD.

How is MCI Currently Treated?

There are no specific treatments for MCI at this time. Initial clinical trials of drug treatment for memory symptoms of MCI have been largely unsuccessful (Winblad et al., 2004) in delaying dementia onset, although individuals with an APOE e4 genotype may gain some temporary benefit from taking acetylcholinesterase inhibitors such as donepezil (Petersen et al., 2005). The utility of using cholinesterase inhibitors remains controversial because of factors such as cost, inconsistent benefit, and both immediate side effects such as gastrointestinal symptoms and vivid dreaming and longer term side effects such as bradycardia or syncope (Gill et al., 2009; Park-Wyllie et al., 2009). Studies of new medication therapies are ongoing.

Medical management of MCI symptoms (Winblad et al., 2004) consists, at best, of control of vascular risk factors, treatment of coexisting conditions such as depression or hypothyroidism, and phasing out anticholinergic drugs that can exacerbate memory symptoms. Some physicians with expertise in dementia recommend medications such as donepezil for MCI patients, while others focus more on encouraging active lifestyles and good nutrition to support general health.

How Might a Healthy Lifestyle Benefit Individuals with MCI?

People with MCI are often very aware of their difficulties, and many are interested in making lifestyle changes or learning coping strategies that may affect their outlook and symptom severity (Winblad et al., 2004).

Neither researchers nor clinicians can be sure of how any particular lifestyle change will affect progression of MCI. However, the feeling that there is nothing that can be done can be disabling in its own right. Positive, well-grounded, interventions may help individuals with MCI avoid "excess disability" (i.e., doing worse over time than actually necessary for the brain condition) as a result of lowered mood and motivation and giving up activities that a person has always enjoyed.

Lifestyle changes to ward off AD are commonly discussed in the media and promoted in product advertising, but these sources do not provide an adequate basis for making important lifestyle decisions. Individuals with MCI may find it harder than cognitively normal older adults to weigh the value of these options, given their cognitive changes. Health professionals and aging services programs can make a positive contribution by offering organized lifestyle enhancement approaches that can be objectively evaluated.

Cognitive Activity and MCI

Cognitively active lifestyles have been linked to a slower rate of cognitive decline and reduced risk of AD (Fratiglioni, Paillard-Borg, & Winblad, 2004). At least two large-scale studies (Verghese et al., 2003; Wilson et al., 2002) found similar associations between cognitive activity and dementia risk when subjects with mild memory impairments were included in data analyses, suggesting that associations between cognitive activity and dementia may hold true for MCI patients as well as cognitively normal older adults. However, a more recent follow-up from one of these studies suggests a more complicated interaction between cognitive activity, cognitive deficit, and rates of cognitive decline (Wilson et al., 2010). It is important to recognize that the frequency and types of mental activities that may be optimal for sustaining cognitive skills have not been clearly established for either cognitively healthy older adults or those with MCI.

To our knowledge, there are no published interventions that have aimed to increase cognitive activities in persons with MCI in the home or other everyday settings, but a few investigations have provided training in specific cognitive skills. Table 21.1 shows results from four training studies for individuals with MCI. All showed some benefits for participants who received active training compared to control conditions, although not all found significant cognitive improvements.

Belleville et al. (2006) reported the strongest objective cognitive benefits, as well as improvements in subjective well-being, based on training on three specific memory tasks. Rapp et al. (2002) also provided memory training, but they did not see any immediate cognitive benefits compared to a control condition. At a 6-month follow-up, the trained group did better on one memory task. In this study, too, participants who received training reported improved subjective well-being. A short-term group intervention by Kinsella et al. (2009) focused on improving everyday memory through general memory education and practice with both external aides and mnemonic strategies. Significant benefits in performance on prospective memory tasks (e.g., remembering to ask for an appointment card) and knowledge of memory strategies persisted for 4 months after the intervention ended for the intervention group compared to a wait-list control. Finally, Barnes et al. (2009) studied a computerized cognitive exercise program (a special version of the Posit Science Brain Fitness program, see Zelinski et al., Chap. 3) compared to a control condition involving other more traditional forms of cognitive activity. Small benefits of training were noted on two of many cognitive measures.

These investigations show that persons with MCI may benefit from specific cognitive training, but it is important to note that samples were small, and two of the four studies had no follow-up after the end of training to show how long the benefits of training persisted. These studies did not attempt to measure everyday function, and they did not determine whether individuals who received training were more or less likely to develop dementia in later years.

Table 21.1 Cognitive training studies for persons with MCI

References	Sample	Training	Measures	Outcome
Belleville et al. (2006)	*Trained*: 28 amnestic MCI, 17 controls with normal cognition *Untrained*: 8 MCI, 8 controls	8 weekly 2-h sessions, in groups of 4–5; 2 sessions computer-assisted attention training; 4 sessions episodic memory training (e.g., face–name association, text memory)	Prepost only *Primary*: Three episodic memory tasks (face–name, word list, short story) *Secondary*: Subjective memory and well-being questionnaires	Significant improvement with training on face–name recall (effect size=0.59) and word list recall (effect size=0.65), for both MCI and control groups. Greater improvement with younger age and higher education Improved subjective memory and well-being No prepost gain for untrained groups
Kinsella et al. (2009)	*Trained*: 54 amnestic MCI, randomly assigned to a memory intervention group ($n=26$) vs. a wait-list control group ($n=28$). Five in each group withdrew	5 weekly group sessions, 1.5 h each, for participants and family members; practice with external memory aids, mnemonic strategies (e.g., categorization, visual imagery), and general wellness education	Assessed at baseline and at 2 weeks and 4 months postintervention; prospective memory tasks, self-rated Multifactorial Metamemory Questionnaire	Significant improvement with training on prospective memory tasks and in knowledge and use of memory strategies Some benefits persisted at 4 months postintervention No change in self-appraisal of everyday memory
Rapp, Brenes, and Marsh (2002)	19 MCI: nine trained, ten untrained	6 weekly 2-h group meetings. One relaxation training session. Five sessions of training in mnemonics (categorization, chunking, loci, etc.)	Prepost and 6 month follow-up 4 episodic memory tasks (word list, grocery list, names and faces, story) Subjective memory questionnaires, Memory Controllability Inventory, Profile of Mood States	No prepost training benefits on memory tests, but trained group did better on word list at 6 months Trained group had better perceived memory ability and stronger belief in potential for improvement

(continued)

Table 21.1 (continued)

References	Sample	Training	Measures	Outcome
Barnes et al. (2009)	47 MCI patients, randomly assigned to training ($n=22$) or control group ($n=25$). 77% completed the study	Special version of the Posit Science training program vs. "comparable computer-based tasks" (reading newspaper, audio book, computer game). 90–100 min/day, 5 days/week for 6 weeks	Prepost only RBANS[a] and seven other standard cognitive tasks	No training effect on RBANS total scores, but marginally significant benefit on delayed memory ($p=0.07$) in trained subjects and significant improvement in spatial span scores

[a]Repeatable Battery for the Assessment of Neuropsychological Status

Physical Exercise and MCI

Encouraging adequate levels of physical exercise is one of the most promising approaches for sustaining cognitive abilities in normal aging (see Boot and Blakely, Chap. 2), and there have been a few controlled trials of exercise interventions for persons with MCI.

In a recent study conducted in Australia (Lautenschlager et al., 2008), 170 adults 50 years or older who had memory concerns were randomly assigned to a physical activity group or a usual care group. One hundred of these volunteers had objective evidence of MCI on a cognitive screening battery, and remainder had normal cognitive scores. The usual care group received educational information about memory loss, stress management, healthy eating, alcohol consumption, and smoking, but they were given no information about physical activity. The physical activity group received the same educational information, but in addition, they were encouraged to get at least 150 min of moderate-intensity physical exercise (like walking) per week for a period of 24 weeks and to record their activities in a diary. Behavioral support to increase adherence to the physical activity regimen was also provided, including a workshop, manual, newsletters, and phone calls related to the benefits of exercise, goal setting, and potential barriers. On cognitive testing at 6, 12, and 18 months, the physical activity group performed slightly better in the areas of memory, language, and visual-perceptual skills compared to the usual care group. The finding that cognitive benefits persisted for 12 months after the intervention ended is important, as if the fact that participants increased their exercise and sometimes sustained it with no direct training and relatively little program support. An additional important finding was that participants with MCI showed as much benefit from this physical exercise intervention as those with normal cognition at baseline.

Another recent study (Baker et al., 2010) focused on a smaller sample but provided more intensive exercise training. Thirty-three sedentary older adults (age 55–85 years) with amnestic MCI were randomly assigned to either an aerobic exercise intervention or a stretching control group. The aerobic group exercised at 75–85% of heart rate reserve using a treadmill, stationary bicycle, or elliptical machine for 45–60 min/day, 4 days/week for 6 months. The control group performed stretching activities for the same amount of time. Exercises for both groups were supervised by a trainer for the first eight sessions and once per week for the remainder of the study. Participants tracked their activities and heart rate in a daily exercise log. At the end of the 6-month period, aerobic exercise was found to improve executive control processes, especially for women. In women only, aerobic exercise reduced cortisol (a stress hormone) levels and improved insulin sensitivity, which could potentially improve glucose uptake in the brain. The investigators were uncertain why results were more positive in women than men, but they noted that women had poorer cardiovascular status (e.g., higher body fat, higher cholesterol levels) at the start of the study and may therefore have had more room to improve.

These MCI interventions are complemented by a growing literature on exercise interventions for persons diagnosed with AD. Several benefits of sustained exercise for AD patients have been documented, and protocols have been developed for training caregivers as exercise partners or coaches, such as the reducing disability in Alzheimer disease (RDAD) program developed by Linda Teri, Rebecca Logsdon, and colleagues (Logsdon & Teri, 2010; Teri et al., 2003). Such approaches may also prove useful for persons with early-stage cognitive deficits such as MCI.

Applied Cognitive Wellness Programs

The Mayo Clinic at Rochester, MN, is offering a behavioral rehabilitation intervention for individuals with amnestic MCI. Extrapolating from techniques that have proven effective in rehabilitation of traumatic brain injury, this program focuses on training in the use of a portable day calendar and note-taking system to support everyday memory. An initial report (Greenaway, Hanna, Lepore, & Smith, 2008) described outcomes of an open trial with 24 MCI patients and their caregiver partners in which each pair received 12 1-h training sessions over the course of 6 weeks. Dementia severity ratings remained stable across prepost measurement, and based on partner/caregiver ratings, MCI clients' memory-related activities of daily living improved after training. This intervention, called HABIT (Healthy Action to Benefit Independence & Thinking), has since been expanded to include physical and relaxation exercises, cognitive maintenance activities, and an emotional support group and is being offered on a fee-for-service basis. A controlled trial of the HABIT intervention is also planned.

Another multimodal intervention program has been described by Olazarán et al. (2004). Twelve persons with MCI, 48 with mild AD, and 24 with moderate AD enrolled in a year-long "global stimulation" intervention. One half were randomly assigned to a psychosocial-only program, with standard senior day-care type activities, while the other half received a cognitive-motor intervention that entailed twice weekly group sessions of 3.5 h involving reality orientation, cognitive exercises, activities of daily living training, and psychomotor exercises. Cognitive status remained stable at the 6-month assessment for participants receiving the psychomotor intervention, while those in the psychosocial-only group declined on cognitive measures. Depression scores remained stable over 12 months for most of the cognitive-motor intervention group, but worsened for nearly half of those in the psychosocial-only condition. There were no differences between the two groups on ratings of everyday function. Results were not reported separately for persons with MCI vs. AD, and because a combination of supportive activities was provided, the benefits of particular program components (e.g., cognitive exercises vs. psychomotor activities) are unknown.

In the United States, day-care programs for persons with early-stage dementia or other cognitive problems are increasing in popularity. Most combine games or other cognitive stimulating activities with socialization and light forms of exercise. The chapter by Fritsch et al. (Chap. 22) describes preliminary evaluation results for some of these programs.

Table 21.2 Take Charge program structure

One-year program
Individualized activity care plans for exercise and cognitive stimulation – "personal trainer" approach
Brief focused education on healthy diet and stress management
Participation in community-based group activities encouraged as part of activity care plans
Longitudinal monitoring of exercise, mental activity, everyday cognitive function, subjective memory ratings, and mood

Table 21.3 Take Charge time line and intervention modules

Intake session
Exercise and diet module
  14 weeks (seven bimonthly sessions)
  National Institute on Aging (2006) exercise guidelines and American Heart Association (2006) diet guidelines
  Short talks and demonstrations on diet
Cognitive activity and stress management module
  16 weeks (eight bimonthly sessions)
  Cognitive goal – minimum of 30 min of novel information processing activity most or all days per week
  Brief stress management training (e.g., "mini-meditation" techniques)
  Three sessions of training in techniques to remember names and faces
Minimal intervention phase (2–3 months)
Final session (outcome measures and program evaluation)

The Take Charge Pilot Program

Objective and Design

Take Charge was designed to offer a "personal trainer" approach to memory wellness for persons diagnosed with MCI (see Table 21.2). Individualized activity plans were developed to increase aerobic exercise and to boost engagement in cognitively stimulating everyday activities. Adherence to the plans was supported by twice-monthly meetings with a professional experienced in geriatrics and dementia. These meetings also provided educational information on diet and stress management and training in one important aspect of everyday memory (face–name recall). Aiming for sustainability, the program was designed to capitalize on activities that people had enjoyed for many years and to help them engage more often, or in new ways, in these activities, in addition to developing new activities if desired. Table 21.3 shows the general time line and intervention modules.

The objective of the Take Charge pilot study was to determine the feasibility of the Take Charge approach, its key intervention components (Diet and Exercise module and Cognitive Activity and Stress Management module), and the assessment tools. There was no control condition in this initial phase.

Participants

Participants were 38 volunteers recruited from four memory diagnostic clinics (three in small to medium-size cities, one in a rural setting). All had been diagnosed with amnestic MCI and were 60 years or older, English-speaking, able to hear and see well enough to participate in project activities, and able to travel to participate in the project sessions. All had a close family member (usually a spouse) who provided information on participants' cognitive skills and everyday functioning and sometimes attended sessions. At the start of the project, none of the volunteers had a major psychiatric disorder, neurological condition, or medical illness severe enough to prevent them from participating. Eight individuals did not complete the study (3 developed significant medical illnesses, 1 died, 1 moved, and 3 opted out for other reasons).

The 30 volunteers who completed the year-long study ranged in age from 60 to 89 years (median = 76 years). There were 16 women and 14 men, all non-Hispanic white. Education ranged from a high school degree to graduate or professional degrees. All but three participants were retired, and most rated their health as "good."

Project Staff and Training

Each site had a single staff member who provided the Take Charge programming. One was a clinical nurse practitioner, two were social workers, and the fourth was a program director for a community agency providing support to persons with dementia. All had extensive experience in working with older adults with dementia.

Two half-day training meetings were provided to review the rationale and procedures of the study and to practice program components that required a standardized administration (e.g., face–name training). The initial training sessions were followed by scheduled conference calls and additional e-mail or telephone communications.

Getting Started: Intake and Module Selection

Participants were first contacted by telephone to explain the study and verify their interest. At the initial intake session, a consent form, a short activities interview, a health questionnaire, and the geriatric depression scale (GDS, Yesavage et al., 1982) were completed by the participant. A close family member (usually a spouse) provided ratings of participants' everyday cognitive skills (Everyday Cognition Questionnaire, Farias et al., 2006) and ability to do higher-level functional activities such as taking medications or managing finances (Instrumental Activities of Daily Living scale Lawton & Brody, 1969).

At the end of the initial session, the two Take Charge modules were described (one focusing on cognitive activity and stress management, the other on physical activity and diet), and participants were asked to choose which they would like to work on first.

Cognitive Activity and Stress Management Module

The 8-session, 16-week module on cognitive activity and stress management focused on cognitively stimulating activities and education about ways to manage everyday stress.

The aims of this module were to:

- Increase participants' knowledge of cognitive activities that have been associated with good cognitive abilities in later years.
- Assist participants in sustaining adequate levels of cognitive activity, or if needed, to gradually increase cognitive activity to levels associated with healthy cognitive aging.
- Provide strategies and practice in face–name recall.
- Increase participants' knowledge of common symptoms of stress and provide tools that may help in managing or reducing stress levels.

Table 21.4 shows the activities at each 2-week session for this module. Participants completed several questionnaires specific to this section (see Table 21.5) at the first meeting for this module. On the Cognitive Activity Questionnaire, participants indicated how often they engaged in each of 50 everyday cognitive activities currently or recently. Items on a Novel Information Processing factor derived from this questionnaire formed the focus of Take Charge intervention. Participants' current patterns of cognitive activity were reviewed in this first session, and barriers to being mentally active were identified and discussed. A daily log for tracking "brain activities"

Table 21.4 Cognitive activity and stress management module

Session	Curriculum
1	Complete memory and cognitive activity questionnaires; stress questionnaire Introduce and practice with cognitive activity log form
2	Healthy aging: Why are cognitive activity and stress management important? Review of cognitive activity log. *Choose cognitive activity goals and plan*
3	Discuss list of "stress buster" recommendations Relaxation exercise: controlled breathing and progressive relaxation Discussion of cognitive activities
4	Relaxation exercises: "mini-meditation" and mental imagery Discussion of cognitive activities. *Revise cognitive activity plan as needed*
5	Discussion of cognitive activities Names and faces training – part 1
6	Discussion of cognitive activities. *Revise cognitive activity plan as needed* Names and faces training – part 2
7	Discussion of cognitive activities Names and faces training – part 3
8	Review of cognitive activity log Complete postintervention questionnaires (cognitive activity, stress) Participant feedback on the cognitive activity and stress management module

Table 21.5 Assessment tools for the cognitive activity and stress management module

Measure	Description	Source
Cognitive activity questionnaire	Fifty common activities, rated for frequency of current engagement	Adapted from Hultsch, Hertzog, Small, and Dixon (1999)
Barriers to brain activity	Self-rating of factors that may limit engagement in cognitive activities	Developed for Take Charge
Memory self-efficacy questionnaire	Self-ratings of memory for different types of information	Zelinski and Gilewski (2004)
Everyday stress questionnaire	Self-report of stressful life events and current symptoms of stress	Holmes and Rahe (1967) plus stress symptom checklist from Mental Health America FactSheet (1998)
Geriatric depression scale, short form	Fifteen symptoms of depression, self-rated	Yesavage et al. (1982)

was introduced and practiced, and participants were asked to use the log to monitor their cognitive activities for the 2-week interval before their next session.

At the second session in the Cognitive Activity and Stress Management module, goals for being cognitively active were discussed and identified. Generally, participants were asked to select one or two activities that they would like to do more often. Many of the targeted activities were ones which the participant had enjoyed in the past but had discontinued or currently engaged in with low to moderate frequency. Some participants opted to enroll in continuing education classes, attend lectures or concerts, or attend other organized educational or cultural activities that are available in their communities as part of their Take Charge plans. The goal of the cognitive activity intervention was for all participants to be engaging in *a minimum of two Novel Information Processing activities on a daily or near-daily basis by the end of the 16-week module*. This equals or exceeds the frequencies of cognitively stimulating activities that have been associated with reduced dementia risk in studies of older populations (Verghese et al., 2003; Wilson et al., 2002).

Sessions 3 and 4 added education and practice with stress management tools. A list of "stress buster" recommendations was reviewed, and simple exercises for stress reduction (controlled breathing with progressive relaxation, simplified meditation exercise, and mental imagery) were introduced and practiced.

The final three sessions in Cognitive Activity and Stress Management module provided brief, systematic training in strategies for enhancing face–name associations based on current research in cognitive rehabilitation (Belleville et al., 2006; Clare, Wilson, Carter, Roth, & Hodges, 2002). A five-step strategy for face–name association was introduced and modeled by the Take Charge staff person, and participants practiced learning a small number of names of persons shown in photos. Spaced retrieval techniques were used to encourage remembering over progressively longer time intervals within a session, and home practice was also encouraged.

In the 2 weeks preceding the final session of this module, participants were again asked to monitor their cognitive activity using the daily "brain activity" log form, and at the last session, they completed the questionnaires for this section.

Although active programming for cognitive activity and stress reduction ended at this point, participants were encouraged to continue their cognitive activities and any changes they had made to manage everyday stress.

Exercise and Diet Module

All participants completed a health screening form at the Take Charge intake session, and for those who indicated potential problems such as heart conditions or gait instability that might affect safety to exercise, written permission was obtained from the participant's primary care providers before they enrolled in the Exercise and Diet module.

The 7-session, 14-week module on exercise and diet was adapted from the "Eat Better and Move More" program (Wellman et al., 2004) sponsored by the Administration on Aging and implemented in multiple senior community sites across the country. The main adaptations for Take Charge were as follows: (a) our program was given in an individual rather than group format; (b) although walking was encouraged as a relatively safe and versatile form of exercise, other forms of aerobic exercise could be included in exercise plans; and (c) some of the "mini-lectures" provided in the program guide for "Eat Better and Move More" were replaced by new educational components. Table 21.6 shows the schedule of activities for every 2 weeks.

The aims of this module were to:

- Increase participants' knowledge of exercise and diet habits that have been associated with good health in later years, including healthy brain function.
- Assist participants in sustaining adequate levels of aerobic exercise, or if needed, to gradually increase aerobic exercise to recommended levels.

Table 21.6 Diet and exercise module

Session	Curriculum
1	Complete exercise and diet questionnaires Introduce and practice with exercise log form
2	Healthy aging: Exercise recommendations (National Institute on Aging, 2006) Review of exercise log. *Choose exercise goals and plan*
3	Diet recommendations (American Heart Association, 2006) Discussion of exercise activities
4	Tips for measuring portion size Discussion of exercise activities. *Revise exercise plan as needed*
5	Fruits and vegetables; antioxidant nutrients Discussion of exercise activities
6	Fish and omega-3 fatty acids; "good fats" Discussion of exercise activities. *Revise exercise plan as needed*
7	Review of exercise log Complete exercise and diet questionnaires (postintervention) Participant feedback on the exercise and diet module

- Provide participants with tools to monitor portion size and to recognize specific food groups and nutrients that have been associated with healthy cognitive aging.

At the first session in the Exercise and Diet Module, participants completed the following questionnaires specific to this section: Physical Activity Questionnaire, Nutrition Questionnaire, and Barriers to Being Active quiz. All were adapted from the "Eat Better and Move More" program. A log form for monitoring daily exercise was introduced, and examples and practice in using this form were provided. Participants were asked to use this log form to track their current physical activities for the 2-week interval between the first and second sessions.

At the second session in the Exercise and Diet module, exercise goals were discussed, using the National Institute on Aging (NIA) guidelines (2006) and available literature on exercise effects on cognition in older adults. The goal was for participants to engage in at least *30 min of moderate-intensity exercise (i.e., increasing breathing and heart rate) for five or more days a week* by the end of the 14-week module. This was the level of aerobic exercise recommended by the NIA for older adults, and it equals or exceeds levels previously associated with cognitive benefits in older populations (e.g., Larson et al., 2006; Yaffe, Barnes, Nevitt, Lui, & Covinsky, 2001).

Participants who reported that they were already exercising regularly at recommended levels were encouraged to continue their current activities and to consider additional forms of exercise (e.g., balance or flexibility training) to complement their aerobic activities. For more sedentary individuals, preferred forms of exercise were identified, and participants were asked to select one or two activities that they would like to increase in frequency or intensity. The pace of increased activity was individualized, and for participants who were sedentary, increases of approximately 10% per week in exercise frequency or duration were recommended. The Take Charge staff member worked with the participant to select exercise activities, to translate goals into specific recommendations for each 2-week interval, and to problem-solve regarding barriers (e.g., loss of transportation, unavailability of an exercise partner) to continuing exercise. Walking for exercise was encouraged, but many other activities could be substituted, including sports or physical tasks such as gardening or household chores. Some participants enrolled in exercise programs for older adults in their area as part of their Take Charge plan.

In sessions 3 through 6, there were brief educational presentations and discussions on an identified topic (see Table 21.6). Educational information emphasized the value of certain food sources for heart health and *potential* value for brain health. At each session, the Take Charge staff member asked participants to describe any dietary changes made in the intervening 2 weeks and to estimate their typical daily consumption of key food items.

In the 2 weeks before the final session of this module, participants were asked to monitor their exercise activity using the daily log form. At the final session, participants were again asked to complete questionnaires specific to this section. Although active programming for exercise and diet ended at this point, participants were asked to continue to track their physical exercise informally and to continue any dietary changes they had made to achieve and maintain an appropriate weight and to incorporate "brain healthy" foods.

Project Outcomes

The main outcomes of this project are summarized below. It is important to remember that this was an open trial of a pilot program with no control or comparison condition.

- When given a choice about whether to begin working on cognitive activity vs. physical activity, most participants (22 of 30, or 73%) chose to work first on boosting cognitive activity. This suggests a high degree of enthusiasm for increasing mental stimulation in meaningful ways.
- Nearly all participants (93%) rated the Cognitive Activity and Stress Management module as helpful, and most (87%) reported an increase in their cognitive activity as a result of participating. This was reinforced by their specific reports (on the 50-item activity list) of how often they engaged in particular novel information-processing activities at the end, compared to the beginning, of the module. Most reported that name–face memory training was helpful, at least "a little." When asked to say what was hardest about this module, 47% listed remembering the names and faces, 33% listed keeping track of activities, 17% identified doing the activities as hardest, and 4% had other responses.
- Two thirds of the participants reported reduced stress as a result of participation in the program. Nine of the ten who did not find the stress management information helpful reported low stress levels at baseline. The median score of 2 on the GDS did not change from baseline to the 1 year retest, but the percentage of participants with elevated baseline depression scores (≥ 5) declined from 18 to 4%. These results suggest that the program may have had a beneficial impact on the emotional well-being of those participants who needed it the most.
- There was less enthusiasm (and less behavior change) for the Exercise and Diet Module. Although 66% of participants described the module as helpful, only 38% reported that they had increased their physical activity as a result of participating. This was borne out by their reports of the amount of time they spent in vigorous physical activities at the end, compared to the start, of the module. Some participants were already very physically active at the start of the study, and others were clearly sedentary. Neither of these subgroups markedly changed their rate of physical activity. When asked to describe what was hardest about this module, 47% of the participants reported that doing the physical activities was hardest, another 47% listed keeping track of their activities as hardest, and 6% had other responses.
- Take Charge did not administer cognitive tests to assess for change in memory or other cognitive abilities. Participants' subjective ratings of their everyday memory abilities improved only slightly (not statistically significant) from baseline to 1 year. The same was true for informants' ratings of participants' memory and other cognitive skills. At baseline, the mean memory rating provided by spouses and other close family members on the Everyday Cognition (eCog) questionnaire indicated mild to moderate decline in participants' everyday memory compared to 10 years earlier. At 1 year (1–3 months after active Take Charge programming ended) the mean observer-rated memory score was nearly identical. Ratings of participants' independence in performing higher-level everyday

activities indicated that participants had either no impairment or mild impairment in these activities at baseline and at the end of the project year, with nearly identical mean scores at both times.
- All but one participant reported that they would recommend Take Charge to others. What they liked best about the program was attending the sessions with the project staff member (endorsed by 60%), which provided opportunities to talk on a one-to-one basis; gains in knowledge and personal awareness (endorsed by 23%); and specific training or information gained (endorsed by 13%). When asked what they would like to see changed about the program, 57% reported no changes needed and 23% indicated that they would like to have fewer logging requirements or fewer forms to complete.

Lessons Learned and Looking Ahead

Comments, Cautions, and Recommendations

A strength of Take Charge was that participants' MCI had been identified by a thorough diagnostic workup. Their deficits, though mild, were confirmed by cognitive testing, patient and caregiver reports, and medical assessment to rule out reversible causes. If participants for wellness interventions are selected on the basis of self-report alone, or a brief cognitive screen, there is the risk that instability of mild memory impairments could be mistaken for program-related improvements in prepost comparisons.

Many volunteers for cognitive wellness programs are already very active physically or cognitively or both. Although there are likely to be few risks from participating in memory clubs or programs like Take Charge, it can be hard to demonstrate reliable program-related gains for persons who already have an active and engaged lifestyle. A major challenge is to make cognitive-wellness intervention programs appealing, appropriate, and accessible for less-active individuals who may benefit the most from this type of intervention (Barnes, 2010). Understanding "change readiness" of program volunteers is an area that has been neglected in most cognitive wellness programs so far, and it is likely to be important (Lautenschlager, 2010).

Simple test–retest results from programs such as Take Charge provide valuable information about the appropriateness of assessment tools, intervention procedures, participant acceptance, and feasibility. For example, we did not know in advance whether older adults with MCI would be willing and able to commit to a 1-year intervention. However, specific benefits cannot be claimed for this program in the absence of a comparison or control condition. A next step could be to randomly assign older persons diagnosed with MCI to Take Charge vs. a usual care group provided with information on exercise, diet, cognitive activity, etc., but no specific training and no regular meetings with a healthcare provider. Another option would be to randomly assign individuals to either an individualized activity care plan program such as Take Charge or a group program (e.g., a "memory club").

The strong endorsement by participants of the one-on-one format suggests that an individualized cognitive support program may be a valuable alternative to group formats, at least for some individuals. Because the Take Charge staff members all had extensive clinical or programmatic experience in the fields of aging and dementia, their time and support were valuable indeed. Whether an individualized care-plan program would work as well with less experienced staff (e.g., students or nonprofessional volunteers) cannot be determined from this project.

Although the Take Charge volunteers reported subjective benefits from participating, as well as increases in their involvement in specific everyday cognitive activities, family member informants described their everyday cognitive and functional skills as stable, on average, at 1 year. Is this a good outcome? Given that these individuals' MCI was diagnosed at memory clinics and that at least 16–18% would be expected to develop dementia within 1 year (Gauthier et al., 2006), the fact that none developed dementia may be encouraging. Given the open study design and small sample, however, this could be due to chance. Adding cognitive tests to the prepost protocol would provide objective measures of cognitive change. Adding quality of life measures may be even more important for future cognitive wellness programs.

A final caution concerns the selection of cognitive activity interventions for persons with MCI (or early-stage dementia). Many cognitive wellness programs emphasize learning new skills or doing unfamiliar tasks. Because AD and other dementias undermine new learning abilities, it may be important to temper this emphasis on novelty with strengthening of familiar activities that provide cognitive stimulation. To try to increase the odds that cognitive activities might continue after the study ended, one goal of Take Charge was to help participants engage more fully in hobbies or pursuits that they had once done more often and had enjoyed. Several participants resumed complex activities (e.g., playing the cello, writing poetry) that they had stopped years ago and reported great pleasure in rediscovering their talents. Whether a building-on-existing-strengths approach is more (or less) beneficial than focusing on new learning for individuals in early stages of progressive cognitive change is a question that needs to be explored.

What the Future May Hold?

Memory gyms, personal trainers for cognition, and a plethora of commercial products marketed for cognitive enhancement are all possibilities for the future. What is needed is for research to catch up with the natural experiment in "brain fitness" that is taking place in this country and elsewhere.

Several large scale clinical trials of multifaceted interventions to support cognitive function are now underway. The Finnish Geriatric Intervention Study (FINGER) is a population-based program for older adults that combines nutrition education, exercise, cognitive training, social activity, and monitoring of chronic disease (Kivipelto, 2010). The Multi-Domain Alzheimer Preventive Trial (MAPT) in France is a controlled trial of cognitive training plus exercise, social activity, and health prevention information designed for older adults with cognitive or physical frailty (Ousset, 2010). In the United States, the Mental Activity and Exercise (MAX) trial (Barnes, 2010) is one of several promising projects. These investigations and new interventions in the planning phase will add greatly to our knowledge about the value of social- and activity-based programs in helping older adults with or without MCI to develop and sustain their cognitive skills.

Acknowledgments Take Charge would not have been possible without the help of project staff members Teresa Fleming, Tammy Pence, Philomena Poole, and Mary Reines; physicians and social work staff at participating memory diagnostic clinics, including Ronald Kodras, Thomas Loepfe, Mark Sager, Robert Smith, and Marie Hornes; and financial support from the Helen Bader Foundation to the Wisconsin Alzheimer's Institute for the memory clinic network and dementia outreach efforts. The persistence and efforts of Take Charge participants are also greatly appreciated.

References

American Heart Association. (2006). Diet and lifestyle recommendations revision 2006: A scientific statement from the American Heart Association Nutrition Committee. *Circulation, 114*, 82–96.

Baker, L. D., Frank, L. L., Foster-Schubert, K., Green, P. S., Wilkinson, C. W., McTiernan, A., et al. (2010). Effects of aerobic exercise on mild cognitive impairment. *Archives of Neurology, 67*, 71–79.

Barnes, D. E. (2010). The Mental Activity and Exercise (MAX) trial: A randomized, controlled trial to enhance cognitive functioning in older adults with cognitive complaints. *Alzheimer's & Dementia, 6*(Suppl. 1), S145.

Barnes, D. E., Yaffe, K., Belfor, N., Jagust, W. J., DeCarli, C., Reed, B. R., et al. (2009). Computer-based cognitive training for mild cognitive impairment: Results from a pilot randomized, controlled trial. *Alzheimer Disease and Associated Disorders, 23*, 205–210.

Belleville, S., Gilbert, B., Fontaine, F., Gagnon, L., Ménard, E., & Gauthier, S. (2006). Improvement of episodic memory in persons with mild cognitive impairment and healthy older adults: Evidence from a cognitive intervention program. *Dementia and Geriatric Cognitive Disorders, 22*, 486–499.

Bruscoli, M., & Lovestone, S. (2004). Is MCI really just early dementia? A systematic review of conversion studies. *International Psychogeriatrics, 16*, 129–140.

Clare, L., Wilson, B. A., Carter, G., Roth, I., & Hodges, J. R. (2002). Relearning face-name associations in early Alzheimer's disease. *Neuropsychology, 16*, 538–547.

Farias, S. T., Mungas, D., Reed, B. R., Harvey, D., Cahn-Weiner, D., & Decarli, C. (2006). MCI is associated with deficits in everyday functioning. *Alzheimer Disease and Associated Disorders, 20*, 217–233.

Fratiglioni, L., Paillard-Borg, S., & Winblad, B. (2004). An active and socially integrated lifestyle in late life might protect against dementia. *Lancet Neurology, 3*, 242–253.

Gauthier, S., Reisberg, B., Zaudig, M., Petersen, R. C., Ritchie, K., Broich, K., et al. (2006). Mild cognitive impairment. *Lancet, 367*, 1262–1270.

Gill, S. S., Anderson, G. M., Fischer, H. D., Bell, C. M., Li, P., Normand, S. L., et al. (2009). Syncope and its consequences in patients with dementia receiving cholinesterase inhibitors: A population-based cohort study. *Archives of Internal Medicine, 69*, 867–873.

Greenaway, M. C., Hanna, S. M., Lepore, S. W., & Smith, G. E. (2008). A behavioral rehabilitation intervention of amnestic mild cognitive impairment. *American Journal of Alzheimers Disease and Other Dementias, 23*, 451–461.

Holmes, T., & Rahe, R. (1967). Holmes-Rahe social readjustment rating scale. *Journal of Psychosomatic Research, 11*, 213–218.

Hultsch, D. F., Hertzog, C., Small, B. J., & Dixon, R. A. (1999). Use it or lose it: Engaged lifestyle as a buffer of cognitive decline in aging. *Psychology and Aging, 14*, 245–263.

Kinsella, G. J., Mullaly, E., Rand, E., Ong, B., Burton, C., Price, S., et al. (2009). Early intervention for mild cognitive impairment: A randomized controlled trial. *Journal of Neurology, Neurosurgery, and Psychiatry, 80*, 730–736.

Kivipelto, M. (2010). Finnish Geriatric Intervention Study to prevent cognitive impairment and disability (FINGER). *Alzheimer's & Dementia, 6*(Suppl. 1), S146.

Larson, E. B., Wang, L., Bowen, J. D., McCormick, W. C., Teri, L., Crane, P., et al. (2006). Exercise is associated with reduced risk for incident dementia among persons 65 year of age and older. *Annals of Internal Medicine, 144*, 73–81.

Lautenschlager, N. (2010). The importance of self efficacy for the adoption and maintenance of physical activity in older adults with memory complaints. *Alzheimer's & Dementia, 6*(Suppl. 1), S145.

Lautenschlager, N. R., Cox, K. L., Flicker, L., Foster, J. K., Bockxmeer, F. M., Xiao, J., et al. (2008). Effect of physical activity on cognitive function in older adults at risk for Alzheimer disease. *Journal of the American Medical Association, 300*, 1027–1037.

Lawton, M. P., & Brody, E. M. (1969). Assessment of older people: Self maintaining and instrumental activities of daily living. *Gerontologist, 9*, 176–186.

Logsdon, R. G., & Teri, L. (2010). An evidence-based exercise and behavior management program for dementia care. *Generations, Spring*, 80–83.

National Institute on Aging. (2006). *Exercise: A guide from the National Institute on Aging*. Bethesda: National Institute on Aging. Retrieved July 30, 2009, from http://www.nih.gov/nia.

Olazarán, J., Muñiz, R., Reisberg, B., Peña-Casanova, J., del Ser, T., Cruz-Jentoft, A. J., et al. (2004). Benefits of cognitive-motor intervention in MCI and mild to moderate Alzheimer disease. *Neurology, 63*, 2348–2353.

Ousset, P. J. (2010). The multi-domain Alzheimer Prevention Trial (MAPT): A new approach for the prevention of Alzheimer's disease – characteristics of the study population. *Alzheimer's & Dementia, 6*(Suppl. 1), S146.

Park-Wyllie, L. Y., Mamdani, M. M., Li, P., Gill, S. S., Laupacis, A., & Juurlink, D. H. (2009). Cholinesterase inhibitors and hospitalization for bradycardia: A population-based study. *PLoS Medicine, 6*(9), e1000157.

Perri, R., Carlesimo, G. A., Serra, L., Caltagirone, C., & Early Diagnosis Group of the Italian Interdisciplinary Network on Alzheimer's Disease. (2009). When the amnestic mild cognitive impairment disappears. Characterisation of the memory profile. *Cognitive and Behavioral Neurology, 22*, 109–116.

Petersen, R. C., & Morris, J. C. (2005). Mild cognitive impairment as a clinical entity and treatment target. *Archives of Neurology, 62*, 1160–1163.

Petersen, R. C., Thomas, R. G., Grundman, M., Bennett, D., Doody, R., Ferris, S., et al. (2005). Vitamin E and donepezil for the treatment of mild cognitive impairment. *New England Journal of Medicine, 352*, 2379–2388.

Rapp, S., Brenes, G., & Marsh, A. P. (2002). Memory enhancement training for older adults with mild cognitive impairment. *Aging and Mental Health, 6*, 5–11.

Teri, L., Gibbons, L. E., McCurry, S. M., Logsdon, R. G., Buchner, D. M., Barlow, W. E., et al. (2003). Exercise plus behavioral management in patients with Alzheimer disease: A randomized controlled trial. *Journal of the American Medical Association, 290*, 15–22.

Verghese, J., Lipton, R. B., Katz, M. J., Hall, C. B., Derby, C. A., Kuslansky, G., et al. (2003). Leisure activities and the risk of dementia in the elderly. *New England Journal of Medicine, 348*, 2508–2516.

Wellman, N., Friedberg, B., Weddle, D., Cuervo, L., Sanchez, N. K., Rosenzweig, L., et al. (2004). *Eat better & move more: A guidebook for community programs*. Miami: National Resource Center on Nutrition, Physical Activity & Aging, Florida International University. Retrieved July 30, 2009, from http://www.aoa.gov/youcan/EBMM/ebmm.asp

Wilson, R. S., Barnes, L. L., Aggarwal, N. T., Boyle, P. A., Hebert, L. E., Mendes de Leon, C. F., et al. (2010). Cognitive activity and the cognitive morbidity of Alzheimer disease. *Neurology, 75*, 990–996.

Wilson, R. S., Bennett, D. A., Bienias, J. L., Aggarwal, N. T., Mendes De Leon, C. F., Morris, M. C., et al. (2002). Cognitive activity and incident AD in a population-based sample of older persons. *Neurology, 59*, 1910–1914.

Winblad, B., Palmer, K., Kivipelto, M., Jelic, V., Fratiglioni, L., Wahlund, L. O., et al. (2004). Mild cognitive impairment – beyond controversies, towards a consensus: report of the International Working Group on Mild Cognitive Impairment. *Journal of Internal Medicine, 256*, 240–246.

Yaffe, K., Barnes, D., Nevitt, M., Lui, L. Y., & Covinsky, K. (2001). A prospective study of physical activity and cognitive decline in elderly women: Women who walk. *Archives of Internal Medicine, 161*, 1703–1708.

Yesavage, J. A., Brink, T. L., Rose, T. L., Lum, O., Huang, V., Adey, M., et al. (1982). Development and validation of a geriatric depression screening scale: A preliminary report. *Journal of Psychiatric Research, 12*, 37–49.

Yesavage, J. A., O'Hara, R., Kraemer, H., Noda, A., Taylor, J. L., Ferris, S., et al. (2002). Modeling the prevalence and incidence of Alzheimer's disease and mild cognitive impairment. *Journal of Psychiatric Research, 36*, 281–286.

Zelinski, E. M., & Gilewski, M. J. (2004). A 10-item Rasch modeled memory self-efficacy scale. *Aging and Mental Health, 8*, 293–306.

Chapter 22
Early Memory Loss Clubs: A Novel Approach for Stimulating and Sustaining Cognitive Function

Thomas Fritsch, Kathleen A. Smyth, Maggie S. Wallendal, Kristin Einberger, and David S. Geldmacher

Abstract In this chapter we describe a particular intervention, Early Memory Loss Clubs, that we believe exemplify the type of intervention needed for those with Alzheimer's disease and related disorders (ADRD). We summarize the current status of medical management of ADRD and provide a brief introduction to non-pharmacological approaches to ADRD intervention and management.

Introduction

Earlier contributions to this edition have highlighted the growing body of research suggesting that, as people age, cognitive function can be stimulated and even enhanced by influencing mutable (i.e., changeable) life-style factors and conducting behavioral interventions. There is now compelling evidence that *active engagement* throughout the life-course – pursuing mentally stimulating activities, having close social networks, and exercising regularly – can lower a person's risk for developing Alzheimer's disease and related disorders (ADRD) (Friedland et al., 2001; Fritsch et al., 2005; Karp et al., 2006), or perhaps even slow rates of cognitive decline (Barnes, Mendes de Leon, Wilson, Bienias, & Evans, 2004; Wilson et al., 2003; Yaffe, Barnes, Nevitt, Lui, & Covinsky, 2001). Epidemiological investigations (e.g., Karp et al., 2006), neuro-imaging work (e.g., Scarmeas et al., 2003), and animal studies (e.g., Hamm, Temple, O'Dell, Pike, & Lyeth, 1996) all support this hypothesis.

T. Fritsch (✉)
Parkinson Research Institute, Aurora Sinai Medical Center,
945 N. 12th Street, Suite 4602, Milwaukee, WI 53233, USA

University of Wisconsin-Milwaukee, Helen Bader School of Social Welfare, P.O. Box 786, Milwaukee, WI 53201, USA

Department of Neurology, Case Western Reserve School of Medicine, 10900 Euclid Avenue, Cleveland, OH 44106, USA
e-mail: tfritsch.pri@gmail.com

In spite of this heartening evidence, most researchers and policy makers agree that the number of new cases of dementia will explode in the next several decades. In 2010, the estimated prevalence of all dementias was 5.1 million (Hebert, Scherr, Bienias, Bennet, & Evans, 2003). That value is predicted to increase to 13.2 million by 2050. Our healthcare system may very well buckle under the weight of new cases which will require more trained practitioners; sufficient numbers of hospital and nursing home beds for acute and long-term care; and reimbursements to cover sky-rocketing costs. Coupled with its devastating impact on those with dementia, their families, and society, ADRD could be considered the medical and social scourges of the twenty-first century. It is clear that we should be prepared for this epidemic with novel, creative, efficacious, and economically viable interventions that will help to maintain the quality of life (QOL) for persons with dementia and their care partners.

Medical Management of ADRD

Typically, management of ADRD has centered on the use of drugs such as donepezil (Aricept®, Eisai, Inc.) and other cholinesterase inhibitors, and memantine (Namenda®, Forest Pharmaceuticals, Inc.), an NMDA glutamate receptor inhibitor. However, this approach has limitations. In one meta-analysis,[1] the authors reviewed 96 publications representing 59 unique studies of cholinesterase inhibitors and memantine (Raina et al., 2008). While these agents were shown in the individual studies to have consistent effects in the domains of cognition and global assessment, the overall effect size[2] based on a summary of results across all the studies was small. Further, most of the studies were of short duration, usually following subjects for up to 6 months. The authors of this review concluded that while treatment of dementia with cholinesterase inhibitors and glutamate inhibitors can result in statistically significant effects, the clinical importance of the effects is only marginal (Raina et al.). Nonetheless, other outcome measures, such as time spent in caregiving, favor treatment and may be of more direct impact on families facing dementia (Sano, Wilcock, van Baelen, & Kavanagh, 2003). Regardless of their perceived degree of effectiveness, most experts recognize that these medications are best used in combination with non-pharmaceutical interventions.

While the National Institute on Aging's Alzheimer's Disease Education & Referral Center web site (http://www.alzheimers.org/clinicaltrials/recs.asp, June 30,

---

[1] A meta-analysis is a comprehensive review of articles, all concerned with a specific topic, in which statistical techniques are used to estimate the *overall magnitude* of the intervention being considered.

[2] Effect sizes (ESs) are standardized indicators of the strength of an effect associated with an intervention, e.g., increases in scores on a cognitive test after treatment with a particular medication. Cohen's *d* is the most commonly used measure of ESs. In the social sciences, small, medium, and large ESs are, respectively, 0.20, 0.50, 0.80 (Cohen, 1992).

2010) lists over 70 clinical trials now being conducted to help prevent or treat ADRD, it takes many years for effective agents to move from the investigational stage to actual use in clinical care. The limited effect of current drug treatments and the long wait for development of new agents both underscore the need for interventions that are not based solely on the traditional medical model. But the paucity of pharmacological treatments is not the only motivation for the development of alternative forms of intervention.

The Non-Pharmacologic Movement

The notion that ADRD can be treated using interventions that are *not* based primarily on medicine is not new. As Kitwood and Bredin (1992) noted more than 15 years ago, before the availability of prescriptive pharmacotherapy, perhaps the most fruitful approach to developing a clinical response to ADRD is to view it as an interplay between neurologic impairment, which sets upper limits on performance, and the psychological and social-psychological nature and experience of the person affected. This approach acknowledges that those who have face-to-face contact with the person with ADRD as well as the pattern of social relations in which the person with ADRD operates contribute considerably to their health and well-being. Novel approaches of this type continue to emerge which, in combination with pharmacologic interventions, could help sustain a higher QOL for persons with dementia for a longer time. This synergy of different interventions could be powerful. It has been suggested that if we could delay the onset of dementia symptoms by 5 years, the prevalence of ADRD could be cut by half (Brookmeyer, Gray, & Kawas, 1998). Thus, multi-disciplinary management and treatment of ADRD represent "fertile soil" in which new ideas about interventions and treatments for ADRD may germinate. These non-pharmacologic approaches seem to hold much promise (Acevedo & Lowenstein, 2007).

Early Memory Loss Clubs

One particular form of non-pharmacologic intervention for Alzheimer's is becoming extremely popular, emerging at a grass-roots level all across the country. It is known by many different names, but is most commonly referred to as "early memory loss (EML) club" or "memory club." One reason for the emergence of these clubs may be the realization that programs commonly offered at senior day care centers are neither appealing to nor appropriate for persons with early-stage memory loss. EML clubs vary greatly in their approaches. Some are best described as "cognitively based stimulation programs" (Brookdale Foundation, 2010). Others are more aptly termed "out and about" programs. In the latter form, persons with memory loss gather together to go on stimulating outings, such as field trips to museums, zoos, and art shows, or dining together as a group.

The memory club model we focus on here was inspired by the widely used Brookdale cognitive stimulation model, developed by Einberger and Sellick (2007) who are currently activity directors at the Fairfield Senior Center near Davis, CA. The central theme of the Brookdale-inspired model is that mental exercise can benefit persons with ADRD. With financial support from the New York-based Brookdale Foundation, Einberger and Sellick published a manual[3] which provides step-by-step instructions for setting up a Brookdale-inspired club. Here we briefly summarize the intervention.

The EML Intervention

The Brookdale-inspired model, which we evaluated, involves having persons with early memory loss/mild cognitive losses gather together at a Continuing Care Retirement Community (CCRC), senior center, or library for 4 h once or twice per week. The emphasis is on doing meaningful activities that "exercise" various domains of cognitive functioning. A club facilitator, usually someone with expertise working with people who have memory loss, such as a social worker,[4] is present for each of the 4-h sessions to guide the flow of activities, provide feedback, encourage participants, and facilitate the program. Lunch is served at mid-day, providing opportunities for socializing. Strong feelings of camaraderie are believed to emerge as participants get to know one another through their once- or twice-per week contacts. Indeed, the social networks that are formed during these group meetings seem to contribute to increases in well-being reported by participants (Brown, 2000). Each club also uses light exercise, e.g., stretching, walks around the campus, or Tai Chi, to stimulate the body as well as the brain.

In 2007, a conference was convened in Milwaukee, WI, to outline and establish the critical elements of the Brookdale-inspired cognitive stimulation model we evaluated. Based on their considerable experience facilitating memory clubs, the conference team outlined ten core "pillars" of the program, shown in Table 22.1. A more detailed description of the program can be found in Einberger and Sellick (2007).

---

[3] Einberger and Sellick (2007). Copies of the manual can be obtained, free of charge, from the Brookdale Foundation by calling 212-308-7355.

[4] Successful club facilitators have come from a variety of educational backgrounds. Social workers, recreation therapists, teachers in the field of aging, and speech therapists are perhaps best suited to be club facilitators. Facilitators should have, at minimum, a bachelor's degree that provides them with knowledge and experience regarding how to interact with elders, especially those with cognitive impairments.

Table 22.1 The ten pillars of the program

Camaraderie
Social interaction
Laughter/humor
Family support
Physical exercise
Mental exercise
Creative work
Engagement with the environment
Memory techniques
Education about memory loss

Enthusiasm for the EML Approach

As of this writing, there are approximately 46 Brookdale cognitive stimulation programs funded across the country (Brookdale Foundation, 2010). Countless other clubs have also sprung up. In Wisconsin, for example, where the memory club concept seems to have taken root, we know of 14 active clubs (Nowak J., April 14, 2010, personal communication). As is frequently the case with grass-roots interventions, the sudden and widespread interest in and implementation of memory clubs *preceded* scientific inquiry into their effectiveness. In this instance, we have clearly placed the proverbial cart before the horse. Why do we find ourselves in these circumstances? First, the predicted increase in new cases of ADRD over the next 40 years provides a powerful motivation to explore alternative therapies for ADRD. Second, the empirical findings showing that mental, social, and physical activity lower the risk of dementia was so compelling that people working on the front lines of dementia care began thinking about ways to translate the findings into interventions for those already affected by ADRD.

Thus far, however, the strongest endorsement for the implementation of memory clubs has come from: the club facilitators; persons with memory loss who participate in the clubs; their respective care partners; and some funders, all of whom strongly believe that the programs are efficacious. Further, the waves of "baby boomers," who are now moving into their retirement years, are known for their drive to "take charge" and participate in the care and management of their own health problems (Marks, Katz, & Smith, 2009). Memory clubs provide such an opportunity.

Early Memory Loss Clubs: The Importance of Empirical Evaluation

As impressive as the spread of memory clubs is, it is essential to verify that the beliefs about the clubs' efficacy are valid. Why? Federal, state, and local funding – critical to sustaining these programs – will only be available if efficacy of the groups can be demonstrated. Funding is also dependent on agencies' demonstrated willingness to implement the programs. With good reason, administrators often will not implement programs unless efficacy can be shown through research.

How Should EML Clubs Be Evaluated?

Carrying out a program evaluation study can be a demanding task. Practitioners, while highly skilled in working on the "front lines" of care, may be unprepared to consider all the details involved in research. They may have little or no research background, and may lack the appropriate resources to do research. It is much easier to design an evaluation research study than to carry it out.

Usually, researchers start with a "strong" research design in mind, one which would allow them to confidently say, "This program works. We have shown it through a rigorous program of well-conceived research, using appropriate measures, and guided by a rationally derived theoretical model."

However, different study designs provide different levels of confidence about the quality of a study and whether or not it has positive causal effects (Harbour & Miller, 2001) (see Table 22.2). And, especially in the field of applied research, researchers must confront a myriad of practical problems and challenges not encountered in laboratory research that frequently take them farther away from the ideally designed study they had initially hoped to conduct.

Meta-analyses of randomized control trials (RCTs). When considering the effectiveness of an intervention, systematic reviews and meta-analyses of RCTs are thought to provide the *most compelling line of evidence* (Harbour & Miller, 2001). However, at present, there are far too few studies of EML clubs to even consider conducting a meta-analysis of RCTs.

RCTs. RCTs are studies in which individuals agreeing to take part in the study are *randomly* assigned to one or more treatment/intervention conditions, or to a "control" condition in which no treatment or intervention is given. These types of studies are highly regarded by researchers, because the process of randomization is believed to "wash out" other differences between the groups, so that changes can be more confidently attributed to the intervention. Researchers, therefore, feel comfortable in claiming that the intervention *caused* the desired effect.

A variation of the RCT design involves the use of a "wait list." Here, participants are again randomly assigned to an intervention or control condition, and those in the

Table 22.2 Study designs, rank-ordered by "strength"[a]

Meta-analyses of randomized control trails
Randomized control trials (RCT)
Observational studies
Pre/post-test without control group

[a]Modified from Harbour and Miller's (2001) list

control group do not get the intervention while it is being evaluated. However, they are told that they will also have the opportunity to receive the intervention, but will have to wait a certain amount of time before they can receive it. Once the formal evaluation is completed, those on the "wait list" are offered the opportunity to receive the intervention. This approach seems more equitable since both groups receive the treatment intervention at some point in time. However, because ADRD are characterized by declines in cognitive and physical function, the control group may continue to decline while waiting for treatment. This delay could negatively affect them in the short- and long-term, because earlier treatment of dementia seems to be associated with better outcomes (DeKosky & Marek, 2003).

Observational/Correlational studies. This design ranks lower on the hierarchy of research methodologies considered by Harbour and Miller (2001). In observational/correlational studies, data are gathered using at least two measures, and the researcher examines whether there is an *association* between them. For example, one could ask, "Does the amount of time spent doing memory club activities, say memory games (measure 1) correlate with performance on an outcome measure, say scores on the Mini-Mental State Exam (measure 2) (MMSE; Folstein, Folstein, & McHugh, 1975)?" While it would be exciting to see a statistically significant positive correlation – suggesting that the more time spent doing memory games, the better (higher) the MMSE score – a careful evaluation that all other causes of the relationship have been ruled out is necessary. For example, better performance on the MMSE may simply be a reflection of skills which allow a person to do relatively better doing the memory games. In this case, the direction of causality is said to be reversed. Or a third factor, for which the researchers have not accounted, could be causing *both* variables to behave in certain specific ways. For example, club participants who spend more time doing memory games may differ in terms of their education levels. If this is not known, it is not possible to claim to know whether these differences in educational attainment vs. the memory club activities are the critical element that is preserving their cognitive performance, as measured by MMSE scores. Causal inferences cannot generally be drawn from a correlational study.

The pre/post-test design. The third design commonly used in program evaluation studies is the pre/post-test design with no control group. In this case, a measurement of the outcome of interest is taken *before* and *after* the intervention is given. Since subjects are being tested twice, they essentially serve as "their own controls," and differences between people are essentially washed out. This design falls low on the hierarchy of research designs, because it is extremely difficult to show that it was the intervention, and not some other exposure or experience during the period between the two measures, that accounts for any change in the post-test measure as compared to the pre-test measure. The design is strengthened to the degree that relevant variables that could be affecting performance on the outcome are measured and taken into account when analyzing findings. In spite of its weaknesses, this design is favored in applied research because it is relatively simple to implement and is easily understood by participants and community research partners.

What do the Current Studies Show?

The literature on Brookdale cognitive stimulation or other types of memory clubs is sparse at best. Most of the research that we can point to is only tangentially related to the topic of memory club program evaluations, and comes from studies of cognitive stimulation programs that are *not* embedded within the structure of a memory club.

What does this research show? An early meta-analysis of 52 studies, conducted by Floyd and Scogin (1997), determined that memory training interventions have relatively little effect on objective measures of memory performance. The mean effect size for subjective memory functioning was Cohen's *d* of 0.19 (small), but the mean effects size for objective memory measures was Cohen's *d* of 0.66 (medium to large). Sitzer, Twamley, and Jeste (2006) reviewed two types of cognitive stimulation interventions: restorative interventions (interventions attempting to restore function to previous levels through repetition, reminiscence, spaced retrieval techniques, etc.) and compensatory interventions (new ways of performing cognitive tasks, such as organizing to-be-remembered items into categories). The analysis, based on a total of 17 studies, provided a more optimistic appraisal of cognitive stimulation interventions than those of Floyd and Scogin (1997). When considering both restorative and compensatory programs together, the authors reported an effect size (Cohen's *d*) of 0.47 (medium). However, for restorative interventions, an effect size of 0.56 (medium to large) was reported. For compensatory interventions, the authors calculated a smaller effect size, 0.36 (small to medium) (Sitzer, Twamley, & Jeste, 2006). Complicating the analyses, however, was the fact that different studies often used a mixture of these strategies.

There are only two studies in the literature that address the impact of structured memory clubs on memory and cognition. In the first study (Werner, 2000), 31 community-dwelling memory club members from Jerusalem, Israel, with a mean age of 80, participated in the program evaluation. They were assessed with the MMSE every 4 months for 1 year.

The memory club was directed by a gerontological social worker and a clinical psychiatrist. The club's focus was on social and cultural activities, as well as on memory training activities, such as reminiscence and the use of computer programs. A goal was to train better encoding operations (making "external" to-be-remembered items "internal") and retrieval operations (finding to-be-remembered items which were previously encoded and stored in memory). The clubs met for two to three sessions per week, each lasting 4 h. Overall cognitive functioning was assessed with the MMSE.

Different sub-sections of the MMSE were used to measure encoding of information and retrieval of information. Language was measured by how many animals could be named from memory in 1 min. There was also a recall test of ten words.

Results indicated a significant decrease (worsening) in overall MMSE scores from baseline (median = 22.4) to 1-year follow-up (median = 19.9). However, there were no statistically significant declines in the encoding score based on a sub-set of

MMSE items, nor in the animal naming or word recall scores. These latter findings indicate that functioning was *maintained* in some cognitive domains over the course of the study period. Rather than being a sign of intervention failure, the preservation of memory and language functions in neurodegenerative illnesses over the course of 1 year suggests that the intervention was a success. The authors concluded from their findings that memory function can be maintained by participation in a structured memory club. Although exactly what was responsible for the reported effect cannot be established by this study, it may have been the social and cultural aspects of the club that helped participants maintain their memory. However, because there was no control group, and because the authors did not adjust their significance level to account for the number of differences they tested for, this study must be considered with caution.

In the second study, conducted in Madrid, Spain, the authors reported on a cognitive-motor intervention in 84 patients with mild cognitive impairment (MCI), mild AD, or moderate AD, all of whom were being treated with a cholinesterase inhibitor (Olazarán et al., 2004). A strength of this study is that research volunteers were randomly assigned to either an experimental group (EXP) that received a cognitive-motor intervention in addition to psycho-social support or a control group (CON) that received psycho-social support only. The intervention involved 103 sessions of cognitive exercises over a 1-year period. The EXP intervention consisted of: (a) a welcome period; (b) reality orientation; (c) cognitive exercises; (d) training in ADLs; (e) coffee breaks; (f) psychomotor exercises and workshops; and (g) a "closing."

Subjects were tested using several outcome measures: the MMSE; the ADAS-Cog, a measure commonly used in drug studies to assess important cognitive domains; the Functional Activities Questionnaire (FAQ), measuring ability in Instrumental Activities of Daily Living (IADLs); and the Geriatric Depression Scale (GDS). These measures were taken at baseline, 3, 6, and 12 months. There were no differences on the measures at baseline, suggesting that the process of randomization was successful in balancing the groups. There was one exception: EXP-group members had significantly better ADAS-Cog scores at baseline than CON-group members.

Results showed that compared to the CON-group, the EXP-group members maintained their cognitive function at 6 months, whereas the CON-group members declined from baseline to 6 months. After 6 months, both groups declined in cognitive function. Further, group differences were not observed at the 12-month observation. Results also showed that compared to EXP-group members, the CON-group members had significantly better GDS scores than EXP-group members at 6 months. However, at the 12-month evaluation, EXP-group members reported significantly worse GDS scores than at 6 months and baseline. The authors concluded that, among persons with cognitive deficits treated with dementia medications, an intervention consisting of cognitive-motor and psycho-social support resulted in benefits in terms of mood and cognition (Olazarán et al., 2004).

To summarize, meta-analyses of cognitive stimulation programs that are not embedded within the framework of a memory club suggest that cognitive stimulation may have small to moderate benefits for people with memory impairments. The studies that actually tested various forms of a memory club provide weak, but encouraging evidence that structured clubs in which cognitive stimulation is a core component may also be beneficial. Because of the rapid growth and implementation of these clubs across the country, and the dearth of empirical evidence supporting their efficacy, we initiated a pilot study of our Brookdale-inspired cognitive stimulation memory club.

Evaluation of The Milwaukee Brookdale-Inspired Cognitive Stimulation Club (MCSC)

Research goals. In this study, the research goals were to:

1. Examine changes over time in several neuropsychological and psycho-social characteristics of the participants
2. Assess associations between amount of time spent participating in MCSC activities that "exercise" different domains of cognition and objectively measured cognitive performance on standardized tests
3. Examine the content of the curriculum in terms of what types of mental activities were favored by club facilitators
4. Survey care partners about their perceptions of the benefits of the club and whether they felt the program's cost was reasonable

Hypotheses. Predictions relating to each research goal are outlined below.

1. For research goal 1, the rationale for the hypothesis was as follows. Because our intervention provided ongoing and active stimulation for mind and body, and offered opportunities for social interaction with other memory-impaired older adults, it was predicted that decline in cognitive function and well-being would be slowed or perhaps even prevented over the course of the 1-year intervention. Specifically, the hypothesis was that individuals with diagnosed memory impairments would *maintain* their baseline level of cognitive and psycho-social functioning.
2. For research goal 2, it was predicted that there would be positive associations between the amount of time spent doing various classes of activities and better functioning in the cognitive domains these activities were designed to "exercise."
3. For research goal 3, no a priori hypotheses were formulated. The curriculum was developed by the club facilitators over the course of several meetings. No expectations were articulated as to the types of activities that would and would not be favored. It was expected that some classes of activities would be favored by the club facilitators, but there was no basis upon which to predict *which* activity classes would be favored.
4. For research goal 4, evaluating care partners' perceptions of satisfaction with the EML club and its costs, care partners consistently *expressed*, prior to formal evaluation, that they were very satisfied with the Brookdale-inspired memory

club. This led to a hypothesis that the survey data would reflect satisfaction rather than dissatisfaction on our measures.

Research methods. To evaluate the MCSC, a pre/post-test design without a control group was used. Baseline measurements were gathered prior to the intervention, and at 6 and 12 months after the intervention. Although an RCT with wait list would have been an ideal design, it was not possible to conduct this type of study. This was due in part to the fact that, in scope, the study was intended to be an exploratory pilot.

Measures. Measures needed to be selected carefully for a number of reasons. Some measures are insensitive to slight changes in memory and thinking which older adults may be experiencing during the course of participation in the club. Further, some measures are prone to "floor effects," i.e., most respondents score very low on the measure because it is too difficult or the occurrences being asked about are relatively rare. In this case, changes over time cannot be detected. Anticipating this problem, three measures were used for each cognitive domain. The intent was to standardize the three measures of each cognitive domain and then combine them, thus reducing the problem of floor effects (as done in Wilson, Gilley, Bennett, Beckett, & Evans, 2000). Table 22.3 shows a summary of measures used in the study. Some of the measures proved to be poor choices for the intended evaluation purposes because they were too difficult for the population (Trails B); had floor effects CES-D); or took too long to administer (Trails B).

The research that was conducted suggested that modification of the assessment battery would be necessary in future studies. The importance of keeping batteries short to reduce subject frustration and stress and increase the likelihood that they will agree to follow-up assessments became more and more apparent as the study progressed. We also recognize that for ethical reasons, it is necessary to avoid overburdening research volunteers with an excessively long battery which may tire them or cause them anxiety.

The memory measures used in the study were all single learning measures; subjects were presented with a list of words or numbers, or a short paragraph, and asked to recall them. In hindsight, it would have been preferable to use a multi-trial learning test, such as the Hopkins Verbal Learning Test (HVLT) (Benedict, Schretlen, Groninger, & Brandt, 1998). In the HVLT, respondents are presented with a list of words and asked to recall it. The same list is then presented 2 more times. This affords the possibility of distinguishing between true memory problems (because subjects are given multiple trials to learn the list) vs. attentional problems (poor learning on a one-trial test could have been the result of a failure to pay attention during presentation of the words, i.e., during the "encoding" phase).

Table 22.3 Neuropsychological measures

Memory (paragraph recall; CERAD word list learning; forward digit span)
Visuo-spatial function (clock drawing; R-BANS copy; CERAD figure copy)
Language (confrontation naming; animal naming; vocabulary)
Processing speed (Stroop; Timed Months of the Year Backwards; Cancel H)

From a pragmatic standpoint (e.g., ease of administration; low burden on research volunteers; lack of floor and ceiling effects), the measures of processing speed (i.e., speed of "mentation" or thinking) were appropriate, as were the measures we selected to assess visuo-spatial function (i.e., visual abilities). Among tests of visuo-spatial function, the clock drawing test, in which research volunteers are asked to draw a clock and set the hands at 2:45, is probably preferred by most neuropsychologists. Unfortunately, many visuo-spatial tests rely on motor function because respondents must first look at a complex picture and then copy it using paper and pencil. This places demands on motor function, which can be affected by strokes or Parkinson-related symptoms. Our measure of vocabulary from the Wechsler Adult Intelligence Scale-III (WAIS-III) (Wechsler, 1997) is often used as a surrogate for intelligence, which can be useful when interpreting performance on other tests. Other language measures included a verbal fluency test and a test in which subjects are shown line drawings and asked to name the object in the picture. The latter tests were easy to administer and research volunteers were able to understand the directions and take the tests as directed.

Pre and postassessments of club participants were done in person by trained graduate students. Appropriate training, with reliability testing, is strongly recommended when persons collecting neuropsychological data are not professional psychometrists. A review of the data collected revealed unanticipated errors that additional training would probably have prevented or minimized. For example, interviewers sometimes failed to probe for more information (e.g., "Can you tell me more about that?") when administering the Wechsler Vocabulary Test, which invalidated the measure for some subjects. Care partner data were gathered in person, via telephone, and via mail-out surveys. For the care partners, mail-out surveys yielded the best compliance (63% return rate). It may be that care partners are so busy with their caregiving tasks that a phone call, even if relatively brief (30 min and scheduled in advance), is difficult to respond to due to shifting caregiving demands, which often arise unexpectedly.

One option that simplifies data collection and puts relatively less burden on club participants (and only on their care partners) is to use the Everyday Cognition Informant/Care Partner Form (or, ECog) (Farias et al., 2008). In this test, data collectors (or subjects themselves) are asked to think about the subjects' cognition now, but in relation to their cognition 10 years ago. This instrument assesses the domains of memory, language, visual-spatial and perceptual abilities, and various executive functions. La Rue (2011) used the ECog in a cognitive support intervention for individuals with MCI. The ECog was easy to use, compliance was high, and the researchers were able to gather solid data in a parsimonious way.

Preliminary Results: Cognitive and Psycho-Social Outcomes

The sample. Fifty-five research volunteers met the criteria for participation in the study and assisted us in our research. At baseline, persons in the sample averaged 77 years-of-age ($SD = 9.0$) and were highly educated (mean years of education completed = 15; $SD = 2.6$); their global cognitive status, assessed using the MMSE, indicated mild impairment (mean MMSE = 25.4; $SD = 2.4$). Research participants were able to perform most IADLs (mean IADL score = 10.7, $SD = 2.8$; range of possible scores: 0–14, with high scores indicating better function). The gender distribution was 54.5% women ($n = 30$) and 45.5% men ($n = 25$). Most subjects had been participants in the club prior to the study's inception. The mean time in the club prior to implementation of our evaluation study was 1.3 years ($SD = 0.9$), with a range of less than 2 months to just under 3½ years.

Data were collected on a number of potential control variables. Variables that were significantly correlated with any of the study's outcome measures were used as covariates or control variables in our analyses.

Data challenges and analyses. In the preliminary analyses reported here, three outcome measures were examined: depressive symptomology (CES-D), delayed paragraph recall (Logical Memory Test from the Wechsler Memory Battery), and self-rated health. We found clear "floor effects" for our measures of delayed paragraph recall and depressive symptoms. Also, the "shapes" of the data distributions for many variables were not normal (i.e., "bell-shaped"), which is a requirement for many types of statistical analyses. This led us to use a special class of statistics that accounts for these problems ("non-parametric" statistics).

Results

Data from Memory Club Research Volunteers (Goal 1)

Only *age* and *baseline IADL* scores were significantly correlated with any of the three outcome measures at baseline. Persons who were younger at baseline had significantly lower depression scores, and those with poorer baseline IADL functioning had significantly poorer paragraph recall at baseline. Thus, age and IADL scores at baseline were used as control variables in the analyses of depression and paragraph recall, respectively, to account for their effects when interpreting results.

With time as the independent variable (IV) and CES-D the dependent measure (DV), we found that there were *no statistically significant changes in depressive symptoms over time* (i.e., 1 year) among our subjects. Because *age* was a significant correlate of baseline CES-D, we stratified the CES-D analyses by two age groups, ≤79 and 80+. There was no evidence of change in depressive symptoms over time in either of the two age groups.

With *delayed paragraph recall* scores as the DV, we found, again, that there were *no statistically significant changes in scores over time* among our subjects. Stratification by IADL score (low vs. high) did not reveal any substantive differences in delayed paragraph recall scores.

We also examined the relationship between *time* as the IV and *self-rated health scores* as the DV. *There were no statistically significant changes in health scores over time* among our subjects. Since none of the covariates we identified were correlated with the global health outcome measure, it was not necessary to stratify the analyses.

The hypothesis for Goal 1, that participation in a memory club results in *maintenance* of memory and well-being over the course of a year, was supported. These preliminary results suggest that there may be benefits of participation in one version of the Brookdale EML program. We saw that, across three domains of function (depression, memory, and health), persons *maintained* their levels of function over 1 year of observation. This finding may suggest that participation in a memory club results in *maintenance* of memory and well-being over the course of a year.

Results from this preliminary analysis of the data must be interpreted with caution. Given the small sample sizes in these analyses, there may have been insufficient statistical power to find true differences if they existed. All else being equal, the smaller the difference, the larger the sample size needed to detect it. In longitudinal studies, analyses must be viewed and interpreted with caution. Because of the "rolling entry" of participants into the memory club over the course of 1 year, some individuals had already been in the club for some time before the study began. This *time in the program* was not taken into account in the preliminary analyses reported here.

A major problem is the issue of subject attrition (drop-out). With time, some subjects can no longer participate in the study because: they have died; their cognition prevents further participation; they lose interest; or they are lost-to-follow-up (they cannot be located for testing). Each of these types of attrition complicates interpretation of results. If most of the subjects who dropped out of the study did so because their cognition declined to a point where they could no longer participate in testing, the remaining sample is essentially biased: those with the best skills and abilities would be retained in the analyses, giving a distorted sense that the intervention was highly effective. The drop-out rate in the study was 12.5% at 6 months and 28.6% at 12 months when compared with baseline.

Club facilitators noted that, after months of doing very well, some participants' abilities suddenly declined dramatically. The neuronal/cognitive reserve hypothesis may explain the rapid decline in some research volunteers who had previously maintained their cognition. Compared to others, highly intelligent, well-educated and affluent people – such as many of our research volunteers – are thought to have had the chance to develop more cognitive and neurologic resources to cope with neurological insults to the brain, such as the progressive deterioration produced by ADRD (Richards & Deary, 2005). It has been hypothesized that such people are better able to live with ADRD because they have a more comprehensive set of resources or "reserves" which can be called upon to compensate for the physiological brain changes associated with ADRD. However, at some point, compensation is no longer possible; at this point, they experience rapid decline.

These first-ever findings, reporting on the effectiveness of our specific Brookdale-inspired EML Club model, allow us to be cautiously optimistic that aspects of the intervention may be accomplishing their intended purposes. We hope to gain further insights into the effect of the intervention by examining the data in greater detail, using methods (e.g., multi-level modeling) that will specifically address some of the problems we have noted above.

Associations between Specific Activities and Cognitive Outcomes (Goal 2)

Little is known about the possible relationship between doing specific activities and experiencing specific cognitive outcomes. For example, is there a positive correlation between doing memory exercises and memory performance. Or, does performing spatial activities have an impact on actual visuo-spatial function? To explore this question, a licensed neuropsychologist coded activities in the club curriculum according to the cognitive domain they seemed to drawn on most heavily. The selection of domains was based on previous work (Farias et al., 2006) and rational consideration of the activities. Ten activity domains were deemed as relevant: (1) *recent episodic memory*, i.e., memory for personally experienced events which occurred recently; (2) *recent semantic memory*, i.e., memory for newly learned factual information; (3) *remote episodic memory*, i.e., memory for personally experienced events which occurred in the remote past; (4) *remote semantic memory*, i.e., memory for factual information learned in the remote past; (5) *language and verbal skills*; (6) *visuospatial skills*; (7) *executive functions,* i.e., the ability to plan, organize, and focus on relevant facts which require attentional shifts; and (8) *reasoning.* Two other domains that were non-cognitive were (9) *social activities* and (10) *activities involving light exercise*. Each club facilitator was asked to keep track of the time devoted to each activity used during each club session. A form was provided to code the amount of time (in minutes) devoted to doing each respective activity.

This research goal has proven the most labor-intensive. It required club facilitators to make note of the amount of time they were devoting to each activity type in real time. Even with training, we noted that this task was difficult for the facilitators to perform. Data are still in the process of being prepared for analysis. Thus, the results of these analyses will be reported in the future.

Content of the Curriculum (Goal 3)

An important question, for which data have not yet been published, is *What types of activities* are most effective in achieving EML club goals? Preliminary results showed that the *distributions* of different classes of cognitive activities chosen for the curriculum and used during class time favored *remote semantic memory.*

Because the research literature suggests that the ability to form and recall new memories is compromised during the progressive course of ADRD, it follows logically that relatively *more* activities should be directed toward the formation of new episodic and semantic memories. Our program facilitators were responsive to this idea. However, we have not yet analyzed our data to determine whether these types of activities can be shown to maintain participant's scores on standardized tests of episodic and semantic memories over time.

The EML club facilitators' *perceptions* of a sample of curriculum activities used during weeks 35 through 45 of our 50-week program evaluation were also examined. The club facilitators' perceptions of benefits to the group are important data, since facilitators see the activities "in action" on a regular basis.

Club facilitators universally favored several specific activities, tapping different domains of cognitive functioning. For a complete list of activities used in the curriculum, contact Ms. Einberger, who may be reached at the address provided in the acknowledgments section. In Table 22.4, we provide a list of some of her favorite activities. Along with J. Sellick, K. Einberger developed the EML concept.

Care Partner Perceptions of the Club (Goal 4)

We also gathered data from 32 care partners regarding their perceptions of the program and its benefits, as well as their perceptions of the cost of the clubs relative to the gains they observed in their relatives.

The data presented in Table 22.5 summarize care partner's satisfaction with the club. Considering the results in the aggregate, there seems to be a consensus that the clubs were well designed, beneficial, and worthy of recommendation to others.

Cost data are also reported here, and results of the survey are encouraging. The data showed that, on average, care partners endorsed statements such as: "The cost

Table 22.4 Care partners' perceptions of the clubs (*M* Mean; *SD* standard deviation)

On a scale of 1–5, with 1 = strongly disagree, 2 = disagree, 3 = neutral, 4 = agree, and 5 = strongly agree, scores for the satisfaction questions were as follows:	
Overall I am satisfied with the Memory Club	$M=4.5$ ($SD=0.6$)
The club has benefited my spouse/relative	$M=4.5$ ($SD=0.6$)
The club has given me opportunities to recover from caregiving	$M=3.7$ ($SD=1.1$)
The club should be changed or modified in certain ways	$M=2.7$ ($SD=1.0$)
I would recommend the Memory Club to others	$M=4.5$ ($SD=0.7$)

Table 22.5 Some of K. Einberger's favorite early memory loss (EML) club activities

Ten things: Name ten or more inventions of the past 50 years that have changed the way we do things. Next week, name ten or more inventions that club participants think may be invented in the next 50 years to make our lives easier

Consensus survivor: If you were stuck on a deserted island in Bora Bora and could only have ten things, what would they be? This activity is to be done in small groups. First, the small groups brainstorm possible answers; subsequently, they are asked to come to a consensus

A–Z: Participants have to think of something in a specific category that begins with each letter of the alphabet. Two categories we have used were *The A–Zs of Social Activities* and *Things That Make You Happy*

Gratitude letter: Club participants write a letter of gratitude to someone who has had a positive influence on their lives. The letter doesn't need to be mailed – but this is an effective way to think about all we have for which we may be grateful

is about right given the benefits received"; and that most of the participants surveyed felt the program provided assistance that was "More than they expected." Hopefully, these data will be of interest to administrators during our present "tight" economic times, where programs are being cut based on the assumption that persons cannot afford them or will not participate.

Working Effectively with Community Partners When Doing Research

Applied research – i.e., research that is conducted in the "real world" rather than in a laboratory – presents unique challenges that must be thoughtfully considered before initiating a new study. Nonetheless, applied research is critical if we are to understand whether or not findings from basic research studies, conducted in highly controlled environments (such as a research laboratory), can be *translated* or *applied* to real world contexts. In our case, we would want to know whether the epidemiological, neuroimaging, and animal studies, documenting the benefits of mental, physical, and social engagement on cognition, have any applicability in the structured contexts of memory clubs.

In their essay on opportunities and challenges of intervention research, Pillmer, Czaja, Schulz, and Stahl (2003) note, somewhat paradoxically, that there is a tradition of cross-fertilization and communication among gerontological scientists and practitioners. However, later in that same essay, they allude to anecdotal evidence indicating feelings of animosity between gerontological researchers and practitioners. In our experience studying EML clubs, we have encountered both sides of this coin. However, with some effort, preparation, patience, and a willingness to learn – on both the part of researchers and practitioners – we believe that most challenges can be overcome to produce results that are of interest to researchers and useful to practitioners and the persons they serve. Anyone interested in evaluating community-based interventions is likely to find the special issue of *The Gerontologist* (Volume 43, Special Issue), prepared by Pillmer et al. and other authors, which covers many of the issues involved in community participatory work in detail, extremely helpful. Klein and Parks (2007) provide a discussion of data collection challenges, and possible solutions, when doing applied gerontological research.

Conclusions About EML Clubs

EML clubs are being developed and implemented across the United States. The state of Wisconsin, in particular, seems to be at the forefront of formalizing clubs and implementing them. On the one hand, this is good. EML clubs seem to be attracting and retaining members, which can be seen as a measure of client satisfaction. As summarized in this chapter, EML clubs are also grounded in scientific findings that (indirectly) justify their use. However, to establish their efficacy, *more rigorous scientific evaluation is needed.*

Even if effectiveness of the clubs can be demonstrated, sustainability will remain an ongoing problem: In an informal poll, we asked four EML sites to estimate the total costs to them and participants in terms of materials, staffing, lunches, resource materials, rent, etc., to run a club for 1 year. The mean cost, based on data reported from three sites and adjusted to reflect two sessions per week, was $33,215. The mean revenue from the three sites over the year was $28,321.

Promoting the clubs is vital to sustainability. One approach is to make appointments with local physicians, neuropsychologists, gerontologists, and front-line care providers at memory clinics for face-to-face meetings to promote your program. An introductory letter to the physicians may help, followed by a scheduled (short) meeting. One thing that has proven helpful is the creation of bookmarks that have all of the relevant information on them. This way, the care provider does not have to write information about a club's location and contact information for each new patient. He or she may simply recommend the program and hand out a bookmark. Keeping the clinicians well stocked with these promotional materials is advisable, and can serve to remind them on an on-going basis about the existence of your program.

In sum, EML clubs are extremely popular, and it is widely believed that they are effective. But at this point in time, there are not enough studies to support claims about effectiveness. On a positive note, we know that there is a hunger for information about the efficacy of EML programs. Only one RCT addressing EML clubs has been conducted to date. As positive findings emerge from more and better studies, the credibility of EML clubs will be enhanced.

As researchers and practitioners interested in evaluating EML clubs, we must embrace the notion of the "strong" research design. Specifically, rigorous and well-conceived plans for RCTs of EML clubs must be developed. Without such plans, EML clubs will be only a temporary "flash" on the practice scene, and then fall by the wayside, as has been the case with so many other interventions for persons with ADRD.

High Quality EML studies should include the following:

- Specific inclusion and exclusion criteria
- Expeditious methods of consenting research volunteers
- A mechanism to provide control-group members with something that is likely to be beneficial (e.g., mailings of materials written especially for persons with early-stage memory loss), but does not overlap with elements of the EML intervention
- Outcome measures that are appropriate to the individuals involved in the study
- Data on relevant control variables
- Long-term follow-up with research volunteers to determine the duration of any effects that are found
- A unified or common curriculum, for which a detailed written manual has been developed, so that the results of different studies can be easily compared and replicated

A design such as this requires planning, flexibility in working with research partners, patience, and creative thinking. Only with results from rigorous studies will EML clubs flourish.

Acknowledgments The authors gratefully acknowledge the assistance of Asenath LaRue, Ph. D., Paula Hartman-Stein, Ph. D., and Linda R. Rechlin, B. A., who provided review and comment during the preparation of this manuscript. The Helen Bader Foundation (Milwaukee, WI; http://www.hbf.org) provided financial support to conduct the study. Other financial support was provided by the Parkinson Research Institute, Aurora Sinai Medical Center, Milwaukee, WI. Finally, the authors thank the research volunteers with ADRD who participated in our study of memory loss programs, and who made our research and preparation of this chapter possible.

References

Acevedo, A., & Lowenstein, D. A. (2007). Nonpharmacologic cognitive interventions in aging and dementia. *Journal of Geriatric Psychiatry and Neurology, 20*, 239–249.

Barnes, L. L., Mendes de Leon, C. F., Wilson, R. S., Bienias, J. L., & Evans, D. A. (2004). Social resources and cognitive decline in a population of older African Americans and whites. *Neurology, 63*, 2322–2366.

Benedict, R. H. B., Schretlen, D., Groninger, L., & Brandt, J. (1998). Hopkins Verbal Learning Test – Revised: Normative data and analysis of inter-form and test-retest reliability. *The Clinical Neuropsychologist, 12*, 43–55.

Brookdale Foundation. (2010, April 14). 2010 Brookdale national group respite sites. Retrieved from http://www.brookdalefoundation.org/Respite/RespiteForms/BrookdaleRespiteList2010.pdf (August, 2010).

Brookmeyer, R., Gray, S., & Kawas, C. (1998). Projections of Alzheimer's disease in the United States and the public health impact of delaying disease onset. *American Journal of Public Health, 88*, 1337–1342.

Brown, R. (2000). *Group processes: Dynamics within and between groups.* Malden: Blackwell.

Cohen, J. (1992). A power primer. *Psychological Bulletin, 112*, 155–159.

DeKosky, S. T., & Marek, K. (2003). Looking backward to move forward: Early detection of neurodegenerative disorders. *Science, 302*, 830–834.

Einberger, K., & Sellick, J. (2007). *How to plan and implement an early memory loss program.* New York: The Brookdale Foundation.

Farias, S. T., Mungas, D., Reed, B. R., Cahn-Weiner, D., Jagust, W., Baynes, K., et al. (2008). The measurement of everyday cognition (ECog): Scale development and psychometric properties. *Neuropsychology, 22*, 531–544.

Farias, S. T., Mungas, D., Reed, B. R., Harvey, D., Cahn-Weiner, D., & Decarli, C. (2006). MCI is associated with deficits in everyday functioning. *Alzheimer Disease and Associated Disorders, 20*, 217–223.

Floyd, M., & Scogin, F. (1997). Effects of memory training on the subjective memory functioning and mental health of older adults: A meta-analysis. *Psychology and Aging, 12*, 150–161.

Folstein, M. F., Folstein, S. E., & McHugh, P. R. (1975). Mini-mental state. A practical method for grading the cognitive state of patients for the clinician. *Journal of Psychiatric Research, 12*, 189–198.

Friedland, R. P., Fritsch, T., Smyth, K. A., Koss, E., Lerner, A. J., Chen, C. H., et al. (2001). Patients with Alzheimer's disease have reduced activities in midlife compared with healthy control-group members. *Proceedings of the National Academy of Sciences of the United States of America, 98*, 3440–3445.

Fritsch, T., Smyth, K. A., McClendon, M. J., Ogrocki, P. K., Santillan, C., Larsen, J. D., et al. (2005). Associations between dementia/mild cognitive impairment and cognitive performance and activity levels in youth. *Journal of the American Geriatrics Society, 53*, 1191–1196.

Hamm, R. J., Temple, M. D., O'Dell, D. M., Pike, B. R., & Lyeth, B. G. (1996). Exposure to environmental complexity promotes recovery of cognitive function after traumatic brain injury. *Journal of Neurotrauma, 13*, 41–47.

Harbour, R., & Miller, J. (2001). A new system for grading recommendations in evidence based guidelines. *British Medical Journal, 323*, 334–346.

Hebert, L. E., Scherr, P. A., Bienias, J. L., Bennet, D. A., & Evans, D. A. (2003). Alzheimer's disease in the U. S. population: Prevalence estimates using the 2000 U. S. Census. *Archives of Neurology, 60*, 1119–1122.

Karp, A., Paillard-Borg, S., Wang, H., Silverstein, M., Winblad, B., & Fratiglioni, L. (2006). Mental, physical and social components in leisure activities equally contribute to decrease dementia risk. *Dementia and Geriatric Cognitive Disorders, 21*, 65–73.

Kitwood, T., & Bredin, K. (1992). Toward a theory of dementia care: Personhood and well-being. *Aging and Society, 12*, 269–287.

Klein, C. K., & Parks, C. A. (2007). Listening to seniors: Successful approaches to data collection and program development. *Journal of Gerontological Social Work, 48*, 457–473.

La Rue, A. (2011). Supporting cognition and well-being in older adults with mild cognitive impairment: A pilot intervention. In P. E. Hartman-Stein & A. LaRue (Eds.), *Enhancing cognitive fitness in adults*. New York: Springer.

Marks, B. L., Katz, L. M., & Smith, J. K. (2009). Exercise and the aging mind: Buffing the baby boomer's body and brain. *The Physician and Sportsmedicine, 37*, 119–125.

Olazarán, J., Muñiz, R., Reisberg, B., Peña-Casanova, J., del Ser, T., Cruz-Jentoft, A. J., et al. (2004). Benefits of a cognitive-motor intervention in MCI and mild to moderate Alzheimer disease. *Neurology, 63*, 2348–2353.

Pillmer, K., Czaja, S., Schulz, R., & Stahl, S. (2003). Finding the best ways to help: Opportunities and challenges of intervention research on aging. *Gerontologist, 43*(Special Issue I), 5–8.

Raina, P., Santaguida, P., Ismaila, A., Patterson, C., Cowan, D., Levine, M., et al. (2008). Effectiveness of cholinesterase inhibitors and memantine for treating dementia: Evidence review for a clinical practice guideline. *Annals of Internal Medicine, 148*, 379–397.

Richards, M., & Deary, I. J. (2005). A life course approach to cognitive reserve: A model for cognitive aging and development? *Annals of Neurology, 58*, 617–622.

Sano, M., Wilcock, G. K., van Baelen, B., & Kavanagh, S. (2003). The effects of galantamine treatment on caregiver time in Alzheimer's disease. *International Journal of Geriatric Psychiatry, 18*, 942–950.

Scarmeas, N., Zarahn, E., Anderson, K. E., Habeck, C. G., Hilton, J., Flynn, J., et al. (2003). Association of life activities with cerebral blood flow in Alzheimer disease: Implications for the cognitive reserve hypothesis. *Archives of Neurology, 60*, 359–365.

Sitzer, D. I., Twamley, E. W., & Jeste, D. V. (2006). Cognitive training in Alzheimer's disease: A meta-analysis of the literature. *Acta psychiatrica Scandinavica, 114*, 75–90.

Wechsler, D. (1997). *Wechsler Adult Intelligence Scale-III (WAIS-III)*. San Antonio: Psychological Corporation.

Werner, P. (2000). Assessing the effectiveness of a memory club for elderly persons suffering from mild cognitive deterioration. *Clinical Gerontologist, 22*, 3–14.

Wilson, R. S., Bennett, D. A., Bienias, J. L., Mendes de Leon, C. F., Morris, M. C., & Evans, D. A. (2003). Cognitive activity and cognitive decline in a biracial community population. *Neurology, 61*, 812–816.

Wilson, R. S., Gilley, D. W., Bennett, D. A., Beckett, L. A., & Evans, D. A. (2000). Person-specific paths of cognitive decline in Alzheimer's disease and their relation to age. *Psychology and Aging, 15*, 18–28.

Yaffe, K., Barnes, D., Nevitt, M., Lui, L., & Covinsky, K. (2001). A prospective study of physical activity and cognitive decline in elderly women: Women who walk. *Archives of Internal Medicine, 161*, 1703–1708.

Chapter 23
Implementing the "I'm Still Here"™ Approach: Montessori-Based Methods for Engaging Persons with Dementia

Cameron J. Camp, John Zeisel, and Vincent Antenucci

Abstract In this chapter, we describe an approach to providing meaningful activities that engage persons with dementia: the "I'm Still Here"™ Approach. Our approach focuses on remaining strengths and abilities in persons with dementia, rather than focusing on their deficits – a central tenet of the "I'm Still Here"™ Approach. It is useful to see activities programming for persons with dementia on a continuum, ranging from working with a single person and a single skill to community-based events for small or large groups. This continuum is the organizational tool we use for this chapter.

Introduction

Two salient themes ran through the proceedings of a conference on cognitive fitness for older adults a few years ago. The first was that caregivers everywhere were focusing their energy, research, and attention on maintaining residents' optimal physical and mental health throughout their lives with many care giving institutions receiving funding for their efforts to prevent or delay the onset of dementia. Efforts to find the best sources of nutrition and the best physical and cognitive exercise regimens were prominent. Many of these are represented in chapters in this volume, and are worthy of praise. Another theme that ran through the conference was unspoken but clearly present and is reflected in the following comment:

Alzheimer's disease or any other form of dementia is viewed in much the same way that a surgeon views death – a defeat.

C.J. Camp (✉)
Director of Research, Linda-&-Cameron, Inc.,
7274 Hollyhock Lane, Solon, OH 44139, USA
e-mail: Cameron@lindaandcameroninc.com

Forgotten was the fact that regimens designed to provide good nutrition and good exercise for the mind and body, and a good quality of life, are just as vitally important for persons with dementia and their caregivers as for persons attempting to prevent or delay dementia.

In this chapter, we describe an approach to providing meaningful activities that engage persons with dementia. While we present specific recommendations for ways to construct and present such activities, the critical feature of this chapter is the underlying philosophy of treatment for persons with dementia: the "I'm Still Here"™ Approach. It is a conscious decision on our part to call providing such activity "treatment," not "care." In our opinion, it is critical that nonpharmacological interventions for persons with dementia be viewed as treatment. Often the argument is made that nonpharmacological interventions cannot cure the underlying causes of dementia (e.g., Alzheimer's disease, vascular disorders, Lewy bodies, etc.) and therefore are not treatment; but the same is true of current pharmacologic interventions. Should pharmacologic interventions also not be considered treatment?

In our society, providing "treatment" conveys a different meaning than providing "care." Treatment is generally regarded as the province of medicine, and the goals of treatment are to cure or reduce the symptoms of a medical problem. It is hoped that if treatment is successful, the "patient" will have a better quality of life, but such a distal outcome generally is regarded as beyond the more proximal goal of medical intervention, i.e., fix the immediate "medical" problem. Ironically, in a medical approach treatment is no longer the focus once the "patient" is viewed as "terminal." "Palliative care" is then provided, focusing on providing the best quality of life to persons who are in their last days. We contend that quality of life needs to be a major focus of treatment throughout the course of dementia – not just at the end of life – as well as a focus for any other illness.

Pharmacological approaches for treating symptoms of dementia first involve attempts to improve cognitive functioning. If a person with dementia takes a cholinesterase inhibitor and/or a similar drug, the theory goes, memory deficits associated with dementia will improve, concomitant improvement will occur in problematic behaviors associated with dementia, and these will in turn improve quality of life. The following extreme example makes evident the problem from the point of view of the "patient."

Imagine a person with dementia in a long-term care facility is prescribed a drug designed to improve cognition, and that the drug works spectacularly well. The reoriented resident goes to the nurses' station and says, "I am much better now, and don't need to be here. I wish to go home." Those familiar with long-term care can generate a number of scenarios for what might happen next, especially if the resident becomes insistent. The most likely scenario is that the staff administers another drug to calm down the "problem" resident and control the "agitated" behavior – her insistence that she is cured.

Nonpharmacological treatments based on the "I'm Still Here"™ Approach can reduce problematic behaviors associated with dementia, not by trying to improve cognition but by focusing on improving the quality of life of the person with dementia. The following steps begin the quality of life improvement sequence: First, when we encounter problematic behaviors in persons with dementia, we ask "Why is this happening?" If we answer "Because the person has dementia," the question and answer produce a circular argument: "Why is this happening? – Because the person has dementia. How do we know the person has dementia? – Because this is happening" (Camp & Nasser, 2003). The answer cannot be: "Because he has dementia," because this answer does not explain the cause of the problematic behavior, and worse, focuses attention on the symptoms of a problem rather than addressing its cause. "Treatment" of the symptom often involves a pharmacologic formula: "If we see someone who presents symptom X, we prescribe Y drug." Camp and Nasser (2003) describe a systematic method for assessing causes of problematic behaviors in persons with dementia, with concomitant (and generally nonpharmacological) interventions associated with specific underlying causes of problematic behaviors. These interventions include Montessori Programming for Dementia (MPD; Camp, in press) to design engaging activities that provide optimal levels of stimulation. When a person with dementia is engaged in meaningful activity, this person cannot also be exhibiting problematic behavior. This approach to providing activities now has been thoroughly integrated into the "I'm Still Here"™ Approach, as we will discuss shortly.

Our approach focuses on remaining strengths and abilities in persons with dementia, rather than focusing on their deficits – a central tenet of the "I'm Still Here"™ Approach. Focusing on a person's strengths encourages us to see the person rather than his or her disability. Human beings are not defined by our illnesses. I have a cold or cancer. This does not change who I am: focusing on strengths forces us to examine the possibility and acknowledge the reality that persons with dementia can express themselves, relearn, and even acquire new skills and esthetics (see Chap. 19). If persons with dementia feel safe, wanted, and useful contributing members of a community, they have a better quality of life and exhibit fewer "problem behaviors." We all share these needs, whether or not we have dementia, because we share a common humanity.

For this reason alone it is incumbent on all of us to design activity that enables these basic needs to be met in persons with dementia, focusing on their strengths, and accommodating their disabilities regardless of their stage of dementia. Doing so involves activity across a range of levels, from training specific skills or subskills in specific individuals with dementia to creating entire communities that support persons with dementia, as described in the "It Takes a Village" section of Caulfield's chapter.

When persons with dementia have their basic human needs met, problematic behaviors are significantly reduced. Persons *living well* with dementia who enjoy a good quality of life have no need to display apathy, aggression, anxiety, or agitation – the infamous "Four A's" of dementia (Cohen-Mansfield, Libin, & Marx, 2007; Zeisel, 2009). Just as Maria Montessori was able to eliminate property destruction in impoverished children in Rome by providing them with engaging activity in a safe environment that supported learning while providing respect and dignity, so we can significantly reduce problematic behavior in persons with dementia by attending with respect and dignity to their needs for engaging activity in an atmosphere conducive to learning.

The Neuroscience Behind the "I'm Still Here"™ Approach

Our brains – all our brains even with Alzheimer's – are capable of a great deal more than we expect of them. Healthy brains contain 100 billion neurons – as many neurons as stars in our galaxy. With dementia, people may have anywhere between 60 and 90 billion neurons – still a great many. With dementia, only certain parts of our brains are affected, with other areas still working well – such as the part associated with procedural learning. The brain's emotional center, the amygdala, may even be working overtime to make up for losses in the logical executive function frontal lobe. Barry Reisberg's retrogenesis theory holds that people living with dementia lose skills inversely to the sequence these skills developed in the growing child. Grasping an object is developed early, thus is lost late. Expressive language skills are developed later in childhood, thus lost earlier. If this theory holds, hard-wired attributes of our brains, held even before birth, are never lost in dementia.

Creativity also remains vibrant in dementia – with one caveat: the creativity expressed is without constraints because the *comparator*, the brain's brake system, does not function as well as the other creative drivers – the interpreter and the actors.

And then there is multitasking. We now know that even the young have more automobile accidents when they text while driving – not even they can truly multitask. The lack of this skill among those living with Alzheimer's contributes to problem behaviors being suppressed when engagement kicks in.

Let's take these one at a time. There are at least two learning systems that our brains employ to develop the skills we need to survive. The first, episodic memory, is damaged early in dementia. It is increasingly difficult for a person to remember specific experiences – actually to lay down new experiences in their brain – as dementia progresses. These might include a message someone asked them to transmit to another, or even an experience like going to a restaurant. These might be forgotten as quickly as they are experienced. But the second learning and memory technique, procedural learning, is still functional. Procedural learning is what we all use to remember physical skills like playing golf, whipping homemade mayonnaise with a whisk, or finding our way home. Procedural learning takes continual practice. Tennis great Roger Federer practices his strokes all the time, enabling him to maintain his number one ranking for as many years as he has. People with dementia engaged in activities they find meaningful tend to do them over and over with pleasure – thus learn them procedurally.

The brain's amygdala – its emotional center – remains vibrant throughout much of the Alzheimer's journey. It may even grow in importance as a compensatory mechanism for the loss of executive function skills – the skills needed to organize a sequence of actions into a single coherent action like the many steps it takes to brush our teeth or get dressed. Because of this, people along the entire Alzheimer's journey have exquisite perceptions and expression of visual and dramatic arts including poetry. They express the hard-wired instinct of caring for others – for other people or for sick birds – more directly and with greater engagement than others who stop themselves – thinking such expressions silly or weak.

Examples of hard-wired skills and abilities include finding our way by recognizing landmarks (Koziol & Budding, 2009) and responding to another person's touch. Music and dance are hard-wired; it is not necessary to teach a baby to move rhythmically in response to music – whether this is called the Mozart effect or just hard wiring. Hard-wired abilities such as these remain alive in the brains of people living with Alzheimer's because they are so deeply rooted; they are evolved survival skills that even dementia cannot touch. The hard-wired skill of caring for others is one of the most powerful. Just ask someone with dementia to help you and almost immediately they will stop crying or being anxious to help you solve your problem. This instinct also makes volunteering and helping others a particularly meaningful Montessori-based "I'm Still Here"™ activity.

Creativity in the brain has three major drivers: the left lobe *interpreter* which creates holistic images and stories to explain what the person perceives, the *actors* which move about the brain depending on the action, and the *comparator* which puts the brakes on creative actions by comparing actions to the interpretation made earlier and to contextual factors. In dementia, the brain's interpreter continues to make up stories and develop images as can be seen by the sometimes sensible and sometimes fantastic stories people with Alzheimer's generate. Their *actors* continue to work as well, as can be seen in people with dementia walking, painting, singing, and generally *"doing things"* whether or not the action seems to make sense in the particular context. What does not work so well as the journey of dementia progresses is the brain's *comparer*, the organs tasked with correcting actions if they fail or do not make sense to the person. But this last element is not so important in terms of creativity. Without it, a person still has imagination and the drive to act on their image of the world around them. These creative abilities serve as a firm basis for many of the activities in the Montessori-based and I'm Still Here™ Approach.

Finally, we come to multitasking or rather our fundamental inability to multitask. If we are not totally engaged with a task, we can carry out another at the same time – or rather in the moments between focusing on the task at hand. But when we are totally engaged, such as when we face an emergency or are engrossed in a passionate scene in a film, we cannot do anything else. The same is true for those living with dementia. When they are engaged in a meaningful activity, they cannot also be anxious, agitated, aggressive, or apathetic – the four "A"s of Alzheimer's. The measure of success of the approach presented in this chapter is both positive and negative at the same time; positive because engaged persons clearly have a better quality of life; negative because engaged persons are not exhibiting "problem" behaviors. When measuring engagement, therefore, we must always measure the positive qualities along with the absence of the negatives.

Applying the "I'm Still Here"™ Approach: Application to Activities Programming

Last year, a staff member in charge of activities programming for persons with dementia at a Hearthstone Alzheimer Care residence noticed a baby bird that was abandoned and hungry while walking to work. She carefully wrapped the bird in her jacket and brought it to the residence where residents with dementia gathered around the bird and went to work. First, a veterinarian was called by residents to determine how to care for and feed the young bird. Residents took turns feeding the bird bits of dog food with tweezers. They provided water for the animal and named him "Jacob." The bird was made comfortable while a staff member found a facility on the web for rehabilitating animals and sending them back into the wild. Eventually, an outing was scheduled to bring Jacob to the rehabilitation facility, and a fond farewell was organized. Residents and staff together created an illustrated memory book (Bourgeois, 2007) of Jacob's time at the residence to remind residents of their part in his rescue.

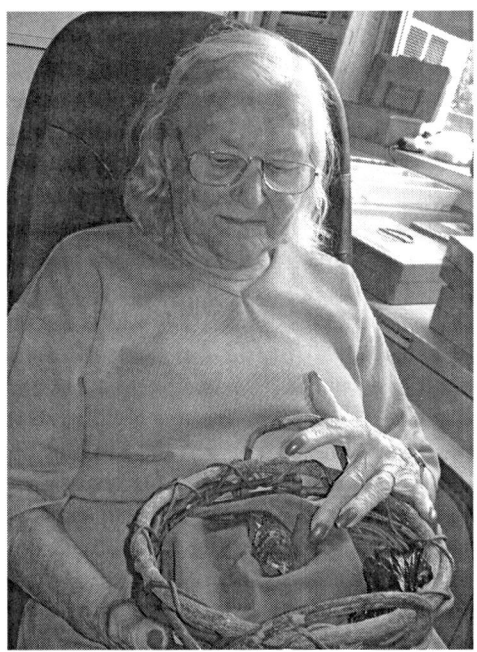

At another Hearthstone residence, an activities program director heard about an equestrian riding school nearby which specialized in providing riding experiences for children with physical disabilities – hippotherapy. She contacted the school, and asked if older adults with dementia and some physical disabilities could take part in their program. Five engaged persons with dementia eventually enjoyed their own hippotherapeutic experience – a horseback ride.

At still another Hearthstone residence, older adults with dementia practiced making phone calls to a local casino as an activity using a prepared script. When they felt ready they called the casino manager to ask if the casino would be willing to donate used decks of playing cards. The manager agreed to do this, and an outing was organized to pick up the decks from the casino. Upon returning, the older adults sorted the cards into full decks, packaged them, and mailed them to servicemen and servicewomen overseas for use during their off duty time.

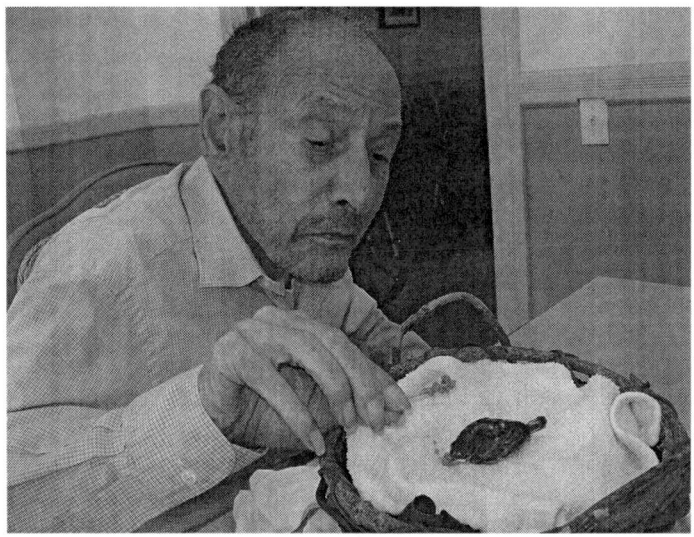

Hard-wired caring emotion naturally engages resident in feeding injured bird

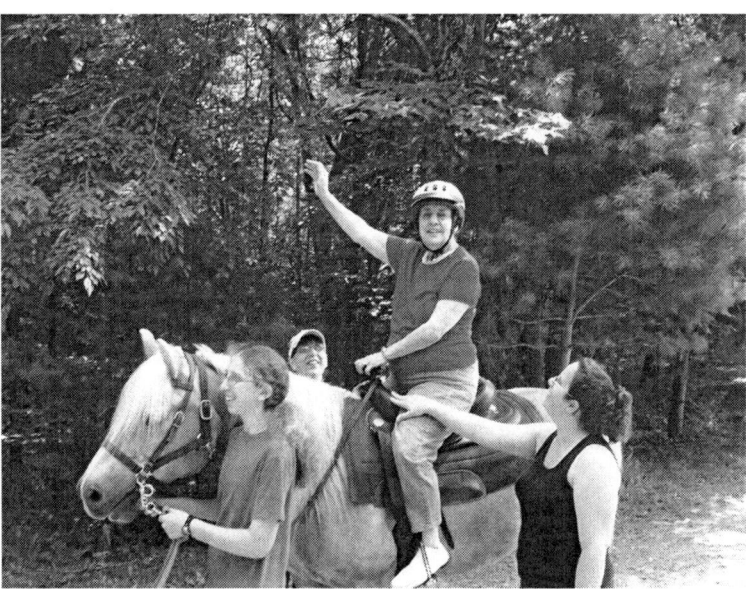

Riding a horse is procedurally learned and pleasurable

These are examples of activities that are the product of a different way of thinking about dementia – the "I'm Still Here"™ Approach. This approach to dementia treatment starts with the assumption that a person with dementia is a person – one who happens to have a chronic and debilitating illness. As we say in our training for caregivers, "There is no 'we' and 'they.' There is only 'us.'"

It is useful to see activities programming for persons with dementia on a continuum, ranging from working with a single person and a single skill to community-based events for small or large groups (Table 23.1). This continuum is the organizational tool we use for this chapter. We will discuss each stage in detail, but think for a moment about the implications of this illustration. An idea, theme, or event grows into a series of opportunities for a person to pursue individual interests while participating – *and succeeding* – at different cognitive levels. Each short-term opportunity can connect and extend over a long period of time if the person wants, as would a hobby or vocation. The backdrop for this approach extends from the individual's residence to the entire community.

The *I'm Still Here*™ Activity Continuum is not intended as a rigid, step-by-step process in which individuals advance from left to right. Rather the continuum illustrates how to see activities as a progression that flows from narrow to broad in terms of community. Individualized Skill Building is the most personalized stage in the progression, while attending a community event is the most social or collective stage. A community-based event may spark interest in learning a related procedure, or it may inspire a Montessori-based activity. Likewise, participation in a Montessori-based activity may require following a specific procedure, and then lead to participating with others who have a shared interest. Thus, the Continuum shows activities in a social, community-based context and how activities programming can and needs to be flexible and dynamic to provide quality of life rather than mere task completion.

Personalized Skill Building

Personalized Skill Building (PSB) involves training procedures to create, recover, or strengthen specific skills a person requires to complete an activity. PSB builds on the fact that learning can take place in dementia. The implications of this are powerful in that old skills may be relearned and new ones acquired following the onset of dementia. This is accomplished through focusing on and utilizing remaining strengths in persons with dementia, such as the desire to improve with practice; motor learning; and hard-wired emotions like caring for an injured bird.

Essentially PSB works as follows: First identify a target goal, such as learning to play golf and then develop a set of PSB procedures to help the individual acquire or regain the skills necessary to reach the target goal. Using task analysis skills familiar to occupational therapists and to persons working in human factors, the activities professional identifies each individual skill or step necessary to accomplish the target goal. In the example of learning to golf, a first target goal might be to properly grip the golf club. How might this proceed?

First, it is important that the presenter herself knows how to properly execute the goal behavior before asking the person with dementia to try it. While this may seem obvious, we have learned from experience that it can be a problem. A student was working with an adult day care client who had been a golf instructor but had

Table 23.1 I'm Still Here™ Activity Continuum (©Hearthstone Alzheimer Care, 2010; used with permission)

Individualized skill building	Montessori programming for dementia	Interactive living events	Performance and large social events	Community-based events
Holding a utensil safely	Following a recipe for guacamole	Cooking club; catering committee	Cooking demonstration in the residence Party catered by residents	Culinary arts class
Practice reading aloud	Take turns reading jokes; discussing comedy	Clown troupe/comedy Club	Vaudeville Routine Stand-up comedy night	Attend circus/comedy act
Gripping a golf club	Putting practice	Golf Enthusiast Club	Lessons from guest golf pro	Attend pro golf tournament

advanced dementia with expressive language difficulties. The client did not take part in most activities presented to him at the center, pacing silently instead throughout the day for the most part. Though not familiar with golf, the student thought that if she let the client see her hitting a plastic golf ball with a golf club, it might arouse his interest. Leading him to the back yard, she teed up the ball and got ready to strike it with the club. The former instructor approached the student, placed his hands over hers, saying "You'll slice" (a golf term meaning that if she had hit the ball with her original grip, the ball would not have traveled straight,) while adjusting her grip. Since we recommend that persons with dementia be given a demonstration of what is to be done before asking these persons to perform a procedure, it is important to give an accurate or appropriate demonstration.

After making sure you know what you are doing, provide external cues to assist in the learning process. This might involve coloring the places on the golf club where the hands are to grip it, placing tape or color where a walker needs to be gripped; putting sand paper on the button to press to make a CD player play a recorded message from a relative (for a person with low vision); etc. Diagrams and/or verbal instructions also can be used, but direct tactile and visual communication works best. If printed text is to be used we recommend a large type size (e.g., 48 point), a sans serif font (such as Arial), and bold lines. The best test of whether a text is appropriate is to simply ask the person with dementia to read it aloud.

It may also be necessary to modify materials to accommodate physical or cognitive challenges. Just as spoons or other utensils with oversized handles can be acquired to facilitate their use by persons with motor skill deficits, so the golf club might have to be modified so that it can be gripped more effectively by the person with dementia. It is important not only to perform a task analysis but also to determine which physical or cognitive challenges face the person with dementia and determine means to overcome or circumvent such challenges. It is important to respect the person's abilities and disabilities. Discussion with physical and occupational therapists regarding use of assistive or adaptive devices and technologies is a useful way to learn about this approach, which involves viewing activities programming as a means of infusing rehabilitation practices within all aspects of daily routines for caregiving (Camp & Mattern, 1999).

The training regimen or schedule to be employed must be selected next. This involves how often and in what context the PSB training needs to take place to achieve desired effects. One training schedule that has proven effective in allowing persons with dementia to learn and reach goals is called spaced-retrieval, or procedural interval learning (Camp, 2006a; Malone et al., 2007, Zeisel, 2009). For example, someone with dementia forgets to look at a prepared diagram of the correct golf grip before holding the club; a goal would be to teach her to pick up and look at the diagram first. Using spaced-retrieval to draw on the person's procedural learning abilities, you can help the individual learn by practicing the target response ("I look at the diagram") in very short intervals at first, and then gradually increasing the intervals. Assuming that looking at the diagram leads to using the grip as illustrated in the diagram, with practice over time, the diagram becomes less necessary and the target goal procedure becomes increasingly automatic. Note that task analysis does not end with analyzing the steps necessary to display an ability or accomplish a task successfully. It also involves determining which steps are not being executed appropriately by the person with dementia, determining the cause of the problem(s), modifying procedures to allow success, training the new procedures, analyzing the results, and making further modifications as needed. This iterative process needs to be implemented repeatedly over time, especially if a person's skills deteriorate due to physical decline or illness.

There may be many separate steps necessary to complete an overall task, even a simple one, such as putting a golf ball. Gripping the club is only the first step. Putting involves hitting the golf ball with the putter, using the right amount of force when hitting the ball, aiming the ball, and possibly picking up or retrieving the ball before and after striking it. Each skill must be practiced, either separately or chained in sequence (e.g., learn to grip the club; after this is available, learn to use the club to strike the golf ball, etc.). In addition, fundamental abilities such as grip strength might have to be developed or improved prior to work with gripping a golf club. Again, activities programming using this approach can be seen as an extension of rehabilitation methods applied to activities (Camp, 1999a; Camp & Mattern, 1999).

The key thing to remember is that employing the "I'm Still Here"™ Approach, just as with the Montessori educational approach, activities are never viewed as "busy work." There is always a purpose for any activity, with the end goal clearly in mind. Each activity is one step in a sequence of steps leading toward a goal. The columns in Table 23.1 show how an ultimate goal might extend from an ISB to a community-based event. We will examine this progression "across the columns" next.

Montessori Programming for Dementia

The Montessori-based approach to activities has been shown to result in high levels of positive engagement and reduction of negative affect and problematic behaviors (Camp et al., 1997; Camp, Judge, Orsulic-Jeras, & Schneider, 2000; Camp & Skrajner, 2004; Judge, Camp & Orsulic-Jeras, 2000; Orsulic-Jeras, Judge & Camp, 2000). Based on the teachings and educational philosophy of Maria Montessori (Lillard, 2005; Montessori, 1964), this approach can be applied to individual or group activities and can be adapted to different levels of cognitive ability (Camp, 2006b). In essence, any activity can be made Montessori-based by following some key principles and concepts.

At the heart of the approach is enabling the individual to have control over, and success in, his or her environment by breaking down activity tasks into steps, using guided repetition, providing feedback, and progressing from simple to complex and concrete to abstract. Maria Montessori created an environment in which her students' abilities could be maximized; Montessori-based activities for persons with dementia capitalize on relatively spared memory systems. Using hand-held props that Montessori called "manipulatives" during activities bolsters learning and enhances successful participation. Other key Montessori principles applied to activities

Table 23.2 Elements of the Montessori-based programming paradigm (© Hearthstone Alzheimer Care, 2010; used with permission)

The Montessori-Based Programming Paradigm	
Give up	Embrace
Right and wrong way to conduct an activity	Engagement is the measure of right and wrong
Check off each component of an activity to make sure everything was "accomplished"	Respond to the person and remain flexible
Schedule (of activities)	Routines (of everyday life)
Task as end	Task as means to an end
"I need to run it"	"They run it"
"The" leader	The "group" leads
Entertainment	Engagement
Failure free (activities)	Errorless (interaction) with occasional chance to fail and to learn from it
It's my activity; If it does not "work," I have failed; if it does, I have succeeded	It's their activity; others' success is my success
Activity(ies) – keep them busy	Life – all the decisions related to linked things to do

programming for persons with dementia include clearly inviting individuals to participate and offering choices, always demonstrating an action before asking a person with dementia to perform it, and extensive use of external cues. Research reveals that, when these key principles are effectively followed, difficult behaviors give way to constructive engagement for the duration of the activity. Additional elements of Montessori-Based Programming for people with dementia are shown in Table 23.2, and contrasted with "standard" approaches to activity programming for dementia.

To maximize the effectiveness and positive impacts of Montessori-based activity programming for residents and staff, it is necessary to adapt to changing interests among individuals and groups and to think creatively about extending activities over longer periods of time to maintain continuous positive engagement. The I'm Still Here™ Continuum provides a model for doing exactly that.

In our previous golf example, the next step after a person learns to grip a putter appropriately is to provide a larger purpose by giving the person practice putting a golf ball into a target, such as an electronic device simulating a hole on a putting green that can return the ball as well. With practice, and if the procedures and materials are set up appropriately, the person with dementia indeed will improve in putting.

Of course, as with any individual, there has to be a motivation for practicing a behavior such as putting. In many facilities, persons with dementia engage in activities not so much out of a particular interest, but to please staff members. Persons who are interested in neither doing an activity nor pleasing staff express their preferences by leaving activities, never coming to activities, "outbursts," and the 4 "A"s of Alzheimer's – agitation, aggression, anxiety, and apathy. Self-determination in selecting activities or deciding on most any other aspect of daily living is usually minimal or nonexistent for residents with dementia in long-term care. It is necessary to understand the person with dementia – her background, past preferences, occupation, hobbies, and interests in order to make activities meaningful to the individual, not simply as a means of pleasing or appeasing staff, but as a truly purposeful endeavor.

An example might speak louder than theory. In an assisted living residence, in the hopes that a former occupation could be linked to an activity for a resident, a former mailman was asked if he would like to deliver mail to other residents. The resident responded that he had delivered all the mail that had ever been required of him, and that he was now retired, and that he did not want to deliver another letter – he had "served his time." Another resident at a Hearthstone residence who showed no interest in taking part in activities was a sports fan. Activities were created for him that involved sorting teams into their respective leagues, such as labeling Boston Red Sox players as American League, while the Saint Louis Cardinals players were separated and placed in the National League basket. While knowing an individual's past can be useful, only tailoring an activity to a person's current interests will engage him.

The golf pro will definitely be engaged if he practices to compete in a putting contest with other residents, or if he sees himself on a putting green at a golf course outside of the facility when the winter turns into spring and summer. Learning to hold a utensil such as a knife or spoon as an ISB that can lead to following a recipe for making guacamole, involving slicing open an avocado, mashing the avocado, mixing in lime juice, and serving to others. Each step could be practiced individually, and ultimately combined in expanding sequences. The end result is guacamole to enjoy with friends.

Detailed descriptions of how to construct numerous Montessori-based activities for dementia are provided in a number of manuals (Camp, 1999b; Camp et al., 2006; Hearthstone Alzheimer Care, 2010; Joltin, Camp, Noble, & Antenucci, 2005). As always, such activities are open-ended in that any activity can be expanded vertically (made more challenging or less challenging) or horizontally (similar or related activities can be used). In addition, these activities can be expanded socially, to include more persons and/or larger social agendas. That is the essence of the next columns in Table 23.1, which we will now discuss.

Interactive Living Events

A natural extension of Montessori-Based Activity Programming is to focus activities toward an extended or broader purpose. Research demonstrates that persons in early to middle stages of dementia can successfully lead activities for other persons with dementia (Camp & Skrajner, 2004; Skrajner & Camp, 2007), present Montessori-based activities to preschool children (Camp et al., 1997, 2004), and exercise degrees of autonomy in their daily lives beyond present day stigmatized expectations. Whether choosing to participate as a leader, artistic contributor, commentator, or some other role, each individual can contribute and help to build a greater sense of community – with or without dementia. This research has also revealed a great deal about preparing activities, setting them up, and presenting them to capitalize on the existing abilities and strengths of persons living with dementia.

Interactive Living Events (the third column in Table 23.1) involve a series of Montessori-based activities centered on a broader theme or objective. Participation requires a higher level of involvement analogous to participating in an organized community event or club in which everyone has a role and contributes to the effort. It involves working together and being part of a team. This level of participation leads to a sense of purpose and fulfillment among participants. Interactive Living Events (ILEs) provide a way to create opportunities for individuals with cognitive impairments to participate and meaningfully contribute to a social group to which they wish to belong.

In our golf example, a group of persons who took part in a putting competition began to meet regularly as a "Golf Enthusiasts' Club." Members choose the name of their club – one that is meaningful to them. The club reads golf magazine articles, looks at videos of classic golf matches, visits golf courses in the area, and holds other golf competitions. Like in any other club, there are officers, rules, a club charter – all developed by club members. In a similar way, the resident who learned to grip utensils and prepare guacamole joins a group of like-minded individuals to form a Cooking Club and Catering Committee.

Most people were parts of groups at work, as well as belonging to formal or informal groups in neighborhoods, communities, or places of worship. Naming similar groups "committees" or "task forces" in dementia care provides connectivity to these past associations. In addition, providing meaningful activity for these groups shows respect to persons with dementia. When the group of residents set up a committee with a mission to support members of the armed forces, they felt empowered. A group of residents called the casino, traveled there to collect old decks of playing cards, put together full decks of cards, and sent them overseas to servicemen and servicewomen. They truly fulfilled their group's mission.

Performance and Large Social Events

Many creative activities and Interactive Living Events lend themselves to a performance event, column 4 in Table 23.1. A cooking demonstration for staff organized by the Cooking Club would be a performance as well as a catered party for family members. Holding such an event generates a host of related subactivities such as menu planning, selecting recipes, purchasing and preparing ingredients, setting up and decorating the room for the event, and creating materials for audience members. Performance events provide a sense of shared purpose for participants while enabling guests, family members, and staff to witness their family members succeeding in ways that they perhaps never believed possible. Such a demonstration is a powerful way to destroy negative stereotypes, myths, and defeatist attitudes surrounding Alzheimer's disease and dementia.

The manual "Living the 'I'm Still Here'™ Lifestyle" (Hearthstone Alzheimer Care, 2010) provides a wide variety of examples of such events. Just as the postman who did not want to deliver mail demonstrated the need to fit a specific Montessori-based activity to a specific individual, so social events must fit the culture of a community. Camp (in press) describes how an activity such as an ice-cream social, familiar to residents with dementia in long-term care facilities in the US, is an utterly foreign concept in Australia. There, a comparable social event might be a "sausage sizzle," unless you are dealing with an aboriginal Australian indigenous population. Then, the "sausage sizzle" becomes a "camp cookout," including the slicing and cooking of kangaroo tails.

Putting on a golf green could be elaborated to a golf pro visiting the residence to chat with the golf enthusiasts' club members and give golf lessons. A chef might come to the cooking or catering group to give a cooking lesson. The Ladder to the Moon™ theater club described in Chap. 19 is another example of this level of programming, and indicates where ARTZ and Artists for Alzheimer's® programming described in Chap. 19 can fit within our model. It is an important initial link between residents with dementia and the larger community outside of their residence.

Community-Based Events

The social culmination of the I'm Still Here™ Activities Continuum is the Community-based Event. Imagine a cultural, sporting, spiritual, or historical event seamlessly attended by residents with dementia along with members of the community at large. Going to a golf tournament and to a cooking class at a culinary institute are ways in which our previous examples of activity programming and extended into the community. In such settings, individual differences are an asset, and persons with dementia experience the moment and contribute as any other attendee. In New York City, a large group of residents with dementia from a number of Hearthstone residences combined to take a boat tour around Manhattan Island. One resident with dementia was chosen by the boat's activity director to give the champagne toast to the boat's crew. She did so with panache. A trip to Bermuda is in the planning stage for a group of residents with dementia.

The final extension of the "I'm Still Here"™ Approach is described in Chap. 19 with regard to the ARTZ: Artists for Alzheimer's® *It Takes A Village* Program. Community organizations with trained staff enable people living with dementia access to any number of events: artistic, social, entertainment, athletic, spiritual, and political. It is our hope that on a grand scale and over time, these events will help change public perceptions about Alzheimer's disease and dementia for the better. The stigma of this disease presents a major barrier to providing people with dementia the dignity they deserve. In communities where this training becomes widespread, a village providing numerous supportive opportunities for engagement with the larger world can evolve. It is our hope that the stigma, learned helplessness, and excess disabilities imposed upon persons with dementia will be replaced by a focus on the person, who happens to have dementia. By demonstrating the ability to progress from the small beginnings of Individualized Skill Building (ISB) to connection with a supportive external community, we as a society can begin to change for the better, as well.

References

Bourgeois, M. S. (2007). *Memory Books and other graphic cuing systems: Practical communication and memory aids for adults with dementia*. Baltimore: Health Professions Press.

Camp, C. J. (1999a). Memory interventions for normal and pathological older adults. In R. Schulz, M. P. Lawton, & G. Maddox (Eds.), *Annual review of gerontology and geriatrics* (Vol. 18, pp. 155–189). New York: Springer.

Camp, C. J. (Ed.). (1999b). *Montessori-based activities for persons with dementia: Volume 1*. Beachwood, OH: Menorah Park Center for Senior Living.

Camp, C. J. (2006a). Spaced retrieval: A case study in dissemination of a cognitive intervention for persons with dementia. In D. Koltai Attix & K. A. Welsch-Bohmner (Eds.), *Geriatric neuropsychological assessment and intervention* (pp. 275–292). New York: Guilford Press.

Camp, C. J. (2006b). Montessori-Based Dementia Programming™ in long-term care: A case study of disseminating an intervention for persons with dementia. In R. C. Intrieri & L. Hyer (Eds.), *Clinical applied gerontological interventions in long-term care* (pp. 295–314). New York: Springer.

Camp, C. J. (in press). Origins of Montessori programming for dementia. *Non-Pharmacologic Treatments for Dementia*.

Camp, C. J., Judge, K. S., Bye, C. A., Fox, K. M., Bowden, J., Bell, M., et al. (1997). An intergenerational program for persons with dementia using Montessori methods. *The Gerontologist, 37*, 688–692.

Camp, C. J., Judge, K. S., Orsulic-Jeras, S., & Schneider, N. M. (2000). Montessori-based activities in adult day care. *Activities Directors' Quarterly for Alzheimer's and Other Dementia Patients, 1*(1), 1–8.

Camp, C. J., & Mattern, J. M. (1999). Innovations in managing Alzheimer's disease. In D. E. Biegel & A. Blum (Eds.), *Innovations in practice and service delivery across the lifespan* (pp. 276–294). New York: Oxford University Press.

Camp, C. J., & Nasser, E. H. (2003). Nonpharmacological aspects of agitation and behavioral disorders in dementia: Assessment, intervention, and challenges to providing care. In P. A. Lichtenberg, D. L. Murman, & A. M. Mellow (Eds.), *Handbook of dementia: Psychological, neurological, and psychiatric perspectives* (pp. 359–401). New York: Wiley.

Camp, C. J., Orsulic-Jeras, S., Lee, M. M., & Judge, K. S. (2004). Effects of a Montessori-based intergenerational program on engagement and affect for adult day care clients with dementia. In M. L. Wykle, P. J. Whitehouse, & D. L. Morris (Eds.), *Successful aging through the life span: Intergenerational issues in health* (pp. 159–176). New York: Springer.

Camp, C. J., Schneider, N., Orsulic-Jeras, S., Mattern, J., McGowan, A., Antenucci, V. M., et al. (2006). *Montessori-based activities for persons with dementia: Volume 2*. Beachwood, OH: Menorah Park Center for Senior Living.

Camp, C. J., & Skrajner, M. J. (2004). Resident-assisted Montessori programming (RAMP): Training persons with dementia to serve as group activity leaders. *The Gerontologist, 44*, 426–431.

Cohen-Mansfield, J., Libin, A., & Marx, M. S. (2007). Nonpharmacological treatment of agitation: A controlled trial of systematic individualized intervention. *The Journals of Gerontology; Series A; Biological Sciences and Medical Sciences, 62*, 908–916.

Hearthstone Alzheimer Care. (2010). *Living the "I'm Still Here"™ lifestyle*. Woburn, MA: Hearthstone Alzheimer Care.

Joltin, A., Camp, C. J., Noble, B. H., & Antenucci, V. M. (2005). *A different visit: Activities for caregivers and their loved ones with memory impairment*. Beachwood, OH: Menorah Park Center for Senior Living.

Judge, K. S., Camp, C. J., & Orsulic-Jeras, S. (2000). Use of Montessori-based activities for clients with dementia in adult day care: Effects on engagement. *American Journal of Alzheimer's Disease, 15*, 42–46.

Koziol, L. F., & Budding, D. E. (2009). *Subcortical structures and cognition*. New York: Springer.

Lillard, A. S. (2005). *Montessori: The science behind the genius*. New York: Oxford University Press.

Malone, M. L., Skrajner, M. J., Camp, C. J., Neundorfer, M., & Gorzelle, G. J. (2007). Research in practice II: Spaced-retrieval, a memory intervention. *Alzheimer's Care Quarterly, 8*(1), 65–74.

Montessori, M. (1964). *The Monstessori method*. New York: Schocken Books.

Orsulic-Jeras, S., Judge, K. S., & Camp, C. J. (2000). Montessori-based activities for long-term care residents with advanced dementia: Effects on engagement and affect. *The Gerontologist, 40*, 107–111.

Skrajner, M. J., & Camp, C. J. (2007). Resident-assisted Montessori programming (RAMP™): Use of a small group reading activity run by persons with dementia in adult day health care and long-term care settings. *The American Journal of Alzheimer's Disease & Other Dementias, 22*(1), 27–36.

Zeisel, J. (2009). *I'm still here: A breakthrough approach to understanding someone living with Alzheimer's*. New York: Penguin.

Chapter 24
Kirtan Kriya Meditation: A Promising Technique for Enhancing Cognition in Memory-Impaired Older Adults

Dharma Singh Khalsa and Andrew Newberg

Abstract This chapter reviews some of the predictors and markers for Alzheimer's, focusing on stress for the breadth of its impact and because it is an amenable target for treatment. We then describe a low cost and easy to learn meditation technique, Kirtan Kriya, that can not only lower stress, but preliminary evidence suggests it also increases cognitive ability among those with incipient Alzheimer's Disease.

Humankind's New Problem

"It's easy to overlook the remarkableness of aging," exclaimed the renowned gerontologist, Ken Dychtwald (2010). He pointed out that for 99% of the history of humankind, average life expectancy at birth was less than 18 years of age. Long before they reached what we would consider old age, people during that time died first of infectious diseases, accidents, or violence. Over the last thousand years, life expectancy climbed from 25 years, reached 47 by the turn of the twentieth century, sky-rocketed to 78 by the twenty-first century, and is still climbing. Currently, the age group with the greatest population increase is centenarians.

At the time that the Constitution of the United States was being ratified, arthritis, heart disease, and dementia were seldom, if ever problems that physicians were called upon to treat, in part because lifespan was too short for these conditions to emerge as medical problems. Beginning of the last century, however, something unprecedented has been happening. Advances in sanitation, public health, food science, pharmacy, medicine, and wellness-oriented lifestyles, have resulted in an eleven-fold increase in the number of Americans of 65 years or older age, from 3 to 33 million. The US Census Bureau predicts that number will increase to 70 million by the year 2035.

D.S. Khalsa (✉)
Alzheimer's Research and Prevention Foundation, Tucson, AZ, USA

Center for Spirituality and the Mind, University of Pennsylvania, Philadelphia, PA, USA
e-mail: drdharma@alzheimersprevention.org

While the increase in lifespan enjoyed by many people is to be applauded, increasing longevity brings with it a major problem: the dramatic increase in the incidence of cognitive decline, dementia, and particularly, Alzheimer's disease (Alzheimer's Association, 2010). Today there are 5.3 million people with Alzheimer's disease in the United States with a price tag of $148 billion a year, not counting the over ten million unpaid caregivers. Alzheimer's is the sixth leading cause of death. More telling however, is the fact that Alzheimer's disease is now the number one worry of aging baby boomers, surpassing cancer and heart disease.

Predictors and Markers of Alzheimer's

Age. The best predictor for Alzheimer's disease (AD) is advancing age. As a person gets older, the probability of having AD increases. However, significant cognitive decline is not a normal part of aging.

Subjective cognitive impairment (SCI). SCI describes the experience of healthy older adults who have the feeling that their memory is not functioning as well as it should, but for whom the subjective symptom cannot be verified objectively by clinicians. Where clinicians used to dismiss this complaint, it has recently emerged as an early marker for AD (Reisberg, Shulman, Torossian, Leng, & Zhu, 2010). These researchers reported that, over a 7-year period, study participants who had SCI progressed to mild cognitive impairment (MCI) and AD at a higher rate than those who did not. Of those without SCI at the start of the study but who did decline to MCI or AD over its course, mean time to decline was 3.5 year longer than for SCI subjects. In patients without pure cognitive complaints, such as those with multiple sclerosis, there is a relationship between depression, fatigue, SCI, and objective neuropsychological functioning (Kinsinger, Lattie, & Mohr, 2010).

Mild cognitive impairment. Individuals with MCI have cognitive problems that exceed what is expected for their age and background but are not severe enough to meet the criteria for the diagnosis of dementia. MCI is a risk factor for developing AD or other dementias and is often considered a preclinical stage of dementia (see Chap. 21).

Medical conditions. Medical conditions that are high risk factors for AD include cardiovascular disease, high cholesterol, Type 2 diabetes, high blood pressure, smoking, and obesity. Many of these factors are modifiable via medications and lifestyle changes; undertaking such modifications may decrease the likelihood of developing both heart disease and cognitive dysfunction. Although epidemiologic studies show associations with these factors and AD risk, randomized clinical trials have not clearly demonstrated yet that odds of getting dementia actually decrease with treatment or lifestyle changes.

Stress. Stress occurs when a person is unable to cope with the demands placed upon him/her. When his/her ability to perform is exceeded by the demand, stress ensues. Individuals have different levels of tolerance to stress, and different responses at different times in their lives. Although well documented in the research literature, the effect of chronic stress is an under-discussed and underappreciated aspect of maintaining brain fitness in an aging population. The next section offers historical and recent research results that show why stress management is so important to brain health.

Stress and the Brain

In the first author's personal and clinical experience, chronic, unrelenting stress may be near the top of the list of today's lifestyle factors that impact the cause and possibly the progression of AD. Why? Stress stimulates the adrenal glands to release the hormone cortisol, which then flows throughout the blood stream. Cortisol suppresses the immune system function. Stein-Behrins and Sapolsky (1992) found that illness and aging are times of decreased ability to handle stress.

Cortisol also shortens the lifespan of cells and of the organism overall. The lifespan of a normal, healthy cell is controlled by its telomeres, a segment of DNA at the tip of the chromosome. Telomeres are believed to have a protective function, like the plastic tip of a shoe lace that prevents the lace from unraveling. Telomeres prevent chromosomes from losing genetic information needed in the replication process. Each time the cell divides, the telomere is shortened, until at last the telomere length is insufficient for the cell to replicate itself and it eventually dies. However, there is an enzyme, telomerase, which can rebuild the DNA sequence at the end of the chromosome and thus lengthen the telomere. Choi, Fauce, & Effros (2008) found that exposure to cortisol was associated with a reduction in telomerase activity in human T lymphocytes. By acting on telomerase, cortisol affects cell life. When cortisol reduces telomerase activity, the telomeres in the DNA shortened precipitously and, in turn, the shortened telomeres accelerate aging and illness. People with both chronic stress and AD are in double jeopardy in regard to their cells, as Lukens, Van Deerlin, Clark, Xie, & Johnson (2009) found, because telomere length in peripheral blood is already diminished in individuals who have AD.

Of most interest here is the research into the direct role of stress and cortisol on the development of dementia. Early life stresses, such as abuse and neglect at a young age, result in the development of inflammation in the hippocampus, the brain structure that is fundamental to learning and commonly the site of initial deterioration in AD. Although causal linking has not yet been established, this early-age inflammatory process could potentially contribute to AD pathology (Anda et al., 2006; Bornstein, Copenhaver, & Mortimer, 2006).

Newcomer et al. (1999) found decreased memory performance in healthy humans who were injected intravenously with stress-levels of cortisol. In a longitudinal study conducted over a period of 30 years, Crowe, Andel, Pedersen, and Gatz (2007) found a higher risk of dementia in individuals who reported a high incidence of work-related stress. Wilson et al. (2003) showed that Alzheimer's disease is higher in people with a stress-prone personality. Peavy et al. (2007) showed that stress produced more reactivity and higher levels of cortisol with subsequent worse effects on memory function in older individuals who had a genetic risk for the development of AD (i.e., ApoE4 positive).

The hormone cortisol has been shown to kill brain cells in the hippocampus, the brain structure fundamental to learning and sometimes considered to be the memory center of the brain (Sapolsky, 1992; McEwen & Sapolsky, 1992). Prolonged exposure to stress leads to loss of neurons, particularly in the hippocampus (Lupien, McEwen, Gunnar, & Heim, 2009).

In both humans and animals, reactions to stress – and also regulation of many other body processes, including digestion, mood, immune function, energy – are controlled by means of communications among a set of structures in the midbrain called the hypothalamic-pituitary-adrenal axis, or the HPA axis. If the functioning of the HPA axis becomes impaired, the ability to regulate the body functions just listed is also impaired. A connection between cognition in the older adult and the HPA has been found. For example, MacLullich et al. (2006) showed that a smaller anterior cingulate cortex (ACC) is associated with an impaired hypothalamic-pituitary-adrenal axis (the HPA axis) regulation in healthy elderly men. The ACC plays an important role in rational cognitive functions, including focusing attention and decision-making. It is a central station for processing stimuli and assigning appropriate control to other areas in the brain. It is involved in learning and problem-solving tasks. Hence, the Alasdair et al. finding associating diminishment of the ACC to impaired stress regulation is especially significant.

To summarize, chronic, unmanaged stress causes excessive cortisol release from the adrenal gland into the blood stream. This cortisol then travels to the hippocampus, where it causes brain cell death and shuts off the inhibition of production of further cortisol from the adrenal gland. The excess of cortisol causes inflammation and hippocampal neuronal cell death, and also accelerates aging by decreasing telomere length, which in turn may lead to more inflammation, cardiovascular disease, cancer, and Alzheimer's.

Stress Response Versus Relaxation Response

Humans and most animals exhibit a stress response when facing a situation whose difficulty is beyond their perceived ability. Humans also possess a counterbalancing capability, the relaxation response. The main difference between the two is that the stress response may occur as a result of environmental stimulation, but the relaxation response requires the individual to take action.

The stress response and the relaxation response were first demonstrated by Walter Hess in 1949 by stimulating two discrete areas of the hypothalamus in the brain of a cat. Table 24.1 shows that these two phenomena are opposites of each other.

The relaxation response was popularized by Benson in 1975. This is a relaxed, self-healing state, and requires positive action to experience. In addition to the effects listed in Table 24.1, it is said to activate the body's natural healing mechanism. There are four requirements to enter it (Benson, 1975):

1. A comfortable position.
2. A quite environment.

3. A tool or mental device.
4. A specific attitude.

The comfortable position can be achieved by simply sitting on a chair, or on the floor in a comfortable, cross-legged posture. The environment should be quiet with an absence of distraction. The next two requirements to enter into a relaxation or basic meditative state are perhaps the most important. The tool can be any thought, sound, phrase, or object on which one focuses. Examples include a chosen word such as "one," or "peace," or an object such as the breath flowing in and out. The attitude has to do with not becoming attached to any thoughts that enters consciousness, but rather to acknowledge them and then go back to the chosen focus. So it is an attitude of accepting that one's mind will wander in spite of the desire to focus, and of not being harsh with oneself when it happens.

The relaxation response is a way to manage stress. Meditation is closely related to this technique, sharing both the four requirements listed above and also outcomes in regard to stress management. There are at least 13 physiological effects of basic meditation that have been observed (Khalsa, 2001). In addition to the four listed in Table 24.1, these include decreases in the stress hormones epinephrine, norepinephrine, and cortisol; decrease in lactic acid, which signifies a decrease in anxiety level; decrease in lipid peroxidase, which reveals a decrease in free radical formation; an increase in the hormone DHEA; increase in the sleep and antiaging hormone, melatonin; enhanced immune system function, and a reduction in inflammatory molecules.

Meditation is frequently, if not always, associated with positive psychological changes (See Kaszniak's review, chapter 5). These changes, in turn, are related to telomerase activity in immune cells (Jacobs et al., 2011), which has the potential to promote longevity in those cells, as explained above. Older adults who learned and continued to practice Transcendental Meditation® (TM®) were indeed found to have the highest survival rates 3 years after completion of a study that compared the effects of TM®, relaxation training, mindfulness, and no treatment (Alexander, Langer, Newman, Chandler, & Davies, 1989).

Neuroimaging studies of meditators with such scanning techniques such as magnetic resonance imaging (MRI), positron emission tomography (PET), and single photon emission computed tomography (SPECT) have provided evidence that meditation has direct benefits on the brain. These include increased activity in the hippocampus (Lazar, Bush, Gollub, & Fricchione, 2000), increased cortical thickness (Lazar et al., 2005), diminished loss of brain volume with age (Newberg et al., 2001) and enhanced activity in the prefrontal cortex (Newberg et al., in press). This last finding is especially significant because the prefrontal cortex is associated with attention, concentration, focus, decision-making, and short-term memory.

Table 24.1 Walter Hess's (1968) discovery of the stress response

	Stress response	Relaxation response
Blood pressure	Increased	Decrease
Pulse	Increased	Decrease
Respiratory rate	Increased	Decrease
MVO_2 or oxygen demand	Increase (rise)	Decrease (drop)

This extensive menu of benefits from meditation is available at a relatively low cost (patient's time) and generally no side effects, resulting in a high benefit-to-cost ratio, not only for the patient, but for society.

The forms of basic and more advanced meditation are legion, and some require the investment of many years of practice to master. However, one form of particular interest is Kirtan Kriya (KK) meditation because it can be performed even by those whose memory has some impairment, and the benefits accrue from the very first practice session, based upon preliminary evidence from our research. Before describing the research on which these claims are based, the next section describes the KK practice.

Kirtan Kriya Meditation

Kirtan Kriya is a 12-min singing exercise in the Kundalini yoga tradition that people have been practicing for thousands of years. A *kirtan* is a song. *Kriya* refers to a specific set of movements. In the Eastern meditation tradition, kriyas are used to help bring the body, mind, and emotions into balance, thus creating healing. The Kirtan Kriya form of meditation is meant to be practiced for greater attention, concentration, improved short-term memory, and better mood.

KK brings together several modalities of behavior: singing or chanting, finger movements (mudras), visualization, and sequence tracking. Hence, it is a multifaceted, multisensory exercise that engages several areas of the brain. The complexity of the method thus absorbs attention to such a degree that the likelihood of distracting thoughts entering the mind is greatly diminished. KK shares the four requirements listed above for the relaxation response and basic meditation. It applies the standard meditation behaviors for posture, eye direction, and breath as well. The technique is described by Khalsa (2001).

Posture. The individual can sit comfortably in a chair with their feet flat on the floor. Alternatively, one can sit on the floor with legs crossed, although older adults are not likely to choose this option. The essence of the posture is to be comfortable and sit with spine straight with only the natural curvature.

Breath. The practitioner simply breathes naturally as the meditation unfolds.

Eyes. Eyes are closed.

The chant or mantra. The chant uses the sounds, Saa, Taa, Naa, Maa. These ancient primal sounds from Sanskrit, taken together, mean "my true identity" or "my highest self." The tune to which these sounds are sung is the first four notes of the familiar children's song, "Mary had a Little Lamb." That is, the notes are "Mar-y had a." See Fig. 24.1.

The mudras or finger movements. The thumb is touched to each of the other four fingers in sequence. Both hands perform the same mudra set simultaneously. Figure 24.1 illustrates.

24 Kirtan Kriya Meditation: A Promising Technique for Enhancing Cognition …

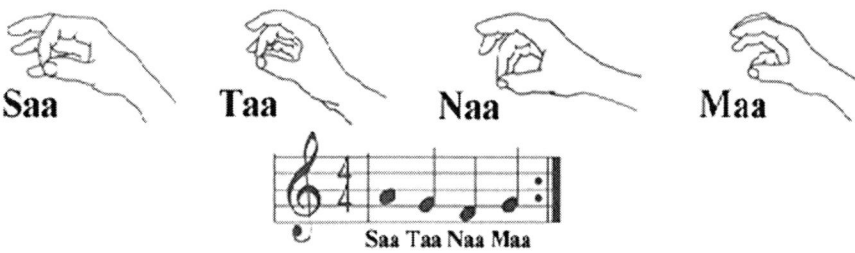

Fig. 24.1 Tooch fingers on sequence as you sing the sounds

Fig. 24.2 Visualize the sound entering the top of the head and out the forhead

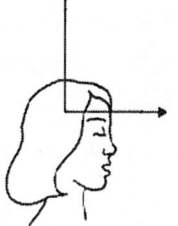

L Form of Concentration

On Saa, touch the index fingers of each hand to the thumbs.
On Taa, touch your middle fingers to your thumbs.
On Naa, touch your ring fingers to your thumbs.
On Maa, touch your little fingers to your thumbs.

Always go forward in sequence: thumb to index finger, middle finger, ring finger, and pinky; never go backwards.

The visualization. Visualize energy coming down from above into the middle of the top of the head, proceeding straight down into your brain, and then changing to a lateral direction so that this force comes out of your head at a point in the middle of your forehead, in the center lined up with the nose (the spot referred to as "the third eye" in some Eastern traditions). Hence, the energy is visualized as following the path of a capital letter L. One may think of this action as sweeping through like a broom. See Fig. 24.2.

The sequence

1. Chant the sounds *Saa Taa Naa Maa* while also performing the mudras with the fingers of both hands. At the same time, visualize the L coming into and leaving the head. With each syllable, imagine the sound flowing in through the top of your head and out the middle of your forehead (your third eye point).
2. For 2 min, sing in your normal voice.
3. For the next 2 min, sing in a whisper.

4. For the next 4 min, say the sound silently to yourself.
5. Then whisper the chant for 2 min, and then out loud for 2 min, for a total of 12 min.
6. To come out of the exercise, inhale very deeply, stretch your hands above your head, and then bring them down slowly in a sweeping motion as you exhale.

The first author has made a video demonstrating the KK meditation, which can be seen by going to www.alzheimersprevention.org/kkmeditation.

Effect of KK Meditation on Brain and Cognition

According to Kundalini yogic tradition, there are several mechanisms by which Kirtan Kriya conveys its benefits. The use of the tongue in Kirtan Kriya during the chanting is believed to stimulate the 84 acupuncture meridian points on the roof of the mouth in a certain permutation and combination that sends a signal to the hypothalamus, as well as to the brain itself. How this works on a chemical level is theoretical, but the first author conjectures that practicing KK may rejuvenate the brain synapse by increasing important brain chemicals, such as acetylcholine.

The dense nerve endings in the fingertips, lips, and tongue are associated with a high level of representation in the motor and sensory areas of the brain. Therefore, when the practitioner utilizes the fingertips in conjunction with the sound, specific areas in the brain, as seen on SPECT scans, are activated. Khalsa, Amen, Hanks, Money, and Newberg (2009) showed particular cerebral blood flow changes during the practice of Kirtan Kriya. As shown in Fig. 24.3 the frontal lobes exhibited

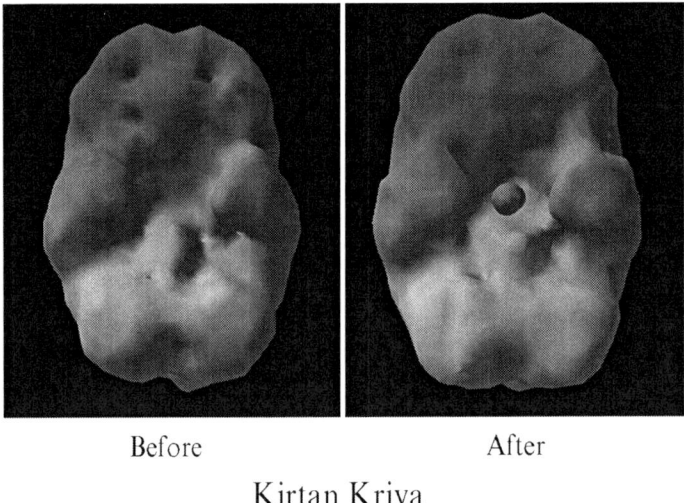

Before   After
Kirtan Kriya

Fig. 24.3 SPECT scan before and after Kirtan Kriya: brain healing in action

Preventing Alzheimer's in 12 Minutes a Day?

Up

Posterior Cingulate Gyrus

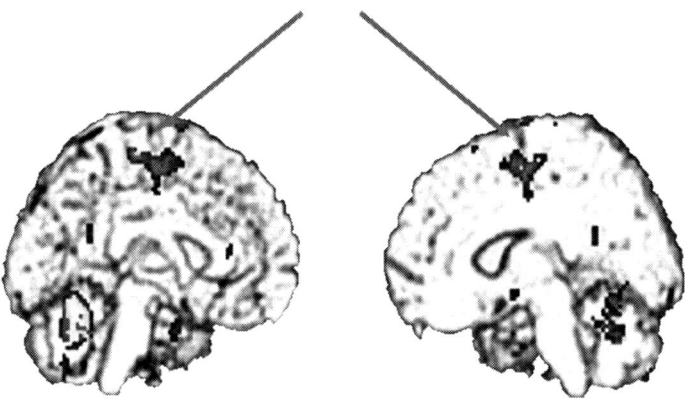

Fig. 24.4 Activation of the posterior cingulate gyrus (Source: Khalsa et al. (2009) "unpublished data")

increased cerebral blood flow. The posterior cingulate gyrus was activated (Fig. 24.4). This is significant, because the posterior cingulate gyrus is one of the first areas that demonstrate decreased activity on a scan when one develops Alzheimer's disease. One might therefore conjecture that consistent practice of the KK meditation and the concomitant activation of the posterior cingulate gyrus, potentially lead to a decreased risk for cognitive decline and Alzheimer's disease. Long-term studies involving clinical outcomes as well as brain imaging will be needed to determine whether this conjecture is true. At present, exploratory studies are showing some intriguing cognitive benefits when Kirtan Kriya is practiced on a regular basis.

Newberg, Wintering, Khalsa, Roggenkamp, and Waldman (2010) described positive effects of Kirtan Kriya on cognitive function and cerebral blood flow in subjects with memory loss. Significantly, this is the first study in which the KK meditation has been explored in people diagnosed with memory impairment although it is not the first study of people with memory loss; Alexander, Langer, Newman, Chandler, and Davies (1989) also included subjects with dementia in all treatment groups, including the TM group. In our preliminary study, participants who complained of memory loss symptoms were recruited, and either practiced KK for 12 min per day (the experimental group) or listened to music for an equal amount of time (the comparison group). The 15 experimental participants ranged in age from 52 to 77 (mean 64, SD 8). Their MMSE scores ranged from 16 to 30. Seven had mild age-associated memory impairment (i.e., SCI), five had MCI, and three had a diagnosis of AD and moderate impairment. However, one of those with AD, whose MMSE score was 16, was found to be incapable of following the directions for performing the meditation, and her data was not included further in the results. Thus, 14 participants constituted the final experimentation group, two of whom had AD.

The experimental group participants were individually instructed in how to perform the KK meditation. The training began with a 20-min video of one of the investigators explaining and demonstrating the technique. In this video and in further instructions to participants, the visualization component was not included. Then the participant was told to perform KK for a 12-min period while being supervised by one of the researchers. Participants were told to perform the 12-min KK practice daily for 8 weeks, and provided a CD to help guide them. The CD was a recording of the audible aspects, plus some background music as an aid in the rhythm.

The comparison group comprised two people with MCI and three with age-associated memory impairment (SCI), for a total of five participants who ranged from 56 to 79 years old (mean 65, SD 10). The mean MMSE score was 29 (SD 1). They were to listen daily to a CD on which had been recorded 12 min of two Mozart violin concertos.

The participants in the experimental group kept a practice log revealing a high degree of compliance (75%, on average). Participants were scanned (SPECT) both on the first day at which they had been instructed, and at the follow-up session after 8-weeks of at-home practice. They were also given a battery of neuropsychological tests on both occasions.

The testing revealed a significant improvement in scores on a verbal fluency test, animal naming, and a test of divided attention, trailmaking, Part B. Both of these neuropsychological tests tap into executive functioning skills.

Subjectively, the experimental participants also reported improvement in their overall memory functioning. Given Reisberg et al.'s (2010) findings about SCI, this may be significant, as individuals with SCI may be at higher risk for progression to MCI and later Alzheimer's disease.

As stated above, this is the first study of the effects of the Kirtan Kriya meditation on people who are experiencing memory loss, and it revealed that KK had a positive effect in enhancing cerebral blood flow and improving cognitive functioning. Previous studies of meditators using attention-focusing practices other than KK have revealed activations in brain structures in the frontal lobe and ACC. Previous studies of meditators using mantras (not KK) have revealed changes in the temporal lobe.

As can be seen in the scans below in Fig. 24.5, from Newberg, Wintering, Khalsa, Roggenkamp and Waldman (2010), KK practice produced a difference in activation in the frontal lobe, posterior cingulate gyrus, and anterior cingulate gyrus, both the first time the subjects practiced the meditation on the day of instruction, and more prominently after 8 weeks of doing the meditation only 12 min a day. MacLullich et al.'s (2006) result reported earlier on the association between the ACC and the body's ability to regulate stress, we speculate that enhancing activity of the anterior cingulate gyrus could improve hypothalamic-pituitary-adrenal axis function, and normalize the stress response so that not much of cortisol bathes the hippocampus.

Changes in the Anterior Cingulate Gyrus

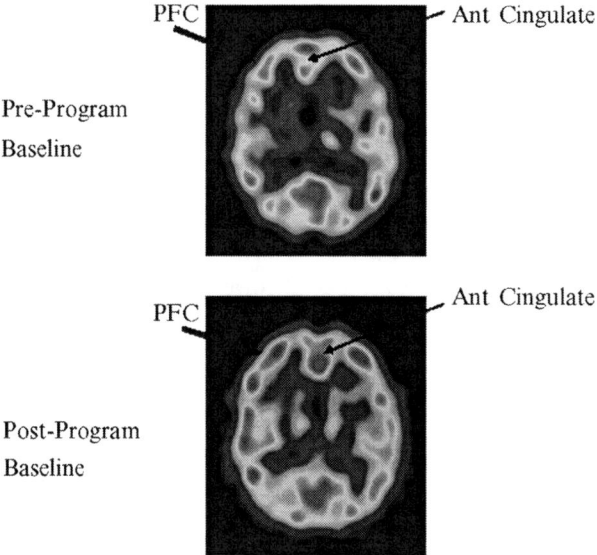

Fig. 24.5 Enhanced cerebral blood flow in the anterior cingulate gyrus

Conclusion

Mitigating the biochemical effects of stress on the body and brain is an important, although rarely discussed, target of prevention for Alzheimer's disease. Meditation has been shown to be helpful in lowering anxiety and stress as well as a variety of other positive health outcomes. However, some meditation techniques appear to be unattractive to older adults and too complex to be utilized by those whose memory is already compromised.

This chapter described a form of meditation, Kirtan Kriya, that has been successfully used in preliminary studies by this population at risk for Alzheimer's disease. Participants reported that it was enjoyable and subjectively beneficial, including a perception of improved cognition. Directed to practice it daily over a period of 8 weeks, participants did indeed practice it 75% of the days, on average. Newberg, Wintering, Waldman, Amen, Khalsa and Alavi (2010) found objective evidence of cognitive benefit as well. Hence, the Kirtan Kriya meditation appears to also improve a number of aspects of psychological well-being.

Most noteworthy are the facts that this was a self-directed training program using a CD, after only a brief one-on-one instruction; the amount of time necessary was only 12 min a day for 8 weeks for these results to be observable; it is both a practical and a low cost intervention; and it has no side effects, and does not interfere with medications. Our preliminary findings suggest KK meditation is a promising intervention for enhancing cognition in older adults with mild memory impairment that warrants further research and possible inclusion in complementary treatment protocols.

First Author's Final Comment

Yogi Bhajan, Ph.D., Master of Kundalini Yoga who brought KK to the West, was once asked: "Sir, does meditation prevent dementia?" "Not only does it prevent dementia" he replied, "But it takes you to another dimension." In Khalsa's opinion, this other dimension is one where the regular practitioner of KK will discover optimal health, psychological well-being, and brain longevity.

References

Alexander, C., Langer, E. L., Newman, R., Chandler, H., & Davies, J. (1989). Aging, mindfulness and meditation. *Journal of Personality and Social Psychology, 57*, 950–964.

Anda, R. F., Felitti, V. J., Bremner, J. D., Walker, J. D., Whitfield, C., Perry, B. D., et al. (2006). The enduring effects of abuse and related adverse experiences in childhood. A convergence of evidence from neurobiology and epidemiology. *European Archives of Psychiatry and Clinical Neuroscience, 256*, 174–186.

Association, A. (2010). *Alzheimer's disease facts and figures*. Chicago, IL: Alzheimer's Association.

Benson, H. (1975). *The relaxation response*. New York, NY: Morrow.

Bornstein, A. R., Copenhaver, C. I., & Mortimer, J. A. (2006). Early-life risk factors for Alzheimer disease. *Alzheimer Disease and Associated Disorders, 20*(1), 63–72.

Choi, J., Fauce, S. R., & Effros, R. B. (2008). Reduced telomerase activity in human T lymphocytes exposed to cortisol. *Brain, Behavior, and Immunity, 22*(4), 600–605.

Crowe, M., Andel, R., Pedersen, N. L., & Gatz, M. (2007). Do work-related stress and reactivity to stress predict dementia more than 30 years later? *Alzheimer Disease and Associated Disorders, 21*(3), 205–209.

Dychtwald, K. (2010). *Keynote presentation*. American Society on Aging Annual Conference, Chicago, IL.

Hess, W. R. (1968). Nobel prize received in 1949 for the discovery of the functional organization of diencephalon as a coordinating center of visceral function. [Article in Polish]. *Wiadomosci Lekarskie, 21*(19), 1791–1792.

Jacobs, T. L., Epel, E. S., Lin, J., Blackburn, E. H., Wolkowitz, O. M., Bridwell, D. A., et al. (2011). Intensive meditation training, immune cell telomerase activity, and psychological mediators. *Psychoneuroimmunology, 36*(5), 664–81.

Khalsa, D. S. (2001). *Meditation as Medicine*. New York, NY: Atria.

Khalsa, D. S., Amen, D., Hanks, C., Money, N., & Newberg, A. N. (2009). Cerebral blood flow changes during chanting meditation. *Nuclear Medicine Communications, 30*, 1–6.

Kinsinger, S. W., Lattie, E., & Mohr, D. C. (2010). Relationship between depression, fatigue, subjective cognitive impairment, and objective neuropsychological functioning in patients with multiple sclerosis. *Neuropsychology, 24*(5), 573–580.

Lazar, S. W., Bush, G., Gollub, R. L., & Fricchione, G. L. (2000). Functional brain mapping of the relaxation response and meditation. *Neuroreport, 11*, 1581–1585.

Lazar, S. W., Kerr, C. E., Wasserman, R. H., Gray, J. R., Greve, D. N., & Treadway, M. T. (2005). Meditation experience is associated with increased cortical thickness. *Neuroreport, 16,* 1893–1897.

Lukens, J. N., Van Deerlin, V., Clark, C. M., Xie, S. X., & Johnson, F. B. (2009). Comparisons of telomere length in peripheral blood and cerebellum in Alzheimer's disease. *Alzheimer's & Dementia, 5*(6), 463–469. doi:10.1016/j.jalz.2009.05.666.

Lupien, S. J., McEwen, B. S., Gunnar, M. R., & Heim, C. (2009). Effects of stress throughout the lifespan on the brain, behaviour and cognition. *Nature Reviews. Neuroscience, 10*(6), 434–445.

MacLullich, A. M., Ferguson, K. J., Wardlaw, J. M., Starr, J. M., Deary, I. J., & Seckl, J. R. (2006). Smaller left anterior cingulate cortex volumes are associated with impaired hypothalamic pituitary adrenal axis regulation in healthy elderly men. *The Journal of Clinical Endocrinology and Metabolism, 91*(4), 1591–1594.

McEwen, B., & Sapolsky, R. A. (1992). Stress and cognitive function. *Endocrine Reviews, 7,* 284–301.

Newberg, A. B., Alavi, A., Baime, M., Pourdehnad, M., Santanna, J., & D'Aquili, E. G. (2001). The measurement of regional cerebral blood flow during the complex cognitive task of meditation: A preliminary SPECT study. *Psychiatry Research. Neuroimaging, 106,* 113–122.

Newberg, A. B., Wintering, N., Khalsa, D. S., Roggenkamp, H., & Waldman, R. W. (2010). Meditation effects on cognitive function and cerebral blood flow in subjects with memory loss: A preliminary study. *Journal of Alzheimer's Disease, 20,* 517–526.

Newberg, A. B., Wintering, N., Waldman, M. R., Amen, D., Khalsa, D. S., & Alavi, A. (2010). Cerebral blood flow differences between long-term meditators and non-meditators. *Consciousness and Cognition, 19*(4), 899–905.

Newcomer, J. W., Selke, G., Melson, A. K., Hershey, T., Craft, S., Richards, K., et al. (1999). Decreased memory performance in healthy humans induced by stress-level cortisol treatment. *Archives of General Psychiatry, 56*(6), 527–533.

Peavy, G. M., Lange, K. L., Salmon, D. P., Patterson, T. L., Goldman, S., Gamst, A. C., et al. (2007). The effects of prolonged stress and APOE genotype on memory and cortisol in older adults. *Biological Psychiatry, 62*(5), 472–478.

Reisberg, B., Shulman, M. B., Torossian, C., Leng, L., & Zhu, W. (2010). Outcome over seven years of healthy adults with and without subjective cognitive impairment. *Alzheimer's & Dementia, 6*(1), 11–24.

Sapolsky, R. (1992). *Stress, the aging brain, and the mechanisms of neuron death.* Cambridge, MA: Bradford.

Stein-Behrins, B. A., & Sapolsky, R. (1992). Stress, glucocorticoids and aging. *Aging Clinical and Experimental Research, 4,* 197–210.

Wilson, R. S., Evans, D. A., Bienias, J. L., Mendes de Leon, C. F., Schneider, J. A., & Bennett, D. A. (2003). Proneness to psychological distress is associated with risk of Alzheimer's disease. *Neurology, 61*(11), 1479–1485.

Chapter 25
Brain Brightening: Neurotherapy for Enhancing Cognition in the Elderly *

James Lawrence Thomas

Abstract With increasing longevity, the absolute number and relative proportion of persons with dementia will become a significant problem in society. Neurotherapy offers a non-pharmacological treatment to enhance the functioning of frontal lobe functioning which usually is reduced as one grows older. This chapter presents preliminary evidence for the use of currently available biofeedback technology that has exciting promise to improve cognition in individuals with mild decline.

Introduction

The term *brain brightening* refers to doing neurotherapy with older adults in order to enhance their cognitive abilities. *Brain brightening* seems to have been coined by Thomas Budzynski in his 1996 paper on this subject (Budzynski, 1996). It has, however, been adapted by many to include a number of possible interventions for the same overall purpose, i.e., helping older individuals improve cognitive functioning. In this chapter, the term brain brightening refers to the use of neurofeedback and neurotherapy for improving cognitive functioning in the elderly.

I will first give a brief overview of biofeedback, and then explain the basics of neurotherapy and neurofeedback. Some background in describing the underlying concepts of the electrophysiology of the brain will be necessary in order to understand some of the research in this area. Then the research on brain brightening will be noted, as well as directions for the future.

*** James Lawrence Thomas, Ph.D.,** Clinical Psychologist and neuropsychologist; faculty, NYU Medical Center.

J.L. Thomas (✉)
NYU Langone Medical Center, New York, NY, USA
e-mail: nurosvcs@aol.com

Biofeedback in general. Biofeedback is a method of treatment in which the patients are trained to become aware and learn to control their own physiology in order to improve physical and psychological health. For example, a patient who is trained to control his/her temperature can help such diverse disorders as headaches, hypertension, anxiety, tinnitus, as well as enhance general relaxation (Schwartz & Andrasik, 2003). There are several modalities of biofeedback treatment, and some of these might be of interest for the treatment of the older adults. Training a person in heart rate variability might be beneficial for those with cardiac conditions. Temperature training could also benefit patients who need a method of overall relaxation or for disorders mentioned earlier. In all cases, biofeedback trains people to monitor and control aspect(s) of their own physiology to improve their health. Training the EEG or brain waves is the modality of biofeedback considered in this chapter.

In all biofeedback procedures, specialized equipment measures the physiology of various modalities, which in turn are fed back to the patient (usually on a computer screen) so that the patient knows what is going on with regard to his or her physiology. For example, in temperature training, the degrees of the body where the sensor is (typically on the finger) can be displayed on the computer screen so that the patient can see if the temperature is raised by specified exercises, such as imagining that the hand is getting warmer. Modern biofeedback instruments are quite sensitive, and in the case of temperature training, the resolution is to the 100th of a degree. Thus, even small changes can be seen on the computer in a graph or other visual display. Biofeedback for heart rate variability measures a detailed and complex spectral frequency of the heart rate over a range of values; this kind of physiological information is understood only by cardiologists. Muscle tension is measured in microvolts (millionths of a volt). The EEG is also measured in microvolts, and one possible display is to see one's own brain waves in microvolts pass in front of you while learning how to control them.

A substantial amount of training is necessary in order to learn how to use this kind of equipment, and there are several different systems one can choose (e.g., Thought Technology, Nexus, J & J Engineering). Each has detailed and complex software. Some biofeedback systems do all the modalities mentioned above (Thought Technology and Nexus) while others specialize in neurofeedback (e.g., BrainMaster, and pirHEG). Still other forms of neurotherapy deal with aspects of treatment that do not deal with feedback *per se*, but train the brain waves in a direct stimulation method (e.g., MindAlive). In this chapter, the term neurotherapy is used to indicate all forms of training the brain with specialized equipment such as noted earlier.

Neurotherapy is any method of training the brain to enhance the functioning of the patient. This can include neurofeedback (also known as EEG biofeedback), as well as hemoencephalography (HEG), and audio–visual entrainment (AVE), or stimulation (AVE or audio–visual stimulation, AVS). In all these cases, equipment is used in the treatment.

Neurofeedback consists of training the patient to control their brain waves. Ordinarily, this means training the patient to become aware of and learn to train his or her brain waves or electroencephalograph, also known as EEG. Thus, neurofeedback is also called *EEG Biofeedback*.

25 Brain Brightening: Neurotherapy for Enhancing Cognition in the Elderly

Brain physiology. Everyone has electricity all over their body, and in the brain this electrical activity is measured in terms of its brain waves; the unit of measure is microvolts. Brain waves occur in different frequencies, and are understood in cycles per second, or in hertz (abbreviated Hz). All frequencies occur in all parts of the brain, but in different conditions of the brain, the distribution of the frequencies can take on specific proportions. The slowest brain wave frequency is Delta, 0.5–4 Hz, and next is Theta, 4–8 Hz. Alpha is often considered 8–12 Hz, beta is from 12–30 Hz, and gamma is from about 30–45 Hz. Be aware that different researchers define these bands in different ways. Here, is a table that may help make this clear.

Brain wave	Frequency band (Hz)	Characteristic
Delta	0.5–4	Slow waves, often associated with sleep
Theta	4–8	Dreamlike or slow processing
Alpha	8–12	Relaxation, brain idling
Beta	12–30	Active thinking
Gamma	30–45	Very active processing, can be related to intelligence

The frequencies of the brain waves are measured at certain locations or sites. There is a system of location called the 10–20 system which specifies the sites where brain waves are measured. For example, Cz is at the top of the head; Fpz is in the middle of the forehead, about an inch up from the midpoint between your eyebrows. Frontal sites include Fz, F3, and F4, and posterior sites include P3, P4, and PZ. Thus, one protocol could be to train Fz 12–18 Hz up and 4–7 Hz down (or "inhibit") at the same time. This could be used for many ADD children, because Theta is often too high and beta is too low at Fz (midway between Fpz and Cz). Successful training of these frequencies to be more normal can reduce the typical ADD symptoms (Levesque, Beauregard, & Mensour, 2006). In order to determine precise protocols for doing neurofeedback, it is common to assess the patient's brain waves with a quantitative EEG (QEEG).

Quantitative EEG. The technology of the electroencephalogram (EEG) has progressed far beyond the original invention of the EEG by Berger (1929), so that the electrophysiological data is now analyzed in very sophisticated ways; only the simplest presentation can be made here.

To give an idea as to how complex this is, consider that the QEEG method measures all frequencies (Delta, Theta, alpha, beta 1, beta 2, beta 3, gamma) at each of the 19 sites, plus all possible pairs of sites in terms of the connectivity variables of Coherence, Asymmetry, and Phase, plus the whole right side of the brain and the whole left side. The result is some 2,500 variables. This complex brain wave data is analyzed by a computer program and compared to people the same age, and the result is called a *quantitative EEG*, or QEEG. These are compared to the normative database which contains the data for all ages; therefore, the patient in question is compared to those members of the database which are the same age. Of importance are the deviations the patient has compared to the norms with respect to all these variables. What is so fascinating about the complexity of this data is that the QEEG patterns are lawful and describe certain pathologies in a reliable way. Thus, a child with attention deficit disorder (ADD) has a certain number of patterns that are typical, such as a high Theta/beta ratio in the frontal area of the brain. However, there are several specific electrophysiological patterns in children with ADD (Chabot, de Michele, Prichep, & John, 2001). Dementia, affective disorder, traumatic brain injury, and obsessive-compulsive disorder all have distinctive patterns to their QEEG. Collecting data for a QEEG database is complex and needs to be done in a very careful way since this database will be used in comparing patient brains to see if they correspond to certain kinds of brain dysfunction. A detailed history of this process can be found in recent work by Thatcher & Lubar, (2009); Thatcher, (1999, 2000).

Some methods involve collecting the QEEG data under different conditions – eyes closed, eyes open, and doing several cognitive tasks. In this way, we can understand how the brain is functioning under different cognitive tasks and then train the brain while doing those tasks in order to correct that cognitive function. One important researcher in this area, Kirtley Thornton, has shown that QEEG data collected under different eyes open conditions of cognitive functioning (e.g., memory, reasoning, visual and verbal attention) are different than in the eyes closed condition (Thornton & Carmody, 2005). This may lead to different kinds of neurotherapy interventions than those described here. For example, one might be able to target the enhancement of memory functioning specifically in some elderly people with this methodology.

Neurofeedback protocols will often have the patient learn how to inhibit the slow waves (such as Delta and Theta) and increase the more active waves, such as high alpha and beta. If fact, this is a pattern found in the elderly – excessive slow waves (Delta and Theta) in the frontal region, and not enough beta in most areas of the brain (Budzynski, Budzynski, & Tang, 2007).

Brain changes in older adults. Cognitive decline in the older adults may likely be associated with a drop in cerebral blood flow as one ages (Gur, Gur, Obrist, Skolnick, & Reivich, 1987; Hagstadius & Risberg, 1989; Kaufer & Lewis, 1999). Alongside this, there is likely an increase in slow waves throughout the brain, but with such disorders as mild cognitive impairment (MCI), there will be an excess of slower brain waves (i.e., increases in Delta and Theta) in the frontal region (Prichep et al., 1994). With nonpathological cases, however, there is a lot of variability (Budzynski et al., 2007). For those with the beginnings of dementia, the presence of frontal slow waves is more likely. Therefore, it would appear logical that if one could reduce the amount of slow waves and enhance the more active or "thinking" waves (beta and high alpha), there might be an enhancement of cognition. Likewise, it is known that cerebral blood flow drops in the frontal region of the brain in the elderly, and more so in those with cognitive problems and dementia. If there is a method of enhancing frontal lobe blood flow, it could potentially improve cognition.

The overall task in neurotherapy is to modify abnormalities in the brain and see if such methods improve functioning. One issue that can be raised is: Why should changing the brain waves make any real difference in functioning? Or why should changing the blood flow change anything, assuming this phenomena can be done in the first place? I would assert that changing the brain waves and improving cerebral blood flow can change the functioning of the entire brain because everything is very connected in the brain. References below give support to this.

Possible synaptic growth. In 1988, Diamond (1988) found that there were differences between rats placed in enriched environments and those that were not. The number of structurally modified dendrites and increased branching of the enriched brains suggests that providing stimulating environments can enhance brain physiology. It appears that stem cells can generate new nerve cells in the hippocampus (Kemperman & Gage, 1999). Thus, it appears to be possible that providing stimulating procedures can enhance development in the brain. Whether this can happen with elderly patients is an empirical question.

EEG biofeedback (aka neurofeedback) is when the patients are trained to control their own brain waves, or what is called the EEG (electroencephalograph). The patient often obtains a quantitative EEG in order to identify where the brain waves need to be trained, or changed. The electrode is then placed in one or more areas, and the patient is displayed a feedback so that the dysfunctional frequencies are trained down, and the "good" waves are trained up. The display can be the brain waves themselves (good for some patients), or a display generated by the computer. The patient is asked to keep the animation going (for example), and by operant conditioning the patient trains his/her brain waves to be more normal.

Neurofeedback is considerably more complex than most other biofeedback modalities, and is the newest modality in the field of biofeedback. Nonetheless, there is a fair amount of research regarding its effectiveness (see Monastra, 2005; Thompson & Thompson, 1998, 2003; Lubar et al., 2003; Yucha & Montgomery, 2008). Neurofeedback has been shown to be effective for ADD, chronic pain, traumatic brain injury, and other brain disorders (Yucha & Montgomery, 2008). Frank Duffy, a well-known neurologist, stated in a special issue of the journal *Clinical Electroencephalography* (2000) devoted to neurofeedback that "if any medication had demonstrated such a wide spectrum of efficacy, it would be universally accepted and widely used" (p. v).

What is also of importance is that there seem to be actual changes in the brain as a result of neurofeedback. In a study by Levesque, Beauregard, & Mensour, (2006), pre- and post-fMRI and neuropsychological tests were done with a neurofeedback treatment group and controls of ADHD children in a randomized, double blind, placebo controlled study. Both the children and the therapists were blinded to whether they received the treatment or not. The treated children improved in functioning and in neuropsychological test scores, and their brain physiology improved in the predicted areas according to the post-fMRI. So, it appears that neurofeedback can change the brain. Several substantial volumes supporting the effectiveness of neurofeedback with a variety of populations can be consulted for research in this area (Budzynski, Budzynski, Evans, & Abarbanel, 2009; Evans, 2007; Evans & Abarbanel, 1999; Thompson & Thompson, 2003; Egnar & Sterman, 2006; Sterman & Egnar, 2006; Thatcher, 1999), as well as a frequently updated bibliography by Hammond (2010).

Neurotherapy is a broader term, which includes neurofeedback as well as some other modalities which have to do with training the brain. As mentioned above, neurofeedback involves giving feedback to the patient, while neurotherapy can be any method of training the brain. We will briefly deal with AVS, AVE, and hemoencephalography.

Neurotherapy can be considered any type of therapy that aims to help the patient by way of brain training. Thus, AVE involves training the brain to enhance certain frequencies by way of flashing lights embedded in a pair of glasses. The visual entrainment protocols can involve a complex series of frequencies designed to have therapeutic effects.

AVS and AVE consists of flickering LED lights embedded in glasses presented to the patient, along with sound vibrations through ear phones. The frequencies can vary according to EEG frequencies (e.g., Delta, alpha, beta). Sometimes the AVS device is programmed to vary the frequencies according to what is believed to be optimal for a given purpose. For example, if low beta (15–18 Hz) is thought to be beneficial for a patient, this frequency might be programmed so that the patient sees lights flicker at 15–18 Hz and hears the 15–18 Hz rhythm in the ear phones. Research has shown that entraining these frequencies can enhance the same frequencies in the brain and its effects can last for a long period of time (Collura & Siever, 2009). Sometimes a variety of frequencies are programmed, so that the flickering lights can go through a range of Delta flickering lights, then ramp up to alpha and beta, then go back down to Delta. In a clinical study, Budzynski & colleagues, (2007) did some "brain brightening" AVE sessions with ten older adults, and there were improvements on many of the measures from the MicroCog computerized cognitive battery.

HEG biofeedback trains the patient to control the cerebral blood flow in the frontal lobes. An infrared camera sensor is placed on the forehead which reads the cerebral blood flow (actually a close correlate of the blood flow), and the patient learns to control the blood flow by the display being watched. In the case of the pir HEG, the display is a movie – any DVD the patient wishes to see. If the frontal lobe blood flow and temperature remains high, the patient can continue to watch the movie. When the temperature drops (believed to be in the anterior cingulate gyrus), the movie stops, and by focusing on a bar graph display, the cortical activity increases such that the movie starts again.

The HEG method of neurofeedback is a new kind of treatment, and there is little research as to its effectiveness, and none to my knowledge with older adults. This biofeedback system was originally designed for migraine headache treatment, and has shown promising results (Toomin & Carmen, 2009). Carmen (2004) took 100 migraine patients who had been through many previous treatments, including many trying several medications, with little success. Positive results were usually seen in six HEG sessions, and over 90% of the patients reported significantly positive results, according to their own report. I am including this method of neurofeedback because it is specifically designed to train the cerebral blood flow of the frontal lobes to increase, and this has been known to be an important area of brain functioning in the elderly. You will recall that a typical problem in the elderly is the reduced frontal lobe blood flow. This methodology may become an important part of future treatment for elderly cognitive enhancement.

Research on Brain Brightening

There is a limited literature on neurotherapy for older individuals with regards to cognitive enhancement. Budzynski in 1996 presented a case study in which he employed neurofeedback and AVS which helped reduce cognitive and memory symptoms. Budzynski & Budzynski, (2000) presented another case study of a 76-year-old man who had a history of two cardiac bypass surgeries, an angioplasty, pacemaker implantation, hearing problems, and self-reported cognitive problems. The assessment given to him was the MicroCog Battery (Powell et al., 1993) before and after treatment. The patient received 30 sessions of neurofeedback, primarily suppressing frontal slow waves (2–12 Hz) combined with 14 Hz AVS at the start of each session. He also did the 14 Hz AVS at home each day for 20 min. At the 20 session point, the patient had his regular hearing exam, and the physician was surprised to find that his hearing improved, whereas previously the patient's hearing had always worsened with each exam. The post-training assessment revealed that there was a reduction in slow wave activity in the frontal area (i.e., 1–7 Hz), an increase in 7–9 Hz, and an increase in all the scaled scores from the MicroCog except the Spatial Processing and Reaction Time scales.

Rozelle & Budzynski, (1995) reported on using neurofeedback with a 55-year-old man approximately 1 year after his left frontal stroke. The medical evaluation revealed his stroke was in the left temporal-parietal area, and his symptoms included hesitant speech, word finding, paraphasia, lack of balance and coordination, poor short-term memory, poor concentration, anxiety, depression, and tinnitus. A QEEG revealed he had increased left hemisphere Theta. The patient was trained to increase 15–21 Hz over the sensorimotor strip and 4–7 Hz down. All the above noted symptoms showed improvement.

In one study reported by Budzynski et al. (2007), part of the Ponce de Leon Project, the authors administered neurofeedback and AVS to two elderly volunteers. One of these volunteers, an 80 year woman, was tracked carefully. After 20 neurofeedback sessions which also utilized AVS, her Wechsler Memory Scale-Revised scores showed significant improvement after treatment and at follow-up on the General, Visual, and Delayed Recall scales.

In another study reported in Budzynski, et al (2007), 31 volunteers ages 53–87 received AVS 3 days per week over 3 months. The AVS EEG frequencies were randomly presented between 9 and 22 Hz, and sessions were 20 min each. Pre- and post-measures consisted of MicroCog and the Buschke Remembering test (Buschke, 1973). Improvement was seen on the Buschke measure and seven of the nine MicroCog measures for the AVS group. Other interesting results were reported, however. Some participants experience a period of confusion for 15–30 min following the AVS session.

Frederick & Berman (2009) did a study with 26 subjects with frontal-temporal lobe dementia, 15 of which were assigned to neurofeedback treatment, and 11 to the control condition. Those in the neurofeedback group received 30 or more sessions, with video, audio, and tactile reinforcers. Pre- and post-measures of neuropsychological tests as well as QEEG were done. Improvements in the treatment groups were found in visual and verbal memory, and ratings by self and a significant other in executive functioning. One conclusion by the authors was that neurofeedback would more likely be effective in cases of very early dementia.

The above noted research and case studies represent beginning efforts in the possible value of using neurotherapy to treat cognitive decline in older adults. There are significant limitations in the above papers, but there is enough evidence to consider developing more extensive research proposals to see if neurotherapy can contribute to the prevention of dementia if caught early enough in the disease process. It is worth noting that in most of the Budzynski articles, neurofeedback sessions are begun with audio–visual stimulation or entrainment. A likely reason is that AVS/AVE seems to increase frontal cerebral blood flow. That is why I included the HEG method of neurofeedback, because HEG specifically trains the patient to increase frontal blood flow. But there are some limitations to what we can expect from neurotherapy with dementia. Frederick & Berman, (2009) concluded in their work that if the pathological process in dementia has progressed too far, there is little likelihood that neurotherapy will be helpful; however, neurofeedback may prove useful in the very earliest stages of cognitive decline.

A final aspect of neurotherapy is worth mentioning. In dealing with patients learning to control their physiological and/or brain functioning, being psychologically minded is not necessary. Indeed, one is able to control one's own physiology without having any psychological insights. For some patients, this could be very attractive and could be especially important in treating those with limited language abilities with respect to the therapist, or those who are not comfortable with the usual psychological treatment situation. In addition, training one's own brain physiology by watching movies is another attractive feature of doing neurotherapy.

Implications of Integrating Neurotherapy into Health Care

It is hoped that as research accumulates supporting neurotherapy as a modality in health care, this will result in lowering overall medical costs for the elderly. Some dementias may be stopped, other cases may have a more benign course, and still others may progress as they do now. With future studies examining these treatment paths, it is likely that neurotherapy and biofeedback will prove to be cost-effective and humane. This will necessitate that professionals master this technology and acquire the specific knowledge of the medical conditions under question. Let us hope that future psychologists and other mental health professionals may be able to attain these skills.

Concluding Remarks

Given the above applications of neurofeedback in the treatment of cognitive decline, it is worthwhile that well-designed studies be conducted to see if these modalities can improve the health of older adults. Substantial methodological weaknesses are admitted in the above studies and case reports, such as lack of control groups, and minimal pre- and postcognitive assessment. But, there is evidence that such work can be beneficial. The result would be improved health and lower medical care costs.

Appendix: Resources

A. Major manufacturers of biofeedback equipment. Those who manufacture biofeedback equipment are listed here. In most cases, this kind of equipment can only be sold to licensed health professionals. These companies also provide training in the use of the equipment.

1. Thought Technology: www.thoughttechnology.com, (800) 361–3651. The largest biofeedback equipment maker in the world; systems are multimodality.
2. J & J Engineering: www.jjengineering.com, (888) 550–8300; systems are multimodality.
3. Nexus: www.stens-biofeedback.com, (800) 257–8367; systems are multimodality.
4. Brain Master: www.BrainMaster.com, specializes in neurofeedback, and supports several of the most popular systems. (440) 232–6000.
5. MindAlive makes audio–visual stimulation and entrainment systems. www.MindAlive.com, 1-800-661-MIND or (6463).
6. PirHEG (Hemoencephalography): Dr. Jeffrey Carmen, www.stopmymigaine.com, 315-682-5272.

B. Biofeedback and Neurofeedback Organizations

1. The Biofeedback Certification Institute of America (303-420-2902, BCIA@resourcenter.com) organization certifies practitioners on biofeedback (Board Certified in Biofeedback, or BCB) and neurofeedback (BCN). They also publish some training materials and books.
2. The Association for Applied Psychophysiology and Biofeedback (AAPB) is the principle professional organization for biofeedback. 10200 W 44th Ave, #304, Wheat Ridge, CO 80033, USA. www.aapb.org, 303-422-8436, aapb@resourcenter.com.
3. International Society for Neurofeedback and Research, www.isnr.org. This is the main professional organization for neurofeedback. They have an annual conference in the Fall; the website has a list of professionals offering neurofeedback, as well as articles.

C. Important Texts in Biofeedback and Neurofeedback.

Introduction to quantitative EEG and neurofeedback. This is a dense and technical book on neurofeedback and related modalities, in theory, the underlying electrophysiology, and practical applications. This volume has very little about dealing with the elderly Budzynski, Budzynski, Evans, & Abarbanel, (2009).

Biofeedback: A practitioner's guide. This is the main text in the field of biofeedback, and contains detailed explanations of the equipment, physiology of the disorders most commonly treated, extensive review of the literature, as well as ethical and office practices for professionals. It is currently under revision with the fourth edition coming out probably in 2011 Schwartz & Andrasik, (2003).

The neurofeedback book. This book is the most thorough text on neurofeedback book to date, written by experienced neurofeedback practitioners, a psychologist, and psychiatrist, with a detailed background in neuroanatomy and neurophysiology presented Thompson & Thompson, (2003).

Evidence-based practice in biofeedback and neurofeedback Yucha & Montgomery, (2008). In this short book, disorders in biofeedback and other behavioral interventions are reviewed and rated according to the Chambless and Hollon, (1998) level of efficacy. Ratings by these authors do not necessarily agree with others rating the utility of biofeedback (e.g., Schwartz & Andrasik, 2003, p. 107).

References

Berger, H. (1929). Uber das Elektroenkephalogramm des Menschen. *Archiv für Psychiatrie und Nervenkrankheiten, 87,* 527–570.
Budzynski, T. (1996). Brain brightening: Can neurofeedback improve cognitive process? *Biofeedback, 24*(2), 14–17.
Budzynski, T., & Budzynski, H. (2000). Reversing age-related cognitive decline: Use of neurofeedback and audio-visual stimulation. *Biofeedback, 28*(3), 19–21.
Budzynski, T., Budzynski, H., Evans, J., & Abarbanel, A. (Eds.). (2009). *Introduction to quantitative EEG and neurofeedback: Advance theory and applications.* New York, NY: Academic.
Budzynski, T., Budzynski, H., & Tang, H. (2007). Brain brightening. In J. R. Evans (Ed.), *Handbook of neurofeedback.* New York, NY: Haworth.
Buschke, H. (1973). Selective reminding for analysis of memory and learning. *Journal of Verbal Learning and Verbal Behavior, 12,* 543–550.
Carmen, J. (2004). Passive infrared hemoencephalography: Four years and 100 migraines. *Journal of Neurotherapy, 8*(3), 23–51.
Chabot, R., de Michele, F., Prichep, L., & John, E. (2001). The clinical role of computerized EEG in the evaluation and treatment of learning and attention disorders. *Journal of Neuropsychiatry and Clinical Neuroscience, 13*(2), 171–186.
Chambless, D., & Hollon, S. (1998). Defining empirically supported therapies. *Journal of Consulting and Clinical Psychology, 66,* 7–18.
Collura, T., & Siever, D. (2009). Audio-visual entrainment in relation to mental health and EGG. In T. Budzynski, H. Budzynski, J. Evans, & A. Abarbanel (Eds.), *Introduction to quantitative EEG and neurofeedback.* New York, NY: Academic.
Diamond, M. (1988). *Enriching heredity: The impact of the environment on the anatomy of the brain.* New York, NY: Free.
Duffy, F. (2000). The state of EEG biofeedback therapy (EEG operant conditioning) in 2000: An Editor's opinion. *Clinical Electroencephalography, 31*(1), v–vii.
Egner, T., & Sterman, M. B. (2006). Neurofeedback treatment of epilepsy: from basic rationale to practical application. *Expert review of neurotheapeutics, 6*(2), 247–257.
Evans, J. (Ed.). (2007). *Handbook of neurofeedback.* New York, NY: Haworth.

Evans, J., & Abarbanel, A. (Eds.). (1999). *Quantitative EEG and neurofeedback*. New York, NY: Academic.

Frederick, J., & Berman, M. (2009). Efficacy of neurofeedback for executive and function in dementia. *Presentation at the international conference on Alzheimer's disease*, Vienna, Austria

Gur, R., Gur, R., Obrist, W., Skolnick, B., & Reivich, M. (1987). Age and regional cerebral blood flow at rest and during cognitive activity. *Archives of General Psychiatry, 44*, 617–621.

Hagstadius, S., & Risberg, J. (1989). Regional cerebral blood flow characteristics and variations with age in resting normal subjects. *Brain and Cognition, 10*, 28–43.

Hammond, C. (2010). Comprehensive bibliography of neurofeedback (arranged by topic). Retrieved Nov 2010 from http://www.isnr.org/ComprehensiveBibliography.cfm.

Kaufer, D., & Lewis, D. (1999). Frontal lobe anatomy and cortical connectivity. In B. Miller & J. Cummings (Eds.), *The human frontal lobes* (pp. 27–44). New York, NY: Guilford.

Kemperman, G., & Gage, F. (1999). New nerve cells for the adult brain. *Scientific American, 1999*, 48–53.

Levesque, J., Beauregard, M., & Mensour, B. (2006). Effect of neurofeedback training on the neural substrates of selective attention in children with attention-deficit/hyperactivity disorder: A functional magnetic resonance imaging study. *Neuroscience Letters, 394*, 216–221.

Linden, M., Habib, T., & Radojevic, V. (1996). A controlled study of the effects of EEG biofeedback on cognition and behavior of children with attention deficit disorder and learning disabilities. *Biofeedback and Self Regulation, 21*(1), 35–49.

Lubar, J. (2003). Neurofeedback for attention deficit disorders. In M. Schwartz & F. Andrasik (Eds.), *Biofeedback: A practitioner's guide* (3rd ed., pp. 409–437). New York, NY: Guilford.

Mendez, M. F., & Cummings, J. L. (2003). *Dementia: A clinical approach*. Philadelphia, PA: Butterworth-Heinemann.

Monastra, V. (2003). Clinical applications of EEG biofeedback. In M. Schwartz & F. Andrasik (Eds.), *Biofeedback: A practitioner's guide* (3rd ed., pp. 438–463). NY: Guilford.

Monastra, V. (2005). Electroencephalographic biofeedback (neurotherapy) as a treatment for attention deficit hyperactivity disorder: Rationale and empirical foundations. *Child and Adolescent Psychiatric Clinics of North America, 14*(1), 55–82.

Powell, D., Kaplan, E., Whitla, D., Weintraub, S., Caitlin, R., & Funkenstein, H. (1993). *MicroCog: Assessment of cognitive functioning*. San Antonio, TX: Psychological Corporation.

Prichep, L., John, E., Ferris, S., Reisberg, B., Almas, M., Alper, K., et al. (1994). Quantitative EEG correlates of cognitive deterioration in the elderly. *Neurobiology of Aging, 15*, 85–90.

Rozelle, G., & Budzynski, T. (1995). Neurotherapy for stroke rehabilitation: a case study. *Biofeedback, 20*(3), 211–228.

Schoenberger, N., Shiflett, S., Esty, M., Ochs, L., & Matheis, R. J. (2001). Flexyx neurotherapy system in the treatment of traumatic brain injury: An initial evaluation. *The Journal of Head Trauma Rehabilitation, 16*, 260–274.

Schwartz, M., & Andrasik, F. (Eds.). (2003). *Biofeedback: A practitioner's guide* (3rd ed.). New York, NY: Guilford.

Siniatchkin, M., Hierundar, A., Kropp, P., Khunert, R., Gerber, W., & Staphani, U. (2000). Self-regulation of slow cortical potentials in children with migraine: An exploratory study. *Applied Psychophysiology and Biofeedback, 25*, 13–32.

Sterman, M., & Egner, T. (2006). Foundation and practice of neurofeedback therapy for epilepsy. from basic rationale to practical application. *Applied Psychophysiology and Biofeedback, 31*(1), 21–35.

Thatcher, R. (1999). EEG database guided neurotherapy. In J. R. Evans & A. Arbarbanel (Eds.), *Introduction to quantitative EEG and neurofeedback*. San Diego, CA: Academic.

Thatcher, R. (2000). EEG operant conditioning (biofeedback) and traumatic brain injury. *Clinical Electroencephalography, 31*, 38–44.

Thatcher, R., & Lubar, J. (2009). History of the scientific standards of QEEG normative databases. In T. Budzynski, H. Budzynski, J. Evans, & A. Abarbanel (Eds.), *Introduction to quantitative EEG and neurofeedback*. New York, NY: Academic.

Thompson, L., & Thompson, M. (1998). Neurofeedback combined with training in metacognitive strategies: Effectiveness in student with ADD. *Applied Psychophysiology and Biofeedback, 23*(4), 243–263.

Thompson, M., & Thompson, L. (2003). *The neurofeedback book*. Wheat Ridge, CO: AAPB.

Thornton, K., & Carmody, D. (2005). Electroencephalogram biofeedback for reading disability and traumatic brain injury. In L. Hirshberg, S. Chiu, & J. Frazier (Eds.), *Child and Adolescent Psychiatric Clinics of North America: Emerging interventions* (Vol. 14, Number 1). Philadelphia, PA: Saunders.

Toomin, H., & Carmen, J. (2009). Hemoencephalography: Photon-based blood flow neurofeedback. In T. Budzynski, H. Budzynski, J. Evans, & A. Abarbanel (Eds.), *Introduction to quantitative EEG and neurofeedback*. New York, NY: Academic.

Yucha, C., & Montgomery, D. (2008). *Evidence-based practice in biofeedback and neurofeedback*. Wheat Ridge, CO: AAPB.

Part V
Gaining Through Giving Back:
Programs with A Positive Societal Impact

Chapter 26
Neurons in Neighborhoods: How Purposeful Participation in a Community-based Intergenerational Program Enhanced Quality of Life for Persons Living with Dementia

Daniel R. George

Abstract This chapter discusses a community-based, non-pharmacological intervention for persons with dementia who engaged as weekly volunteers with students at The Intergenerational School (TIS) in Cleveland, Ohio, over a 5-month period. Concurrent quantitative and qualitative methods were used to investigate the meaning of quality of life (QOL) for persons with mild-to-moderate dementia, and to evaluate through a randomized control trial design whether an intergenerational volunteering program would enhance QOL for participants. Quality of life, a conceptual category that approximates the degree of well-being felt by an individual or group, was defined expansively, encompassing five variables that have been strongly associated with QOL in previous studies: cognitive functioning, stress, depression, sense of purpose, and sense of usefulness. Thus, while cognition was viewed as indispensable to QOL, it was part of a larger biopsychosocial constellation of variables believed to play a role in the wellness of aging persons.

Introduction

In the short story "Fortitude" by Kurt Vonnegut, a doctor named Frankenstein keeps an elderly woman named Sylvia Lovejoy alive with an elaborate network of machinery that has replaced all of her vital organs with tubes and prosthetic devices. Frankenstein and an assistant operate the master console, sending bursts of chemicals

D.R. George (✉)
Department of Humanities, College of Medicine, Penn State Milton S. Hershey Medical Center, 500 University Drive, Hershey, PA 17033, USA
e-mail: drg21@psu.edu

into a tripod that holds Sylvia's synthetic brain to keep her stimulated and content. Perfectly healthy, but dreadfully lacking human contact, Sylvia grows lonely and discreetly begins asking others to hasten her demise.

Vonnegut's story asks us to consider our core definitions of human wellness. In our hypercognitive Western culture, we attach great value to the brain, and spend large amounts of time – and dollars – trying to keep it properly stimulated. Video games, brain-train products, drugs, supplements, crossword puzzles, Sudoku, and myriad other approaches have all been heralded for their ostensible contribution to the enhancement of cognitive functioning of older adults. While using these approaches almost certainly contributes to mental acuity to some degree, these types of reductionist solutions focus exclusively on one aspect of wellness – cognition – and are often undertaken through isolated patterns of consumption. But as Vonnegut's story intimates, wellness in the late-life course is not just about stimulating bundles of neurons. Our brains are one component of our embodied self, which exists as part of a family, a neighborhood, a community, and a natural environment. Real commitments to wellness must look beyond the brain to the whole person, and consider the enormous power of community-based solutions to maintaining a vital and purposeful existence – even for those affected by memory loss.

Theoretical Background

Biopsychosocial Approach to Brain Aging

In recent decades, hope for countering the decrements of brain aging has been consolidated largely in the reductionist promise of pharmacological, biotechnological, or consumption-based solutions to halt or slow the progression of neurodegenerative conditions. However, the inability to yet understand the etiology of Alzheimer's disease (AD) – thought to be the leading cause of dementia worldwide – or to develop pharmacological treatments that consistently, safely, and cost-effectively curtail neurodegeneration or promote cognitive functioning, combined with the imminent demographic realities of an aging world, has given greater impetus to the development and assessment of community-based psychosocial interventions that promote social engagement in the late-life course, such as intergenerational volunteering.

Proponents of biopsychosocial research regard illness as the common final pathway resulting from interacting systems at the cellular, tissue, organismic, interpersonal, subjective, and environmental levels. Multiple factors at each level has a relative weight in facilitating, sustaining, or modifying the course of diseases, varying from illness to illness, from one individual to another, and even between two different episodes of the same illness in the same individual (Engel, 1977; Porcelli & Sonino, 2007). The cognitive and functional deficits of aging do not occur just in isolated brains, as reductionist research would have it, but rather in living human beings who are members of families, neighborhoods, communities, and a local and global ecology.

There is growing evidence in the dementia field that the progression of neurodegenerative conditions such as AD is influenced by personal histories, social interactions, and social contexts across the lifespan (Ferraro & Shippee, 2009; Kitwood, 1997; Shonkoff, Boyce, et al., 2009; Stein, Schettler, Rohrer, Valenti, 2008). Indeed, multiple studies indicate that at least some of the negative consequences associated with dementia may be mitigated or delayed by a biopsychosocial approach to treatment that respects and supports the individual personhood of those with dementia, and which facilitates growth and development in the late-life course (Cohen-Mansfield et al., 2006; Kitwood, 1997; Thomas, 2004). It is increasingly accepted that even something as simple as the way medical conditions are named can affect the way individuals, family members, and society perceive and experience those conditions, and can have harmful or beneficial effects on individual outcomes (Karkazis & Feder, 2008; Kleinman, 1988; Sontag, 1978; Whitehouse & George, 2008).

Quality of Life and Brain Aging

As mentioned, this study defined QOL as a dynamic, multi-faceted concept that included such biopsychosocial factors as cognitive functioning, stress, depression, sense of purpose, and sense of usefulness. While QOL resists universal definition and remains a largely idiosyncratic concept that varies from person to person, research has established a constellation of features that are commonly implicated in the QOL of the elderly. For instance, previous studies have found that QOL tends to decline with age and has been found to be generally – though not directly – associated with measurable, objective properties such as pain, physical decline and comorbidities, cognitive loss, psychosocial stress, recent hospitalization, and loss of activities of daily living that can be assessed using standardized self-report questionnaires or rating scales (Cigolle et al., 2007; Rabins & Black, 2007; Seymour et al., 2008).

However, qualitatively oriented studies undertaken in multiple cultural contexts have shown that psychosocial and cultural factors such as social relationships, social roles, pastimes and activities, subjective health, psychological outlook and well-being, opportunity to help others, personal satisfaction, home and neighborhood, finances and independence, sense of purpose, sense of usefulness, and life-meaning are important domains of QOL for the elderly (Bowling, 1995; Levasseur et al., 2004; Okamoto & Tanaka, 2004; Puts et al., 2007).

Taken together, these types of studies suggest that an excessive focus on cognitive functioning does not capture the biopsychosocial complexity of individual wellness and QOL, and that we should not be content with interventions that merely "stimulate neurons" without meaningful context. Indeed, it is clear that community-based approaches that act through the many biopsychosocial pathways that affect QOL must be an essential component to maintaining wellness for aging persons.

Setting the Scene

An Aging World

Population aging portends a drastic rethinking of resources and values, and human communities will, undeniably, be challenged to adapt to new demographic realities and accommodate unprecedented numbers of elders in coming decades. As advancing age is the major risk factor for dementia, with a doubling of risk every 5 years after the age of 65 (Jorm et al., 1987; Kawas, 2003), an inevitable outcome of the "graying" of populations is that millions more people around the world will be affected by various age-associated neuropathologies that contribute to the development of dementia and other morbidities. Dementia incidence is already beginning to rise precipitously, not just in industrialized nations, but also in low and middle income countries, where over half of the world's elderly live (Ferri et al., 2005). Global estimates suggest that 35.6 million people have dementia today, and the number is estimated to double every 20 years, to 65.7 million in 2030, and 115.4 million in 2050 (ADI, 2010).

Intergenerational Solutions

In the absence of a powerful pharmacological fix for AD, there has emerged a renewed interest both in promoting QOL for those presently living with dementia, and in developing non-pharmacological interventions that can act through various biopsychosocial pathways to promote QOL and perhaps postpone the onset and progression of dementia. There has also been an encouraging shift toward future solutions that are local and community-based. In the early twenty-first century, interest has grown in developing and evaluating local programs that bring different generations together to purposefully collaborate in supporting and nurturing one another – a social process that can break down structural barriers and reduce the stigma associated with dementia. The resolution adopted by the UN Second World Assembly on Aging in Madrid, Spain, has specifically recognized "the need to strengthen solidarity among generations and intergenerational partnerships […] and to encourage mutually responsive relationships between generations" (United Nations, 2002: Article 16). Consequently, intergenerational programs can now be found in a wide range of settings such as churches, schools, child/adult day care programs, neighborhoods, nature centers, universities, community centers, community organizations, and other societal venues (Ayala et al., 2006).

Biopsychosocial Benefits of Intergenerational Relationships

While clear benefits have long been observed in the interaction between older and younger family members, the modern challenge in a world where nuclear families are increasingly rare has been to replicate intergenerational programs between nonbiologically related older and younger persons to achieve the positive outcomes historically observed in filial intergenerational exchange. A small but emerging evidence base in the literature demonstrates that there may be reciprocal benefit for nonbiologically related youth and adults who form intergenerational relationships through local programming, but most existing data have been derived from cross-sectional and retrospective observational studies, and only a few intergenerational volunteering programs have been critically evaluated to measure their direct benefits on the QOL of persons with dementia.

Existing research demonstrates that older adults in intergenerational programs have experienced a range of biopsychosocial benefits, including increased engagement and increased interactions (Camp, Zeisel, & Antenucci, 2010); improvements in health status and well-being (de Souza, 2003); generational closeness, comfort, and empathy (Hayes, 2003); increased activity, strength, and cognitive ability (Fried et al., 2004); mutually supportive interactions and the creation of meaningful relationships (Gigliotti et al., 2005); positive affect, confidence, and enhanced self-esteem supporting personhood (Jarrott & Bruno, 2003; Jarrott & Bruno, 2007); lower levels of negative forms of engagement (Lee et al., 2007); increased social capital (de Souza & Grundy, 2007); and better psychological functioning (Chung, 2009). There is also evidence that children who participate in intergenerational programs may benefit both socially and cognitively from interactions with elders (Hayes, 2003), be more likely to rate their health as good (de Souza & Grundy, 2007), and demonstrate gains in the knowledge of dementia and more positive perceptions of older persons (Chung, 2009; de Souza & Grundy, 2007).

Given this relative dearth of data, researchers have been encouraged to bring innovative methodologies to bear in assessing local intergenerational interventions; however, employing rigorous research designs has been considered challenging, time consuming, complicated, and expensive. There are few studies that make use of randomized designs to measure the effects of intergenerational programs (de Souza, 2003), and no known studies that assess the effects of such programs on QOL.

This study reports results of a 5-month intervention in Cleveland, Ohio, USA that used concurrent quantitative and qualitative methods to investigate the meaning of QOL for persons with mild-to-moderate dementia, and to evaluate whether an intergenerational volunteering program would enhance QOL for participants. Before sharing the results of the study, it will first be necessary to provide an overview of the two community organizations that partnered to provide a shared intergenerational space for the intervention presented in this chapter.

The Study

The Intergenerational School and Judson Park

Research was undertaken in partnership with The Intergenerational School (TIS), an organization that fosters intergenerational interaction between its 175 students and older adults in the Northeast Ohio community, and Judson Park (JP), an assisted living facility. Both organizations are located in Cleveland and have partnered together since 2002. Full results have been reported elsewhere (George & Whitehouse, 2010; George & Singer, 2011)

The Intergenerational School serves approximately 200 largely poor, African-American students from the city and is structured around the ideology that people of all ages can learn alongside each other throughout their lifespan. Students are placed in multi-age classrooms based on individual learning needs where they learn in their own way and at their own pace, moving along six developmental stages: emerging (K-1), beginning (1–2), developing (3), refining (4), applying (5–6), and leadership (7–8), and advancing to the next learning stage at any point during the school year if they meet the necessary benchmarks.

This ideological commitment to multi-age learning extends to older persons in the local community who are invited to serve as "mentors" with the students. The school is the first known educational institution in the world to create a formal mentorship role for persons with dementia, and each of its 11 classrooms makes routine visits to local assisted living homes, including JP. On these trips, the students interact with nursing home residents through art, song, literature, and storytelling, and, in many cases, relationships build throughout the year. By fostering a learning environment that eschews the formal labeling process for both students and older persons with dementia and which facilitates intergenerational relationships, TIS has created a demedicalized, person-centered social space – one in which learning disabilities and age-associated memory impairments alike are de-emphasized.

Judson Park is situated on a wooded hillside border separating the city and the outer ring suburb of Cleveland Heights in the historic Ambelside neighborhood and overlooks the urban skyline of Cleveland. The organization sits less than a mile away from University Circle, a cultural and educational center in Cleveland containing the Cleveland Art Museum, Severance Hall (home of the Cleveland Orchestra), the CWRU campus, the Cleveland Botanical Garden, and University Hospitals. Proximity to these local institutions and to TIS (which is 1 mile away) has enabled JP to form partnerships linking its 400 residents to a variety of rich and diverse cultural and educational opportunities.

Demographically, JP residents are predominantly of European origin and middle-to-upper class, and the facility targets potential residents in more affluent surrounding suburbs. The average age at entry is approximately 84, and nearly 20% of JP residents have had some affiliation with Case Western Reserve University. In the late 1990, JP was the first site in Northeast Ohio registered in The Eden Alternative (Thomas, 1994, 1999), a movement in which eldercare homes commit to making organization-wide attempt to deinstitutionalize and personalize their services, creating lively, liveable habitats for human beings rather than sterile medical institutions, and engaging residents, frontline staff, and family members in the process. The ultimate biopsychosocial aim of this "culture change" is the creation of environments that encourage meaningful, purposeful interactions and relationships between residents, staff, and the community, which are ultimately viewed as protective against the loneliness, helplessness, idleness, and boredom that can afflict the aged.

The Intergenerational School and JP have been collaborative partners since the summer of 2002. This partnership was forged, in part, by Silvia Kruger, a veteran teacher at TIS, who brought her class to JP to swim in the indoor pool at the facility. After several sessions, the children began sharing books they had brought to the pool with JP residents on an outdoor patio. The meaningful relationships that formed over the course of these book-sharing sessions led to Mrs Kruger's class formalizing a relationship with JP as part of their curriculum in the 2002–2003 school year. Each month, they made visits to record biographies with JP residents in the assisted living unit. Together, TIS and JP have combined through their various intergenerational partnerships to create the type of supportive community spaces envisioned by the UN in which older volunteers affected by dementia can feel solidarity with younger generations through meaningful social engagement. No systematic evaluation has yet been undertaken to measure the benefits to older adults that may result from this intergenerational interaction, hence the impetus behind this study.

Study Design

Two classes at TIS were selected as host sites for the intervention: a class with children aged 5–6 and a class with children aged 11–14. Both classrooms contained 16 students. Fifteen participants were recruited from JP based on IRB-approved inclusion criteria (over 50 years old; diagnosis of mild-to-moderate dementia; basic literacy; willingness to read children's book; ambulatory or can be easily transported) and exclusion criteria (severe depression or anxiety; problems working with children, agoraphobia) and randomized into intervention and control groups using a random number generator (see Fig. 26.1).

Baseline data on cognitive functioning (Mini-Mental State Exam, MMSE), stress (Beck Anxiety Inventory, BAI), depression (Beck Depression Inventory, BDI), and sense of purpose and sense of usefulness (single-item questionnaire) was collected in November and December 2007. The intervention commenced on 9 January 2008 and lasted until 7 May 2008 at which time post-intervention data was collected. Concurrently, ethnographic observation took place throughout the duration of the study. All participants in the control and intervention groups took part in formal and informal interviews and participated in respective focus groups. Approximately equal amounts of time were spent visiting the homes of persons in both the intervention and control groups, and equal time was spent conducting structured and unstructured interviews with all participants.

The Community-Based Program

Each Wednesday during the 5-month study, participants were transported to and from TIS on a wheelchair-accessible bus provided by JP. All participants in the intervention group were involved in direct volunteering experiences with children

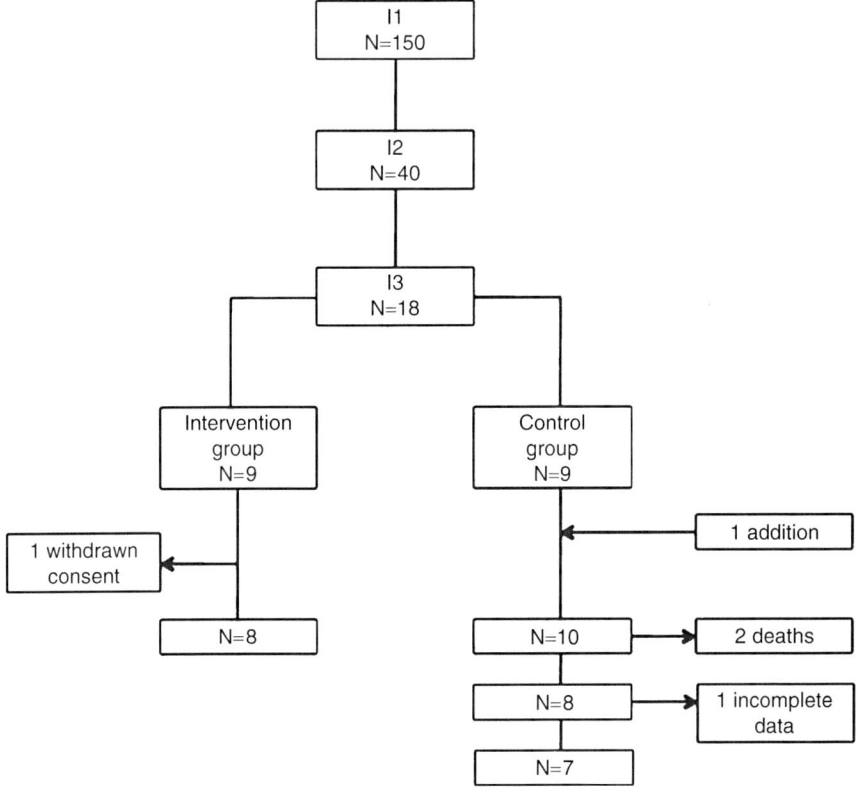

Fig. 26.1 Profile of randomization process at Judson Park

aged 5–14 years. In offsetting weeks, participants alternated between hour-long visits with the younger classroom during which they interacted with children and engaged in singing and small-group reading and writing activities, and an older classroom where they broke into smaller groups with 2–3 students and participated in intergenerational life-history reminiscence sessions. Curriculum for these sessions was codeveloped by the author, the intergenerational coordinator at TIS, the TIS principal, and the two teachers whose classes served as hosts. All activities were explicitly narrative-based, in that they involved an intergenerational exchange of narrative, whether through the sharing of personal stories, books, songs, or collaborative craft-making. Based on the growing literature on intergenerational activities alluded to above, it was believed that narrative-based activities would best enable the formation of relationships between elders and students.

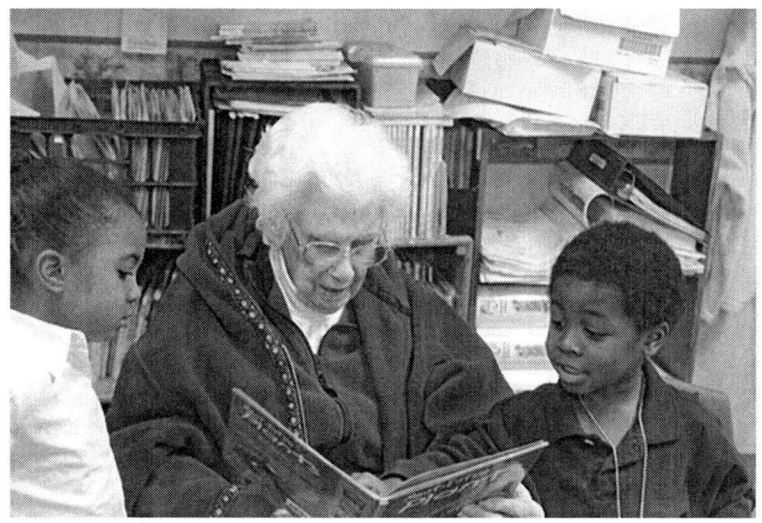

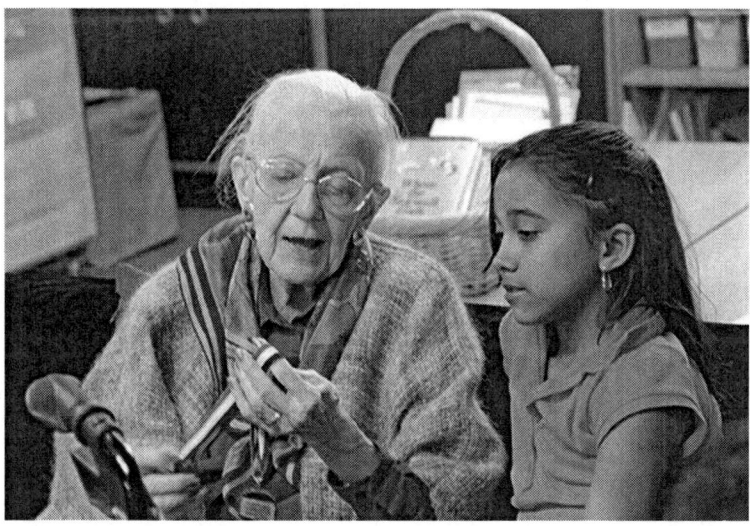

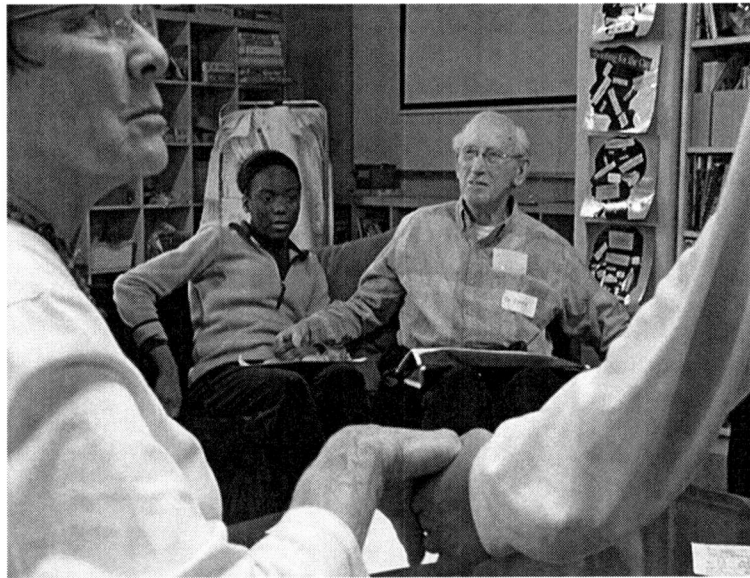

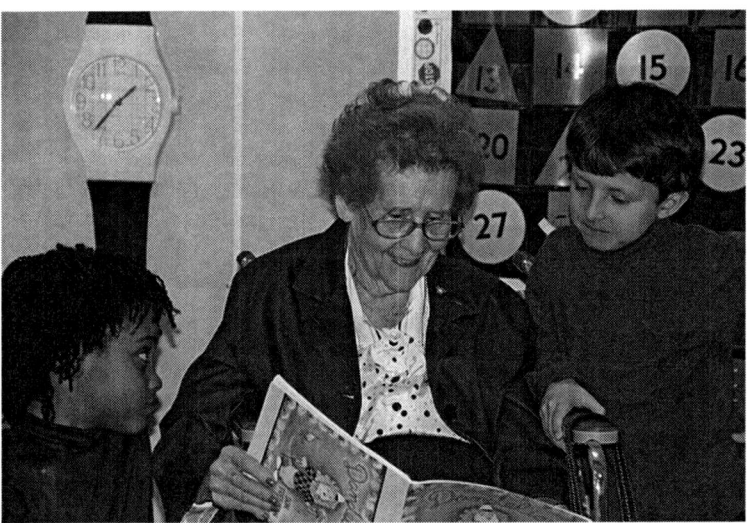

The control group met eight times at JP for a peer education seminar called "Successful Aging: Reclaiming Elderhood" for a total of approximately 12 h. Workshops facilitated by JP staff focused on the following themes: learning, wellness, love, creativity, spirituality, life options, ethics and beauty, and life quality. Control group participants were given eight homework assignments between each session that were intended to take 1 h each to complete; ultimately, the output of volunteer hours for the JP group was equal to the intervention group at TIS.

Statistical Analysis

Change scores between baseline and post-test data in the intervention and control groups were computed for all five variables. Additionally, the data set contained demographic information on gender, age, education, and marital status. Continuous variables for change scores on cognitive functioning, stress, and depression were summarized with means and compared using one-way analysis of variance. A Levene's test for equality of variances was run for each of the three continuous variables for both the control and intervention groups, and was rejected for cognitive functioning, stress, and depression. Therefore, a non-parametric approach was taken. New dichotomous variables were created (e.g., decline vs. no decline or improvement), and two-tailed Fisher's exact probability tests were run for cognitive functioning, stress, and depression. To analyze the data on sense of purpose and sense of usefulness, a chi-square test was initially run but was deemed inappropriate because of the small numbers in the study. As with cognitive functioning, stress, and depression, binaries were created for sense of purpose and usefulness (e.g., decline in sense of purpose/usefulness and no decline or improvement) and analyzed by running a two-tailed Fisher's exact probability test.

Qualitative Analysis

A modified grounded theory approach (Strauss, 1987) was employed in the analysis of final qualitative data. Transcripts of all narrative interviews and focus groups were typed into two separate Word documents, and a third document was created from ethnographic field notes written over the 10-month study. These transcripts were read multiple times and coded at the end of the study using the data analysis software NVivo. The coding framework drew on preliminary pilot data, the aforementioned existing research on intergenerational volunteering and QOL, as well as emergent themes and structure that developed as the research progressed. Codes from the three documents were merged into a single file.

To better understand the relationship between the themes that emerged from the three data sets, one-page summary analyses were prepared for all major codes; this involved reading through each section, noting the range of conceptual issues raised by the coded extracts, and looking for thematic interactions and overlaps between codes, while also considering so-called "deviant cases" that challenged emergent themes (Mays & Pope, 2000). Axial coding was performed on the data, and codes were manually grouped under broader, more sophisticated thematic categories based on perceived relationships and causality. In seeking analytic depth in the process of writing up the theoretical conclusions drawn from axial coding, the literature on intergenerational interventions was revisited. Once a final analysis was drafted, data was discussed with colleagues from other disciplinary backgrounds who tested and challenged emergent findings.

Results

Quantitative Results

Table 26.1 shows the results of the statistical analysis. As the study was small, it was surprising to observe a significant decline in stress from baseline to post-testing in the intervention group, which decreased by 2.50 points on the BAI while a mean increase in stress of 3.14 was observed in the control group during that same interval (see Fig. 26.2). This difference was statistically significant using the Mann–Whitney

Table 26.1 Summary results of statistical analysis[a]

Variable	Intervention ($n=8$)	Control ($n=7$)	P-value
Stress change, mean ± SD	−2.50 ± 1.41	+3.14 ± 6.46	0.01
Cognitive functioning change, mean ± SD	−0.75 ± 2.86	−2.14 ± 1.34	0.12
Sense of purpose change, mean ± SD	0.00 ± 0.535	−0.43 ± 0.535	0.28
Depression change, mean ± SD	+0.50 ± 1.41	−2.57 ± 10.5	0.31
Sense of usefulness: change, mean ± SD	0.00 ± 0.926	−0.29 ± 0.756	0.61

SD standard deviation
[a]Fischer's exact probability test

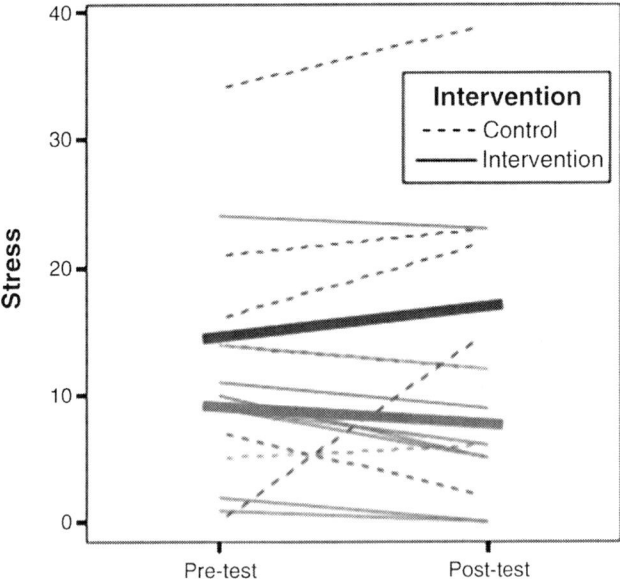

Fig. 26.2 Each of the 15 lines represents a single participant in the study over a 5-month period. Participants in the control group ($n=7$) are represented by a *dotted blue line*, while participants in the intervention group ($n=8$) are represented by a *continuous red line*. The *bold lines* represent averages for each group. The Beck Anxiety Inventory, a self-assessed instrument, was used to measure stress on a 40-point scale, with 40 representing high levels of stress-anxiety and 0 representing low levels

U test with exact p-values (S statistics = 73.0, $p = 0.0485$). Comparison of the dichotomous variable for decline in stress was done using a two-sided Fisher's exact test, and was also significant (Fisher's exact probability $p = 0.0070$), indicating that people in the intervention group were more likely to experience a decline in stress relative to baseline.

On measures of cognitive functioning, the intervention group showed no significant difference in decline relative to the control group, with the mean score decreasing by 0.75 points from baseline to post-testing on the MMSE versus the control group, whose mean score dropped 2.14 points during the same interval. The intervention group showed no significant difference in decline in depression relative to the control group, experiencing a slight mean increase of 0.50 points on the BDI while the mean control group score dropped 2.57 points.

The intervention group showed no significant increase in sense of purpose relative to the control group, experiencing no mean decline in sense of purpose (0.00 points), while the mean score of the control group declined but not significantly so by 0.43 points. The intervention group showed no significant increase in sense of usefulness relative to the control group, experiencing no mean decline (0.00 points), while the control group declined but not significantly so (0.29 points).

Qualitative Results

Qualitative data from formal narrative interviews, focus groups, and ethnographic field notes were pooled, and 30 themes were coded during initial analysis. The 15 major themes that emerged from initial pilot data were also present in the pooled study data, which yielded an additional 15 themes. Secondary analysis and axial coding condensed these 30 total themes into 11 larger themes that clustered around three broader conceptual meta-categories representing the main biopsychosocial pathways through which intergenerational volunteering affected QOL: perceived health benefits, sense of purpose and sense of usefulness, and relationships (see Table 26.2).

Table 26.2 Summary of qualitative themes

Quality of life	
Main themes	Sub themes
Perceived health benefits	Reduced stress and depression
	Youthful energy
	Cognitive stimulation
Sense of purpose and sense of usefulness	Role continuation
	Reminiscence
	Joy of teaching children
Relationships	Physical touch
	Proxy grandchildren
	Racial reconciliation
	Acceptance
	Reciprocity

Perceived Health Benefits

Participants, caregivers, and staff made reference to direct health benefits derived from intergenerational volunteering that appeared to enhance participant QOL, and such changes were also observed during longitudinal ethnographic observation of participants at JP and TIS. These benefits were couched in idiosyncratic ways. Some acknowledged that the process of learning new facts as well as thinking and responding to students helped them stay cognitively stimulated. As one volunteer put it:

> I like the questions the older students ask because it has caused me to reach back and think about things I haven't thought about in a long time—my younger years, what's the first time you did this or that.

Others described the drastic improvements in mood that resulted from encountering the youthful energy and interpersonal warmth of the students they worked with:

> It is energizing…the younger kids especially, but, you know the older ones, both age groups make you feel very wanted. They want to be with you, they fight for your attention, and they struggle with each other to get your full attention.

Still others identified the basic biopsychosocial benefits of simply laughing and having fun with children who did not judge them on the basis of their cognitive incapacities, thereby alleviating the social pressure many participants felt when among their peers. As one volunteer said:

> [Children] are more free. The older you get the more you have to think about what you have to say and all that kind of thing. Kids are much more spontaneous. They're fun. They're not all serious and you don't have to think about every word you said, and it gives you a nice warm feeling to interact with them […] it gets me out of my head.

Sense of Purpose and Sense of Usefulness

All aspects of the qualitative data strongly suggested that serving as "mentors" to students imbued participants with a sense of purpose and sense of usefulness that enhanced their QOL. Interactions with students provided an opportunity for participants to reprise meaningful professional roles in their late-life course and thereby evince remaining strengths and capacities in a context that valued their life experiences and gave them opportunities to feel useful and altruistic. As one volunteer said of the students:

> They really are getting a feel for how to share and listen in a conversation. In my life, I always talk to people about movies, plays, books, politics, and take in different opinions. It's good that we're helping build that kind of curiosity and skills so that they can do the same as they get older. That's how you stay active and keep your mind in good shape. And it needs to be done. And I think it's great, you know, what people are really trying to do. It's very important.

Participants also felt that engaging in structured reminiscence about their lives and addressing other topical issues in their interactions with children was a purposeful way to broaden the minds of their student partners and convey important lessons that would give the students greater opportunity to succeed in life. One of the more severely affected volunteers in the study seemed to allude to this point when she said:

> They're under a certain 'they can't do this and they can't do that', or 'they can do this or they can do that'. I think that is the most important thing: that they have to come 'across the street' so to speak. I don't know what to call it now. But it's the whole thing to keep going and not with an, well, I don't call it academic, but they have to learn these different things that happen. I think I can help them a lot…and if we can do that, then I think it is a situation that can be helpful and healthful.

Relationships

There was a clear emphasis from participants that QOL is a concept deeply reliant on maintaining affirming relationships. Volunteering at TIS enabled participants to gain access to a nonmedicalized community in which meaningful and affectionate relationships could be constituted with children from the local community who simply accepted them without regard for their diagnosis of dementia. As one volunteer – a woman who had previously been affected by episodes of acute memory loss and aphasia exacerbated by overlapping medications – put it:

> [Before visiting TIS] I could not find words to say […] and at that point I could hardly get through a sentence. And there was this feeling of not being able to talk. So it was terrible. I thought I might as well quit. I was really down in the dumps about the whole thing. But the nice part of it is that the children in that group seem to be perfectly willing to accept me in the way that they accept everybody else, and isn't that a neat thing?

These relationships were built not only through the aforementioned reminiscence sessions and other classroom activities, but also in more embodied ways, such as through physical touch. Further, it emerged that students at TIS were perceived as "proxy grandchildren" by many of the participants in the study. Some volunteers explicitly stated that the students they worked with reminded them of their children and grandchildren; as one woman said:

> I love being around the younger ones 'cause I don't see many of those any more. And I enjoy being with the older ones too, I guess, although they're a little younger than my grandkids.

This psychological association served to deepen relationships, while also helping to reconcile major differences in age and race. During the life history sessions in the older classroom, one woman learned that a student partner lived on the same street that she had grown up on decades ago:

> I got a big kick out of when people were discussing one thing or another, where they lived or something or other, I don't know, and some little kid I said I used to live in [the Cleveland suburb] South Euclid and she said 'I lived here', and I said 'oh that's where one of my friends used to live'. I thought that was all very interesting because you think that's not something that could happen in your neighbourhood – that someone nice of a different race and culture could move into your house. So it was really something worthwhile for me to learn.

Finally, a theme of reciprocity was prevalent in the qualitative data, suggesting that participants felt their intergenerational relationships were of mutual benefit both for themselves and for the students they mentored. One of the more severely affected women said at the end of the study:

> For heaven's sakes, we're trying to help children and we can still be doing this! That's the most important thing: it helps both sides of the picture!

Discussion

The results suggest that intergenerational volunteering enhanced the QOL of intervention group participants as demonstrated by a significant decrease in stress in the quantitative data and the emergence of multiple biopsychosocial benefits in the qualitative data. This finding is especially salient to dementia treatment because multiple mechanisms have been found linking elevated stress with increased risk of AD and an exacerbation of cognitive decline (Lupien et al., 2005; Wilson, Evans, Bienias et al., 2003). That a community-based intervention as widely accessible as intergenerational volunteering could potentially act on a major risk factor for dementia and contribute to overall QOL is a finding that should be taken seriously by the long-term care field and by caregivers of persons with mild-to-moderate dementia. One cannot posit a causal role for intergenerational volunteering in the reduction of stress, but the preliminary findings in this study warrant larger more robust studies that might confirm this association or explore the actual mechanisms through which stress might be lowered through engagement with children.

These results also strengthen the notion that solutions to the challenge of aging populations must be inclusive, not just of reductionist pharmacological and biotechnological approaches that strive to enhance longevity and improve cognition, but also of community-based strategies that promote wellness and QOL. This seems particularly true for persons living with dementia who may be perniciously affected by the stigma and isolation of their condition.

Previous authors (Sabat, 2003) have noted that for many people living with dementia – and especially those living in caregiving institutions – it is increasingly rare to be asked to help another person. Consequently, most social interactions are confined to "patient–physician" or "patient–caregiver" relationships in which there is little opportunity to feel reciprocity, to share their personal stories, or to realize and pursue goals, or find avenues through which to experience enhanced self-worth or establish a worthy social identity.

For persons who have spent their lives delineating and achieving meaningful goals only to find themselves confined to a nursing home, the feeling of being bereft of purpose and ostensible value can be overwhelmingly and appropriately saddening (Sabat, 2003). Being able to serve as a volunteer with children over the 5-month intervention created a meaningful role in community for the participants in this study. The forming of relationships with older and younger children with whom the volunteers felt empowered to teach inverted the patient–physician dyad that so often defined their interactions at JP, placing emphasis on remaining strengths and capacities while enabling the re-enactment of meaningful professional and familial roles and the constitution of a relevant social identity through narrative-based activities. The alembic TIS environment engendered a host of positive dispositional changes in volunteers that ultimately enhanced QOL.

There are numerous limitations to the research reported. The intervention was situated in a unique environment (TIS) with an ethos of intergenerational learning, which calls into question the generalizability of the data and underscores the need for more experimental research nested in a range of intergenerational environments. The study also possessed a relatively small number of participants, and the sample had demographic characteristics unrepresentative of the population at large. There was also an obvious weakness in the control group since participants in this arm could not be confined to a clinical setting making it impossible to control for any intergenerational interactions they might have had in their spare time.

Moreover, it is acknowledged that any conceptualization of QOL – including the five-domain definition established in this study – has inherent limitations, and is perhaps best understood as an idiosyncratic rather than normative concept. Lastly, intergenerational interventions must not be promoted as a proscriptive solution to the formidable global challenges wrought by both dementia and changing demographics. Besides the fact that not all persons with dementia are in possession of the cultural resources that would allow them to invest their time in late-life volunteer activities, every individual is equipped with a different repertoire of personal resources that have been acquired through differing life experiences. These experiences define one's personality and coping styles, which may or may not be conducive to intergenerational volunteering with children. The successful aging movement must not ignore the diverse ways in which people age, the range of limitations faced by many aging individuals that might affect their capacity to "engage," and the many idiosyncratic pathways to achieving QOL at the end of one's life.

Future Research

Future studies might enlist more participants, and critically assess a diverse spectrum of community-based intergenerational volunteering experiences with a variety of methods to know which practices lead to the most beneficial outcomes, as well as which types of social institutions are most supportive of the QOL of persons with dementia. Understanding the mechanisms through which such psychosocial interventions as intergenerational volunteering may affect persons with dementia on the cellular level (for instance, exploring an association between engagement and serum cortisol levels, cerebral blood flow, glucose metabolism, serotonin, or blood pressure) may be a particularly fruitful avenue for more biologically orientated research, while comparative inquiry into the effects of active interventions in different cultural contexts may be a more desirable avenue for socially orientated researchers.

Guidelines for Future Intergenerational Programming

For those interested in setting up community-based intergenerational pilot programs, it may be helpful to follow a few well-established guidelines on how to ensure success:

- *Leadership*: Any intergenerational program requires the presence of champions from each partner organization.
- *Consistency*: Good programs will ensure that visits – whether they be once per week or once per month – occur with consistency and are carried out with enthusiasm and adept organization. This enables intergenerational relationships to develop and appreciate over time.
- *Activities and curriculum*: It is effective to use evidence-based methods, such as the narrative-oriented activities in this project (discussions about heritage, holidays/culturally significant customs and practices, oral history interviews, reminiscence, scrapbooking, exercise, arts and crafts, etc.).
- *Age-appropriateness*: While there is no one-size-fits-all approach, good activities should be accessible, mutually stimulating, engaging, purposeful, fun, and age-appropriate for both students and elders.

There also appear to be barriers to quality partnerships:

- Inconsistency of visits.
- Lack of engagement.
- Lack of agreement on what constitutes meaningful activities.
- Scheduling and transportation difficulties.
- Perception that students are entertainment rather than partners.
- Lack of preparation from students who may not have understood the cognitive, physical, and emotional challenges of the elders they work with.

Conclusion

At the end of "Fortitude," Sylvia uses her prosthetic arms to shoot Dr. Frankenstein with a revolver that has been smuggled to her by one of her friends, a beautician who visits her each week. Though he is mortally wounded, it turns out that Frankenstein has built his machine to accommodate two, and that the ultimate aim is not merely to extend life, but to be able to enjoy Sylvia's companionship and "live in such perfect harmony … that the gods themselves will tear out their hair in envy!" As misguided as Frankenstein's vision may be, Vonnegut ends the story by reminding us that human wellness is not just about a race for longevity or cognitive stimulation, but also about preserving relationships over time.

So too must we remember that wellness is not just about the health of a brain, because that brain is one facet of a person who exists as part of a family, a neighborhood, a community, and a natural environment. Real commitments to wellness must look beyond the brain to the whole person, and consider the enormous promise of community-based solutions to contribute to a vital and purposeful existence – even for those affected by memory loss. In both the rapidly aging developed and developing worlds, such interventions that prove cost-effective, capable of improving the QOL of persons with dementia, and which also contribute to community needs will be highly valued, particularly in the continued absence of a pharmacological compound that can affect the onset and progression of age-related dementia.

Acknowledgments This study was undertaken as part of Daniel George's doctoral research in the Institute for Social and Cultural Anthropology at Oxford University, which was supported by the ORS Scholarship Fund. Additional funding for fieldwork and writing was provided by the Takayama Foundation, the Greenwald Foundation, the Fondation Médéric Alzheimer, and Alzheimer's Disease International. Special thanks to Dr. Peter Whitehouse, Dr. Stanley Ulijaszek and Dr. Harvey Whitehouse.

References

Alzheimer's Disease International. (2010). World Alzheimer Report 2010. London: Alzheimer's Disease International.
Ayala, J., Hewson, J., et al. (2006). Intergenerational programs: Perspectives of service providers in one Canadian City. *Journal of Intergenerational Relationships, 5*(2), 45–60.
Bowling, A. (1995). What things are important in people's lives? A survey of the public's judgements to inform scales of health related quality of life. *Social Science & Medicine (1982), 41*(10), 1447–1462.
Camp, C., Zeisel, C., & Antenucci, V. (2010). Implementing the "I'm Still Here"™ approach: Montessori-based methods for engaging persons with dementia. In *Enhancing cognitive fitness in adults: A guide to the use and development of community programs*. New York: Springer.
Chung, J. C. (2009). An intergenerational reminiscence programme for older adults with early dementia and youth volunteers: Values and challenges. *Scandinavian Journal of Caring Sciences, 23*(2), 259–264.
Cigolle, C. T., Langa, K. M., et al. (2007). Geriatric conditions and disability: The Health and Retirement Study. *Annals of Internal Medicine, 147*(3), 156–164.
Cohen-Mansfield, J., Parpura-Gill, A., et al. (2006). Utilization of self-identity roles for designing interventions for persons with dementia. *The Journals of Gerontology. Series B: Psychological Sciences and Social Sciences, 61*(4), P202–P212.
de Souza, E. M. (2003). Intergenerational interaction in health promotion: A qualitative study in Brazil. *Revista de sa´de p´blica, 37*(4), 463–469.
de Souza, E. M., & Grundy, E. (2007). Intergenerational interaction, social capital and health: Results from a randomised controlled trial in Brazil. *Social Science & Medicine (1982), 65*(7), 1397–1409.
Engel, G. L. (1977). The need for a new medical model: A challenge for biomedicine. *Science, 196*(4286), 129–136.
Ferraro, K. F., & Shippee, T. P. (2009). Aging and cumulative inequality: How does inequality get under the skin? *The Gerontologist, 49*(3), 333–343.
Ferri, C. P., Prince, M., et al. (2005). Global prevalence of dementia: A Delphi consensus study. *Lancet, 366*(9503), 2112–2117.
Fried, L. P., Carlson, M. C., et al. (2004). A social model for health promotion for an aging population: Initial evidence on the Experience Corps model. *Journal of Urban Health, 81*(1), 64–78.

George, D. R., & Whitehouse, P. J. (2010). Can intergenerational volunteering enhance quality of life for persons with mild to moderate dementia?: Results from a 5-month mixed methods intervention study in the United States. Journal of the American Geriatric Society. *Journal of the American Geriatrics Society, 58*(4), p 796.

George, D. R., & Singer, M. E. (2011). Intergenerational volunteering and quality of life for persons with mild to moderate dementia: Results from a 5-month intervention study in the United States. *American Journal of Geriatric Psychiatry, 19*(4), 392–396.

Gigliotti, C., Morris, M., et al. (2005). An intergenerational summer program involving persons with dementia and preschool children. *Educational Gerontology, 31*(6), 425–441.

Hayes, C. L. (2003). An observational study in developing an intergenerational shared site program: Challenges and insights. *Journal of Intergenerational Relationships, 1*(1), 113–132.

Jarrott, S. E., & Bruno, K. (2003). Intergenerational activities involving persons with dementia: An observational assessment. *American Journal of Alzheimer's Disease and Other Dementias, 18*(1), 31–37.

Jarrott, S., & Bruno, K. (2007). Shared Site Intergenerational Programs: A Case Study. *Journal of Applied Gerontology, 26*(3), 239–257.

Jorm, A. F., Korten, A. E., et al. (1987). The prevalence of dementia: A quantitative integration of the literature. *Acta Psychiatrica Scandinavica, 76*(5), 465–479.

Karkazis, K., & Feder, E. K. (2008). Naming the problem: Disorders and their meanings. *Lancet, 372*(9655), 2016–2017.

Kawas, C. H. (2003). Clinical practice. Early Alzheimer's disease. *The New England Journal of Medicine, 349*(11), 1056–1063.

Kitwood, T. M. (1997). *Dementia reconsidered: The person comes first*. Buckingham, England: Open University Press.

Kleinman, A. (1988). *The illness narratives: Suffering, healing, and the human condition*. New York: Basic Books.

Lee, M. M., Camp, C. J., & Malone, M. N. (2007). Effects of intergenerational Montessori-based activities programming on engagement of nursing home residents with dementia. *Clin Interv Aging, 2*(3), 477–483.

Levasseur, M., Desrosiers, J., et al. (2004). Is social participation associated with quality of life of older adults with physical disabilities? *Disability and Rehabilitation, 26*(20), 1206–1213.

Lupien, S. J., Schwartz, G., & Ng, Y. K., et al. (2005). The Douglas Hospital Longitudinal Study of Normal and Pathological Aging: summary of findings. *Journal Psychiatry Neuroscience, 30*(5), 328–334.

Mays, N., & Pope, C. (2000). Qualitative research in health care. Assessing quality in qualitative research. *BMJ, 320*(7226), 50–52.

Okamoto, K., & Tanaka, Y. (2004). Subjective usefulness and 6-year mortality risks among elderly persons in Japan. *The Journals of Gerontology. Series B: Psychological Sciences and Social Sciences, 59*(5), P246–P249.

Porcelli, P., & Sonino, N. (2007). *Psychological factors affecting medical conditions: A new classification for DSM-V*. Basel: Karger.

Puts, M. T., Shekary, N., et al. (2007). What does quality of life mean to older frail and non-frail community-dwelling adults in the Netherlands? *Quality of Life Research, 16*(2), 263–277.

Rabins, P. V., & Black, B. S. (2007). Measuring quality of life in dementia: Purposes, goals, challenges and progress. *International Psychogeriatrics, 19*(3), 401–407.

Sabat, S. R. (2003). Some potential benefits of creating research partnerships with people with Alzheimer's disease. *Research, Policy and Planning: The Journal of the Social Services Research Group., 21*, 5–12.

Seymour, D. G., Starr, J. M., et al. (2008). Quality of life and its correlates in octogenarians. Use of the SEIQoL-DW in Wave 5 of the Aberdeen Birth Cohort 1921 Study (ABC1921). *Quality of Life Research, 17*(1), 11–20.

Shonkoff, J. P., Boyce, W. T., et al. (2009). Neuroscience, molecular biology, and the childhood roots of health disparities: Building a new framework for health promotion and disease prevention. *JAMA: The Journal of American Medical Association, 301*(21), 2252–2259.

Sontag, S. (1978). *Illness as metaphor*. New York, NY: Farrar, Straus and Giroux.
Stein, J., Schettler, T., Rohrer, B., & Valenti, M. (2008). *Environmental threats to healthy aging: With a closer look at Alzheimer's and Parkinson's diseases*. Boston, MA: Boston, Greater Boston Physicians for Social Responsibilty: Science and Environmental Health Network.
Strauss, A. L., & Strauss, A. L. (1987). *Qualitative analysis for social scientists*. Cambridge: Cambridge University Press.
Thomas, W. H. (1994). *The Eden alternative: Nature, hope, and nursing homes*. Columbia, MO: University of Missouri Press.
Thomas, W. H. (1999). *The Eden alternative handbook: The art of building human habitats*. Sherburn, NY: Summer Hill.
Thomas, W. H. (2004). *What are old people for? How elders will save the world*. Acton, MA: VanderWyk & Burnham.
United Nations. (2002). *International plan of action on ageing*. Second World Assembly on Ageing, Madrid, Spain.
Whitehouse, P. J., & George, D. (2008). *The myth of Alzheimer's: What you aren't being told about today's most dreaded diagnosis*. New York: St. Martin's.
Wilson, R. S., Evans, D. A., Bienias, J. L., et al. (2003). Proneness to psychological distress is associated with risk of Alzheimer's disease. *Neurology, 61*(11), 1479–1485.

Chapter 27
Experience Corps®: A Civic Engagement-Based Public Health Intervention in the Public Schools

George W. Rebok, Michelle C. Carlson, Jeremy S. Barron, Kevin D. Frick, Sylvia McGill, Jeanine M. Parisi, Teresa Seeman, Erwin J. Tan, Elizabeth K. Tanner, Paul R. Willging, and Linda P. Fried

Abstract The Experience Corps® (EC) program is an innovative, community-based model for health promotion for older adults. Incorporating health promotion into new, generative roles for older adults, it brings the time, experience, and wisdom of older adults to bear to improve academic and behavioral outcomes of K-3 grade children in public elementary schools. The EC program is simultaneously designed to be a cost-effective, high-impact literacy support and social capital intervention for young children that doubles as a potentially powerful health promotion model aimed at improving the cognitive, physical, social, and psychological function of older adults and preventing disability and dependency associated with aging. In this program, older adult volunteers are placed in a critical mass in public elementary schools to perform standardized, meaningful roles developed by the program after selection by the schools' principals as being critical unmet needs. In this chapter, we describe the development and major tenets of the EC model, the science underlying the model and data supporting the effectiveness of this intergenerational intervention for both older adults and children, and policy implications of social engagement programs like Experience Corps for long-term improvements in older adults' health and well-being and practical guidelines for setting up an EC program in the local community.

Introduction

One of the greatest legacies of the twentieth century is that people are living substantially longer. By 2030 the population aged 60 and above is projected to be twice as large as any other age-group, growing from 35 to 71.5 million and representing

G.W. Rebok (✉)
Bloomberg School of Public Health, The Johns Hopkins University, Baltimore, MD, USA
e-mail: grebok@jhsph.edu

nearly 20% of the total U.S. population (National Center for Health Statistics, 2007). With this mass societal aging (Population Division, 2002), people may be living up to one third of their lives after retirement from their primary occupation (Freedman, 1999). This change in our population demands that we rethink how to maximize the health and well-being of our aging population, and how to create meaningful opportunities for a fulfilling life after retirement that may not yet exist.

At the same time, two trends threaten the future of American society: (1) the increasing proportion of older adults living with chronic illnesses who will require economic and social support from a decreasing number of workers, and who will need a prepared, educated younger population to sustain our country's productivity, and (2) the relatively poor quality of education in large, public urban American schools at a time of increasing need to be globally competitive. Therefore, it would be highly beneficial to society to create a program that could reengage older adults as active members in schools and communities in ways that may enhance their health and at the same time provide mentoring to children so that they could receive more differentiated instruction that meets their individual needs enabling them to achieve academic success.

The Experience Corps®, a 15-year-old community-based model of senior service to improve the educational outcomes of children, was designed with previously mentioned goals in mind (Freedman & Fried, 1999; Fried et al., 2004). The Experience Corps model creates a "win–win–win" scenario for older adults, children, and schools by providing older adults the opportunity to use their time, skills, and wisdom to volunteer in low-income, urban elementary schools as mentors of children in grades K-3 for 15 h a week throughout two academic school years (Fried et al., 2004; Glass et al., 2004; Parisi et al., 2009). Experience Corps offers a model for the rapidly burgeoning interest in volunteerism and other forms of civic engagement that seek to expand role options in later life by creating meaningful roles within institutions like the public school system (Butrica et al., 2009; Martinson & Minkler, 2006; Tang et al., 2010). The underlying goal is to create a more active and healthier older population with roles through which they can make a difference in society, a student population having more educational needs met, and as a secondary benefit of Experience Corps design, enhance the ability to create a positive learning environment in the classroom that results in schools having stronger academic performance.

Though social norms have traditionally emphasized the postretirement period as a time of leisure-filled "rolelessness" (Bronfenbrenner, McClelland, Wethington, Moen, & Ceci, 1996), our population of older adults effectively represents an untapped resource, with an abundance of knowledge and skills (human capital) along with attitudes, beliefs, and social networks (social capital) that can contribute to society. Indeed, large majorities of older adults not only have the health and functional ability to continue "giving back" to society, but express a desire to do so (Baltes & Baltes, 1990; Carlson et al., 2000; Tan et al., 2009; Tanner et al., 2011). Growing evidence also indicates that important health benefits accrue from such continued, active engagement in meaningful activities. The benefits of volunteering include better physical health (Barron et al., 2009; Fried et al., 2004; Gruenewald et al., 2007; Luoh & Herzog, 2002; Morrow-Howell, Hinterlong, Rozario, & Tang, 2003), better mental health (Gottlieb & Gillespie, 2008; Hong & Morrow-Howell, 2010; Kim & Pai, 2010; Tang et al., 2010), enhanced subjective well-being (Baker, Cahalin, Gesrt, & Burr, 2005; Greenfield & Marks, 2004; Morrow-Howell et al., 2009), and delayed mortality (Harris & Thoresen, 2005).

This chapter will describe the Experience Corps® program as a civic engagement-based public health model of senior service that seeks to create meaningful, socially-valued roles for older adults while simultaneously serving as a vehicle for health promotion by encouraging greater cognitive, physical, and social activity – all factors that have been shown to promote greater health and well-being and enhance cognitive fitness. We have organized the chapter into three main sections. The first section describes the development of the Experience Corps model and its major tenets, a brief history of program implementation in Baltimore in collaboration with our community partner, the Greater Homewood Community Corporation (GHCC), and how the model has been used to address questions about health promotion and enhancement of cognitive fitness and positive well-being in later life. The second section describes the science underlying the model, drawing on the original design theory (Freedman & Fried, 1999) and research evidence from an initial pilot trial (Carlson et al., 2008; Fried et al., 2004; Frick et al., 2004; Glass et al., 2004; Rebok et al., 2004), two large national demonstration trials, and a recent national evaluation (Hong & Morrow-Howell, 2010), and on the hypothesized outcomes of an ongoing randomized controlled trial of the Experience Corps program in Baltimore City. The third section focuses on policy implications of social engagement programs like Experience Corps for long-term improvements in older adults' health and well-being and practical guidelines for setting up an Experience Corps program in the local community.

The Experience Corps Model

Codeveloped by Dr. Linda Fried (Professor, Johns Hopkins University, and currently Dean of the Mailman School of Public Health, Columbia University) and Mr. Marc Freedman (President, Civic Ventures, Inc.)(Freedman & Fried, 1999), the model was designed to meet the age-appropriate needs of many older adults, to be productive and give back, or – in the terminology of Erik Erickson – to be *generative* and leave a legacy (Erikson, 1982). It was, more specifically, designed as a social model for health promotion and engagement, and to model an intergenerational win–win by increasing physical, cognitive, and social activity among seniors through meaningful, high-impact volunteer roles in public elementary schools. The model in Baltimore implemented rigorously the key elements of EC design (Freedman & Fried, 1999; Fried et al., 2004): meaningful high-impact roles designed to enhance health; intensive service in teams and critical mass to ensure results; and infrastructure to ensure effectiveness and longevity. Specific volunteer roles (e.g., literacy and math support) were developed to support the educational success of young children in public elementary schools (kindergarten through third grade) (Rebok et al., 2004). Multiple roles were encouraged to maximize stimulation of diverse cognitive abilities.

These roles were chosen as the initial focus of the program for several reasons. First, there is a profound and unrealized societal need in the U.S. to improve the educational success of children. We targeted children in the younger grades based on evidence that children not succeeding by the third grade were at high risk of future school failure. For example, children who do not learn to read by third grade are at greater risk for failure at school, dropping out of school, and limited occupational opportunities (Annie E. Casey Foundation, 2010; Crijnen, Feehan, & Kellam, 1998; Kellam & Rebok, 1992; Lloyd, 1978). To quote a recent report from an early education initiative, "Children's success in school and in life must be built on a foundation of seamless learning during their earliest Pre-K-3 school years" (Foundation for Child Development, 2008). It is for that reason that a major goal of the No Child Left Behind Act (NCLB) of 2001 (Pub L No. 107-110 (HR1)) is to ensure that all children are reading at grade level by third grade. NCLB seeks to close the achievement gap between disadvantaged students and their peers and to change the culture of America's schools so that all students receive the support and high-quality, individualized instruction they need to meet higher expectations.

Further, we began in public urban elementary schools because of the perceived need of many of these children for increased adult attention and role models. We theorized, further, that older adults were likely to be more attracted to supporting young children than older ones, at least initially, permitting us to demonstrate the diversity of older adults who could create a critical mass of human and social capital for children and schools (Glass et al., 2004). A large unmet need in many of our schools is a lack of the parental and community support necessary to create success. Volunteerism by older adults in the community can help to meet this need.

At the same time, intentionally embedded into the Experience Corps program design is another level of potential benefits: a health promotion program for the older adults. The rationale for this component is that there is substantial evidence that healthy behaviors, including physical activity, social supports and engagement, and cognitive activity, are important to health and prevention of cognitive decline and disability as people age – even into the oldest ages (Rowe & Kahn, 1987, 2004). However, it has proven difficult to attract older adults to participate in health behavior change programs, particularly for sustained periods of time (Tan et al., 2010). Those who do participate tend to be of higher socioeconomic status (Katula et al., 2007; Stewart et al., 2001); even among these groups, long-term retention is not high. Those with fewer economic means or lower education appear to have both less ability to participate in and/or less access to health promotion programs and optimal health behaviors.

The Experience Corps program recruits, trains, and places men and women 55 years of age and older as volunteers in public elementary schools, serving children in kindergarten through third grade. Those eligible to volunteer must be literate at the eighth grade level, be high school graduates, meet screening criteria for general cognitive status, and pass a criminal background check conducted by the school system. All volunteers must complete a 1-week, 30-h training program to prepare them for serving effectively in their roles within the schools. Specifically, volunteers are trained in supporting literacy and math skill development and motivation for reading; assisting in school libraries; violence prevention, behavior management, and conflict resolution; and other roles. In addition to providing rigorous training sessions, the program works with the schools' Principals and Experience Corps Team Leader to assign the volunteers to classrooms in roles that would meet the school's greatest unmet needs for increasing the success of their students. The program also provides ongoing support, oversight, and in-service training of the volunteers once they are placed in the schools.

The Experience Corps model was designed based on the hypothesis that meaningful, socially-valuable, generative roles could be created for older adults to accomplish the following: (1) attract a large proportion of the older population; (2) demonstrate that an aging society can address unmet societal needs (e.g., improving elementary school education); (3) be a vehicle for enhancing the cognitive, physical, and social health of older adults; and (4) provide a visible intervention to revise our social conceptions of appropriate roles and responsibilities at older ages (Freedman & Fried, 1999). Key elements of the EC program in Baltimore are outlined in Table 27.1 below. Each of the EC program elements described in the Table is designed to maximize the program's attractiveness to schools and older volunteers,

Table 27.1 Core features of the Baltimore Experience Corps program

Productive roles	EC program explicitly works with each school to identify important, unmet needs related to improving children's academic/behavioral performance and to develop meaningful EC volunteer roles to help address those needs (most frequently cited to be literacy and math support, and conflict resolution)
Training	Participants go through a 1-week (5 day) training program explicitly designed to provide them with skills needed to function effectively in the roles they will assume in the schools
Critical mass, teams	A team of 12–20 volunteers is placed in schools; the team structure embeds seniors in a network of similar volunteers, fostering social contacts/support, problem solving and results in greater satisfaction and retention in the program. In collaboration with each school principal, the number of volunteers is determined to provide a critical mass of EC adults to support children's academic outcomes and have sufficient impact to shift outcomes for whole grades
Time commitment	Required commitment of 15 h/week ensures that schools receive adequate, ongoing EC input, allowing for consistency and development of relationships with children and school staff, and that older adults get an adequate "dose" of exposure to the physical, cognitive, and social activities designed to promote health and well-being
Incentive reimbursement	EC volunteers receive a monthly stipend (~$250) to offset volunteer expenses (e.g., transportation, meals). This reimbursement also serves to differentiate EC from traditional volunteering and acknowledge (in a small way) the value of their activities
Infrastructure support	Field and site coordinators provide ongoing support and supervision. They assist with initial team integration into the schools and organized weekly team meetings for problem solving throughout the school year and in-service training in new EC roles
Program flexibility	Multiple different roles are available to volunteers as their interests and skills evolve, allowing for ongoing development of new skills and opportunities for leadership

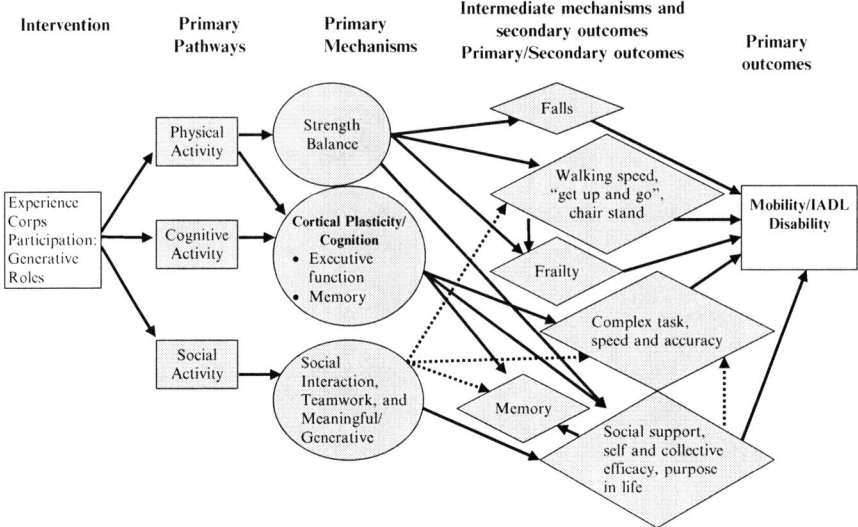

Fig. 27.1 Causal model for the impact of Experience Corps on older adult's outcomes (Fried et al., 2004)

to maximize its effectiveness in enhancing educational outcomes among children, and to promote better cognitive, physical, social, and psychological functioning and health in older adults. The specific benefits we hypothesize will accrue to older adults from participation in the EC program are detailed in Fig. 27.1. Cognitive benefits are expected to occur along multiple dimensions of ability through various volunteer roles and the need to flexibly shift among these roles, and include improved executive function, memory, and enhanced speed of processing. These cognitive benefits, particularly in executive functions, are further expected to generalize to real-life activities of daily living. The expected physical benefits of EC participation include enhanced strength and balance, reduced number of falls, faster walking speed, and decreased frailty leading to improved mobility/IADL functioning. Expected social benefits include an increase in social interaction/integration, an increase in the receipt and provision of social support, and a decrease in loneliness. The anticipated psychological benefits include increased feelings of generativity and usefulness, enhanced personal and collective efficacy, a greater sense of purpose in life and personal growth, more positive views and expectations of aging, greater perceived quality of life, and lower levels of depression.

As noted above, the EC model was designed to train and place a critical mass of older adults, in teams, in public elementary schools to serve in roles identified by principals and teachers as their greatest unmet needs. At the individual child level, the hypothesized mechanisms by which the program is expected to impact the early risk antecedents of poor reading/academic achievement and classroom behavior are shown in Fig. 27.2. Beneficial child outcomes are expected to include reading/academic achievement; behavioral indices, including disruptiveness and conflict; and readiness for learning and motivations/expectations regarding school and learning. It is hypothesized that the deployment of a critical mass of older adults in carefully

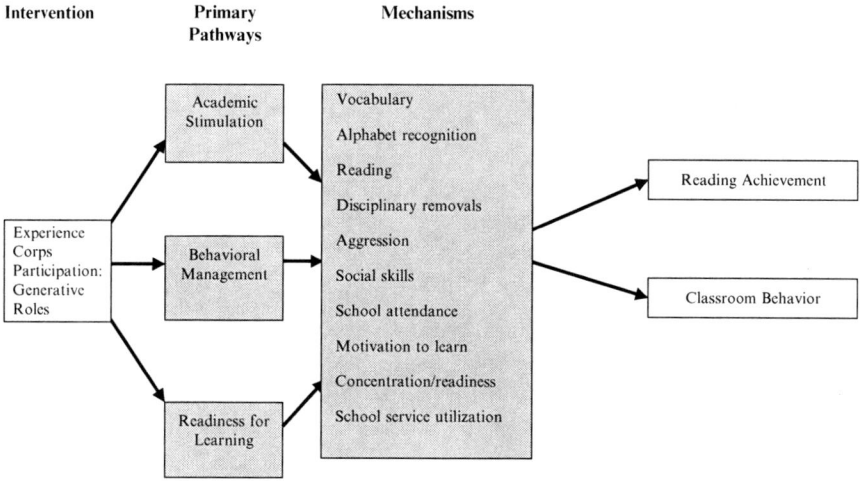

Fig. 27.2 Causal model for the impact of Experience Corps on children's outcomes (Rebok et al., 2004)

designed, generative roles will lead to improvements in the primary outcome of reading achievement (standardized assessments) and the secondary outcome of classroom behavior. If intergenerational programs like Experience Corps were to result in just a small effect on the number of students graduating from high school, such programs would produce a net savings to society (Frick et al., 2004).

Brief History of Experience Corps Program Implementation

National demonstrations. In 1996–1998, the Experience Corps model was implemented in a national demonstration by the National Senior Service Program (NSSP) of the Corporation for National Service, evaluating feasibility and roles for older adults in five U.S. cities (two schools per city). The theorized, previously described model was deemed highly successful by schools, teachers, volunteers, and the funder (Freedman & Fried, 1999; Fried, Freedman, Endres, & Wasik, 1997). Specific observations included: (1) that older adults could be recruited to this high intensity model, with retention rates through the year of 70%; (2) that the idea of "critical mass" was seen as important to impacting outcomes and affecting school climate for whole grades and entire schools and in changing the culture of the schools; (3) that to be able to recruit volunteers for this high intensity commitment, it was essential to offer an incentive stipend of $250 per month to reimburse volunteers for daily expenses associated with travel and school lunches, critical to many older adults living on a fixed income, and offered a metric of high valuation of their roles as volunteers; (4) principals and teachers reported substantial changes in their attitudes toward older volunteers, and became positive about the volunteers' roles in the school; and that essential features were all deemed important.

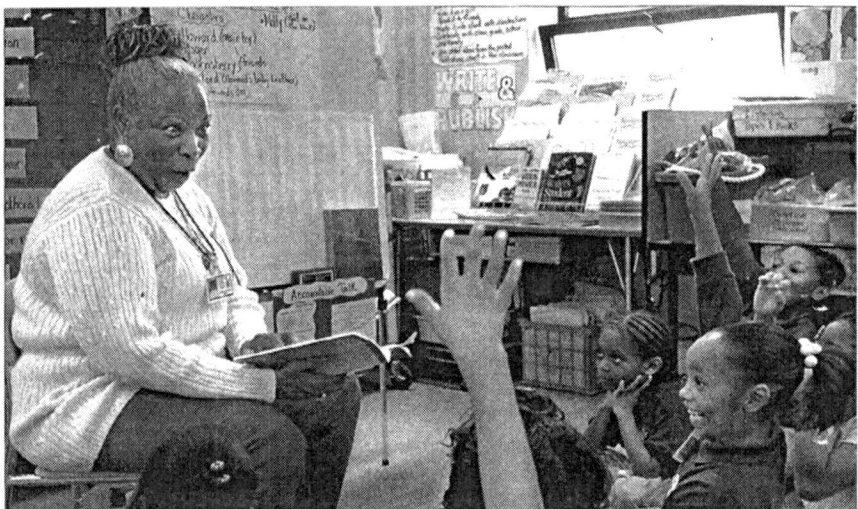

"YOU ARE A FRIEND IN THE CLASSROOM."
AUDREY WEEMS, 70, READING A STORY TO STUDENTS IN A THIRD-GRADE CLASS AT WAVERLY. A MOTHER OF EIGHT, SHE WORKED AT THE SOCIAL SECURITY ADMINISTRATION FOR 35 YEARS, RETIRING IN 2002. WEEMS LEARNED ABOUT THE BALTIMORE EXPERIENCE CORPS PROGRAM THROUGH HER CHURCH.

Fig. 27.3 Photograph of Experience Corps volunteer in a third grade classroom

A second U.S. demonstration was funded from 1998 to 2001, expanding into nine cities, and focusing on refining the literacy support program within the Experience Corps. The Experience Corps is now operating in 20 cities across the U.S. Hong and Morrow-Howell (2010) recently reported results from a quasi-experimental study of multiple Experience Corps sites around the country in which Experience Corps volunteers and a matched comparison group from the Health and Retirement Study (Fonda & Herzog, 2004) were compared. The results showed that after 2 years of participation in the Experience Corps program, participants reported significantly reduced depressive symptoms and functional limitations. There was also a trend toward less decline in self-rated health among Experience Corps participants.

Experience Corps Baltimore City, the focus of this chapter, is a product of the partnership between the Greater Homewood Community Corporation and the Johns Hopkins Center on Aging and Health (COAH), and exemplifies how communities can benefit when academic institutions are involved with the design, implementation, and evaluation of a community development project. This partnership was initiated by the codesigner of EC (Dr. Linda Fried). Started in 1998, GHCC was a local nonprofit community association involved in community development and organizing as well as economic development with a strong focus on childhood education, while COAH was nationally known as a leader in research on healthy aging, and was primarily involved in large, longitudinal observational studies of older adults. The primary goals of the program in Baltimore were to refine theory and practice through research and development, implement a standardized program in the public elementary schools with carefully designed volunteer roles to optimize impact on children and schools, and to evaluate benefits to all constituencies (Fried et al., 2004, 2006). Secondary goals involved developing and refining recruitment and retention methods, ascertaining acceptability of randomization to volunteers and schools, and to study the potential for long-term retention.

The Science: Results from the Baltimore Pilot Trial

Building upon the two feasibility studies (1996–1998 and 1998–2001) and the partnership between GHCC and COAH, we conducted a pilot randomized trial of the effects of the program on the older volunteers, the schools, and the school children in Baltimore City 1999–2000 (see Fried et al., 2004; Frick et al., 2004; Glass et al., 2004; Rebok et al., 2004). During this pilot trial, 148 men and women 60 years and older were recruited and randomly assigned to serve in Experience Corps (or to a wait list/no contact control group). After randomization, 70 volunteers assigned to the program ultimately served in the Baltimore City Public schools. Demographic characteristics of the pilot trial participants and study results are shown in Table 27.2. Health status ranged from excellent to fair, by self report, with 2.5 diseases on average and frequent mobility difficulty at baseline. Volunteers signed up for the program for generative reasons, primarily; e.g., to "make a difference" for children (Tan et al., 2009). In addition to randomly assigning individuals to the program, we also randomly assigned six public elementary schools interested in receiving Experience Corps volunteers to either receive the program or serve as a control school for one year (Rebok et al., 2004).

Follow-up evaluations at the end of the school year, conducted 4–8 months after entry into the program, were focused on determining, in this short-term time frame, whether Experience Corps participation was associated with meaningful improvements in each of the health behaviors which the program was intended to affect: cognitive, physical, and social activity and support. As reported in Fried et al. (2004), we evaluated evidence for change in cognitive activity in Experience Corps participants. We found that there was no significant change in moderate or high-intensity cognitive activities outside the program (e.g., number of books read per month), but those in the program decreased their hours of TV watching while the controls increased this activity ($p=0.02$). Those in the Experience Corps program were, on average, participating 22 h per week and engaged in different activities in the schools. The cognitive activity embedded within this social health promotion program and roles resulted in measurable gains in executive functioning and working memory, with the gains being greatest for older adults who showed executive functioning deficits at baseline (Carlson et al., 2008). Those with executive functioning deficits at baseline showed a 44–51% improvement in executive functioning and memory in the post-intervention follow-up. In another small pilot study (Carlson et al., 2009), eight EC volunteers were matched to nine wait-listed controls,

Table 27.2 Characteristics of the Baltimore Experience Corps older adult participants and short-term change in risk factors and potential intermediate mechanisms; Pilot, by Treatment Group Assignment (1999–2000)

	Intervention group (n=70)		Control group (n=58)		
	Baseline	Follow-up	Baseline	Follow-up	p
Demographics					
Age, years, %					
60–65	29.4		27.3		
66–70	27.9		40.0		
71–75	30.9		21.8		
>75	10.3		5.5		0.23
Sex					
Female	88.6		94.8		
Male	11.4		5.2		0.21
Race					
African-American	97.1		94.7		
Caucasian/other	2.9		5.3		0.66
Education, high school or less[a]	80.9		84.2		0.63
Outcomes					
Activity					
Physical Activity					
More active at follow-up, %		62.7		42.6	0.04
Number of blocks walked/week[b] (mean)	26.7	35.1	20.2	18.4	0.30
Flights of stairs climbed/week[b] (mean)	13.9	16.6	19.7	21.2	0.83
Activity in kilocalories/week (mean)	1,624.1	2,035.8	892.6	933.3	0.20
Strength					
Very good/excellent, %	47.7	64.8	52.4	35.9	<0.03
Feel stronger at follow-up, %		43.6		18.2	<0.02
Fallen in past 12 months	14.8	6.6	10.4	12.5	0.17
Cane use: less often, %		50 (3/6)		20 (1/5)	0.30
Walking speed (m/s)	0.95	0.92	1.06	0.86	0.001
Social activity					
Number of adults one could depend on (mean)	5.3	6.2	5.8	4.3	0.03
Cognitive activity					
High-intensity activities	3.1	3.1	3.1	3.0	0.83
Moderate-intensity activities	2.8	2.6	2.8	2.7	0.73
Low-intensity activities	3.5	3.5	3.5	3.5	0.78
Books read/month (mean)	5.9	5.4	5.6	5.6	0.43
Hours of television/day (mean)	4.6	4.4	4.5	5.3	0.02

(continued)

Table 27.2 (continued)

	Intervention group (n=70)		Control group (n=58)		
	Baseline	Follow-up	Baseline	Follow-up	p
Cognition					
Trail making test					
Part A (s)	68.7	52.8	66.6	56.3	ns
Part B (s)	174.3	160.7	169.6	191.3	<0.05
Word list memory					
Immediate recall	20.7	20.3	21.0	20.8	ns
Delayed recall	5.6	6.1	6.3	6.3	ns
Rey–Osterrieth					
Copy score	19.5	17.9	18.8	17.0	ns
Delayed recall	11.0	12.0	11.4	10.3	0.05

[a]Volunteers with less than a high school education were allowed to participate in the initial pilot study; the current national criteria for program participation include having a high school diploma
[b]Among those who walked any blocks or climbed flights of stairs

and were assessed with functional magnetic resonance imaging (fMRI) while performing an executive functioning task of attention control and inhibition, prior to placement and at the end of the school year. Results again showed short-term gains in a component of executive function along with corresponding increases in neural activation patterns in prefrontal regions that support executive functions. These pilot results provide important support for short-term neural plasticity and the potential of activity-based interventions to improve health and function to increase plasticity in age-vulnerable regions of the brain supporting executive functioning (Carlson et al., 2009).

Fried et al. (2004) reported further pilot evidence for changes in physical and social activity resulting from Experience Corps participation. Sixty-three percent of volunteers assigned to Experience Corps reported that they were more physically active, compared to 43% of controls ($p<0.05$). Although not statistically significant in this small pilot, the mean number of blocks reported walked per week by the intervention group increased 31%, compared to a decrease of 9% among the controls, and there was a 19% increase in stairs climbed versus 8% increase in these two respective groups. There were also reports of 25% increase in kilocalories expended (versus a decrease of 5% in controls) and significantly greater improvements in strength among those in the Experience Corps, compared to controls, providing support for the likelihood of the increase in physical activity having had meaningful effects. There was less decline in walking speed, and a greater decrease in falls and cane use rates in the intervention group compared to controls, although these differences were not statistically significant. The intervention group also reported significant increases in the number of people to whom they could turn to for help (compared to a decline among controls).

It appeared that engagement in this program could be sustained over a significant period of time. Using a five-stage screening approach designed by this program to maximize retention after placement in the schools (Martinez et al., 2006), drop-out of volunteers from the program was quite low during the school year: 2%. At follow-up, 98% of those in the intervention group reported satisfaction with their experience, and 82% stated that they planned to stay in the program 2 or more years. In fact, 80% returned in the following year. Martinez et al. (2006) describe our successful experience in recruiting and retaining older adults in subsequent years of the program.

With regard to child outcomes, we observed improvements in children's academic and behavioral performance (see Rebok et al., 2004). For example, kindergarten children in the Experience Corps schools had significantly greater increases in vocabulary ability than those in the control schools. There was also a significant difference in standardized reading achievement scores for third graders in the Experience Corps schools, where scores for the three schools increased, compared to the control schools. There were meaningful differences observed in behavioral indices over the 4–8 month follow-up period, as well. Based on data collected by the school principals, the number of referrals to their offices for behavioral issues dropped by 50% in two Experience Corps schools and 34% in the third; similarly dramatic drops in office referrals were not reported by the principals of the three control schools.

This small pilot randomized trial of the Experience Corps program offered initial evidence of benefits to the academic and behavioral improvements for children in public elementary schools conferred by placing a critical mass of older adults trained and placed into public elementary schools. Simultaneously, as summarized above, there is evidence suggesting meaningful short-term improvements in important health behaviors among older volunteers participating in the program, compared to controls, including improved executive functioning and memory, enhanced physical activity and strength, and greater social support.

Current Experience Corps Randomized Controlled Trial in Baltimore City

We initiated a large, randomized controlled trial (RCT) of the Experience Corps program being operated in Baltimore City in 2006, funded by the National Institute on Aging (NIA). We sought to capitalize on plans of the City of Baltimore at that time to scale the Experience Corps program up in Baltimore City, and the City's agreement to allow us to conduct a formal evaluation of the impact of this program on older adults' health and function and on schools and children. As a result of this funding, we were able to scale-up this program into a formal process of community-based participatory research, simultaneously evaluating impact on both older adult volunteers and schools.

Two different projects from this trial focus on the older adult outcomes. The first project (see Fig. 27.1) involves a community-based RCT for effectiveness, utilizing strict RCT rules, including intention-to-treat analyses. The hypotheses to be tested are: (1) that EC participation leads, simultaneously, to increases in physical and cognitive activity (along with social activity) sufficient to independently and interactively result in the primary outcome of decreased disability, and secondary outcomes of decreased falls, frailty, and decreased rate of decline in memory; (2) that EC participation across 2 years will lead to sustained benefits in terms of persistent delayed decline in outcomes above, compared to controls, due to benefits from sustained or improved physical abilities, executive function and memory, and greater social networks; (3) that the EC model will provide an effective vehicle for health promotion, effecting a compression of morbidity (via health outcomes affected) if applied at a city-wide or other broad community level, and that the benefits experienced could have broad population-based implications in terms of the health status of our aging population. Additionally, we hypothesize that those most likely to benefit in the short term will be high-risk older adults, including urban African-Americans and those with low socioeconomic status, and that the population-based benefits in health status resulting from EC participation can lead to a diminution in health disparities in older adults (Adler, 2003). In the longer term, we hypothesize potential benefits in health for most of the older adults. A second project evaluates social and psychological outcomes and pathways (see Fig. 27.1) – separately as well as jointly with the first project. A third project conducts a parallel, randomized, controlled trial of the EC program's impact on schools (children and teachers) (see Fig. 27.2). If EC can significantly improve the likelihood of early school success, particularly across whole grades of children (rather than just one or a few children), then it has the potential to affect these lifelong outcomes for individuals and for whole communities and to be highly cost-effective for society (Frick et al., 2004).

A fourth project from this trial, known as the Brain Health Substudy (BHS), will evaluate brain function and structure in a subset of cases and controls, as well as, with the first project, potential cognitive and physical activity mechanisms for these effects. The BHS project builds on the promising results reported earlier showing improved efficiency in brain activation, as indexed on fMRI and executive inhibitory ability. A fifth project, under separate funding from the MacArthur Foundation, seeks to measure the cost-effectiveness of the Experience Corps and its potential to have highly positive effects (e.g., increased productive activity) or negative effects (e.g., increased consumption of ever more medical care resources) on the economy. Documentation of the EC program's economic benefits of the compression of morbidity and to the schools and children is critical (Frick et al., 2004).

Monitoring Fidelity of the RCT

There has been an increased focus on how research-based programs can be effectively implemented in the context of attempts to "scale-up" effective interventions like Experience Corps, while remaining true to the intended purpose or concept underlying the theoretical model – also known as *maintaining fidelity* (Flay et al., 2005; Greenberg et al., 2005). Despite many compelling reasons why fidelity should be monitored and assessed in intervention evaluation, the majority of intervention research studies still do not include a fidelity component in their evaluation.

A meta-analysis of indicated preventive intervention programs (i.e., programs for high-risk populations) found that over two-thirds of the programs were described too broadly to be replicated. Further, few included measurement of intervention fidelity (Durlak & Wells, 1998). With supplementary funding from NIA, we are monitoring intervention/implementation fidelity of the ongoing RCT of the Experience Corps program in the Baltimore City Public School system to document factors that contribute to the fidelity of overall EC program implementation and training and steps that can be taken to optimize intervention fidelity. This effort takes place within the context of theoretically based models for evaluating the older adult, child, and school outcomes (see Figs. 27.1 and 27.2) that can be used both to verify fidelity of program implementation and to test the theory of intervention effects.

Starting Experience Corps in Your Community

Experience Corps has helped connect over 2,000 older adults nationwide to volunteering opportunities in schools across 22 cities in the U.S. To find out more about the ongoing trial and the program and how to start one in your local community, readers can visit The Johns Hopkins COAH website (http://www.jhsph.edu/agingandhealth/) and the national Experience Corps website (http://www.experiencecorps.org). There you will find information about becoming a program affiliate and ten different guideposts that can be used to determine whether your organization is a good match for the program. As indicated on the website, although Experience Corps was developed to improve the academic achievement and overall well-being of children and strengthen the schools working with these children, there is also interest in expanding the program to meet other societal needs.

To start and sustain an Experience Corps program, it is critical to have a strong commitment from the organization sponsoring the project and strong partnerships with public and private organizations in the community that are critical to the program's success (see Guidepost #5 on the Experience Corps website). Resources to collect and analyze data that assess program impact and potential for improvement are also needed. Financial resources are required for start up and sustaining the program over a period of many years. The typical costs for starting up a program in the first year of operation average $100,000, but that amount varies depending on the local community, scope of the project, and size of the school. This amount includes costs for monthly volunteer stipends and administrative costs.

Policy Implications for Elder Health

There is growing interest in civic engagement-based public health interventions for promoting the health and well-being of older adults (Hinterlong, 2008; Kaskie et al., 2008). The current interest in civic engagement and other forms of volunteerism can be seen in new federal initiatives and increased program funding by private foundations (Morrow-Howell, 2010). Of particular import from the point of view of the health of an aging society will be to determine whether changes observed in health behaviors translate into slowed onset and decreased rates of disability and dependency in older adults. However, there has been limited study of the effects of these initiatives, and greater and more sustained efforts are needed to understand their impact. To date, the Experience Corps program has demonstrated significant impact in small-scale pilot investigations (Carlson et al., 2008, 2009; Fried et al., 2004; Frick et al., 2004; Glass et al., 2004; Rebok et al., 2004; Tan et al., 2006), in two national demonstration projects, and in a recent national evaluation (Hong & Morrow-Howell, 2010). As a model of evidence-based health promotion for senior adults, it demonstrates that one can gain personally while giving back to others and produce positive societal benefits. Assuming that even larger benefits will be found from prolonged Experience Corps participation, this program would offer a community-based, social approach to bringing effective health promotion to the vast majority of older adults, and – on a population level – contributing to the goal of a compression of the morbidity now associated with aging (Fries, 1980).

As evidenced by several other chapters in this book, the aging population offers exciting new resources for the development of other community-based, health promotion programs, namely the older adults themselves. We can envision new roles for older adults that include meaningful service in environmental organizations, healthcare facilities, nursing homes, and other community settings. One example of meaningful new volunteer roles is based on the Asthma Club, which we designed to deploy older adults in the Experience Corps program to teach children about asthma and its management (see Reddy et al., 2007). Results showed that older adults can learn and retain information about asthma and that young school children can learn this information from the older adults. This improvement in students' knowledge about asthma through the Experience Corps Asthma Club could help reduce asthma-related morbidity and resulting school absenteeism. This model of equipping older volunteers as public health agents also might help community health promotion efforts and offer new opportunities for civic engagement-based public health interventions.

Further, increased access to national and community service programs may help to begin to address the health disparities in African-American and other disadvantaged groups, and simultaneously address important unmet societal needs (Tan et al., 2009). Estimates from the Current Population Survey of the U.S. Bureau of Labor (U.S. Bureau of Labor Statistics, 2009) indicate that about a quarter (23.5%) of adults aged 65 and older volunteered in 2008, compared with about a third of adults aged 35–44 (31.5%) and 45–54 (30.8%). However, the rates of volunteering among older adults have been increasing steadily for the past 30 years and older volunteers contribute more time than younger volunteers (Morrow-Howell, 2010). On the other hand, older adults with less education, less income, poorer health, and poorer social integration are less likely to volunteer. Nonwhite older adults also are less likely to volunteer, perhaps due to long-standing barriers to economic and health resources and structural barriers related to discrimination (McBride, 2007). However, with few exceptions, flawed research designs and a lack of information about how volunteering is defined, counted, and experienced in diverse individuals and communities make it difficult to draw conclusions (Martinson & Minkler, 2006).

Conclusion

Experience Corps was designed to reach large numbers of older adults when scaled up, and to be attractive to diverse older adults, notably including minority and low socioeconomic status groups at highest risk of health disparities (Fried et al., 2004). With acceptably high retention rates of Experience Corps older volunteers in Baltimore (Fried et al., 2004), this approach of using civic engagement as a vehicle or social context for health promotion has substantial potential for effectively improving health and cognitive fitness of at-risk older adults and maintaining health for those still physically and cognitively able. The combined effects of impact on health of the individual and the potential to involve and retain large numbers of older adults suggest that this could be an important component of a societal strategy for effecting a compression of morbidity for an aging population.

Acknowledgments Funding support for this chapter was provided by the National Institute on Aging under contract P30-AG02133, the Harry and Janette Weinberg Foundation, and the John D. and Catherine T. MacArthur Foundation, We thank the Greater Homewood Community Corporation, Experience Corps National, Civic Ventures, the Baltimore City Public School System, the City of Baltimore, and the Commission on Aging and Retirement Education for ongoing vision and support.

References

Adler, N. E. (2003). Community preventive health services: Do we know what we need to know to improve health and reduce disparities? *American Journal of Preventive Medicine, 24* (3 Suppl), 10–11.
Annie E. Casey Foundation (2010). *Early warning: Why reading by the end of third grade matters.* A KIDS COUNT Special Report from the Annie E. Casey Foundation, Baltimore, MD.
Baker, L. A., Cahalin, L. P., Gesrt, K., & Burr, J. A. (2005). Productive activities and subjective well-being among older adults: The influence of number of activities and time commitments. *Social Indicators Research, 73*, 431–458.
Baltes, P. B., & Baltes, M. M. (Eds.). (1990). *Successful aging: Perspectives from the behavioral sciences.* New York: Cambridge University Press.
Barron, J. S., Tan, E. J., Yu, Q., Song, M., McGill, S., & Fried, L. P. (2009). Potential for intensive volunteering to promote the health of older adults in fair health. *Journal of Urban Health, 86*, 641–653.
Bronfenbrenner, U., McClelland, P., Wethington, E., Moen, P., & Ceci, S. J. (1996). *The state of Americans: This Generation and the next.* NY: The Free Press.
Butrica, B. A., Johnson, R. W., & Zedlewski, S. R. (2009). Volunteer dynamics of older Americans. *Journal of Gerontology Psychological and Social Sciences, 64*, 644–655.
Carlson, M. C., Erickson, K. I., Kramer, A. F., Voss, M. W., Bolea, N., Mielke, M., et al. (2009). Evidence for neurocognitive plasticity in at-risk older adults: The Experience Corps Program. *Journal of Gerontology: Medical Sciences, 64*, 1275–1282.

Carlson, M. C., Saczynski, J. S., Rebok, G. W., Seeman, T., Glass, T. A., McGill, S., et al. (2008). Exploring the effects of an "everyday" activity program on executive function and memory in older adults: Experience Corps®. *The Gerontologist, 48*, 793–801.

Carlson, M. C., Seeman, T., & Fried, L. P. (2000). Importance of generativity for healthy aging in older women. *Aging, 12*, 132–140.

Crijnen, A. A. M., Feehan, M., & Kellam, S. G. (1998). The course and malleability of reading achievement in elementary school: The application of growth curve modeling in the evaluation of a Mastery Learning intervention. *Learning and Individual Differences, 10*, 137–157.

Durlak, J. A., & Wells, A. M. (1998). *Community programs to promote youth development*. Washington, DC: National Academy Press.

Erikson, E. (1982). *The life cycle completed: A review*. New York: Norton.

Flay, B. R., Biglan, A., Boruch, R. F., VCastro, F. G., Gottfreson, D., Kellam, S., et al. (2005). Standards of evidence: Criteria for efficacy, effectiveness, and dissemination. *Prevention Science, 6*, 151–175.

Fonda, S., & Herzog, A. R. (2004). *HRS/AHEAD documentation report*. Ann Arbor, MI: Survey Research Center, University of Michigan.

Foundation for Child Development. (2008). *America's vanishing potential: The case for Pre-K-3rd education*. New York: A Report from the Foundation for Child Development.

Freedman, M. (1999). *Prime Time: How baby boomers will revolutionize retirement and transform America*. New York: Public Affairs.

Freedman, M., & Fried, L. (1999). *Launching Experience Corps: Findings from a two-year pilot project mobilizing older Americans to help inner-city elementary schools*. Oakland, CA: Civic Ventures.

Frick, K. D., Carlson, M. C., Glass, T. A., McGlll, S., Rebok, G. W., Simpson, C., et al. (2004). Modeled cost-effectiveness of the Experience Corps® Baltimore based on a pilot randomized trial. *Journal of Urban Health, 81*, 106–117.

Fried, L. P., Carlson, M., Freedman, M., Frick, K. D., Glass, T. A., Hill, J., et al. (2004). A social model for health promotion for an aging population: Initial evidence on the Experience Corps® model. *Journal of Urban Health, 81*, 64–78.

Fried, L. P., Freedman, M., Endres, T. E., & Wasik, B. (1997). Building communities that promote successful aging. *The Western Journal of Medicine, 167*, 216–219.

Fried, L. P., Frick, K., Carlson, M. C., & Rebok, G. W. (2006). Experience Corps: A social model for health promotion for older adults that, simultaneously, harnesses the social capital of an aging society. *Gesundheit und Gesellschaft Wissenschaft, 1*, 23–35.

Fries, J. F. (1980). Aging, natural death, and the compression of morbidity. *The New England Journal of Medicine, 303*, 130–135.

Glass, T. A., Freedman, M., Carlson, M., Hill, J., Frick, K. D., Ialongo, N., et al. (2004). Experience Corps®: Design of an intergenerational program to boost social capital and promote health of an aging society. *Journal of Urban Health, 81*, 94–105.

Gottlieb, B. H., & Gillespie, A. A. (2008). Volunteerism, health, and civic engagement among older adults. *Canadian Journal on Aging, 27*, 399–406.

Greenberg, M. T., Domitrovich, C. E., Graczyk, P. A., & Zins, J. E. (2005). *The study of implementation in school-based preventive interventions: Theory, research, and practice*. Rockville, MD: U.S. Department of Health and Human Services, Center for Mental Health Services, Substance Abuse and Mental Health Services Administration.

Greenfield, E. A., & Marks, N. F. (2004). Formal volunteering as a protective factor for older adults' psychological well-being. *Journal of Gerontology: Social Sciences, 59B*, S258–S264.

Gruenewald, T. L., Karlamanga, A. S., Greendale, G. A., Singer, B. H., & Seeman, T. E. (2007). Feelings of usefulness to others, disability, and mortality in older adults: The MacArthur Study of Successful Aging. *Journal of Gerontology: Biological and Medical Science, 62*, P28–P37.

Harris, A. H., & Thoresen, C. E. (2005). Volunteering is associated with delayed mortality in older people: Analysis of the Longitudinal Study of Aging. *Journal of Health Psychology, 10*, 739–752.

Hinterlong, J. E. (2008). Productive engagement among older Americans: Prevalence, patterns, and implications for public policy. *Aging and Social Policy, 20*, 141–164.

Hong, S. I., & Morrow-Howell, N. (2010). Health outcomes of Experience Corps: A high-commitment volunteer program. *Social Science & Medicine, 71*, 414–420.

Kaskie, B., Imhof, S., Cavanaugh, J., & Culp, K. (2008). Civic engagement as a retirement role for aging Americans. *The Gerontologist, 48*, 368–377.

Katula, J. A., Kritchevsky, H. B., Guralnik, J. M., Glynn, M. W., Pruitt, L., Wallace, K., et al. (2007). Lifestyle interventions and independence for elder pilot study. Recruitment and baseline characteristics. *Journal of the American Geriatrics Society, 55*, 674–683.

Kellam, S. G., & Rebok, G. W. (1992). Building developmental and etiological theory through epidemiologically based preventive intervention trials. In J. McCord & R. E. Tremblay (Eds.), *Preventing antisocial behavior: Interventions from birth through adolescence* (pp. 162–195). New York: Guilford Press.

Kim, J., & Pai, M. (2010). Volunteering and trajectories of depression. *Journal of Aging and Health, 22*, 84–105.

Lloyd, D. N. (1978). Prediction of school failure from third grade data. *Educational and Psychological Measurement, 38*, 1193–1200.

Luoh, M., & Herzog, A. R. (2002). Individual consequences of volunteer and paid work in old age: Health and mortality. *Journal of Health and Social Behavior, 43*, 490–509.

Martinez, I. L., Frick, K., Glass, T. A., Carlson, M. C., Tanner, E., Ricks, M., et al. (2006). Engaging older adults in high impact volunteering that enhances health: Recruitment and retention in the Experience Corp® Baltimore. *Journal of Urban Health, 83*(5), 941–953.

Martinson, M., & Minkler, M. (2006). Civic engagement and older adults: A critical perspective. *The Gerontologist, 46*, 318–324.

McBride, A. M. (2007). Civic engagement, older adults, and inclusion. *Generations, 30*, 66–71.

Morrow-Howell, N. (2010). Volunteering in later life: Research frontiers. *Journal of Gerontology: Psychological and Social Science, 65*(4), 461–469.

Morrow-Howell, N., Hinterlong, J., Rozario, P. A., & Tang, F. (2003). Effects of volunteering on the well-being of older adults. *Journal of Gerontology B Psychological and Social Science, 58*, S137–S145.

Morrow-Howell, N., Hong, S. I., & Tang, F. (2009). Who benefits from volunteering? Variations in perceived benefits. *The Gerontologist, 49*, 91–102.

National Center for Health Statistics. (2007). *Trends in Health and Aging*. Retrieved April, 2007, from http://www.cdc.gov/nchs/agingact.htm.

Parisi, J. M., Rebok, G. W., Carlson, M. C., Fried, L. P., Seeman, T. E., & Tan, E. J. (2009). Can the wisdom of aging be activated and make a difference societally? *Educational Gerontology, 35*, 867–879.

Population Division. (2002). *World Population Ageing, 1950-2050*. New York, NY: Population Division: Department of Economic and Social Affairs.

Rebok, G. W., Carlson, M., Glass, T. A., McGill, S., Hill, J., Wasik, B., et al. (2004). Short-term impact of Experience Corps® participation on children and schools: Results from a pilot randomized trial. *Journal of Urban Health, 81*, 79–93.

Reddy, D. M., Fried, L. P., Rand, C., McGill, S., & Simpson, C. F. (2007). Can older adult volunteers serve effectively to improve asthma management for children? Experience Corps® Baltimore. *The Journal of Asthma, 44*, 177–181.

Rowe, J., & Kahn, R. L. (2004). Health promotion in the urban elderly: Experience Corps commentary. *Journal of Urban Health, 81*, 61–63.

Rowe, J. W., & Kahn, R. L. (1987). Human aging: usual and successful. *Science, 237*, 143–149.

Stewart, A. L., Verboncoeur, C. J., McLellan, B. Y., et al. (2001). Physical activity outcomes of CHAMPS II: A physical activity promotion program for older adults. *Journal of Gerontology A: Biological and Medical Sciences, 56*, M465–M470.

Tan, E. J., Rebok, G. W., Yu, Q., Frangakis, C. E., Carlson, M. C., Wang, T., et al. (2009). The long-term relationship between high-intensity volunteering and physical activity in older African-American women. *Journal of Gerontology: Social Sciences, 64*, 304–311.

Tan, E. J., Tanner, E. K., Seeman, T. E., Xue, Q.-L., Rebok, G. W., Frick, K. D., et al. (2010). Marketing public health through older adult volunteering: Experience Corps® as a social marketing intervention. *American Journal of Public Health, 100*, 727–734.

Tan, E. J., Xue, Q., Li, T., Carlson, M. C., & Fried, L. P. (2006). Volunteering: A physical activity intervention for older adults: The Experience Corps program in Baltimore. *Journal of Urban Health, 83*, 954–969.

Tang, F., Choi, E., & Morrow-Howell, N. (2010). Organizational support and volunteering benefits for older adults. *The Gerontologist, 50*(5), 603–612.

Tanner, E., Fried, L., Piferi, R., Martinez, I., Gruenewald, T., Parisi, J., et al. (2011). Development of the Hopkins Generativity Index: Assessing generative desire, behaviors, and fulfillment. Manuscript in preparation for publication.

U.S. Bureau of Labor Statistics. (2009). *Volunteering in the United States, 2008*. Washington, DC: Bureau of Labor Statistics, United States Department of Labor.

Index

A
Acetyl L carnitine, 259
Actors learning strategy
   college student's participation, 277–278
   full active experiencing strategy, 278
   memory performance improvement, 277
   mental activity demand, 278
   pilot investigation, 279
ADRD. *See* Alzheimer's disease and related dementias; Alzheimer's disease and related disorders
Aerobic activity, 240–241
Age-associated memory impairment (AAMI), 214
Aging mind
   brain function changes, 68–69
   brain structural changes, 68
   cognitive change, 68
   neurocognitive function, 67
   STAC model, 67–68
Alpha-lipoic acid (ALA), 259
Alzheimer's disease (AD). *See also* Alzheimer's disease and related dementias
   life span, 419–420
   meditation (*see* Kirtan Kriya meditation)
   predictors and markers, 420–421
   stress
      cortisol hormone, 421, 422
      HPA axis, 422
      vs. relaxation response, 422–424
      telomeres, 421
Alzheimer's disease and related dementias (ADRD)
   antioxidants, 250
   creative writing (*see* Creative writing)
   dietary patterns and brain health, 251
   healthy lifestyle strategy, 250
   medical foods and memory shakes, 254–255
   neuronal plasticity improvement, 250
   nutritional supplements
      ALA, 259
      appetized and cooked food, 262
      balanced diet, 261–262
      brain health maintenance, 264, 265
      brain power food, 262–263
      comprehensive assessment, 260
      folic acid deficiency, 257–258
      food medication, 266
      ginkgo biloba (GB), 259
      HCPs, 256
      healthy snacks/meals, 264, 265
      HupA, 259
      hypertriglyceridemia, 263
      niacin deficiency, 258
      O3FA, 258
      resources, 267
      saturated fat intake reduction, 263
      sweetened beverages, 264
      tocopherol, 258–259
      vinpocetine, 259
      vitamin B6, 258
      vitamin B12, 257
      vitamin B1 deficiency, 258
      vitamin D, 257
   oxidative stress, 250
   pathogenesis, 250
   scientific evidence, 249
   specific food groups
      alcohol, 254
      coffee, 253
      dark chocolate, 253
      fruits, vegetables, and legumes, 251–252
      MUFA, 252
      nuts and green tea, 253

Alzheimer's disease and related dementias
(ADRD) (*Continued*)
O3FA, 252
spices, 253
sweeteners, 253–254
whole grains, 252
spelling errors, 180–181
tissue-damaging free radicals, 250
Alzheimer's disease and related disorders
EML club (*see* Early memory loss clubs)
medical management, 382–383
non-pharmacologic movement, 383
American Association of Retired Persons
(AARP), 170–172
Artists for Alzheimer's® (ARTZ)
benefits of participation, 307
benefits of volunteering
Alzheimer programs, 307
evidence-based museum program,
311–312
facts and figures, 310
Massachusetts ARTZ museum
network, 309–310
museums, 308–309
popularity/need/demand, 310–311
research and evaluation, 312–313
professional training, 305
specific cultural access programs, 305
treatment for Alzheimer's symptoms,
306–307
Art, museums, and culture
Alzheimer's disease, 301
ARTZ
benefits of participation, 307
benefits of volunteering, 307–313
professional training, 305
specific cultural access programs, 305
treatment for Alzheimer's symptoms,
306–307
cultural treatment, 302–303
dementia, 303
Fable Art Museum, 303
Hearthstone Alzheimer's Foundation, 322
museum educator and activity director
observation
cinema, 319
circus and the vaudeville arts, 321–322
"It Takes a Village" project, 313–315
Ladder to the Moon process, 317–318
local organizational partner, 315
LTTM, 316
mill nursing home model, 316
poetry, 319–321
nonpharmacologic intervention, 302–303

quality of life, 304
Audio–visual entrainment (AVE), 438
Audio–visual stimulation (AVS), 438–440
Autobiographical writing, 202
Axona, 254, 255

B
Biofeedback technologies
AVE, 438
AVS, 438–440
EEG biofeedback/neurofeedback
brain, changes, 437–438
definition, 435
observed improvements, 439, 440
procedure, 437
HEG biofeedback, 438–439
Brain brightening
biofeedback, 434
brain physiology, 435
elderly, brain changes, 436–437
neurotherapy, 440–441
AVE, 438
AVS, 438–440
EEG biofeedback/neurofeedback,
435, 437–440
HEG biofeedback, 438–439
QEEG, 435–436
Brain fitness
brain plasticity
brain engagement schedule, 52
dystonia, 51
functional or structural plasticity, 50
IMPACT Study, 53–55
information processing quality, 52
neuromodulatory control, 52
plasticity effects, 50–51
positive and negative plasticity, 51
sensory neuroplasticity, 50
buyer beware, 62–63
cognitive reserve, 61–62
commercial products
control groups, 57–58
double-blind randomized clinical trial, 57
far transfer evaluation, 58
practice effect, 57
publication of findings, 59
regular and frequent usage, 60
report findings for older adults, 58
scientific advisory committee, 57
testing to standards, 57
test performance, 58
user-friendly products, 60–61
mental exercise and brain capacity, 45

software, 27, 37, 40
transfer across multiple dimensions, 49–50
transfer of cognitive training
  context transfer, 48
  definitions, 47
  dual-task training/multitasking, 48–49
  everyday functioning measurement, 47
  near and far transfer, 47–48
  performance rehabilitation, 46
  processing speed, 50
  purpose, 46
  temporal, functional and modality transfer, 47–48
  transfer model, 49
  word discrimination, 49
Brain health enhancement
  access to musicality, 327
  cultural expression, 326
  inclusion, key, 328
  international audience, 328–329
Brookdale-inspired cognitive stimulation model, 384–385

C

Calciferol, 257
Cardiovascular endurance, 240–241
Chapbook, 210
Cognitive aging, theater art
  active experiencing principle, 276
  actors learning strategy
    college student's participation, 277–278
    full active experiencing strategy, 278
    memory performance improvement, 277
    mental activity demand, 278
    pilot investigation, 279
  actors teasing behavior, 273
  cognitive measures, 281
  empirical evidence, 274–276
  health care facility, 280
  memory, movement and text, 276
  memory trace durability, 277
  multivariate covariance analysis, 281
  NIA study, 279–280
  role acquisition process, 276
  role learning process, 274
  scene learning instruction, 274
  second NIA intervention, 280
  SPTs, 276
  third NIA intervention, 281–282
Cognitive-behavioral therapy (CBT), 91

Cognitive enrichment hypothesis, 29
  ACTIVE trial, 30–31
  IMPACT trial, 31
  Internet and computer use interventions, 31–33
  video games, 33–34
Cognitive training. *See also* Physical fitness training
  age-related changes, brain structure and function, 25
  cognitive enrichment hypothesis, 29
    ACTIVE trial, 30–31
    IMPACT trial, 31
    Internet and computer use interventions, 31–33
    video games, 33–34
  comparative effectiveness, 37–38
  concurrent discrimination judgment, 26–27
  general *vs.* targeted training: effectiveness and training efficiency, 36–37
  individualized training, 38
  mnemonic techniques, 27
  neural plasticity, 36
  practical recommendations, 40
  quality of life, 26
  technology products, 26
  training and transfer of training, 27–29
  training intervention design, 27
  unresolved issues, 36, 37
  video game interventions, 38–39
Cognitive wellness program
  cognitive health perceptions, 231–232
  development of
    communication methods, 235
    computer-based programs, 235–236
    older adults, 236–237
  Experience Corp, 234
  health behaviors
    gender differences, 233–234
    racial/ethnic groups, 232–233
  SeniorWise study, 234
Community-based intergenerational program
  benefits and QOL enhancement, 462–463
  biopsychosocial benefits, 450–451
  brain aging
    biopsychosocial approach, 448–449
    QOL, 449
  dementia, 450
  guidelines, 464
  intergenerational relationships, 450
  TIS and JP
    eldercare homes, 452
    multi-age learning, 452

Community-based intergenerational program (*Continued*)
  narrative-based activities, 454
  partnership, 453
  perceived health benefits, 460
  qualitative analysis, 457
  quantitative results, 458–459
  relationship maintenance, 461–462
  sense of purpose and usefulness, 460–461
  statistical analysis and results, 457, 458
  study design, 453, 454
  workshops and assignments, 456
Computerized cognitive fitness programs, 235–236
Consumer-based brain fitness programs. *See* Brain fitness
Continuing care retirement community (CCRC), 108
Creative writing
  Alzheimer's disease
    cognitive impairment, 201–202
    life-defining moments, 199–200
    lifelong learning program, 201
    life style modification, 200–201
  aphasia/depression
    behavioral activation approach, 205
    death fears, 204, 205
    psychotherapeutic treatment, 205–206
    Silver sneakers program, 205
    verbal expressive skills, 204–205
  compilation of excerpts, 210
  expressive writing
    alexithymia, 208
    health/psychological benefits, 203–204, 211
    maladaptive cognitions, 204
    working memory capacity, 203–204
  mild cognitive impairment/dementia syndromes, 206–207
  mind-body workshop, 209
  older adults, 211
  role of group leader, 209–210
  structure of, 207–208
  therapeutic writing
    benefits, 210–211
    guided autobiography, 202–203
    types of, 202
    workshops, 206
Creative Writing for Health and Healing, 201
Cyanocobalamin, 257

D

Dancing Heart™ – Vital Elders Moving in Community
  apprentice program, 286
  cognitive, physical, and emotional functioning, 286
  community vitality, 299
  health and quality of life benefits, 286
  innovative role, artists
    enrichment programs, 294
    future explorations, 297
    future programming and community involvement, 297–298
    intergenerational cross-functional teaching, 295
    perspectives, participants, 296–297
    physical and emotional safety, 295
  language of dance, 287–288
  limitations, 298
  real-world health settings, 285
  skepticism to enthusiasm
    anecdotal evidence, 292–294
    benefits of dance, 290–291
    health and emotional benefits, 290
    preliminary findings, 291–292
    working with elders, 288–289
Dietary approaches to stop hypertension (DASH) diet, 251
Digital photography, 74–75
Distinctive processing, 7

E

Early memory loss (EML) clubs
  ADRD patients interest, 385
  applied research, 397
  Brookdale-inspired model, 384–385
  care partner's perception, 396, 397
  clubs promotion, 398
  cognitive and psycho-social results, 392–393
  effect size, 388
  Einberger's club activities, 396
  EML study quality, 398
  evaluation, 386–387
  experimental group (EXP), 389
  MCSC (*see* Milwaukee Brookdale-Inspired Cognitive Stimulation Club)
  MMSE, 388–389
  participation and benefits, 393–394
  remote semantic memory, 395
  specific activities *vs.* cognitive outcomes, 394

Index 493

Elaboration and imagery, 11–12
Exercise Assessment and Screening for You (EASY), 242
Experience Corp (EC), 234
Expressive writing
  alexithymia, 208
  health/psychological benefits, 203–204, 211
  maladaptive cognitions, 204
  working memory capacity, 203–204
External reminders
  calendar, 9
  compensatory benefit, 8
  habit of preparing, next day, 9
  iPhone alarm clock, 9
  laundry, 10
  pill box, 9
  routines/habits of behaving, 8
  rule of thumb, 10
  written appointment schedule, 8

F
Fraboni Scale of Ageism (FSA), 146

G
Gerontology
  goals, 138
  Intergenerational Discussion Group Program (*see* Intergenerational Discussion Group Program)
  lifelong learning and volunteerism, 137–138
Green exercise, 246
Guided autobiography (GAB)
  life review, 187
  older adults, 202–203
  writing prompts, 208

H
HEG biofeedback technology, 438–439
Huperzine A (HupA), 259

I
"I'm Still Here"™ approach
  activities programming
    continuum, 408, 409
    treatment perspective, 407
  aim, 403
  community-based events, 415–416
  ILEs, 413–414

Montessori-based approach, 411–413
neuroscience
  actors, comparator and interpreter, 405
  amygdala, 404
  hard-wired skills and abilities, 405
  retrogenesis theory, 404
performance and large social events, 414–415
PSB, 408, 410, 411
QOL improvement, 402–403
treatment, 402
Institute for Retired Professionals (IRP), 127
Interactive living events (ILEs), 413–414
Intergenerational Discussion Group Program
  college student, 146–147
  community-dwelling older adults, 139
  equal status, 139
  expected outcomes, 140
  experiences, 150–152
  highlights, 139–140
  implications, 147–149
  limitations, 149–150
  older adults
    attitudes toward aging, 145–146, 148–149
    benefits to, 140–141
    cognitively stimulating activities, 148
    experience sharing, 148
    focus group responses, 143
    lifelong learning, 149
    motivation, 143
    multi-method approach, 141
    positive perceptions, 143–144, 147
    recruitment of, 139
    self-report questionnaires, 142
    social and cognitive benefits, 144, 149
    volunteerism, 145, 148
  plenary sessions, 139
  student-older patient interaction, 138–139

J
Journal writing, 202, 203

K
Kent Area Orthography Society (KAOS), 176–178
Kirtan Kriya meditation
  brain and cognition
    cerebral blood flow enhancement, 428–429
    finger and sound, 426
    memory loss patients, 427–428

Kirtan Kriya meditation (*Continued*)
    posterior cingulate gyrus, 427
    tongue usage, 426
  breath and eye direction, 424
  chant/mantra, 424, 425
  movement sequence, 425–426
  mudras/finger movements, 424–425
  posture, 424
  visualization, 425
Korsakoff syndrome, 258

L
Ladder to the Moon Theatre Company (LTTM), 316
Life review
  biographical interventions, 186
  communal process, 185
  consent and negotiation, 193
  core principles
    human memory system, 192
    older adults, 191
    story telling, 191–192
    truth, 192–193
  fact-based questions, 195
  hospice programs, 185
  individual/group intervention, 185
  interpersonal communication, 189
  interview guide, 195–198
  life themes and metaphors, 194–195
  narrative self, 188
  open-ended questions, 195
  reminiscence, 183–184
  resources, 194
  stories, 188
  StoryCorps, 184
  teaching, 186–188
  therapeutic activity, 189–190
  time and legacy, 195
  value-added intervention, 186
Loving-kindness meditation (LKM) training, 94

M
Massed practice, 15
MCI. *See* Mild cognitive impairment
Meditation, mindfulness, cognition, and emotion
  behavioral and neuroscientific research
    attentional blink task, 92
    attention, emotion, or brain structure measurement, 92
    buddhism and science, 91
    cognitive enhancement program, 92
    contemplative science, 91
    emotion regulation, 93
    emotion response process, 94
    LKM training, 94
    MBSR training program, 92–93
    MLI, 91–92
    pain-processing brain area, 95
    relaxation training, 93
    self-reported trait anxiety, 94
    Shamatha Project, 93
    telomerase activity, 95
    top-down or volitional attention control, 93
    vipassana retreat participation, 93
  behavioral and neuroscientific study, 86
  brain region, 88
  CBT, 91
  cognitive enrichment, 86
  community-based cognitive enrichment program, 86
  community-based program, 86
  contemporary psychology, 89–90
  dementia
    Alzheimer's disease, 95–96
    attention task performance, 99
    biological outcome measure, 98
    brain default network activity, 97
    caregiver-administered behavioral intervention, 96
    caregivers education program, 98
    compassionate action/altruism, 97
    depression symptom, 96
    physiological emotional response, 97
    PMR program, 98
    skills-training approach, 96
    somatic complaint, 97
  discomfort/drowsiness, 88
  emotion regulation, 87
  focused attention *vs.* open monitoring, 89
  loving-kindness meditation, 90
  MBSR, 90
  mental continuum, 89
  older adults, community based program, 99–101
  self-centered preoccupation, 89
  self-monitoring skill, 90
  stress symptom, 90
  task-relevant information and suppression, 87
  teaching center and group, 86
  training method, 87
  Wallace statement, 87
Mediterranean diet, 251

Memoir writing, 202
Memory enhancement strategies
  breadth of transfer, 4
  cognitive and life-style interventions, 4
  combining strategies, 17–18
  dementia, 3
  diagnosing the problem, 6–7
  dietary supplement, 4
  elaboration and imagery, 11–12
  exercise, 21
  explicit noticing and rehearsing, 10–11
  external reminders
    calendar, 9
    compensatory benefit, 8
    habit of preparing, next day, 9
    iPhone alarm clock, 9
    laundry, 10
    pill box, 9
    routines/habits of behaving, 8
    rule of thumb, 10
    written appointment schedule, 8
  memorization technique, 4–5
  method of loci, 6
  mnemonics, 18–19
  processing and retrieval principles, 7
  reasoning and speed training, 4–5
  self testing
    effective learning, 14–15
    information retrieval, 13–14
    memory boosting, 14
    regulation-training
      intervention, 14
    successful and unsuccessful
      retrievals, 15
    variety of tasks, 14
  spacing practice
    chateau – castle, 15
    concept learning, 16–17
    performance levels, 16
    problem solving, 17
    scheduling, 15–16
  structure analysis, 12–13
  text learning, 5
  training recollection, 20–21
Memory training. *See* Cognitive training
Memory training peer (MTP) program
  age-related physical and cognitive
    decline, 214
  curriculum
    class exercises, 218
    course content, 218–220
    manual, 220
    mnemonic techniques, 218
    skill-builders, 218
  development
    behavior modification, 216
    cognitive-behavioral approaches, 217
    declarative memory, 216
    educational interventions, 215
    learning theory, 216–217
    low tech, 217
    manualize, script, and stage, 217
    multifactorial memory programs,
      216–217
    pilot program, 217
  implementation
    administrative activities,
      223–224
    characteristics for participants, 221
    national and local venues, 223
    trainers, 222–223
  memory improvement results,
    224–225
  program revisions, 225
  research, 226
  translation and development, 225–226
Mental alertness, 232
Method of loci, 6
Mild cognitive impairment (MCI)
  age-related declines, 214
  cognitive activity, 364–366
  creative writing, 206–207
  definition, 361
  healthy lifestyle, 363
  identification, 362–363
  physical exercise, 367–368
  rehabilitation, 368
  take charge (*see* Take charge
    pilot program)
  treatment, 363
Milwaukee Brookdale-Inspired Cognitive
    Stimulation Club (MCSC)
  goals, 390
  hypotheses, 390–391
  measures, 391–392
  research methods, 391
Mind and Life Institute (MLI), 91–92
Mindfulness-based stress reduction
    (MBSR), 90
Mini-Mental State Exam (MMSE),
  388–389
Mnemonics technique, 18–19, 27
Monounsaturated fatty acids
    (MUFA), 252
Montana Lifelong Learning Institute
    (MOLLI), 129, 131
MTP program. *See* Memory training peer
    program

N

National Institute on Aging (NIA)
  cognitive aging enhancement, 279–280
  Experience Corps program, 480
  personal characteristics, 244
  physical activity, definition of, 241
  RCT, 482
  second intervention, 280
  Synapse, 77
  third intervention, 281–282
National Spelling Bee, 170
Northeast Ohio Senior Spelling Bee
  Center for Healthy Aging, 172
  Cinco de Mayo theme, 174–175
  Derby Day theme, 175
  mental health center's Foundation, 173–174
  preparation classes, 172–173
  venues, 176
Nutrition
  ALA, 259
  appetized and cooked food, 262
  balanced diet, 261–262
  brain health maintenance, 264, 265
  brain power food, 262–263
  comprehensive assessment, 260
  folic acid deficiency, 257–258
  food medication, 266
  ginkgo biloba (GB), 259
  HCPs, 256
  healthy snacks/meals, 264, 265
  HupA, 259
  hypertriglyceridemia, 263
  niacin deficiency, 258
  O3FA, 258
  resources, 267
  saturated fat intake reduction, 263
  sweetened beverages, 264
  tocopherol, 258–259
  vinpocetine, 259
  vitamin B6, 258
  vitamin B12, 257
  vitamin B1 deficiency, 258
  vitamin D, 257

O

Odyssey of the Mind (OOTM). *See* Senior Odyssey program
OLLI. *See* Osher Lifelong Learning Institute
Omega–3 fatty acids (O3FA), 252
Oral history, 187
Oral life review. *See* Life review
Osher Lifelong Learning Institute (OLLI)
  history
    Bernard Osher Foundation, 126
    Classic Mediterranean Cuisine, 133
    Continuing Education, 130
    Elderhostel/Road Scholar Institute Network, 128
    First Night Missoula, 132
    International Wildlife Film Festival, 132
    IRP, 127
    lifelong learning activity, 126
    MOLLI membership or course, 131
    MOLLI mission, 129
    peer-led groups, 131
    UM, 128
    university-affiliated companies, 130
    Wonder Wheels, 133
  intellectually stimulating courses, 125
  responsive organization course, 134

P

Peer-led memory training programs. *See* Memory training peer program
Personalized skill building (PSB), 408, 410, 411
Physical activity
  ACSM and NIA definition, 241
  cardiovascular endurance, 240–241
  EASY tool, 242
  vs. exercise, 241
  health-related fitness, 239–240
  physical fitness definition, 239
  recommendations
    cool-down period, 244
    functional activities, 243
    gaming system, 242
    hobby-like activities, 243
    housekeeping activities, 242
    RDAD, 244
    resources, 244
    safety, 241–242
    Talk Test, 243
    walking, 242
    warm-up period, 243
  strategies, long term success
    behavior management techniques, 246–247
    daily routine, 245
    green exercise, 246
    interesting and choice of activity, 245
    personal characteristics, 245
    program enhancers, 246
    social network, 245

Physical fitness training. *See also* Cognitive training
    aerobic exercise interventions, 35
    brain structure and functioning, 36
    cardiovascular fitness, 36
    cognitive functioning, 34
    combined aerobic and strength training, 35
    practical recommendations, 40
Phytochemicals, 251
Phytonutrients, 251
Practice effect, 57
Prefrontal bilaterality, 69
Productive engagement
    cognitive domains, 74, 75
    digital photography, 74–75
    example stories, study effects, 78
    focal tasks, 74
    quilting, 74–75
Progressive muscle relaxation/autogenic imagery (PMR) program, 98
Prospective memory failures, 8–9

Q
Quality of life (QOL)
    and brain aging, 449
    community-based strategy, 462
    conceptualization, 463
    improvement sequence, 402–403
Quality programming, retirement community
    age-related mental decline, 120
    brain plasticity, 110
    brainstormed topics and activities, 111
    CCRC, 108
    class satisfaction and quality indication
        attendance, 113
        concentration and memory, 116
        intergenerational creative writing class, 114
        Likert scale, 115
        on-site entertainment activity, 114
        performance-based skill, 115
    cognition and well-being
        auditorium-like community room, 117
        brainstorming and planning session, 119
        cognitive maintenance/improvement, 118
        communication skill, 119
        data collection and clerical support function, 119
        descriptive statistics, 117, 118
        feelings about memory scale, 117
        Likert-type response, 117
        memory skill, 118
        memory skill, mood, and social connectedness, 116
        mindfulness, 120
        statistically significant difference, 118
        Thinking Survey, 119
    cognitive fitness, 111
    hallway-word-of-mouth effect, 113
    intellectually challenging program, 108
    intellectually stimulating program, 108
    K2SM programming, 110–111
    lifelong learning program, 107
    memory functioning, 120
    neurogenesis, 111
    physical and psychological health, 110
    program evaluation, 111
    residents' selection of pursuits, 112–113
    self-blame, stress and worry, 109
    self-determination, control, and autonomy, 109
    self-programming, 120
    social change, 109
    staff behavior, 108
    TRACK, 112
Quantitative EEG (QEEG), 435–436
Quilting, 74–75

R
Reasoning training, 4–5
Reducing Disability in Alzheimer's Disease (RDAD), 244
Reminiscence, 183–184, 187
Reverse Cognitive Aging, 26, 28, 32. *See also* Cognitive training; Physical fitness training

S
Scaffolding Theory of Aging and Cognition (STAC), 67–68
Scaffolds
    aging, 70
    intellectually challenging work, 70–71
    juggling training, 71
    neural scaffolding development, 72
    neurogenesis, 70
    scientifically driven interventions, 71
    Synapse Intervention Trial, 72
    targeted skill training, 71

Self testing
    effective learning, 14–15
    information retrieval, 13–14
    memory boosting, 14
    regulation-training intervention, 14
    successful and unsuccessful retrievals, 15
    variety of tasks, 14
Senior Odyssey program
    cognitive optimization, 163
    development of
        Illinois state tournament, 161–162
        individual sessions, 166
        local coaching talent, 165
        local, regional, state association, 165
        local tournaments, 160–161
        long-term problems, 166
        opportunity for competition, 166
        pilot activities, 160
        quantitative and qualitative assessments, 160
        recruit participants, 165
        registration, 165
        regular schedule, 165–166
        resources for spontaneous problems, 166
        sponsors, 165
    goal, 167
    history of
        cognitive intervention, 158–159
        long-term problems, 157–158
        spontaneous problems, 158
        spring tournaments, 157–158
        structural lag, 159
    individual experiences, 163–164
    substantively complex environment, 156
SeniorWise study, 234
Silver sneakers program, 205
Social engagement, 232
Songwriting Works model
    brain health enhancement
        access to musicality, 327
        cultural expression, 326
        inclusion is key, 328
        international audience, 328–329
    cognitive fitness and health program, 354
    cognitive playground, 330–331
    evidence-based model, 333–334
    health and community restoration
        cognitive intelligence, 346–347
        cost effective social innovation, 352–353
        pastoral care, 352
        power of association, 351–352
        WWII Veterans and caregivers, 347–351
    heritage recipies, 331–332
    multivalent stimulation, 353
    music, 325–326
    musical intelligence, 354
    musical mural painting, 329–330
    principles, healthy creative engagement
        access, 341
        authenticity, 343
        celebration, 345–346
        originality, 342
        Providence Health and Services, 341
        reciprocity, 344
        restoration, 344–345
    research
        cognitive benefits of musical improvisation, 339
        cognitive impairment, 335
        cognitive variance, 337
        dignity, 336
        healthcare delivery system, 337
        leaping into aging, 339–340
        musical creativity and brain health, 334
        music therapy intervention, 336
        Olympic Peninsula care center, 335
        speech, song, rhythm and memory, 338–339
Spacing practice
    chateau – castle, 15
    concept learning, 16–17
    performance levels, 16
    problem solving, 17
    scheduling, 15–16
Speed training, 4–5
Spelling clubs and competitions
    age-related changes, 179–180
    Alzheimer's dementia, 180–181
    children and adults
        AARP Spelling Bee, 170–172
        KAOS, 176–178
        morphological analysis, 178
        National Spelling Bee, 170
        overpronunciation, 178
        rote learning, 178
        self-testing, 179
        visualization, 178–179
    Northeast Ohio Senior Spelling Bee
        Center for Healthy Aging, 172
        Cinco de Mayo theme, 174–175
        Derby Day theme, 175
        Mental Health Center's Foundation, 173–174
        preparation classes, 172–173
        venues, 176
    reading, 169

Index

StoryCorps, 184
Structure analysis, 12–13
Subject-performed tasks (SPTs), 276
Successful aging, 231–232
Synapse intervention trial
   aging mind
      brain function changes, 68–69
      brain structural changes, 68
      cognitive change, 68
      neurocognitive function, 67
      STAC model, 67–68
   hypotheses, 76–77
   National Institute on Aging, 77
   pilot study, 77
   productive engagement
      cognitive domains, 74, 75
      digital photography, 74–75
      example stories, study effects, 78
      focal tasks, 74
      quilting, 74–75
   Scaffolding Theory of Aging
      and Cognition, 69–70
   scaffolds
      aging, 70
      intellectually challenging work, 70–71
      juggling training, 71
      neural scaffolding development, 72
      neurogenesis, 70
      scientifically driven interventions, 71
      targeted skill training, 71
   study design
      cognitive assessment, 73–74
      Dallas, Texas, 72
      enrollment and retention, 73
      research arms, 73
      structured recruitment and screening protocol, 72

T

Take Charge pilot program
   benefits, 376–377
   cautions, 377
   cognitive activity and stress management, 371–373
   cognitive enhancement, 377–378
   intake session, 370
   participants, 370
   physical activity and diet module, 373–374
   project results, 375–376
   structure, 369
   time line and intervention modules, 369
The Intergenerational School (TIS) and Judson Park (JP)
   eldercare homes, 452
   multi-age learning, 452
   narrative-based activities, 454
   partnership, 453
   perceived health benefits, 460
   qualitative analysis, 457
   quantitative results, 458–459
   relationship maintenance, 461–462
   sense of purpose and usefulness, 460–461
   statistical analysis and results, 457, 458
   study design, 453, 454
   workshops and assignments, 456
Therapeutic writing
   benefits, 210–211
   guided autobiography, 202–203
   types of, 202
   workshops, 206
The Resident Advisory Committee for Keys (TRACK), 112
Thiamine, 258
Tip of the tongue (TOT), 179
Training recollection, 20–21
Transmission-deficit model, 179–180

U

University of Montana (UM), 128

V

Video game interventions
   aging issues and gaming, 38–39
   cognitive enrichment hypothesis
      Rise of Nations, 33–34
      short-term video game intervention, 33
      transfer of training issue, 34
      visual and attentional abilities, 33
   combined physical and mental exercise, 39
VIVA!, 77

CPSIA information can be obtained at www.ICGtesting.com
Printed in the USA
LVOW100739120812

293955LV00003B/15/P